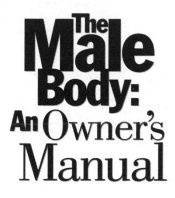

The Male Body:
An Owner's Manual

The **Ultimate**
Head-to-Toe Guide
to Staying **Healthy** and
Fit for Life

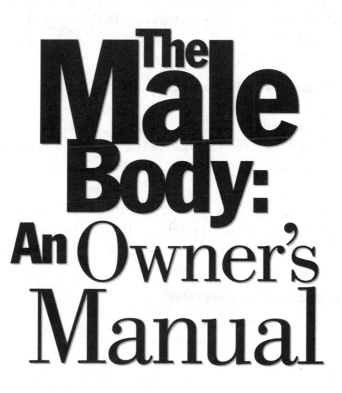

The Male Body: An Owner's Manual

By **K. Winston Caine, Perry Garfinkel** and the **Editors of** Men'sHealth **Books**

Rodale Press, Inc.
Emmaus, Pennsylvania

Library of Congress Cataloging-in-Publication Data

Caine, K. Winston.
    The male body : an owner's manual : the ultimate head-to-toe guide to staying healthy and fit for life / by K. Winston Caine, Perry Garfinkel and the editors of Men's Health Books.
        p.   cm.
    Includes index.
    ISBN 0–87596–297–1 hardcover
    ISBN 0–87596–401–X paperback
    1. Men—Health and hygiene.   I. Garfinkel, Perry.   II. Men's Health Books.   III. Title.
RA777.8.C35   1996   96–18195
613'.04234—dc20

Distributed in the book trade by St. Martin's Press

2   4   6   8   10   9   7   5   3   1   hardcover
2   4   6   8   10   9   7   5   3   1   paperback

OUR MISSION

We publish books that empower people's lives.

RODALE BOOKS

Contents

Entries in gray are illustrated guides to
your body's systems and senses.

Part One
Maximizing Your Machine

Part Two
Body Maintenance

Part Three
The Complete Fitness Guide

✕ Introduction

The problem with the human body is that it lacks push buttons. And knobs. Switches would be useful, too. So would meters and warning lights.

If the body had these things, you can bet we men would be far, far healthier than we are. We can relate to machines. Meter says the fuel mix is too rich? Easy—adjust the food intake. Throw the "energy surge" switch but get no response? Better run analytics on sleep, stress and exercise patterns. Warning light flashing on the thigh? Time to slow down the pace of the run, maybe do some stretches.

The reality is that our bodies don't even have on-off switches. If a man wants to be truly health-savvy, he has to read signals that are both subtle and conflicting—things such as headaches, thirst, fatigue, too-tight pants. As for preventive measures, it's often impossible to tell whether those vitamins or bike rides have any direct effect on your health, be it positive or negative.

Which is why so many men don't bother. It's all just too complicated. "Ignore the pain and carry on!" is our creed. "Who needs doctors!" is our battle cry. "No one is going to tell me how to lead my life!" is our slogan. And so what happens? We break down far earlier than women, and in uglier ways. Heart attacks, strokes, cancer, diabetes, mental burnout: These are primarily the domain of men, not women.

Stupid us. The human body, while awe-inspiring in its complexity, is not nearly as hard to take care of as we may think. In fact, as machines go, it is one fun gizmo to master. *The Male Body: An Owner's Manual* makes taking care of yourself both easy and pleasurable. The underlying message in this book is that subtle changes in your daily routines can add up to a big, positive impact on the length and quality of your life, not to mention enhanced energy and spirit. What kind of choices? Simple ones: a bagel instead of a doughnut. A walk after dinner rather than an hour of television. Laughter rather than anger. Taking a vitamin. Having more sex. Responding to, not ignoring, your body's symptoms. You can do these. Easily.

Like an owner's manual for a car or computer, *The Male Body: An Owner's Manual* focuses on a few key areas: how to use your machine properly; how to maintain it; how to troubleshoot problems; warning signs to watch for. In other words, this is not a repair manual. Why? Our stance is that good health is not merely the absence of disease or injury. Health is also about having a body full of energy, a mind full of creativity and wisdom, a spirit full of adventure and joy. These are our ambitions for you, and what we promise to provide.

We've broken things down into three sections. In part 1, we offer tools for mastering the big-picture health issues in your life: nutrition, stress, sleep, sex, energy. In part 2, we take you on a body-part-by-body-part tour, explaining how to keep each part healthy and strong, along with how they communicate to you. In part 3, we offer a complete fitness guide that features stretches and exercises for virtually every body part.

You may have sworn back in seventh grade that you would never read about the endocrine system again. Well, give us a try. We've done everything we can to make *The Male Body: An Owner's Manual* as lively, funny and useful as possible. Because caring for your body was never meant to be a dour, serious thing—inane television shows about hospitals notwithstanding. Your body is an amazing machine, and making it work stronger and better is about as an important a thing in life as there is. Here's how to enjoy doing it.

Neil Wertheimer
Senior Managing Editor,
Men's Health Books

Part One
Maximizing Your Machine

Nutrition

- **Swear off fat.**
- **Eat more fresh produce.**
- **Eat more beans and whole-grain foods.**
- **Spread out your eating schedule.**

Eating used to be so uncomplicated. You just gathered a bunch of your buddies and set out on your manly duty: risking life and limb to stalk, hunt and, hopefully, kill dinner for the brood. If you were lucky, you and the boys had steak. If the beast was lucky, it had you and the boys.

Today, putting on the feed bag is still a test of survival. But this time, instead of facing down some saber-toothed wildebeest, you're hedging your odds against heart disease. Cancer. Diabetes. Stroke. These and scores of other diseases—everything from acne and arthritis to hair loss and hearing loss—are caused or aggravated by the way you eat.

"Most people don't think of food as medication, but in reality, it's the single biggest medication we're exposed to," says Neal Barnard, M.D., president of the Physicians Committee for Responsible Medicine in Washington, D.C., and author of *Food for Life: How the Four Food Groups Can Save Your Life* and other books on the healing aspects of food. "When you're sitting down for meals, three times a day you are dosing yourself with huge quantities of things that will determine what's coursing through your arteries and blood vessels for the rest of the day."

Old Habits Die Hard

Unfortunately, that could explain why four of the ten leading causes of death in the United States are linked directly to our diet— and why these diseases tend to strike men at higher rates than women.

Guys are used to eating what they want

to when they want to. Meat loaf. Macaroni and cheese. Fritos. Cold pizza . . . even for breakfast, dang it! Count fat grams? Check out serving sizes? Follow the Food Guide Pyramid? Hah! What's next? Asking for directions?

Old habits die hard, and because of that, so do we. But you can have your testosterone and eat well, too. In fact, with a little strategic eating—knowing what, when and how much to eat—you could improve your health and drastically lower your risk of disease with your dyed-in-the-wool taste buds becoming none the wiser.

First, you need to know some of the new rules.

• Our apologies to Mom, but you don't have to eat three square meals a day. In fact, many nutritionists say it's better to have smaller meals more often, or more "grazing periods," throughout the day. By eating the same amount of calories at each smaller meal, you keep your body's chemistry at an even level, which has many terrific health benefits, says Thomas Wolever, M.D., Ph.D., associate professor of nutritional sciences at the University of Toronto.

• Forget about centering each meal around a slab of meat. It's better to eat like a European and treat meat as a side dish instead of the main course.

• Forget about the four food groups. There are now five.

• And forget about the convenience of "convenience foods," packaged snack foods, TV dinners and other products that come from boxes. Some frozen dinners have twice as much fat as you would use to make them at home. Homemade can often be better than factory-packaged.

Fat: How to Cut Back

But if there is one old-fashioned eating habit that we men need to drop most, it's our passion for steak, ribs, pork chops, butter. The typical American man gets about 35 percent of his calories from fat; experts say that figure should be 30 percent at most—preferably much lower. What's more, the fat we consume most is the most dangerous type: Saturated fat, from animal sources such as meats, eggs, cheeses and dairy, clogs arteries and contributes to scads of health problems.

Not that fat is all bad. We need about 30 grams a day to give us energy, build muscles and nerve cells and even keep hair and skin healthy.

"Around every cell is an enveloping membrane that contains a layer of essential fats. One of the many functions this membrane performs is chemical communication with neighboring cells," says Michael Klaper, M.D., director of the Institute of Nutrition Education and Research in Manhattan Beach, California. "One way these cells communicate is by throwing little pieces of their cell membranes back and forth to each other. In this way, cells help regulate tissue functions such as inflammatory reactions, blood flow patterns and so on."

The trouble is that we American guys consume far more fat than our bodies need. And that poses serious health risks. Excess fat intake is a leading contributor to heart disease, the nation's top killer of men. Saturated fat is believed to play a major role in the development of at least one-third of cancers as well as in many other conditions, ranging from impotence to psoriasis.

In addition, fat packs roughly nine calories per gram, compared with only four calories per gram for carbohydrates. What does that mean? Simple: Eating fat is the quickest way to become fat. You can eat more carbohydrates than fat and still end up consuming fewer calories.

Of course, there's more to the fat equation than this. Some fats are better than others.

"All people are afraid of those three letters: *f-a-t*. But the reality is that all fats are not created equal," says Dr. Klaper. While saturated fat, the type that comes from animals, can break more hearts than Don Juan, monounsaturated and polyunsaturated fats, found in vegetables, grains and nuts, can have the opposite effect. These fats can lower cholesterol and counteract some of the negative effects that an-

imal fat has on the body. Here's how to limit the bad stuff and get more of the health-enhancing fats.

Be hip to hydrogenation. Take notice of the word "hydrogenation" on food labels. It refers to an industrial food process in which hydrogen is added to usually heart-healthy unsaturated fats such as soybean oil to give foods longer shelf life as well as the texture of more expensive animal fats. Problem: Because many guys assume vegetable oils are heart-healthy, they think they're in the clear. But according to Alberto Ascherio, M.D., Dr.P.H., assistant professor of nutrition and epidemiology at Harvard School of Public Health, foods labeled "partially hydrogenated" contain a type of fatty acid that can actually do more damage to your body, in his opinion, than saturated fat—even when these foods are labeled "low-fat" or "no cholesterol."

You'll find partially hydrogenated oils in hundreds of foods, but they're especially abundant in fried fast foods, baked goods such as cakes and cookies and packaged snack foods such as crackers. You should avoid, or at least sparingly eat, foods that say they contain partially hydrogenated oils. When replacing saturated fat, use tub margarine instead of stick margarine, says Robert Nicolosi, Ph.D., director of the Center for Cardiovascular Disease Control at the University of Lowell in Massachusetts and former chairperson of the American Heart Association's nutrition subcommittee. Tub margarine has fewer of those harmful fatty acids than stick margarine.

Give frozen foods a cold shoulder. Sorry, guys, but the meat and potatoes of our eating—frozen meat-and-taters TV dinners and other processed foods—is a bad choice. One of these meals can have twice the saturated fat content of a similar meal that you'd prepare yourself, because manufacturers add extra fat to give the food more flavor. Most are also very high in sodium, which can affect blood pressure. For example, frozen pasta primavera has 305 calories, more than 14 grams of fat and

1,410 milligrams of sodium. Homemade has 267 calories, 7 grams of fat and 220 milligrams of sodium.

Although the jury is still out on whether eating low-fat versions of regular foods means you'll lose weight, there are many frozen and packaged varieties available on the market that are low in fat and sodium. So read labels carefully to be sure you're getting the nutrition you want.

Avoid the tropics. All cooking oils get their calories, about 120 per tablespoon, from fat. But some are still better than others, because they get a higher percentage of fat from the heart-healthy polys and monos. Canola, safflower, olive and sunflower are the best choices; they get only a small percentage of their calories from saturated fat, says Dr. Nicolosi. So-called tropical oils such as palm and coconut, along with butter, lard and vegetable shortening, are the worst, since they get most of their calories from saturated fat.

But whatever you use, go easy. Instead of pouring oil into a pan, brush it on with a paper towel, or better yet, use a no-stick pan, which requires no oil. Orange juice makes a great nonfat substitute for cooking oil when preparing a stir-fry, advises Dr. Nicolosi.

Lean your cuisine. Before you cook any meat, trim off all visible fat. Also, remove the fat that rises to the top of soups, chilies, stews and sauces. And when browning meat to use in any of these dishes, drain all of the excess fat from the pan before adding the meat to the rest of the ingredients, says Dr. Nicolosi.

The Building Blocks of Good Nutrition

Leave it to Uncle Sam to regulate what we should eat. But according to the U.S. Department of Agriculture's Food Guide Pyramid, there's a definite eating plan we should strive to follow for optimum nutrition. And here it is.

Grains should be the foundation of your diet, with between 6 and 11 servings each day. A serving is one slice of bread (so a sandwich counts as two servings), half of a bagel or one-half cup of rice or pasta. For more fiber and better nutrition, think whole grain: Brown rice is better than white rice; whole-wheat bread is better than white bread. Bulgur, polenta and barley are also good choices.

Vegetables should account for three to five servings each day, with one serving equal to one cup of raw vegetables or one-half cup of cooked or chopped raw vegetables. Vegetables should be eaten raw or lightly steamed rather than mushy, so you get the most nutrition per bite (boiling tends to remove vitamins and minerals). Again, the more color, the more nutrients: Choose dark green lettuce, such as romaine, over iceberg. Yellow and orange vegetables such as squash and carrots tend to be high in beta-carotene, one of the so-called antioxidants, which counter cell damage that could lead to cancer and heart disease.

Fruits should be eaten two to four times a day. One serving is one-half cup of chopped, cooked or canned fruit, three-quarters cup of fruit juice or one fruit the size of a medium apple. When it comes to eating fruit for good health, variety is also important. Cantaloupe, kiwifruit, strawberries, peaches and citrus fruits are just a few that offer a wealth of nutrients and phytochemicals, says Melanie Polk, R.D., director of nutrition education at the American Institute for

Fiber: Why You Need to Get Roughage

There's no argument that eating like a Kentucky Derby contender can put you in the winner's circle nutrition-wise. Dietary fiber, found in grains such as oats, barley and corn, fills you up, so you actually eat less food. And that's good for us guys, since that spare tire tends to be a testament to our rarely being shy about going back for seconds (or thirds). Moreover, fiber, which is also found in fruits and

Cancer Research in Washington, D.C. Phytochemicals are not nutrients but newly discovered substances in fruits, vegetables and grains that may decrease cancer risk.

Milk, yogurt and cheeses represent the dairy grouping; you should aim for two to three servings a day. Stick to nonfat or low-fat varieties such as a slice of reduced-fat cheese or eight ounces of skim or low-fat milk or yogurt.

Meats, poultry, fish, dried beans, eggs and nuts should supply no more than two to three servings a day. That means if you have a handful of nuts, one cup of cooked dried beans and three ounces of skinless chicken, you have all of the protein you need from this group. Remember that dried beans, such as navy, black, pinto, kidney and garbanzo, are low in fat and high in fiber. Eggs aren't the nutritional bad guys they were once thought to be; although high in cholesterol, they pack a lot of nutrients per bite and can be part of a good diet. If desired, use only egg whites, since they are free of fat and cholesterol. And forget those 16-ounce porterhouse steaks and the triple cheeseburgers: One serving of meat is three ounces, about the size of a deck of cards.

Fats, oils and sweets should be eaten as little as possible. Health experts recommend that you consume no more than 30 percent of your total daily calories as fat. For an even healthier breakdown that limits fat to 25%, get 9 percent or less of your total daily calories from polyunsaturated fat, 9 percent or less from monounsaturated fat and 7 percent or less from saturated fat. For example, if you consume about 2,500 calories per day, your daily total fat intake should be 69 grams or less.

oats, barley and rye called heart-helping because it has bee help lower cholest its name because it dissolves in water to form a gel. "The theory is that since it's soluble, it forms a gel-like material that keeps some of the cholesterol and fat molecules from getting into the interior walls of the intestines, where they are absorbed into the bloodstream," says Dr. Newman. "When these materials aren't absorbed, they are excreted through bowel movements."

In contrast, insoluble fiber, found in vegetables, cereals and grains such as wheat, doesn't gel. Its main benefit is helping to keep us regular. While it's less effective at keeping fat and cholesterol from being absorbed into the bloodstream, it is useful for increasing bulk and speeding the progress of materials through the intestines.

Unfortunately, most guys don't get enough of either, largely because they think they have to eat like Mister Ed. The American Heart Association recommends 25 grams of total dietary fiber each day, what

vegetables, keeps us regular and can help reduce the risk of heart disease by slowing down absorption of all of the fat and cholesterol we consume in foods, says Rosemary Newman, R.D., Ph.D., professor of foods and nutrition at Montana State University in Bozeman, who has studied the nutritional benefits of fiber since the early 1980s.

There are two kinds of fiber, and both are important to a man's health. Soluble fiber is abundant in beans, fruits and grains such as

you'd find in about 15 dried figs or about two cups of cooked dried beans; we tend to get only about 18 grams a day. The obvious way to weigh the scales in your favor is to eat more fiber-rich foods. But here are some easy ways to add fiber to your diet.

Time it right. Since oat bran probably isn't your ideal snack (unless it's oat bran pretzels), you can make the most of what fiber you do consume by timing it right. "My belief is that you should have most of your fiber with your

...tiest meal of the day in order to have it work most effectively," says Dr. Newman. So if you're starting your day with an omelet and bacon, have a side bowl of oatmeal. Pastrami for lunch? Top it off with a pear or two. And if you're feasting on steak, have beans as a side dish.

Get fruity. Of the recommended 25 grams of fiber you should consume each day, experts say that 25 percent, or 6.25 grams, should come from soluble sources. This so-called 25/25 rule is fine if your goal is to keep going to the bathroom regularly. But if you want to use fiber to prevent disease, you ought to double the soluble ante to about 12 grams a day, says Dr. Newman. But if chicken feed isn't your idea of good vittles, reach for some produce: Most fruits and many vegetables contain pectin, a form of soluble fiber. As a bonus, produce also contains phytochemicals believed to help prevent cancer and other diseases (more on these later). Best sources of pectin include citrus fruits such as grapefruit and oranges as well as pears, plums and peaches.

Bowl yourself over. "Perhaps the easiest way to get a five-gram booster is with cereal, since there are so many high-fiber choices," says George L. Blackburn, M.D., Ph.D., associate professor of surgery at Harvard Medical School and chief of the nutrition/metabolism laboratory of the Cancer Research Institute at Deaconess Hospital in Boston. All it takes is one-third to one-half cup of high-fiber cold cereal or one cup of cooked hot cereal.

Not willing to give up your Lucky Charms? You can still have a magically delicious and nutritious breakfast or snack by sprinkling a few tablespoons of oat, rice or

Eating Ethnic

If you don't want to bear the weight of the world on your belly, keep in mind these suggestions from nutritionists at Baylor College of Medicine in Houston the next time you're eating ethnic.

Asian. Asian cuisine, emphasizing vegetables with only small amounts of meat, tends to be among the healthiest—as long as it's not swimming in oil. Avoid anything that says "crispy," "fried" or "tempura" or is breaded, such as General Ts'ao's chicken and sweet-and-sour dishes. Also keep watch for peanut sauces, curry dishes made with coconut milk or heavy cream and dishes with cashews or peanuts (which are often deep-fried before they're added to the meal). Better choices include stir-fry dishes (ask that they be cooked in as little oil as possible), steamed white rice rather than fried rice and dishes that use water chestnuts rather than nuts to add crunch.

Mexican. Avoid deep-fried dishes such as chalupas and chimichangas and foods made with deep-fried tortillas (such as tacos). Instead, stick to chicken, shrimp or bean fajitas or enchiladas. Taco salads can be low-fat, as long as you don't eat the fried shell and you top your salad with fat-free salsa rather than dressing. Grilled chicken and fish dishes are also good choices. Dip your chips in fat-free salsa rather than fat-laden guacamole.

Italian. Think red, not white. Creamy white sauces

wheat bran over those stars, moons and clovers. You'll find bran in health food stores and many supermarkets.

Protein: Too Much of a Good Thing

All of Mom's talk about your needing your protein was a bit misdirected—unless you grew up in Bangladesh. Granted, over 700 million people worldwide are believed to suffer from protein deficiency, but most of them live in developing countries. In the United States, we have the opposite problem: We tend to get too much protein.

"Americans are probably eating twice as much protein as they really need," says Melanie Polk, R.D., director of nutrition education at the

tend to be loaded with fat (fettuccine alfredo, for example, packs close to 700 calories and 40 grams of fat), while marinara and primavera sauces contain about 100 fewer calories and one-third of the fat. And don't think eggplant parmigiana is a great choice just because its main ingredient is a vegetable. The eggplant is dipped in an egg batter, then deep-fried before being added to a casserole of heavy cheese and tomato sauce. An average serving packs close to 1,100 calories and nearly 100 grams of fat.

French. A mixed bag, since French restaurants offer some of the best of both low-fat and high-fat dishes. Grilled fish and other grilled foods as well as trimmed leg of lamb are good choices among the low-fat items. Ask for a little sauce on the side, and remember that sauces based on meat juices, stocks and spices tend to be lighter than traditionally creamier sauces such as béarnaise, béchamel and hollandaise. And keep in mind that croissants have about 12 times more fat than plain French bread.

Cajun. Avoid anything made with roux, a mixture of fat and flour often added to gumbos, étouffées, sauces and gravies. Steer clear of deep-fried hush puppies and seafood; order grilled blackened seafood and poultry dishes instead. Also order white rice or red beans and white rice rather than "dirty rice," which is made with chicken gizzards and livers, ground pork, butter or other fat.

American Institute for Cancer Research in Washington, D.C. "I think the myth that we have to have some protein at every meal is still around."

Protein helps build and repair muscles, and excess protein can be used as fuel in the body. But high-protein foods tend to also be high in fat. Besides, protein interferes with the absorption of certain minerals, such as calcium, and can also overwork your kidneys (since more minerals are excreted in the urine). The protein-rich American diet may be one reason why kidney disease is so prevalent in the United States.

You'll be getting the right amount of protein if you try to limit it to 10 percent of your total calories, according to Daily Value guidelines set by the Food and Drug Adminis-

tration. To do that, avoid eating more than two three-ounce servings of meat, poultry or fish each day.

Carbohydrates: The Energy You Need

Okay, you want to limit your intake of "energizers" such as fat and protein. So how do you fuel your manly self? With carbohydrates, those sugars and starches that your body can easily break down into energy.

"Your body works best when it's running on a high percentage of carbohydrates with small amounts of protein and fat," says Andrea Gardiner, R.D., a registered dietitian in Thousand Oaks, California. Carbohydrates help break down fat; they team up with proteins to form compounds that are essential for beating infections and lubricating joints; and they help keep skin, bones and nails healthy.

Here's how to make the most of your carbs.

Keep them complex. There are two kinds of carbs: simple and complex. Simple carbs are tiny molecules of sugar found in foods such as table sugar, honey and molasses. The most common simple carb is glucose.

Complex carbs, also known as starches, are composed of groups of simple carbohydrates stuck together in long molecular chains. These take longer to digest, a plus for people with diabetes and for those who want long-term energy. Since they also contain fiber, unlike simple carbs, complex carbohydrates fill you up faster, may help decrease your cravings for fatty foods and help remove cholesterol from your body before it's absorbed into your bloodstream.

Start each meal with carbs. The first

thing you should eat at a meal is a complex-carbohydrate food such as pasta, potatoes or noodles, according to Dr. Blackburn. Coupled with eating slowly, this can actually help you eat less food and better control your weight.

Cancer "Phyters"

We'll give Mom this one: You should eat all of your vegetables—every chance you can. That's because most vegetables, as well as fruits and other plant foods such as soybeans, are nutrient-dense, meaning they are extremely rich in vitamins and minerals and have little, if any, fat. This helps keep your immune system strong, so you're more resistant to disease.

As a bonus, fresh produce also contains hundreds of phytochemicals, naturally occurring compounds that help protect plants from the ravages of Mother Nature. In men, these phytochemicals have been found to block cancerous tumors—particularly those of the lungs, bladder, colon, stomach, rectum, larynx and pancreas—before they start.

Men should get a minimum of five (and ideally, as many as nine) servings of fruits and vegetables each day, with a serving usually being one-half cup of chopped, cooked or canned fruit, three-quarters cup of fruit juice, one fruit the size of a medium apple, one cup of raw vegetables or one-half cup of chopped or cooked raw vegetables. But only about 1 in 12 men eats the recommended five portions. In a survey of more than 2,800 people over age 18, the

Buying Fresh

How do you make sure your foods are fresh? Some advice from the U.S. Department of Agriculture:

Meats. Look for the last sales date, not the expiration date, which is usually a week or so later. Meats should look pink and be well-sealed in their packages; dark colors indicate spoilage.

Seafood. Try to get a look at the whole fish. If the fish is fresh, the eyes should be bulging and shiny, not cloudy; the gills should be bright red or pink, not brownish; and the scales should be tight and shiny, not slimy. Press the skin: If it bounces back, the fish is fresh; if an indentation remains, pass on it. And the fish should smell like an ocean breeze but not excessively fishy.

Fatty fish such as salmon and tuna can be stored in a freezer for up to three months. Leaner fish such as cod, flounder and haddock can be frozen for up to eight months. Previously frozen fish should not be refrozen in your own freezer. It should be eaten within two days.

Shellfish. When buying clams, oysters or mussels, make sure the shell is closed tightly or closes when tapped. Lobsters, crabs and crayfish should be lively when you buy them. Be sure your oysters are properly cooked if you:

• Drink more than two drinks a day

• Have liver disease, diabetes, stomach problems or cancer

• Have been a long-term steroid user (as for asthma or arthritis). The oysters may contain bacteria that won't affect others but could be dangerous to you.

Fruits and vegetables. Look for an even color and texture to the skin, without bruises; the food should feel firm to the touch. Realize that organic produce may be slightly more imperfect-looking than highly waxed or polished fruits and vegetables. Organic means that the produce contains no known pesticide residues; other fruits and vegetables may. Try to buy local produce in season. This ensures the freshest foods possible, and they're less likely to have been processed with post-harvest pesticides. Commercially grown foods that have the most pesticides are strawberries, sweet peppers, spinach, peaches, Mexican cantaloupes, celery, apples, apricots and green beans.

average intake of fruits and vegetables was 3.4 servings per day.

Eating this much produce is actually

Spices for Life

How you season your foods can help you see more seasons. Certain spices and flavorings have been found to prevent or cure certain conditions and may even help build immunity. Among the best:

Garlic was used by the ancient Egyptians to treat diarrhea, by the Romans for intestinal and lung problems and by the ancient Jews for local treatment of wounds. Today, it's thought to help prevent high cholesterol, cancer and other conditions, including sore throats, urinary tract infections and even ear infections. It keeps the liver from producing LDL, the so-called bad cholesterol. And since it's rich in certain phytochemicals, garlic is also believed to help prevent or slow cancerous tumor growth. Strive for two cloves a day.

Onions, like garlic, can help prevent and treat many infections and can clear clogged nasal passages by virtue of their pungent aroma. Use them in cooking, or if you can stand it, eat them raw. Or get your onions in salsa, suggests Marilyn Swanson, R.D., a nutritionist and extension food safety specialist at the University of Idaho in Moscow. Spoon salsa over baked potatoes, chicken and other foods.

Hot peppers have a natural decongestant effect on mucous membranes because they contain a chemical known as capsaicin, which stimulates the free flow of mucus and thins heavy mucus. Curry powder, ginger, turmeric, cumin and other spices may have similar effects to varying degrees.

Cinnamon is more than just another tasty spice. Historically, it has been used for treating fever, diarrhea and menstrual problems. (The Egyptians also included it in their embalming mixtures.) Researchers now say that cinnamon has proven benefit as an antiseptic, killing bacteria, viruses and fungi. Like many culinary spices, it also helps soothe the stomach. And an animal study in Japan revealed that it may help prevent ulcers.

calories less (
making you
ceptible to v

So how much is enough? It all depends—on your age, activity level and current weight. So get out your calculator and use one of these formulas to determine the number of calories that's right for you.

• If you're between ages 18 and 30, multiply your current weight by 15.3. Then add 679. So if, for example, you're a 25-year-old man who weighs 180 pounds, that's 180 × 15.3 + 679, or 3,433 calories a day.

• If you're between ages 31 and 60, multiply your current weight by 11.6. Then add 879.

Of course, this calculation is for maintaining weight. To gain one pound per week, eat an additional 500 calories per day; to lose, cut back at least 500 calories a day and increase your amount of exercise.

easier than you may think: Slice a banana over your cereal in the morning, have a side salad and an apple with lunch, add a couple of vegetables to your dinner, and you're there.

How Much Should You Eat?

The average guy over age 30 can expect to gain 1.6 pounds per year, every year. Why? While the average man tends to eat the same amount of food day in and day out, his metabolism slows with age. That means you burn

The Whens and Hows of Eating

Three square meals a day: For many, it's as absolute as the sun rising in the morning. Well, things change. Nutritionists today are advocating anywhere from six mini-meals (with each meal having about half of the food of a full meal) to three small but well-balanced meals and several snacks—ideally fruits, vegetables or nuts—in between. The goal in all cases is the same: to keep your energy level steady by evening out the ebb and flow of nutrients in your system.

Then there is real life. Sitting down at a table for a full meal a few times a day is what we men do. With that in mind, we offer these suggestions for making old-fashioned sit-down meals healthier and more fulfilling.

Appetize yourself. One way to slow the feeding frenzy is to start off with an appetizer that takes longer to eat: half of a grapefruit rather than a glass of juice at breakfast, for example, or a bowl of hot soup or a mixed-green salad instead of a roll at lunch or dinner.

Take your time. Make a point of consuming a food with all of your senses: touch, smell, taste, sight and sound (if the idea of a good crunch appeals to you). Studies show that people overeat when they really don't pay attention to what they're eating (yet another reason why frequent fast-food meals tend to pile on the pounds).

Don't drink during a meal. Alcohol tends to dull your satiety signals, making you more likely to overeat. Besides, it's loaded with "empty" calories, offering little or no nutritional value. And alcohol has seven calories per gram, whereas carbohydrates have only four calories per gram. Our bodies treat alcohol more like fat than like protein or carbohydrates.

Control those condiments. Don't assume you're in the clear with a salad dressing labeled "cholesterol-free." Some have 10 grams of fat per tablespoon. Mayonnaise is nearly all fat, with 11 grams of fat per tablespoon. And since most of us guys use these toppings very liberally, we can easily add as many as 30 grams of fat per day. If you can't control your condiments, consider healthier options such as

Vitamins and Minerals: What You Need

If you eat right, you may not need supplements. But for some men, supplements can contribute to better nutrition and can actually fill the gaps for certain nutrients, such as vitamin E, which is in very few foods.

Keep in mind that vitamins and minerals work as a team and interact to keep you in good nutritional status. If you want to take a supplement, taking a good-quality multivitamin/mineral, along with eating a sound and varied diet, is your best bet, says Diane Grabowski, R.D., nutrition educator with the Pritikin Longevity Center in Santa Monica, California. Such a supplement should contain a mixture of all or most of the essential vitamins and minerals and contain close to 100 percent of the Daily Value for each.

But for protection against the diseases we worry about most, you may need supplements that go beyond the government-established Daily Values. Here's what is typically recommended for the nutrients men need most.

Vitamin C is an antioxidant, meaning that it helps kill free radicals, which can trigger diseases such as cancer. Vitamin C also keeps immunity strong, making you more resistant to disease. The Daily Value for vitamin C is only 60 milligrams, what you'd get from a small glass of orange juice. But many experts recommend 250 to 500 milligrams daily for disease prevention.

Vitamin E has been shown to help prevent heart dis-

fat-free yogurt, nonfat dressing, mustard, ketchup, horseradish, relish and salsa.

Same goes for vegetable dips. While they may sound virtuous, some are just simple mixes of herbs and sour cream or cream cheese, which are loaded with fat and calories. Trick yourself into consuming less by alternating between eating one vegetable with dip and one without. Or better yet, make dips with low-fat sour cream or mayonnaise, or don't dip at all.

Do quality add-ons. Dagwood Bumstead is a comic strip character, so his spare tire can be erased. But if you eat sandwiches like his, you're bound to pack on the pounds quicker than Dagwood can fall asleep on the sofa. Not that you shouldn't build sandwiches higher than Mount Rushmore. Instead of heaping on

ease, but only when taken in amounts of more than 105 international units a day. Many experts suggest shooting for between 30 and 400 international units (but not more than 600 international units) a day. These amounts are impossible to get from food sources, since vitamin E is in very few foods.

Chromium may not be the weight-loss miracle that it was advertised to be, but this mineral can help reduce your risk of diabetes and heart disease by improving blood sugar and insulin levels and lowering cholesterol and triglycerides, a form of fat in the blood. The recommended amount is 50 to 200 micrograms a day; doses of more than 200 micrograms a day should be taken only under medical supervision.

Zinc is possibly the most underrated nutrient there is. It helps keep immunity strong (some say even better than vitamin C) and can heal infections and wounds. The Daily Value is 15 milligrams, but most guys get only about 9 milligrams a day from foods. Look for no more than 15 milligrams in your multivitamin/mineral supplement.

Selenium is a mineral with antioxidant qualities. It has also been shown to protect against heart disease, alleviate arthritis symptoms and even boost mood. For men, the Daily Value of selenium is 70 micrograms a day. If you are considering this potentially toxic mineral, take a supplement containing no more than 100 micrograms.

healthy meals. Ask for a doggie bag at the beginning of the meal, remove the portion that you think is excess and pack it up for the next day, says Polk. You'll get two meals for the price and effort of one—and save on calories, too.

The Bottom Line

Truth is, keeping track of your caloric intake takes a lot of time and effort and may not be worth your while. Counting the number of servings of fruits and vegetables you eat in a day is easier and more important. But even this falls by the wayside when your attention is focused on dealing with tough bosses, overactive kids, broken faucets and tense commutes. So we'll boil down all of the details above to these final two pearls of wisdom.

First, always acknowledge that what you eat is enormously important. Smart eating is about making the right choices. Doughnut or bagel? Apple or chocolate bar? Steak or chicken breast? Pretzels or butter cookies? You know the answers. It's the accumulation of many smart decisions that ultimately helps you to be healthy, lean and well-nourished, says Polk.

Second, take the "variety and moderation" approach to eating. Over the course of a few meals, be sure to mix-and-match all types of foods, advises Polk. If it's red meat for lunch, it's fish or beans for dinner and chicken and pasta the next day. If you have eggs for breakfast one day, make it oatmeal the next. If you eat a variety of healthful foods every day, over time you'll be ahead of the game, even if you occasionally decide to break all of the rules for a meal or two. Single meals won't do long-term harm; it's how your diet adds up over time that counts.

layers of cold cuts, use the opportunity to pile on vegetables such as sprouts, tomatoes, onions, lettuce and red peppers. Just avoid grilled vegetables that are swimming in oil and "melts," which tend to have lots of cheese.

Pass on the side dishes of coleslaw and potato salad made with mayonnaise or dressing. And an ounce of potato chips (about 17 chips) packs about 160 calories and ten grams of fat; pretzels are a better choice, with only one gram of fat. A pickle is also a good low-fat choice, unless you're trying to cut back on sodium.

Take it home. When you're in a restaurant, plan to take home a portion of your meal rather than eating a large dinner all at once. Most restaurant entrées today go well beyond the recommended portion sizes for

⚇ Body Shape

- **Know your physique.**
- **Dress appropriately for your shape.**
- **Exercise according to your body's strengths.**

Ed Lange saw every inch of more than 10,000 men a year and knew all too well that we have many shapes and sizes. But somehow he managed to look beyond tall and lean, short and stocky or bronzed and chiseled. To him, all of us looked the same.

Nude.

"There are no body perfect types here," said Lange, founding director of the Elysium Institute in Topanga, California, the only clothing-optional resort in Los Angeles County. Lange passed away in 1995. "To me, all men and women who are nude are beautiful in form and in shape. With clothes, even the best body shapes can look dumpy and klutzy. But without clothes, even the heaviest men can look smooth and graceful."

True to Type

In our media-saturated, bigger-is-better culture, the average man tends to feel . . . well, if not inadequate, at least a little nondescript. We know in our hearts that nature didn't intend everyone to look like Tom Cruise. Yet on some painful level of insecurity and regret, we're convinced that it's all our fault—that if we had worked out a little more often, lifted a few more weights, we, too, would have the ideal masculine builds of Tinseltown's A-list stars.

But despite the perception that everybody is given a fair jump out of the starting gate, it's really not so. Babe Ruth wasn't cut out to be a sprinter, and if you fit in a size 36 regular coat now, you probably won't be needing a 44 long any time soon. Put another way, you can stuff yourself with pasta, lift weights every afternoon

and watch 12 Schwarzenegger flicks back-to-back, and at the end of the day, you still won't look like the Terminator unless you already have the genetic blueprint for that kind of physique.

This is not to say you're stuck with the hand Mother Nature dealt you. Not entirely, anyway. "The body is incredibly plastic," says Melvin Williams, Ph.D., director of the human performance laboratory at Old Dominion University in Norfolk, Virginia. "While you can't change your bone structure, you can modify what's on those bones through exercise and a proper diet to bring out the best in your body type."

Consider the case of Charles Barkley, star of the Phoenix Suns, who went from weighing 310 pounds during the World University Games in Edmonton, Alberta, more than ten years ago to weighing just 250 now. By eating more fruits and vegetables and less fast food and shifting his training routine to include more fat-melting aerobic exercise, he became lighter, quicker, more mobile. "It's a totally different Barkley," says John Larkin, head basketball trainer during Barkley's days at Auburn University in Alabama.

Body Categories

Each of us has inherited a distinct frame, called a somatotype. Round, heavyset guys who are strong without really trying are known as endomorphs. Mesomorphs are the muscular, male model types. Tall, lean guys who don't have much fat or muscle are known as ectomorphs.

In reality, few of us fit neatly into these categories. A man may have the bulk of an endomorph but the speed and agility of a mesomorph. But if you know what your predominant body shape is, you can customize a workout and dietary program that will make the best use of your natural assets.

The idea of putting a lot of effort into changing our bodies—or, to look at it another way, fighting the changes that begin to happen as we cross the Big 3-0—is something that many men are not comfortable with. Some would say it's all vanity. But is it? "Not at all," says Doug Lentz, director of the Chambersburg Sports Medicine and Rehabilitation Center in Pennsylvania. "It's wanting the most out of what we were given. If you think about it, it's the men who think that their bodies are perfect as they are who are truly vain."

But willingness to change is only half of the battle. The other half is reality. The kinds of changes you make and the way you need to go about them depend to some extent on the body type you begin with.

Endomorphs: Big and Brawny

If you ever watched William "Refrigerator" Perry tear up Soldier Field on Sunday afternoons, then you have a pretty good idea

---

How Does Your Chest Stack Up?

If you think you can pump up your love life by becoming a clone of Mr. Universe, you may be making a huge mistake. Yes, women like men with big pecs, but not as big as you might think.

In a study of 130 men and women, guys rated their own chest sizes as far scrawnier than what they thought women would find attractive, says J. Kevin Thompson, Ph.D., professor of psychology at the University of South Florida in Tampa.

But in reality, the men were closer to ideal than they knew. The chest size that the women said they liked virtually matched the smaller size that the men said they would prefer for themselves.

"These findings suggest that women do not prefer men with huge chests. Most women are attracted to someone who is athletic and physical but not bodybuilder size. So any man who is trying to develop a huge, bodybuilder's chest is probably out of line," Dr. Thompson says.

---

of the endomorph's native advantages.

Although they can't dance like a butterfly, endomorphs are surprisingly swift when

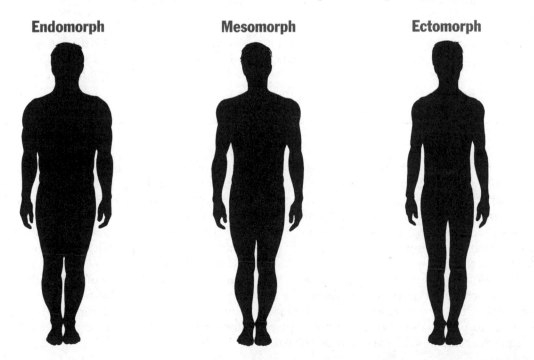

Endomorph   **Mesomorph**   **Ectomorph**

Average Men Don't Wear Plaid

Beyond the fashion basics—clean underwear—many of us are clueless about the do's and don'ts of being a sharp-dressed man. To help you out, here's a handy chart featuring the best fashion tips for each of the three body types from the Fashion Association in New York City and Combe, the maker of Just for Men hair care products.

	Endomorph	Mesomorph	Ectomorph
Goal	Minimize bulk; keep it simple; avoid layering; different textures.	Accentuate your best features without looking arrogant.	Maximize bulk; layer your look—vest over shirt, worn under blazer.
Tie	Big and tall (63"); narrow; neat pattern.	Average (55"), with small, elegant polka dots; bow ties.	Average (55") or big and tall (63"), if you're 6'4" or taller; wide.
Shirt	Create simple lines with vertically striped dress shirts, turtlenecks, banded-collar shirts; loose collar masks a double chin.	Solid polos and sports shirts; any type of dress shirt.	Dark colors and bold plaids, with extra length in the sleeves and tail.
Jacket	Long cut; opt for those with less detail.	Long duster overcoat.	Short styles, such as bomber jacket, give illusion of bulk.
Pants	Pants in stretch fabrics; jeans.	Gabardine wool dress pants, cuffed for smoother line.	Pleats; cargo pants and shorts.
Colors	Dark colors; solids; small-pattern plaids.	Bright colors such as red, pink and light blue.	Plaids; dark colors; avoid solid on solid look (black shirt and black pants).
Hair	Keep it short—long hair draws attention to girth.	Any style is fine; facial hair is often a plus.	Long hair okay, can help conceal long neck.

they're in condition. A low center of gravity and an ability to easily grow strong muscles make a guy with this large body type an instant pal of every neighbor who is moving heavy furniture or boxes. Endomorphs are good at moderate-intensity, long-duration activities such as cycling, alpine skiing, walking and rowing.

Because of a slower metabolism (the speed at which the body processes food), an endomorph has a greater tendency than other body types to put on the pounds. Endomorphs who don't stay in shape are also more prone to

heart disease and to injuries to weight-bearing joints such as the knees and ankles. So it's important that you keep a close watch on your diet and that you are a diligent exerciser, Lentz recommends.

The average American male follows a diet that's 35 percent fat. "That's disastrous for the endomorph," says *Men's Health* adviser Bryant Stamford, Ph.D., director of the Health Promotion Center at the University of Louisville in Kentucky. "Cutting that figure in about half still allows enough fat and affords plenty of variety in the diet."

One Size Fits All?

Just once you'd like to be able to walk into a clothing store and find a sea of trendy threads that fit just right. But too often it seems like men's fashions are designed for everybody except you. So who do the clothing mavens think is buying their stuff? Here's a glimpse at what the "average" man looks like, according to the Fashion Association in New York City.

Height	6 feet
Weight	165 to 175 pounds
Tie length	55 inches
Collar size	15½ inches
Arm length	34 inches
Jacket size	42 regular
Waist	32 inches
Inseam	32 inches
Shoe size	10

Mesomorphs: You've Got the Look

Blessed with broad shoulders, thin waists and natural strength, mesomorphs have basically all of the physical tools to outshine both endomorphs and ectomorphs. "The mesomorph is the guy that everybody probably hates because he has muscle stacked on top of muscle and may not have worked to get it," says Lentz.

Famous mesomorphs include the likes of Dan Marino, Carl Lewis and Deion Sanders, natural athletes who have a high percentage of muscle and little body fat. Men with this body type are naturally swift and dexterous. Because of this, mesomorphs often excel in multiple sports, says Lentz. But long-distance running and swimming probably aren't their favorite activities, because the weight of all of that muscle saps their endurance and lowers their buoyancy in water. Also, though a mesomorph may be somewhat freer with his diet than an endomorph, he is still prone to weight gain and may develop a potbelly if he doesn't pay attention to what he eats. "Just like anyone else, the mesomorph must watch the fat in his diet,"

says Chet Furhman, strength and conditioning coach for the Pittsburgh Steelers.

Ectomorphs: The Skinny on Leanness

This is the Kareem Abdul-Jabbar or Bill Rodgers type: all arms and legs. If you're an ectomorph, you're light, lean and less prone to overuse injuries. You're usually good at long-distance running and a natural at other endurance sports. You move nimbly and seem to have more energy than others. But because you have smaller muscles than other guys, it's harder for you to build up your strength and gain weight. Your thin frame, low body weight and high center of gravity work against you in many contact sports.

Too many ectomorphs get discouraged about their body type, says Lentz. "I hate to see someone selling himself short just because he feels he has been dealt a bad card genetically," he adds. The key to maximizing an endomorphic build? Know your body and focus on what you are blessed with, says Lentz.

Here's the upside: Ectomorphs have high metabolic rates. Even if they're just moderately active, they often get away with eating practically anything without gaining weight. They're also less susceptible to cardiovascular disease.

If your goal is to bulk up, protein and carbohydrate intake is critical to keeping your muscles primed. Also, be sure to get enough magnesium. A study conducted at Western Washington University in Bellingham suggests that getting 500 milligrams of magnesium per day—100 milligrams more than the Daily Value—may double your strength gains when used during a weight-lifting program. Good sources of magnesium include dark green vegetables, nuts, bananas and whole grains.

⚡Energy

- **Get more exercise.**
- **Adopt a positive attitude.**
- **Deal better with stress.**
- **Stay away from energy-draining foods and habits.**

Just 100 years ago, most men led lives of hard physical labor, dawn to dusk. If they were collapsing into bed at the end of the day, their exhaustion was well-earned.

Fast-forward to today, and men are collapsing into bed at night for the opposite reason: not enough physical activity. It is grand irony. Doctors today often recommend more exercise to patients who complain about not having enough energy. Meanwhile, athletes who work out for hours a day seem to be brimming with vitality, and men who earn a living doing physical work rarely complain about fatigue.

If you're dragging around without zip in your shorts, don't fear being alone. One study found that nearly 20 percent of men complain of major fatigue problems to their doctors. Most of these cases can easily be remedied. "Eighty to 90 percent of fatigue felt by men in our society is due not to disease but to very manageable causes," says Harold H. Bloomfield, M.D., psychiatrist and author of *The Power of 5: Hundreds of 5-Second to 5-Minute Techniques to Improve All of Your Life without Wasting Any of Your Time* and *How to Heal Depression.*

This chapter has all of the long-term strategies you need to maximize your vitality, plus quick power boosters you can use whenever you're feeling washed out. Use these strategies to revitalize. Chances are you can rekindle your energy on your own. But if you're still dragging yourself around by the collar after trying these strategies for a few weeks, call your doctor for a thorough evaluation. There might be deep-seated physiological reasons for your fatigue.

Energy and Mind

From a biological standpoint, the energy your body runs on comes from two basic sources: food and oxygen. Digestion breaks down food into amino acids, simple sugars and fatty acids. The primary simple sugar is called glucose; it is the one that your muscles, brain and, for that matter, virtually all of your cells use for fuel.

When work needs to be done—a pencil lifted, an eyelash winked, food digested—cells burn glucose and oxygen in a chemical reaction that creates mechanical energy. Thank your circulatory system for constantly supplying the two fuels and also for carting away the by-products, such as carbon dioxide.

The inference: If you aren't getting enough glucose or oxygen, your energy drops. Deep-breathing exercises often help boost energy, for example, says Leonard Doberne, M.D., a physician in Mountain View, California, who specializes in endocrinology and metabolism. But when guys talk about not having energy, it rarely is because of a shortage of fuel.

What creates the difference between someone who jumps out of bed in the morning enthusiastic and ready to go and someone who drags through the day? Is "energy" something physiological or psychological?

"It's not either/or," explains Dr. Bloomfield. "As men, we are bio-psycho-socio-spiritual beings, and our energy is affected on each of these levels." If our biology is off, or if we're emotionally down or deflated, our energy is going to be lower. "If we're working at a job that's not fulfilling for who we are—let's say we're an artistic personality working in sales—it's going to suppress our energy. And spiritually, if we're not regularly transcending the boundaries of our daily lives and roles, our energy is going to suffer."

When You Need to See a Doctor

Persistent fatigue may be caused by lack of exercise, excessive workload, insufficient sleep or other easily correctable factors, many of which are identified in this chapter. But it can also be a sign of serious illness. Anemia, thyroid problems, mononucleosis, hepatitis, diabetes, lung disease, heart disease and cancer are among the more serious illnesses that may first appear in the form of fatigue. Or the problem may be chronic fatigue syndrome. All of these require a doctor's attention.

Another possible cause of long-lasting low energy is depression. "You need to consider that possibility if you've been to the doctor and he has said that you're in decent medical health and if you know you've done your jogging and tried the tips in this chapter," says psychiatrist Harold H. Bloomfield, M.D., author of *The Power of 5: Hundreds of 5-Second to 5-Minute Techniques to Improve All of Your Life without Wasting Any of Your Time* and *How to Heal Depression*. "You don't have to feel depressed in order to be depressed. The most common symptom of depression presented to doctors is fatigue.

Plugging the Energy Drains

You may be feeling tired from too much exercise, or from not enough. Or from lack of sleep. Or from vitamin deficiency. Or from carrying around too much weight. Or from fighting off a disease or another illness. Or from too much pressure and stress, or from so little challenge that the boredom leaves you feeling fatigued and depressed, says Dr. Doberne.

What saps energy is different for each person. But every cause can be remedied. The trick is to know what is affecting you. Here are some of the most common energy drains and what you can do about them. Recognize what affects you and take action.

Defuse stress. The body's stress reaction—the notorious fight-or-flight response that gears you up for action—is an insidious energy thief. It tenses your muscles, pumps adrenaline into your blood and gets your heart beating faster and harder.

It's exhausting to be preparing for combat all day long. But that's just what intense work pressure, jammed freeways and overdue mortgage payments can do to you. "The complex responses of our bodies to stress," says Dr. Bloomfield, "may lead to the exhaustion of mental and physical energies."

The first step, Dr. Bloomfield suggests, is to "take a good look within yourself and make a checklist. Ask yourself, 'What's bringing my energy down?' "

In making your energy self-assessment, here's an important consideration: Not everyone is Superman, or even Michael Jordan. People's energy levels vary. "Some of us burn regular unleaded, and some burn diesel fuel," says John Douillard, D.C., author of *Body, Mind and Sport: The Mind-Body Guide to Lifelong Fitness and Your Personal Best*, a fitness book based on body types. "It's important to know who you are and, in terms of energy, to accept who you are.

"Some people sprint through the day; others are long-distance runners," says Dr. Douillard. "Some wake up rarin' to go and may feel energy in bursts, then fade. Others may start slowly, then build up and have long-lasting endurance. So make the best of what you naturally have."

Stress management is a big topic. It encompasses the way you look at life, how you manage your time, the goals you set for yourself, the way your parents and your environment have programmed you to operate. (We offer a separate chapter on the subject; see page 25.) Just realize that stress is not an external thing; it is your reaction to the world around you, says Dr. Bloomfield. Change your attitude, take control of your circumstance, and you truly can reduce stress.

If nothing else, take a few minutes several times a day to sit quietly, close your eyes and take a few deep, complete breaths, letting tension slide away. These mental breaks may be enough to give you more energy come evening.

Deflate the spare tire. "Carrying around excess poundage is tiring physically," says Dr. Bloomfield. "It is extra work for your heart and lungs and can be a psychological drain. You'll have a lot more energy if you drop that extra weight."

"But beware of crash diets," warns Dr. Doberne. They may not provide adequate nutrition and may cut your calorie intake too sharply. "A 'fasting' body thinks that it's in danger of starvation and automatically slows metabolism for self-preservation," he explains. This could make you feel even more sluggish and lethargic.

Check out your medications. Get out your magnifying glass and read the fine print that comes with your prescription and over-the-counter medications. "Many medicines can have drowsiness or fatigue as a side effect," says Dr. Doberne. "These include common drugs such as pain relievers and antihistamines as well as cardiac medicines, diuretics and anti-hypertensive drugs." Ask your doctor or pharmacist. And be sure to tell them all of the medications you're taking. Sometimes side effects come from combinations.

Junk the junk food. The typical fast-food meal, consisting of a greasy slab of meat (often with added cheese), fried potatoes and a drink full of sugar, is worse than useless for sustained energy. Fatty foods are the hardest for your body to digest, requiring the most energy. And sugar gives you a quick lift, then drops you to below where you started. So if you need to think or stay awake, steer clear of the cheeseburger, fries and shake, and go for a lean chicken sandwich or the salad bar.

Say good-bye to joe. Caffeine is a stimulator of the central nervous system that can sharpen your mind and senses and banish fatigue—temporarily. It accomplishes this by prodding the system to produce adrenaline and other stress hormones, speeding up your heart and metabolic rates to provide more strength and energy.

Like the effects of stress on the body, however, this ends up being an energy drain. Once the artificial stimulation provided by the caffeine is gone, energy levels plummet, and we feel a need for another jolt.

Bottom line: Don't rely on it. One or two cups of coffee a day for taste is fine. But it's not a good idea to rely on caffeine for energy, says Dr. Douillard. And that's true for whatever source the caffeine comes from: coffee, tea, cola, even chocolate. Too much caffeine can cause nervousness, restlessness, headaches, heartburn and insomnia. In the long run, rely on exercise and a high-energy diet for sustained energy without peaks and valleys.

Quit smoking. "Smokers say that cigarettes give them energy, and in a very limited way, they're right," says Garland DeNelsky, Ph.D., head of the Section of Psychology and director of the smoking cessation program at the Cleveland Clinic Foundation. "Nicotine is a stimulant. But it's not real energy, such as you get from nourishing food."

By stimulating the nervous system, tobacco increases your blood pressure and respiration rate and speeds up your heart. Your body needs more oxygen to handle this heightened activity, but alas, it can't get it. "That's because carbon monoxide from the smoke binds with hemoglobin (a protein that is a component of blood) and lowers the level of oxygen in the blood, so cells and tissues in the body don't get the oxygen they need to produce energy," explains Dr. DeNelsky. In addition, smoking reduces lung capacity, so even when you're not smoking, you can't get as much oxygen as you really need for high-energy performance.

Energy to Burn

Gathered from our experts, here are eight of the most vital ingredients you will need for a high-energy lifestyle.

Get off the couch. Exercise is critical for vitality. A sedentary lifestyle reduces your energy levels. Your heart and lungs become less efficient, so less oxygen gets to the cells and tissues. Metabolism drops, your body burns fewer calories, weight goes on easily, and you feel sluggish and unmotivated.

Exercise reverses this vicious circle. It increases the supply of oxygen to muscles, cells and tissues, revs up metabolism and pumps oxygen-rich blood through your veins, feeding your brain and body with fuel.

But don't overdo it. Too much exercise can be as bad for you as too little, says Dr. Douillard. "Some of us can just walk around the block and have enough. If you have a fast metabolism, you don't need a lot of physical activity to keep your body functioning at its best. But men who more easygoing and complacent need vigorous exercise. We're all different, so being tuned in to who you are and what you need is really important."

Eat a high-octane breakfast. If you want to guarantee pooping out by midmorning, start the day with a large cup of coffee, accompanied by a doughnut or one of those delicious, sticky sweet rolls, preferably filled with sugary jelly, says Dr. Douillard. You'll feel great—until your blood sugar plummets.

A breakfast of whole-grain cereal with skim milk and fruit will keep you going all morning. The protein in the milk will vitalize your brain, and the complex carbohydrates in the cereal and fruit will give you sustained energy until lunch.

Make the most of your prime time. Are you at your best in the early morning? Afternoon? Energy naturally ebbs and flows. Schedule your hardest tasks for those hours when you're at your peak, suggests Dr. Doberne. Be alert to observe your personal energy cycles; not everybody's body clock is exactly the same.

Energize yourself with sex. Does sex energize and restore you, or do you find it depleting? "Particularly as a man gets older," says Dr. Bloomfield, "he may feel better having sex more often but not ejaculating as much. Some ancient Eastern medical texts say that masterfully controlled sex replenishes and revitalizes the life force." Dr. Bloomfield suggests turning sex into sensual "loveplay," including more cuddling and intimacy, rather than focusing exclusively on "the act." "Especially for men over age 40, you don't have to ejaculate every time you have sex," he says.

Get enough sleep. Too obvious to mention? Perhaps—but will you do it? The only way for most of us to get more sleep is to go to bed earlier, but there's always so much to do, so many channels to surf. . . .

If you're serious about increasing your energy levels, there's no better place to start than with a good night's sleep. "In order to have high energy, you have to renew," says Dr. Bloomfield. "All of life is cycles of rest and activity, and the deeper your rest, the more dynamic your energy." Here are five suggestions from Dr. Bloomfield to help you catch enough Zzzs.

- Get regular exercise, in moderation.
- Go to bed at about the same time every night.
- Have a high-carbohydrate bedtime snack.
- Avoid coffee, tea and other caffeinated drinks after 6:00 or 7:00 P.M.
- Just say no to alcohol after dinner. It interferes with sound sleep.

Do what you enjoy. One key to high-energy performance is motivation. If you enjoy what you're doing, the energy will almost certainly be there. So be sure to make time for some really enjoyable activity every day. If your job doesn't fit this definition, then schedule some time to listen to music, read, shoot some baskets or do whatever pushes your personal joy-meter to the top of the charts.

Take breaks. Dozens of studies show that we feel better, and our performance is better, if we take periodic breaks from our work. Most of us operate on 90-minute cycles of concentration. If you find yourself reading the same sentence three times or drifting off to random thoughts, take a 5 or 10-minute break to energize. Go out for a breath of fresh air, stand up and stretch, take a drink of water or just give yourself permission to look out the window for a couple of minutes.

If you feel like you're trying to drive with your brakes on, you may need more than five minutes to renew. Consider taking a vacation. Well, okay, then at least take a day off from work. Go to the beach, the mountains or a museum. Take an afternoon—or an hour. Treat yourself to a walk; read a non-work-related book or a favorite magazine.

Order ginger ale instead. If fatigue is not an issue in your life, it's probably okay for you to have two beers or glasses of wine each day. But those drinks may be having more of an effect than you think, says Dr. Doberne.

Alcohol is a depressant that produces drowsiness as a natural side effect. True, it helps dissolve inhibitions and fosters gregariousness. But as sure as night follows day, the high you feel will be followed by a low, consisting of slowed-down reaction time, drowsiness and foggy, unreliable thinking, says Dr. Doberne. Even though you drink in the evening, the dulling effect can still be there the following day. So if you're complaining of fatigue, try eliminating alcohol and see how you feel, he says.

Fast Energy

Need to get revved up fast? Here are five ways to get a quick surge of energy.

Breathe in power. Take five long, deep breaths, breathing through your nose, suggests John Douillard, D.C., author of *Body, Mind and Sport: The Mind-Body Guide to Lifelong Fitness and Your Personal Best.* To charge the blood with oxygen, breathe slowly from your diaphragm, filling first your belly and then your chest. (There's more blood available in the lower lobes of the lungs for oxygen exchange.)

Follow with five "bellows breaths," faster but still deep, inhaling and exhaling as if you were pushing a bellows in and out. Finish with five more long, deep, slow breaths. Closing your eyes while you breathe adds relaxation, which can help dissolve energy-crunching stress.

Grab 40 winks. A brief nap of five to ten minutes can take the edge off deep fatigue and recharge your batteries.

Take an action break. If you spend most of your time sitting at a desk, get up and get physical for a few minutes. In one study, researchers at Stanford University in California found that four 10-minute exercise sessions yield about the same boost in aerobic capacity as a 40-minute session. So get off your seat and take a brisk walk or a quick jog, or do 10 minutes of stair climbing, cycling or rope jumping.

Have a high-protein snack. "Just a few bites of a healthy, high-protein food may contribute to increased energy, greater attention to detail and alertness, lasting for up to three hours," according to Harold H. Bloomfield, M.D., psychiatrist and author of *The Power of 5: Hundreds of 5-Second to 5-Minute Techniques to Improve All of Your Life without Wasting Any of Your Time* and *How to Heal Depression.* Try a sandwich made with chicken breast, turkey breast or fish; a cup of lentil or bean soup; some nonfat or low-fat yogurt; a few spoonfuls of cottage cheese; a sandwich made with low-fat cream cheese; or a glass of skim milk.

Wash your face. Get up, go the men's room (if you're at work) and splash some cold water on your face and neck. The break in your work, the walk and the cold water will combine to refresh your mind and body.

⬇⬆ Emotions

- **Adopt a resilient attitude.**
- **Understand your instincts.**
- **Transform your anger through appropriate activity.**

Men: cold, calculating, logical, rational, steady, invincible, steely, gritty, oblivious to pain, not swayed by emotion.

Aren't we something?

Truth is, we are expected to exhibit all of the above traits at times. And truth is, none of us is any of these things all of the time. But we are different. Different from women. And that's what makes the male-female dynamic so fascinating and frustrating, says John Gray, Ph.D., author of *Men Are from Mars, Women Are from Venus: A Practical Guide for Improving Communication and Getting What You Want in Your Relationship.*

All of those snips and snails and puppy dogs' tails in male DNA do make us feel and react differently than women. This is why being in touch with our feelings, and understanding how they influence us to act, is so crucial. Our feelings—or lack thereof—govern our relationships, our ability to succeed and navigate the storms of life and our health and overall well-being.

We must express our emotions if we are to maintain health and vigor; we can't bury them. But, notes Dr. Gray, much of the advice that men have been given in the past 20 years about how they need to open up and talk things out is fundamentally wrong. In fact, it's hogwash, he says. The advice is based on studies of what works well for women and ignores the fact that men are different.

Men, Dr. Gray says, instinctively tend to express their emotions through actions rather than through words. We need to understand and respect that, he says. Men sometimes need to talk, but only when they're ready. And that's

usually after they've mulled over a situation and come to terms with it.

In other words, don't take the "sensitive male" persona that pop culture has promulgated in the past decade too seriously. If you have the typical male genetic coding, you are not going to be kind and gentle and open and sharing—at least not all of the time.

We'll explore specific ways that men can best manage their emotions. But first, let's look at what emotions are and how they affect us.

Understanding Emotions

Emotion, says *Dorland's Illustrated Medical Dictionary*, is "any strong feeling state, such as excitement, distress, happiness, sadness, love, hate, fear or anger."

Emotions are complex. They cause changes in body chemistry. And changes in body chemistry bring on certain emotions. It works both ways, usually without any conscious effort on our part. Often we can consciously change our emotions by changing our posture, our type and level of activity and our thinking. A physical problem or defect, though, that causes an abundance or a deficiency of certain brain chemicals can create extreme moods that we cannot effectively control consciously, according to Larry J. Feldman, Ph.D., director of the Pain and Stress Rehabilitation Center in Newark, Delaware, and author of *Feeling Good Again: The Most Powerful Medicine Is What You Can Do for Yourself.*

Much mental illness is biological in origin—that is, it's caused by physiological flaws that create chemical imbalances. But much mental illness is simply the result of poor learned responses to life, says Michael J. Norden, M.D., in his book *Beyond Prozac.* Startlingly, Dr. Norden reports, a major study revealed that nearly half of us between the ages of 18 and 54 have met the criteria for psychiatric illness at some point in our lives, and for a third of us, the illness lasted more than a year.

Is there a benchmark for you to measure your emotional health? Science fails us here, if only because emotions are unquantifiable. But Dr. Feldman does offer this simple list of skills that an emotionally healthy man should have.

- He can manage his thinking.
- He is optimistic.
- He can focus on the needs of others.
- He has self-esteem.

Beyond biology, what determines our emotional balance? There are a number of factors, says mind-body medicine pioneer Bernie Siegel, M.D. Chief among them is our basic learned approach to life: our attitude, how we respond to situations. And tied in to that, he says, are our sense of self-worth and purpose.

Fortunately, says Dr. Siegel, it's never too late to build a better attitude and stronger self-esteem, to find and focus purposefully on a positive mission and to learn better ways to respond to life's stressors.

Develop a Winning Attitude

For a man to feel positive about himself and the world, "he needs to feel he is accomplishing things, doing things, achieving, providing constructively," says Dr. Gray. And as we make the transition from youth to maturity, "what we do needs to have a constructive benefit for others."

Do good deeds. We need to engage in activities that help others in order to develop and maintain a balanced, positive outlook, says Dr. Gray. It can be something as simple as chopping wood for somebody, he adds.

Focus on your greater purpose. "We have bodies," says Dr. Siegel, "so we can do things. And we should ask 'What can I do, more than just earn a living, to contribute love

Ten Twisted Attitudes

Feelings of anxiousness and depression are often the result of illogical thinking patterns. And feelings of anxiousness and depression encourage illogical thought processes.

By identifying the illogical patterns, and by challenging and correcting them as we catch ourselves thinking and speaking them, we can overcome the negative effects they generate, says Margaret A. Caudill, M.D., Ph.D., assistant clinical professor of medicine at Harvard Medical School and author of *Managing Pain before It Manages You.*

Following are ten common twisted attitudes that lead to a downward spiral of thinking, feeling and acting. These and other distorted thinking patterns were first pinpointed by psychiatrist Aaron T. Beck, M.D., in the 1950s and are at the core of commonly used cognitive therapy, which Dr. Beck developed, says Gregory Brown, Ph.D., a research associate in the Department of Psychiatry of the Center for Cognitive Therapy at the University of Pennsylvania in Philadelphia.

All or nothing. Black-and-white thinking. Insisting that things are either/or, one way or the other, and not realizing that nearly always there are many shades of gray, many possible explanations, solutions, choices.

Overgeneralizing. Taking one negative experience and mentally multiplying its effects. Using words such as "always" and "never"; for instance, your company transfers you to another town, and you lament to yourself "I'll never be happy there."

Catastrophizing. Focusing on a small negative to the exclusion of everything else; for instance, your date didn't like the hors d'oeuvres you ordered, and therefore the whole

and compassion to the world?' . . . Decide why you're here, what's important to you, what's the point of all of this. And then go and accomplish it."

Quiet the noise. "You are a satellite dish," says Dr. Siegel. "There are many messages coming to you. You have to decide what to focus on. So you pick up the remote and you pick out a channel and manifest it on your screen. Now the trouble with men, they never focus on one channel. They sit there and fly from one thing to another. They don't focus on 'What has meaning?' "

meal was a disaster. Magnifying negatives. Blowing things way out of proportion.

Discounting positives. Insisting that positive accomplishments or qualities don't count. Rejecting compliments with thoughts like "Not really" or "They're just saying that because they pity me."

Jumping to conclusions or mind reading. When you jump to conclusions, you predict negative outcomes or make negative assumptions based on the flimsiest evidence or no real evidence at all. When you mind-read, you assume you were snubbed because the boss didn't greet you in the hallway.

The Joneses. Comparing yourself unfavorably with people who are more successful than you rather than recognizing how well you've done compared with people who have accomplished less.

Overvaluing feelings. Because you feel incompetent in a certain situation, you decide you are incompetent, for example. Or because you don't like how something feels emotionally, it's bad. Reasoning by emotions.

Tyranny of the shoulds. Scolding (or motivating) yourself or others with "should," "shouldn't," "must," "ought to" and "have to" statements. They make you feel resentful and pressured.

Expansive labeling. Identifying with a shortcoming. Instead of saying "I made a mistake on that," you decide "I am a failure."

Personalizing. Deciding that people don't like you when they reject an idea of yours. Blaming yourself for things you aren't really responsible for.

Pick a positive path. When you are faced with choices, it's important to look deep inside and ask "What feels right?" says Dr. Siegel. Don't ask "What will make me the most money? What will most impress the neighbors?" What's important, he says, is "What will truly make me happiest as my way of contributing to life?" This is not selfish.

Cultivate caring. "If you look at men who are depressed—who have no pride, no self-esteem, no motivation—the most important symptom is that they've stopped caring," says Dr. Gray. "Caring is a very delicate feeling for a man to culture. A man must continue finding things that he cares about, that he's interested in, or he loses his energy and becomes depressed."

Try, try again. "The test for being a successful man is, do you care again? Do you try again?" says Dr. Gray.

"Life is a labor pain," says Dr. Siegel. We get rejected, we fail, we feel pain—all on the way to giving birth to great, fulfilling achievements and to ourselves. "It hurts a lot less," he says, "if we decide 'These are difficulties I choose to confront.' Then we realize that it's not someone else inflicting pain on us but pain we are choosing to go through."

Sweat it out. We can't say it too many times: A program of regular vigorous exercise makes us feel better, helps us think more clearly and causes the brain to release chemicals that make us feel better and make us more resilient. Find an activity you like and do it. (To find out how to do it right, turn to part 3. For some good advice on how to get started, see the tips on page 26.)

Dealing with Feelings

The war of the sexes: Shakespeare managed to build a five-century-long career out of it. Men and women think, feel and react differently. We know this, and yet at times we still get extraordinarily frustrated and confused by the differences.

This is not a unisex world. It is important for men to deal with their emotions in a manly way and for women to understand what men are doing, says Dr. Gray. And never is this more important than when dealing with anger, he adds.

Men, says Dr. Gray, need to retreat to their caves. To be alone. To be quiet. To reflect. To chop wood, to shoot hoops, to work out aggressive feelings and transform them into positive action. It may take a couple of days, he adds.

Women, says Dr. Gray, need to talk, and through talking, they release their energy.

But if a man who is angry is prodded to talk about it, he may become physically destructive, says Dr. Gray. If he's forced to talk before he's ready, "he will stay angry longer than if he had taken some quiet time to think about what's making him angry." Male anger "wants to be put into action," he explains.

"At those stressful times when there is anger, a man should stop talking, and a woman should stop asking him questions, because asking him questions baits him. It pulls him out. It gets him talking about his feelings, which intensifies his feelings, and he tends to act on those feelings. Men put anger into action much faster. Men have much less impulse control than women.

"That's why 90 percent of the people in jail are men," Dr. Gray says. "It's not because women are somehow nobler; it's just that when women hate somebody, they talk about it. When men hate somebody, they hit that person. They steal from that person. They do something based on those feelings of being mistreated."

What to do about it?

Back off. "A wise man," says Dr. Gray, "is able to take emotional energy and back off and think about what those feelings are and what is the most constructive thing he can do with those feelings."

Get active. When you are emotionally upset, do something constructive. "Take your focus off the thing that is upsetting you and shift your energy somewhere else," Dr. Gray suggests. "It could be just throwing a basketball through a hoop, or watching a football game, or working on a hobby—any activity through which the energy can be transformed and redirected." This is how men think about and figure out what they're feeling, he explains.

Overcome fear. Men tend to turn fear into procrastination, says Dr. Gray. "Engage in a hobby or an activity that you have no fear around, one that generates positive feelings," he suggests. "Then when you're feeling confident, come back to the problem at hand."

Give hurt a break. Feelings of hurt can easily move into feelings of anger and revenge, says Dr. Gray. Treat hurt like anger. Mull it over quietly and work it out with constructive physical activity, he says. If you act out your hurt by hurting others, you will always lose.

Don't wait for "I'm sorry." Men want to be right about everything. It's prehistoric, says Dr. Gray; it's a survival thing. And it means we're very, very defensive about our emotions when we express them to the person we are upset with. We tend to remain upset until we receive an apology or an assurance that the offending act won't be repeated. This, however, can sabotage our relationships with women. Instead of waiting for a woman to apologize, says Dr. Gray, we need to learn to dissipate the emotional energy through recreational activities and then forgive and forget.

Even though they complain about it, says Dr. Gray, women want us to be right. "Women don't go around looking for guys who are incompetent," he says. What women don't like, he adds, is when we refuse to apologize for our mistakes or when we demand apologies from them.

Express pride. Let others know you admire them. The best way to support a man is to let him know you appreciate something he does or has done. Men, much more than women, need and appreciate recognition of accomplishments.

Keep a log. Jot down things that evoke strong emotions as they happen throughout the day, urges Dr. Siegel. Then, he says, in the evening or before retiring at night, write out some thoughts about the experience. "I call it writing a poem every day," says Dr. Siegel. This is a healthy way for a man to gain greater awareness of his inner feelings, he says.

Stress

- **Control tension.**
- **Learn to see alternatives.**
- **Exercise physically.**

We're animals: born to run, built to forage across miles of rugged terrain daily. We don't do this, of course. Instead, we sit hunched over our computer keyboards or are engaged in other relatively sedentary or physically monotonous work. But our body chemistry remains in the primitive, primed to stride widely, tiptoe gently and race furiously at any split second to outwit a charging tiger. Sure, we can teach ourselves more positive, enlightened responses to stressful situations. But this primitive chemical reaction will still keep occurring. It is genetic, instinctive.

Back when we lived in caves, and even later when we lived on farms, we burned off stress rather cleanly with intense physical activity. Now we tend to repress it and store it, unhealthfully, in our organs, in our arteries, in our muscles.

"We have incredible amounts of repressed emotion stored up in our bodies. Our memories are stored in our bodies as well. I mean that literally," says mind-body medicine pioneer Bernie Siegel, M.D. The implication: Repressed stress can have physical repercussions such as making your body more susceptible to disease, Dr. Siegel says.

Besides our repressed emotional spikes and frustrations, we face many modern stressors that are seemingly beyond our control: air pollution (both indoors and out), chemical food additives, refined foods stripped of enzymes and nutrients, city noise, impossibly circuitous voice-mail systems and traffic jams, to name just a few.

Stress—physical, mental, emotional and environmental pressure—is not necessarily bad. But too much too often, undissipated, cripples us, notes Margaret A. Caudill, M.D., Ph.D., assistant clinical professor of medicine at Harvard Medical School.

Good stress kicks us into temporary overdrive, quickening our heart and breathing rates, increasing our blood pressure, speeding blood flow to our muscles and more, so we can face or flee danger effectively, according to Dr. Caudill. But if we get stuck in overdrive, we exhaust the body's ability to replenish itself. Chronic stress, says Dr. Caudill in her book *Managing Pain before It Manages You*, leads to the following:

- Reduced immunity to disease
- Constipation and/or diarrhea
- Poor sleep
- Fatigue
- Headache
- Forgetfulness and a short attention span
- Shortness of breath
- Weight gain or weight loss
- More muscle tension
- Depression
- Anxiety
- Increased sensations of pain

We do choose how we respond to stressors. We respond, usually automatically, in ways we have learned to respond, whether healthful or unhealthful. Our responses determine how we feel and function and, to a great extent, are responsible for our health.

We can learn great new, healthy responses that give us more energy and more esteem and, ultimately, make us more resourceful and effective. That's what we'll deal with in most of this chapter. First, though, let's look at exactly how pervasive stress is and what it does to us.

We won't pretend that we have a magic formula for making stress disappear. But we will show you some shockingly simple techniques for effectively managing it. You can choose to adopt them and experience both immediate and long-term benefits.

Get Physical

The first step in dealing with stress effectively—for life—is to take a tip from your caveman ancestors. Try to get out and work out the kinks every day. Find a sport or activity that you enjoy and do it. Make it a habit. If nothing else, walk vigorously for 30 minutes or more a day. Even a brisk 15-minute walk helps, according to David S. Bell, M.D., a family practitioner at the Lyndonville Family Health Center in New York and co-author of *Curing Fatigue.*

And stretch. Stretching relieves tension-bound muscles and flushes muscles and joints with fresh blood and nutrients, keeping them healthy. (Refer to the recommended stretches listed in part 3.)

Exercise improves brain function; increases the output of feel-good brain chemicals, so we feel better both physically and emotionally; dissipates pent-up frustration and aggression; loosens muscles, which eases physical tension; improves digestion; stabilizes blood sugar; reduces blood pressure; and much, much more, according to Susan M. Lark, M.D., who has written a book on dealing with stress.

Here are some exercise tips from Dr. Lark to help you get going, if you don't already have a program.

- Go slowly and gently for the first couple of weeks, increasing your effort gradually.
- Find an attractive location.
- Find your best time. Different people

The Stress Test

This chart, developed by Thomas Holmes, M.D., and his research associates at the University of Washington School of Medicine in Seattle, ranks the stressful events we face. Events with higher numbers (or values) generally elicit greater stress responses than those with lower values. Notice that stressors can be positive as well as negative events.

To check your own stress level, jot down the value of each stressor you've experienced in the past year. Multiply that figure by the number of times you've experienced the stressor during the year, up to four times (if it has occurred more than four times, multiply by four). Finally, add it up.

Dr. Holmes and his researchers have found a clear

Death of a spouse	100
Divorce	73
Marital separation	65
Death of a close family member	63
Jail term	63
Personal injury or illness	53
Marriage	50
Fired from work	47
Marital reconciliation	45
Retirement	45
Change in family member's health	44
Pregnancy	40
Addition to family	39
Business readjustment	39
Sex difficulties	39
Change in financial status	38
Death of a close friend	37
Change to a different line of work	36
Change in the number of marital arguments	35
Mortgage or loan for home or business	31
Foreclosure of mortgage or loan	30
Change in work responsibilities	29

feel better exercising at different times of the day.

- Set aside enough time that you can enjoy your workout without feeling rushed.
- Use your exercise time to unwind from

relationship between stress and health: People with high scores are particularly prone to serious illness. About 80 percent of people with scores higher than 300 get sick soon, as do about 50 percent of those who score between 200 and 299 and about 30 percent of those who score between 150 and 199.

But hold on to your score for a minute. What really matters is not your score but how you respond to the stressors, says Larry J. Feldman, Ph.D., director of the Pain and Stress Rehabilitation Center in Newark, Delaware. A person who is trained in stress management can handle many more stressors. So if your score is high, consider it a warning and a motivator to practice stress reduction rather than a prediction of certain doom.

Son or daughter leaving home	29
Trouble with in-laws	29
Outstanding personal achievement	28
Spouse beginning or stopping work	26
Starting or finishing school	26
Change in living conditions	25
Revision of personal habits	24
Change in the number of troubles with a boss	23
Change in residence	20
Different working hours or conditions	20
Change to a new school	20
Change in church activities	19
Change in type or amount of recreation	19
Change in social activities	18
Mortgage or loan for smaller purchases such as a television	17
Change in sleeping habits	16
Change in eating habits	15
Change in number of family gatherings	15
Vacation	13
Minor violation of the law	11

your daily work and grind.
- Listen to music while working out.
- Always warm up gently and allow time to cool down.
- Wear loose clothes.

Stress Reduction: More Basics

You can't deal with stress effectively if your basic lifestyle is in opposition. Here's how to adjust your days toward a lower-stress existence.

Sleep on it. Getting adequate sleep is essential to beating stress. Most of us need about eight hours to feel rested, says Michael J. Norden, M.D., in his book *Beyond Prozac*. It's simple math: You can't watch the late show every night, then get up with the alarm at 5:00 A.M. or even 6:00 A.M. and have had enough sleep.

How do you know if you're getting adequate sleep? Do you have trouble waking? Are you sleepy during the day? Could you doze off, as they say, at the drop of a hat? Then you're probably not getting the sleep you need, says Dr. Norden.

Adequate sleep means more than a certain number of hours. It also means sleeping at about the same time every day to maintain your body's natural rhythms and cycles.

Starve stress. Okay, okay. We all know we should eat right. But here's where it really hits home. What goes in our mouths day to day will have a substantial effect on our stress levels over both the short term and the long term, says Dr. Norden.

We need a proper balance of nutrients to maintain our bodies' ability to resist disease, repair damage, think clearly and quickly and so on. We don't get that from skipping breakfast, gobbling sugary and greasy snacks, guzzling soft drinks and coffee, grabbing burgers on the run and then getting silly on beer with the guys after work.

When you're feeling under pressure, pay particular attention to the fuels you use. Cut back on stimulants such as coffee and cola. Skip the empty-calorie salty snacks and the menu of white flour/white sugar junk-food temptations ranging from cakes to candies, says Dr. Caudill. They may give you a short burst of energy, but they'll increase your fatigue as the day wears on. Back off from fats and oils a bit. And put the brakes on big-time boozing; it actually runs you down more and interferes with your sleep.

Instead, add snacks of fresh fruits. Drink lots of water. Pack in three daily meals teaming with fresh vegetables, grains and other high-fiber foods. This is the fuel that increases stamina. Dr. Caudill cautions that nutrition is variable from person to person, so be in tune with your body's needs. But a great basis to work from is the U.S. Department of Agriculture's Food Guide Pyramid. (For complete details, see "The Building Blocks of Good Nutrition" on page 4.)

But be realistic. If you decide to shift your diet to the healthy side, do it gradually, so the change is bearable and so you can notice and track the positive effects without feeling overcome by deprivation.

"If you're eating vegetables and exercising and meditating and buying books and tapes so that you won't die, stop," says Dr. Siegel. "Because you're going to be very upset someday. If that's your motivation, you may as well have the steak, sleep late and save the money, because you are going to die. The reason to do these things is to enjoy life more now, because they make you feel better now."

The Art of Relaxation

We can truly train our bodies and minds to relax, according to Larry J. Feldman, Ph.D., director of the Pain and Stress Rehabilitation Center in Newark, Delaware, and author of the book *Feeling Good Again: The Most*

Powerful Medicine Is What You Can Do for Yourself. Try it.

One particularly effective way is to consciously change how we breathe, Dr. Feldman says. But other simple calming measures—going for a walk, calling a friend—may be enough to change our brain chemistry for the better.

How? By consciously relaxing the body and/or the mind, we signal the brain to begin producing a cocktail of relaxation chemicals that, in turn, cause us to relax even more, says Dr. Feldman. Doing this on a regular basis evokes many long-term, positive physical and mental changes and much greater tolerance of stress. Dr. Feldman teaches a process for this called the relaxation response, which centers on concentrated breathing. It can easily be learned, says Dr. Feldman.

Here are some other relaxation techniques.

Progressively relax. Alternately tense and relax each part of your body, starting with your toes and working your way up to your scalp. Combine the tensing and releasing with your in/out breathing, suggests Dr. Caudill. For instance, curl the toes on your right foot as you breathe in, then relax them as you breathe out. Then flex your right foot toward your head, breathing in; then release, breathing out. Then tense your right leg from the knee downward on the breath in and relax it on breath out. Then tense your right hip and buttock as you breathe in, relaxing as you breathe out. Move to your left toes and up to your left hip before progressing the rest of the way up your body.

Breathe through your shoulder. Or wherever you feel tension, says Dr. Caudill. Imagine drawing your breath through the tense area. Breathe out through the same area. Exhale the tension with the breath and picture it disappearing in the air. Some counselors suggest imagining that your in-breath is a healing color or warm, golden light and your out-breath is red or black tension leaving the area and dissipating in the air. You can picture breathing through your neck, your forehead, any tense part of your body.

Sound out tension. So-called New Age music recordings are designed to be soothing, notes Dr. Caudill. Many record stores offer tapes and compact discs of calming nature sounds: a babbling brook, the seashore, a rainstorm. Changing the soundtrack can instantly transform a tense atmosphere.

Soak it away. Hot water relaxes tense muscles and soothes the soul. Try a hot pool, a Jacuzzi or hot springs. Or just draw a steamy bath and soak. (But this caveat: A hot soak doesn't mix well with some health conditions, particularly circulatory problems. If you have chronic health troubles, ask your doctor about this first, cautions Dr. Caudill.)

Get an Attitude

"The optimist is right. The pessimist is right," wrote Ralph Waldo Trine in his 1897 book *In Tune with the Infinite: Fullness of Peace, Power and Plenty.* "Each is right from his own particular point of view, and this point of view is the determining factor in the life of each."

How we view our circumstances from moment to moment—the stories we tell ourselves in the running dialogue in our minds—affects our moods and anxiety levels.

A resilient attitude disarms stress, says Dr. Siegel. "If something adverse happens and all of the people in your life tell you 'God is redirecting you, something good

The Relaxation Response

It's hard to believe that something as simple as focusing on your breathing for a few minutes a day can cause profound, beneficial physical changes.

While yogis had claimed this for thousands of years and some doctors had speculated about it as early as the nineteenth century, modern medicine uncovered the precise principle at work—without any religious dogma—in 1968. It was Herbert Benson, M.D., Ph.D., of Harvard Medical School, who identified the relaxation response.

Students challenged Dr. Benson to monitor people meditating (transcendental meditation was popular at the time) and test for physiological changes. Dr. Benson resisted at first but eventually gave in.

He found that meditators experienced immediate, beneficial changes in physiology. As his studies progressed, he discovered more: that people who evoke the relaxation response daily for 30 days or longer begin to experience an overall decrease in anxiety and depression and increased confidence in their ability to cope with any pitch life throws them.

To evoke the relaxation response, Dr. Benson found, one must simply do the following:

1. Focus on a repetition, such as your breathing and/or a word, gently blocking out the rest of the world.

2. When any other thought comes along, acknowledge it, let it go and gently return to focusing on the repetition.

Dr. Benson feels that one 30-minute session a day is optimum. But shorter sessions of 3 to 5 minutes may be better, says Larry J. Feldman, Ph.D., director of the Pain and Stress Rehabilitation Center in Newark, Delaware, and author of *Feeling Good Again: The Most Powerful Medicine Is What You Can Do for Yourself,* particularly if you do several short sessions throughout the day. And, he notes, it's easier for most people to schedule 3-minute sessions.

Dr. Benson found that you could even practice the relaxation response while exercising. The key here is to focus on your exercise rhythm, your rhythmic breathing or a calming word of your choosing and to gently discard disruptive thoughts as they impinge.

will come of this,' just think about that for a minute," he says. "That changes your entire life. Difficulties are opportunities. They are opportunities for redirection." Clearly, winners don't view setbacks as end-all catastrophes. But that kind of thinking is part of the plague of stress. We must rebuke it and replace it and learn survival behavior.

Challenge negatives. When you find yourself despairing, agonizing, complaining or feeling victimized, give your thoughts the equivalent of a military inspection. Examine them for illogical reasoning. And correct it when you find it, says Dr. Caudill. (For help, you might turn to "Ten Twisted Attitudes" on page 22. It describes illogical thought patterns that often send us plummeting.)

Police your self-talk. Bite back when your inner dialogue is getting out of line. Let it know who's in control. Alter it when it's pummeling you. Insist that it be open to fresh, positive possibilities and that it tell the whole truth, not just some nasty, negative angle it's cornered. Judge thoughts not as good or bad, says Dr. Caudill, but as effective or ineffective. Weed out the ineffective ones.

Change things. Identify and pinpoint stressors in your life. See if you can reduce their negative impact—maybe by altering them, maybe by discarding them, maybe by facing them differently. Deal with the underlying causes of stress, advises Mort Orman, M.D., author of *The 14-Day Stress Cure*.

Seize the moment. Practice simple time management: Prioritize. Buy an organizer and use it. Plan your days and weeks on paper, listing the priority tasks. Adjust as needed based on importance and urgency and not just on urgency alone, which is often a temptation. And just as important as scheduling work tasks is scheduling time for fun and rewards and, of course, relaxation, says Dr. Caudill.

Solve your problems. Identify a problem on paper in a sentence or two. That alone often defuses the tension, noted Dale Carnegie in his 1940s classic *How to Stop Worrying and Start Living*. It brings the problem down to size instead of allowing it to be some big, mysterious pressure looming in the background. You can't begin to solve a problem until you've identified it.

Practice decision making like the pros. After identifying a problem, Carnegie taught, seek the cause of the problem. Then gather as much information as possible about it, as impartially as you can. List all possible solutions. Pick the best one and act on it, he said. Then—and this is the magical part—let it go. You've done the best you can. So quit worrying about the problem. You can always start the process over if the solution doesn't work out well.

Organize your workload. Prioritize and schedule tomorrow's work before you quit for the day, advised Carnegie. Then, he said, you don't feel chased by the clock, harassed by an unmanageable, unpredictable workload. Frank Bettger went one step further in his classic salesman's manual of the 1940s, *How I Raised Myself from Failure to Success in Selling*. He said we should organize the next week's work before leaving the office on Friday. Then we hit the ground running on Monday while most other people are floundering.

Take breaks. If you sit at a desk, get up and move and stretch every 30 minutes or so to keep muscle tension from building up. Reward yourself with short breaks when you complete each major task. Take a fresh-air break or a 5-minute walk, or get a cup of herbal tea. Find healthful rewards you enjoy and indulge yourself with them.

Don't lose your balance. Most of us know the importance of having hobbies or favorite activities to distract us from the demands of our work schedules. But sometimes we make the mistake of choosing hobbies that are really extensions of our office life: for example, the computer programmer who designs video games in his free time, or the journalist who writes screenplays at night.

We certainly wouldn't tell you not to advance your career with outside activities, but if the words "tax deduction" enter your mind, you need a different hobby. Look for something completely removed from your business activities.

Sex

- **Slow down.**
- **Enjoy touch more and orgasm less.**
- **Communicate better.**

The GQ guy and the gorgeous babe meet, buy dinner, head to her place (or his) and make cataclysmic love. Lush, energetic music charges the air and surges to crescendo after crescendo. They moan. They gasp. After about 70 seconds of undressing, caressing, rocking and rolling beneath a light sheet, the woman sobs, screams, shakes in ecstasy. The man collapses atop her, then rolls onto his back.

The woman carefully clutches the sheet to her breasts and reaches for a pack of cigarettes. Exhaling streams of smoke, they tell each other how great they were. And then, within hours, they're at it again, with either each other or someone else.

Thank you, Hollywood. Thank you, pulp novels. Thank you, Madison Avenue. Thank you for an audiovisual noisescape so layered with exaggerated and distorted sexual imagery that most of us don't know what is what anymore.

The fact is, everybody else isn't having better, louder, longer, more frequent sex than we are. They aren't boffing neighbors, co-workers and acquaintances behind our backs and then getting it on with their wives or girlfriends every night.

The fact is, according to the comprehensive *Sex in America* survey conducted by researchers at the University of Chicago, the majority of adult Americans make the beast with two backs only a few times a month or a few times a year—or don't do it at all. And the rest of us? There truly is a lucky eight ball. Eight percent of us, or barely 1 in every 13 guys, make it four times or more a week. And 25 percent of us do it two times a week.

What about all of those swinging The fact is, married and cohabiting couples have lots more sex than folks who are truly single.

No matter what our frequency or our marital status, we can have better, more intense, more pleasurable sex, starting right now. Here's how, broken down into eight steps.

Step 1: Adopt an Attitude

First off, realize that your primary sex organ is not the monster in your pants but the amazing malleable matter between your ears. How you think about sex is everything.

Your attitude, approach, beliefs, expectations, choices and reactions all reside in your mind, says San Francisco Bay–area psychotherapist and sexologist Jack Morin, Ph.D., author of *Erotic Mind.* So when you're seeking better sex, the first thing to look for is some great mind-sets. Do as follows.

Make sex a symphony, not a horse race. Slow down. You're not trying to get to the finish line. In fact, the longer you prolong the process of getting there, the more senses you can involve, and the more stimulation and excitement you have to enjoy, savor and remember, says Dr. Morin. Take detours. Take rests. Lose the race. Vary the pace. Use slow, teasing, dallying, probing strokes and moves much of the time. Pause between them and enjoy the sensations they provoke. Enjoy the journey; it's the real adventure. It's where the most enduring pleasure is found.

Forget formulas. Sex is not a series of how-to steps to be followed in order, for set amounts of time, as though you had a manual and stopwatch in your hands, says Dudley Seth Danoff, M.D., senior attending urologic surgeon at Cedars-Sinai Medical Center in Los Angeles, in his book *Superpotency.* Instead, he says, loosen up. Go with intuition and inspiration. Be spontaneous.

Lose control. Despite perceived—and sometimes actual—expectations, the male is not the sexual entertainment director. It's not up to you to set the pace and keep the show rolling. Become a participant. Lose yourself and let the show develop its own script.

And while we're at it, don't make her orgasm your overriding concern and responsibility, says Dr. Morin. The *Sex in America* researchers found that only 29 percent of women come every time, yet 40 percent of women are physically happy with their sex lives. The moral? Provide an opportunity, but don't hang all of your bets on it and don't count yourself a loser if it doesn't happen.

Give and ye shall receive. Much of the pleasure is in giving and in watching and sensing your partner's response, notes John D. Perry, Ph.D., psychologist, sexologist and co-author of *The G-Spot*.

Shift your focus. Away from the genitals, away from orgasm, onto touch and feeling. Sense your senses, not just your penis; your penis will follow. "Practice this while masturbating," says Dr. Morin. "Touch yourself all over, not on just your genitals. Explore and experiment. Find other areas that are also pleasurable to touch."

Make the most of memories. Recall and analyze your greatest sexual experiences, says Dr. Morin. "Pay attention to your most exciting fantasies," he suggests. "What is going on? What story is being told here?" Are there ways to incorporate some of the exciting elements into your current sex life?

Get back to nature. At its primal base, sex is an animal activity. In her book *Sexual Pleasure*, Barbara Keesling, Ph.D., says, "It's okay to growl, grunt, bare teeth, even howl."

Step 2: Master the Hunt

Before you can put some of these mind-sets into practice, you must find a willing partner. And, of course, we can help with that. (This section is not required reading if you are currently in a long-term relationship. You may, if you like, skip ahead to step 3. Just remember that we're here if you ever need us.)

One-night stands are not very fashionable, to say the least. Want a Hollywood reference?

When Harry Met Sally is a more likely scenario than *Body Heat*.

The *Sex in America* survey found that only 14 percent of couples in relationships that last less than a month do the wild thing within the first two days of meeting. And interestingly, only 1.4 percent of couples who eventually get married have sex within the first two days of meeting. But the study also found that close to 40 percent of couples in short-term relationships have sex within the first month of knowing one another. The lessons here? Expect to invest some quality time. If you're looking to get married, expect to invest more quality time.

The *Sex in America* survey goes on to say that your chances of getting lucky get better when you hang at bars or private parties or you're at work; almost half of short-term couples meet that way. But you're most likely to meet someone you'll go to bed with and have a lasting relationship with when you're introduced by a close mutual friend or family member. Still, slightly more than one-third of longer-term relationships are initiated by self-introduction, so clearly, it doesn't hurt to try. And 47 percent of relationships lasting less than a month are the result of self-introduction.

Before you get to a self-introduction, it is likely that you'll do a little ogling. Men ogle.

In an article called "The Fine Art of Ogling," Denis Boyles, a writer for *Men's Health* magazine, notes that if a woman glances back twice, making eye contact the second time, she's saying "I know you're watching me, and I think you're sort of marginally interesting, and I think I'll see what you're made of, buster." And then what?

"If you look away, too stunned or embarrassed to continue ogling, you're scrapple," Boyles says. "A guy too cowardly to stand up for his own ogle isn't much of a man in most women's books. But if you continue to ogle in the face of a double glance, the ball is back in her court. If she looks away, no point. If she smiles, you can figure you've been asked to politely identify yourself, your motives, your marital standing."

The Female Genitals

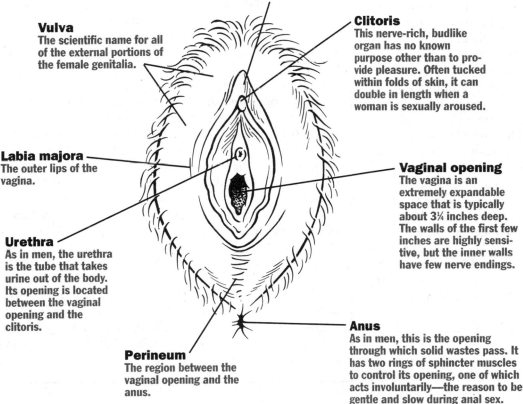

Labia minora
The inner lips of the vagina are also sensitive to sexual touch.

Vulva
The scientific name for all of the external portions of the female genitalia.

Clitoris
This nerve-rich, budlike organ has no known purpose other than to provide pleasure. Often tucked within folds of skin, it can double in length when a woman is sexually aroused.

Labia majora
The outer lips of the vagina.

Vaginal opening
The vagina is an extremely expandable space that is typically about 3¼ inches deep. The walls of the first few inches are highly sensitive, but the inner walls have few nerve endings.

Urethra
As in men, the urethra is the tube that takes urine out of the body. Its opening is located between the vaginal opening and the clitoris.

Perineum
The region between the vaginal opening and the anus.

Anus
As in men, this is the opening through which solid wastes pass. It has two rings of sphincter muscles to control its opening, one of which acts involuntarily—the reason to be gentle and slow during anal sex.

From there, you're on your own. Well, almost. Ten pointers for first dates from those pros at *Men's Health* magazine:

1. Know what you're after. Someone to pal around with? Someone to show off? Someone to sleep with? Someone to marry?
2. Forget weekdays; go out on Fridays. Saturday morning-afters are much less awkward than weekday morning-afters, when we're all rushing to work. And you have all weekend to dig in deeper.
3. Keep it simple. Go to a movie or to a nice but not too fancy spot for dinner.
4. Bathe, brush your teeth and wear clean clothes appropriate to the occasion.
5. If she asks about your past, don't boast. Don't tell her the story of your life and name all of your exes and their neuroses. Mostly, listen to her. Try to find out about her.
6. Don't drink too much. Don't get sloppy, maudlin, out of control, sick.
7. Don't push for sex on the first date.
8. Always pay. Insist on it.
9. Walk her to the door. Don't grope.
10. Do it again, soon.

Step 3:
Warm Up Smartly

Men and women turn on at different speeds. In part, it's a biological thing—more proof that God has a sense of humor. Men blast off. Women need their fires stoked, notes Domeena Renshaw, M.D., in her book *Seven Weeks to Better Sex.* And once men lift off, we feel tremendous momentum. Our engines throb; our pistons are primed for jackhammer pumping. Most women would like some romance, some kissing, some caressing, some stroking. The solution? Sex therapists say it's simple: Men should change.

This is not a small change. But the rewards are great. For many men, it means discovering a whole new way of making love.

William Howell Masters, M.D., and Virginia Johnson, famous for the sexuality studies they conducted in the 1950s and 1960s, taught that men go through four stages of sexual arousal: excitement, plateau, orgasm and resolution. Dr. Keesling and others point out that some men follow this pattern precisely, but many do not. Many have multiple plateaus, and some have multiple sensations of orgasm (though not necessarily accompanied by multiple ejaculations).

Men can gain immeasurable pleasure from lingering between the excitement and orgasm phases and from learning how to go to the brink and then back away without ejaculating, says Dr. Keesling.

Here are eight surefire ways to heighten your desire and excitement and to get her engine purring.

Light her candle. Set the mood. Make

The Right Touch

Rubbing someone the right way is soothing, intimate and a really nice thing to do.

Massage wipes away stress and pumps invigorating oxygen into the muscles. And, says licensed massage therapist Linda Van Ackeren of Santa Fe, New Mexico, deep communication takes place between the giver and the receiver. That makes massage ideal as a communication of love.

Professional massage therapists spend hundreds upon hundreds of hours studying techniques, anatomy, physiology and more. But the beauty of massage is that anyone with two hands (or even one) can communicate love through touch.

Consider using a light oil—scented massage oil, almond oil, even olive oil—to increase sensitivity, says Van Ackeren. Or for less muss and fuss, try regular body lotion or cornstarch.

For a wonderfully sensuous massage, Van Ackeren offers these tips.

- "First," she says, "get centered. Try to feel relaxation in your body." You can't communicate relaxation effectively if you're uptight.
- "You must always touch a person with reverence," she says. The touch needs to be firm but gentle, especially at first. "Firm, so it feels safe and nurturing; soft, so the person you're massaging knows that she can relax, that she's not getting attacked," she says.

the environment, atmosphere, attitude and approach relaxing and conducive to warmth and loving and privacy and excitement. This can be as simple as shutting out distractions and tuning in to her, says Dr. Keesling.

Pay attention! To her. Explore her—all over. Sense her. Use your fingers. Use your tongue. Use your breath. Putting all of your attention on your lover's pleasure is a real turn-on, says Dr. Keesling.

Make love all day. You can start the dance long before undressing. Be affectionate. Be warm. Be cuddly. Be complimentary.

Tell her she's beautiful. Tell her. "But don't lie, though. Focus on what you truly appreciate about her. She needs to feel sexy and

• "Move your hands slowly in long, smooth strokes, all of the way down the area you're massaging and then back up for each stroke," Van Ackeren says.

• Take your time in each area. "Repetitive motions are very relaxing and very calming," she says. Quietly ask for feedback; "Ask if the pressure is okay," Van Ackeren suggests.

• A good place to start is with the back, she says. "It's the broadest body expanse, and because the nervous system runs along the spine, you can affect the whole body by working the spinal region," she explains. "Work the shoulders, the neck, the whole back. These are the areas where I find people hold the most tension."

• If this is an intimate massage with a lover, she says, "feel free to be playful with your touch. But keep it caring and nurturing."

• "The face is a very sensitive area for a lot of people," Van Ackeren says. "Use a gentle, delicate but confident touch when working on the face and jaws."

• Don't forget the scalp, she adds; massage it as though you were washing your hair. "People hold so much tension there," she says.

• Be careful with the hands and feet, but don't ignore them. "It can be really painful if the pressure is too intense. No digging in. Rub. Pull the fingers and toes. Get in between the fingers and toes. Rub the palms in a circular motion. Work out the hands as if you were kneading them," she says.

good about herself and her body in order to relax and feel good about sex," says Dr. Morin.

Touch. Be gentle. Pay attention to where you are touching or being touched and soak up the sensations. Move slowly, slowly, slowly, says Dr. Keesling. Start with her extremities, not with her crotch and breasts. Stroke her arms and legs. Stroke her face.

Don't obsess. An erection isn't everything. It's needed only for humping and pumping. Relax. Let it rise and fall, and don't worry about it. "It's a myth that a man must maintain a rock-hard erection throughout the encounter," says Dr. Morin. "This puts on a lot of pressure, and the erection gets in the way."

Experiment with oils du jour. In porn

stories, a woman's excitement is gauged by her vaginal wetness. Wetness often is a sign of arousal. But in real life, an aroused woman can be dry, while a wet woman can be bored silly. Ample lubrication generally increases everybody's pleasure during intercourse and sex play, says Dr. Keesling.

Playing with lubricants is a healthy way to have fun. Oils, however, dissolve the latex used in condoms and can encourage yeast and bacteria growth in the vagina, says marriage and family therapist Patricia Love, Ph.D., in *Hot Monogamy: Essential Steps to More Passionate, Intimate Lovemaking*, a book she co-authored. So for vaginal lubrication, Dr. Love recommends one of the space-age water-based lubricants that have been developed for sex play. She considers Astroglide one of the best. It's available in many pharmacies and adult stores and by mail order from the manufacturer, BioFilm (call 1-800-848-5900).

Water-based lubricants tend to dry out and get sticky and need to be reactivated from time to time with a splash of water. Saliva will do. A glass of water within reach of the bed is even handier.

P.S.: To truly gauge a woman's arousal level, listen for changes in her breathing, advises Dr. Keesling. Slow, heavy breathing means she's warming up. If she's panting, hot and heavy, she is circling runway O and may be coming in for a landing.

Get oral, Robert. Women appreciate men with clever tongues. The best-selling 1971 sex manual *The Sensuous Man* advised us to "nibble, nip, eat, lick and suck." We are to

(continued on page 38)

A Man's Guide to Sexually Transmitted Diseases

Disease	Number of New Cases in U.S. Annually	How Acquired
Chlamydia	3–5 million	Bacterial infection acquired primarily through vaginal or anal intercourse
Genital herpes	200,000–500,000	Viral infection spread by skin-to-skin contact with the infected area, even when there are no symptoms
Gonorrhea	1.1 million	Bacterial infection of the urethra, rectum, mouth or throat acquired through vaginal, anal or oral sex
Hepatitis B	53,000 (sexually transmitted cases)	Viral infection found in blood, semen, vaginal secretions and saliva; acquired by sexual contact, especially anal intercourse; attacks the liver
HIV/AIDS	N/A (HIV)/90,000 (AIDS)	Viral infection that damages and destroys cells of the immune system; acquired through sex and contact with infected blood
Human papillomavirus (HPV)	500,000–1 million	Viral infection acquired through vaginal, anal or oral sex
Syphilis	120,000	Bacterial infection acquired through vaginal, anal or oral sex or by skin contact with open sores

Symptoms	Treatment	Complications If Not Treated
25 percent of cases in men show no symptoms; symptoms are usually mild, appearing within 2 weeks of exposure, and include abnormal genital discharge, burning during urination and swelling or pain in the testicles.	Antibiotics	Can lead to epididymitis (an inflammation in the scrotum)
Sometimes none; often an itching or burning sensation, lesions; pain in the genital area, legs or buttocks; genital discharge within 10 days of exposure; later developing painful blisters or open sores that heal after several weeks but may reappear.	Antiviral drug reduces frequency and duration of outbreaks; no known cure	Increases risk of HIV infection through open sores
Sometimes none; often mild, appearing within 1–2 weeks and including discharge from the penis or rectum and burning or itching during urination.	Antibiotics, though increasingly penicillin-resistant	Sterility; infected joints, heart valves or brain
One-third of carriers experience no symptoms; symptoms may range from mild to severe and include fever, headaches, muscle aches, fatigue, loss of appetite, vomiting, diarrhea and, in advanced stages, dark urine, abdominal pain and yellowing of the skin and the whites of the eyes.	A vaccine is available; most infections clear up on their own within 8 weeks, though some become chronic	Chronic infections can lead to cirrhosis, liver cancer and death
Sometimes none at first; sometimes flulike symptoms that last for up to a month, beginning 1–2 months following exposure; then the virus becomes dormant, sometimes for years, but continues attacking and weakening the immune system, leaving the individual at risk for all sorts of opportunistic infections and certain cancers.	New antiviral drugs slow its spread	Nearly everyone with HIV eventually develops AIDS and dies of AIDS-related complications
Sometimes none; sometimes produces painless, fleshy, cauliflower-like warts on and inside the genitals, anus and throat.	No known cure; warts can be suppressed by freezing, chemicals or laser surgery but will likely reappear	Occasionally cancers of the penis and anus
Within 3 months of exposure, produces painless sores known as chancres, usually on the genitals; the sores usually disappear within a few weeks. Later, the individual may experience a rash anywhere on the body, mild fever, fatigue, lesions in the mouth or throat, hair loss or swollen glands. Symptoms may come and go for 2 years. Then the disease enters latent stage and is no longer contagious, though it can still do damage.	Penicillin at any stage, though damage will not be reversed	May cause serious damage to the heart, brain, eyes, nervous system, bones and joints

think of the tongue as "a hot electric wire causing a slight shock sensation wherever it touches." It advised us to slide and swirl our tongues all over a woman's body: her neck, her earlobes, her mouth, her nose, her eyelids. To run it "like a tiny paintbrush" along the small of her back and up the insides of her legs. And to ever so slowly wend our way to the clitoris. In the 20-plus years since the book's publication, no group of outraged women has protested, waved signs and shouted "Clitoris first! Clitoris first!" Remember that.

In this age of safe sex, a device called a dental dam is an essential sex toy, suggests Jeffrey Laurence, M.D., senior scientific consultant to the American Foundation for AIDS Research and director of the Laboratory for AIDS Virus Research at Cornell University Medical College, both in New York City. You'll find them in most safe-sex boutiques. "The dental dam is really just a flexible piece of rubber—a six-inch square of heavy latex that's several times thicker than the male condom—that can block the direct spread of bacteria and viruses," he says. Just place the dam over the vagina or anus. It won't stay put on its own, so you'll need to hold it in place while you touch, lick and suck the covered areas. Take care that the side touching the genitals or anus doesn't flip over. The dams cost less than a dollar each and are available unflavored or flavored.

Step 4: Master the Main Act

Masters and Johnson want us to toss out the term *foreplay*. They don't think we should consider playful touching, licking or nipping—or any particular activity—solely as a prelude to sex. It should be part of sex, appropriate at any point in the act.

They're not saying that a prelude is unnecessary, only that strains of the music played then should be repeated during the main movement. Every good symphony has repeated themes.

The main act is like a symphony, with highs, lows, choruses, quiet moments, crescendos and often a thundering climax.

Some lovers lose themselves in the music, prolonging and enhancing the deep state of arousal, pleasure and closeness to the point of achieving an altered, mystical state of consciousness, notes Dr. Morin. They seem to lose track of self and time. That may be the ultimate sexual experience. It doesn't happen every time. And no one has developed a clear road map for how to get there. But these eight steps to heighten pleasure and intimacy during the main movement are a good start.

Make loving a smorgasbord. You needn't jump immediately into intercourse following foreplay, and intercourse needn't be an inevitably culminating act, says Dr. Morin. You can poke around for a little while and then withdraw and spend some time nibbling here and there—and being nibbled. You can trade off and take turns pleasuring one another. You can forgo intercourse altogether and masturbate for each other, or masturbate each other, or reach satisfaction orally. The real key is to relax, enjoy and focus on the depth and multitude of sensations.

Talk it up. Talk during sex. Express your pleasures, fantasies, needs, impressions, says sex therapist Irene Kassorla, Ph.D., in her book *Nice Girls Do*. This exponentially increases intimacy.

Learn to be still. Forgo the friction. Try positions in which the woman controls most movement, such as with her on top, suggests Dr. Morin. Concentrate on the subtle sensations.

Position for success. Start, stop and change positions. Good lovemaking is like a sequence of dances. Work your way through the *Kama Sutra* if you're athletically inclined.

Live and breathe sex. Heavy breathing is a normal physiological aspect of arousal. Trying to suppress it suppresses arousal and enjoyment, says Dr. Renshaw. Deep, easy breaths build arousal more effectively than shallow, short ones. Slowing and deepening your breathing as you approach climax can help you back away from it, says Dr. Morin. Matching your partner's breathing, breath for breath, while lying against her is extremely bonding. So is exhaling on inward thrusts and inhaling as you pull back during intercourse, says sex therapist Marty Klein, Ph.D. For the most explosive ejaculation, try breathing more strongly and deeply during the final approach, fully forcing out each breath from the diaphragm.

Experience G-force.
Stimulate your partner's G-spot and have her do yours. Men have a so-called G-spot just as women do (besides, of course, the ever-important clitoris). Ours is anatomically known as the prostate. According to Dr. Perry, "These spots share a common sensitivity to pressure (not touch). You have to press hard to stimulate them."

These highly sensitive areas are named after Ernst Grafenberg, a German doctor who was the first to make the claim back in 1950. Attention wasn't given to the subject until 1980, when Dr. Perry rediscovered its importance. Dr. Perry suggests that women have an erotic hot spot on the roof of the vagina, about three inches in. Pressing on it, or stimulating it, can cause an orgasm completely independent of clitoral stimulation. Stroke it with your penis or your fingers. Experiment to find it. Its precise location may vary a bit from woman to woman.

In men, the prostate, the frenulum (the ridge of skin running down the underside of the penis just below the head) and the perineum (the area between the base of the testicles and the anus) are all particularly nerve-rich sexual pleasure points.

To heighten your sexual pleasure, encourage your partner to gently press or lightly

Sex by Numbers

In the *Sex in America* survey—purported to be the most balanced, most scientifically randomized survey ever—researchers at the University of Chicago paint the following profile of Americans:

- Ninety percent of us marry or form partnerships by age 29.
- Five percent of married Americans are having affairs.
- Sixteen percent of men have paid for sex.
- Twenty percent of American men have had 1 sex partner since age 18; 21 percent have had 2 to 4; 23 percent have had 5 to 10; 16 percent have had 11 to 20; and 17 percent have had 21 or more. The more educated people are, the more partners they are likely to have over their lifetimes.
- White, college-educated, cohabiting people in their late twenties are more likely to masturbate than anyone else. The youngest people in the study, ages 18 through 24, were less likely to masturbate.
- More than 40 percent of us who are sexually active with three or more partners a year never use condoms; 40 percent of us always do with secondary partners.
- Who catches a venereal disease? Three percent of those who've had 2 to 4 partners; about 10 percent of those who've had 5 to 10 partners; and 28 percent of those who've had 21 or more partners.
- About 90 percent of us have never slept with anyone of another race.
- While the researchers note that other studies have established that people lose track of time and overestimate how long sex lasts, they found that 69 percent of us report that we usually take between 15 minutes and an hour; 20 percent of us say we take an hour or more.

stroke the spot near the base of the scrotum, says Judith Seifer, R.N., Ph.D., president of the American Association of Sex Educators, Counselors and Therapists.

Firm massage of the perineum indirectly stimulates the prostate, says Dr. Perry.

Become a condom connoisseur.
Condoms are not all created equal. But in this age of HIV and other sexually transmitted diseases, they are essential equipment for the man on the make.

Solving the Size Issue

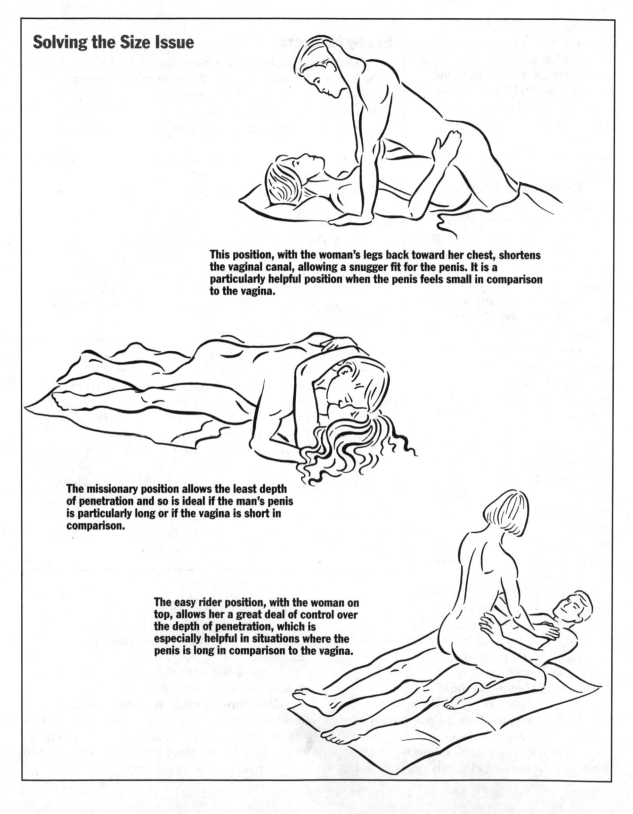

This position, with the woman's legs back toward her chest, shortens the vaginal canal, allowing a snugger fit for the penis. It is a particularly helpful position when the penis feels small in comparison to the vagina.

The missionary position allows the least depth of penetration and so is ideal if the man's penis is particularly long or if the vagina is short in comparison.

The easy rider position, with the woman on top, allows her a great deal of control over the depth of penetration, which is especially helpful in situations where the penis is long in comparison to the vagina.

Some condoms are more comfortable than others, and some allow more sensation and pleasure. *Men's Health* magazine tested a number of condoms on the market, and one of the most highly recommended is the Kimono Micro Thin by Mayer Laboratories. With a thickness measuring less than 0.05 millimeter, it increases the sensation of warmth.

Dr. Laurence doesn't recommend microthin condoms for anal intercourse because they tend to tear easily. In fact, because of the frequency of rupture of both the thins and the regulars, he recommends wearing two regular condoms during anal intercourse.

Any condom will feel better and more sensitive if you lightly lubricate your penis, particularly the head, before putting it on. Use a water-based lubricant such as Astroglide or K-Y Jelly, says Dr. Perry. Oil-based lubes destroy latex.

If you can't find a good variety of condoms in your area, request mail-order catalogs from the following discreet suppliers of sexual paraphernalia: Condomania, 1-800-9-CONDOM (1-800-926-6366) or, by e-mail, http://www.condomania.com; Adam and Eve, 1-800-765-2326; or Stamford Hygienic Company, 1-800-356-6325.

Size up your partner. Women come in all different sizes, too. The average woman prefers the average penis. But what to do if your sizes don't match? Experiment with positions that compensate. (The illustrations on the opposite page show how.)

Step 5: Agree on the Ending

Most male animals copulate quickly, then dash off. Not the boar. He crawls atop a sow, does his thing, then drifts to sleep there. Ever wonder why women sometimes compare men to pigs?

Yes, yes. Once we ejaculate, a sweet heaviness often descends upon our every molecule, our eyes roll backward in our heads, and we can see, touch, hear, smell and sense dreamland through the pleasant haze. And we want nothing more than to go there.

We ejaculate, and boom, we shut down. During the first minute following ejaculation, the penis drops by 50 percent, and buddy, we're done for a while. It's time to recharge.

Not so for Mama Bear. She cools down much, much more slowly. It takes her five to ten minutes. And if you continue clitoral and vaginal stimulation, she won't wind down at all but may have orgasm after orgasm.

So she has just given you an enormous release, and she's hot and bothered, and you roll over and go to sleep. Pig.

See how it looks from the other side of the bed?

Look: Your physiology is different from hers. Now you know. So don't be selfish. Give her a little warmth—some touching and cuddling—for a couple of minutes.

If she is hot and bothered and close but hasn't quite gotten off, do the gentlemanly thing, advises Dr. Keesling. You have two hands and a mouth; use them. Then cuddle. Then nod off. In that order.

Some men find it easier to cuddle if they don't withdraw the penis immediately after ejaculation. This tends to extend the erection and is warm and fuzzy. Plus you get to experience the pleasure of the aftershocks and twitches that follow any earthquake.

Step 6: Communicate Thoroughly

Okay. Was that good for you?

Talking with your intimate partner about sex is essential to a good sex life. "You and your partner must exchange a tremendous amount of information. And much of it changes over time," says Dr. Morin.

Yet for many couples, the communication is nonverbal and results in misunderstandings and incorrect beliefs about each other's preferences and needs.

Talking about sex, says Dr. Morin, is tough for nearly everybody. But it serves useful purposes. Besides helping us to learn the other person's needs and desires, it is a way of communicating compliments and building one another's sexual confidence.

The keys to effective sexual communication, Dr. Morin says, include the following.

Avoid the no-no's. Three don'ts: (1) Don't berate your partner; (2) don't compare your partner with other lovers; and (3) don't talk about your sex life to a mutual friend. (Instead, pick someone you trust who isn't close to your partner and ask him to maintain total confidentiality.) Violating any of these three no-no's undermines a partner's confidence and self-esteem and kills trust and joyfulness in a sexual relationship, says Dr. Morin. The damage is difficult to undo.

If you're happy and you know it, say "Amen!" Give positive feedback, says Dr. Morin. Regularly. Say "I like that." "That feels wonderful." And so on.

Watch the timing and the tone. Discuss difficulties when you're feeling close, but not during sex. And do so in nonjudgmental language. Don't accuse or blame. Listen. Ask questions. Don't let yourself get defensive, says Dr. Morin.

Put that in writing. If talking is just too awkward, write. Lovingly, says Dr. Morin.

Step 7: Be Sexually Healthy

We talk at length about how to overcome a flagging sex drive and erection difficulties and about the effects of medication, poor diet and a poor general fitness level on a man's sexual equipment in the chapter on the penis (page 257).

The fact is, your physical fitness quo does affect your sexual fitness quo. Men who are physically active are more sexually active—at all ages. Aerobic exercise seems to be the real libido builder. And sex itself is a beneficial physical activity: It reduces stress, eases headaches and combats arthritis pain. A 170-pound man burns an average of 5.25 calories per minute during sex. Even if you have sex for ten minutes, that's almost 53 calories gone for doing something you love to do.

In addition to aerobics, easy-to-do Kegel exercises strengthen the muscles involved in sexual pleasure. (For step-by-step instructions, see page 266.)

Step 8: Get Exotic

The myth-shattering *Sex in America* tells us that masturbating, having frequent thoughts of sex and using erotica are components of a sexually active lifestyle, not the domain of the sexually deprived or depraved.

We harbor many guilt-ridden misconceptions about what is "normal" simply because we cannot see behind most bedroom doors.

"A lot of people's peak sexual experiences are naughty or kinky or off-color," says Dr. Morin. "This is part of what makes it fun for many people. This is a natural part of human sexuality."

Dr. Morin says we get into danger zones of perverse or unacceptable sexual behavior when we:

• Lose the ability to distinguish between fantasy and reality. "If a man can make a clear distinction between fantasy and behavior, then nothing he fantasizes is perverse. There are no limits. Fantasy is fantasy."

• Compulsively engage in behaviors that bring negative consequences and we become unable to change or stop.

• Engage in nonconsensual acts. "If a person is in a position to consent to sexual behavior and does consent, even if it is kinky, then we don't have a problem," says Dr. Morin.

Healthy couples, says Dr. Morin, do play. They do use toys, costumes and fantasies—even whips and chains, if they like. And *Sex in America* documents that more than 40 percent of men purchase some type of erotic material or device each year (but only 16 percent of women do).

An unintimidating way to shop is by catalog from a reputable company that ships discreetly. For starters, we suggest Good Vibrations (1-800-289-8423), Eve's Garden (1-800-848-3837) and Xandria Collection (1-800-242-2823).

⟦?⟧Symptoms

- **Pay attention to your body.**
- **Don't confuse the symptom with the underlying cause.**
- **Don't pretend you're Superman.**

There's an old joke about a farmer who sees his neighbor clobbering a mule over the head with a plank of wood. "Why are you doing that?" the farmer asks. "I'm trying to get his attention," answers the neighbor.

Don't mean to insult, but many of us are like that mule. Our bodies constantly send out messages. Important messages. And what do we do? We ignore them. For some reason, it's part of the male image to work and play "hurt"—to ignore things such as fatigue, headache, runny noses, bruises, sore muscles, gut pain. Sure, we'll pop painkillers or cold remedies when symptoms reach the point of affecting our performance. But that just masks the symptom. We rarely take the time to think about what's going on inside, even when our bodies howl for attention.

For the more obstinate among us, only a huge plank whacked against the backside will wake us up: a heart attack, or passing out unexpectedly, or suddenly being unable to stand up in the morning.

Why be this way? We men are far smarter than mules. This is not to suggest that you study medical texts or enroll in an evening anatomy course. Our point is that you make a very subtle shift in your attitude—namely, when your body speaks to you, take the time to listen.

What it has to tell you can be of paramount importance. Despite the advances in medical technology and research, men still live an average of seven years less than women. There are a couple of reasons for this.

Foremost are the inherent health risks of being a man. For example, prior to age 65,

men suffer heart attacks at almost three times the rate of women. One in three American males ages 18 to 74 suffer from high blood pressure, a primary risk factor for heart attack, yet we're less likely than women to be checked for high blood pressure.

In addition, there's the macho ethic that tells us to suffer in silence, tune out pain and consider our bodies as nothing more than vehicles to get us from one place to another—which is why women visit doctors more often than men and their health problems are detected and treated long before we become aware of ours.

It pays to listen to your body. And the sooner you begin, the better.

The Amazing Talking Body

Okay, so it doesn't talk in words. The fact is that your body is communicating with you all of the time. "You feel either comfortable or uncomfortable; you hurt or you feel good," says John W. Zamarra, M.D., founder and director of the cardiac rehabilitation program at Placentia-Linda Community Hospital in Placentia, California. "If you're not feeling comfortable, something is wrong. That is why it's called 'dis-ease.' "

"If you rest when you're supposed to rest and eat when you're supposed to eat, you should be feeling energy and a sense of well-being all of the time," says Michael Grossman, M.D., a family physician in El Toro, California, who specializes in preventive medicine. "If you're not, you know that something is wrong. Then you have to determine what is causing the problem."

When something goes wrong, your body usually provides an obvious message. "Pain and discomfort are the only means the body has of communicating a problem to us directly," says Dr. Zamarra. But all communication is two-sided. Your body can send you message after message, but you have to do your part by listening and thinking about what you hear.

Learn the language. Pain is the most common message that your body sends. It has thousands of variations and locations. (For a detailed look at pain and how to conquer chronic pain, see page 54.) But your body's vocabulary is endless and also includes pressure, fever, cold, chills, swelling, burning, bleeding, diarrhea and dizziness.

Play detective.
Sometimes your body lets you know exactly what's up: "Hey, that food you gave me last night was too spicy. That's why I woke you up with heartburn." Other times it's more subtle; you may need some time to figure out whether your head hurts because you're hungry, tired, tense or suffering from eyestrain or because you just need some fresh air.

Turn to the experts.
Most of us are not medical practitioners trained in the fine art of reading symptoms. That's why we buy books like this one. Get at least one good-quality book on medical symptoms. When something odd occurs, look it up and consider all possibilities, suggests Dr. Zamarra. Then contact your doctor to confirm your suspicions.

But trust yourself. No book or person will ever be able to tell better than you can how and what you feel. No one knows better your baseline feeling of well-being or any of the usual small deviations from that normal, balanced state. Only you know when something really feels off and needs attention, says Dr. Zamarra. And you must remain open and objective to your feelings, he adds.

Knowing an Emergency

"In my opinion, if you go to the emergency room two or three times in your adult life for false alarms, it's well worth it," says John W. Zamarra, M.D., a cardiologist and founder and director of the cardiac rehabilitation program at Placentia-Linda Community Hospital in Placentia, California. "Statistics show that 40 percent of people who have heart attacks are cases of sudden death, with no reported symptoms until that moment. You just collapse out of the blue."

So if you think you might be in trouble, don't tough it out; don't worry about making a fool of yourself. "If you don't want to be a statistic, the only thing to do is to err on the side of safety and go," says Dr. Zamarra.

According to experts, here are nine reasons to make a run for the ER.

Severe chest pain. A strong discomfort in the chest, usually in the center and often radiating to the neck or left arm, might be signaling a heart attack. You may feel pressure, squeezing, heaviness or fullness in your chest, or you may have difficulty breathing. If you also experience fear and anxiety, plus dizziness, sweating, nausea, vomiting or weakness, you need immediate help, especially if any of these symptoms lasts for more than a few minutes or repeatedly occurs, says Dr. Zamarra.

Sudden shortness of breath. If you're not asthmatic and you suddenly experience shortness of breath that lasts for more than a half-hour, chances are it's your heart—angina, heart failure or a heart attack, says Dr. Zamarra. If you wake up short of breath in the middle of the night, it could be pulmonary edema, another major medical emergency.

Sudden loss of coordination, speech or vision. These are stroke symptoms, says Dr. Zamarra. If you are having a stroke, you need the fastest possible medical attention. The sooner you get help, the better your chances of recovery.

Sudden change in heart rate. If you are over age 50, a sudden increase or decrease in heart rate for no apparent reason is a danger signal, says Dr. Zamarra. If your pulse

Your Response Options

When something is bothering us, we have basically four choices.

1. Leave it alone. This is the famous wait-and-see approach that doctors also take in

dips under 40 beats per minute and stays there and you feel weak, faint or dizzy, it's an emergency. A pulse over 125 beats per minute, again for no apparent reason, can also be life-threatening for an older person if it persists.

Severe abdominal pain. If you have some diarrhea and the pain moves around or subsides and then returns, you can afford to wait a while and see what happens. But if the pain is constant for more than an hour, is accompanied by fever or is in the lower right part of your abdomen, you could have appendicitis, requiring immediate attention.

Rectal bleeding. A few drops of blood, especially if it's bright red, is probably just from hemorrhoids. But if there's a lot of blood and it's black, or if your stool is kind of tarry black, that comes from bleeding in the upper intestine, which needs to be treated right away.

Fever above 104°F. If you know exactly what the cause is, are being treated and are in touch with the doctor, you can stay at home if those are your instructions. Otherwise, head for the emergency room.

Back pain that isn't clearly muscular. Back pain that is independent of movement or position can be caused by a kidney infection. It's usually accompanied by pain on urination, blood in the urine or increased frequency of urination. You need to be on antibiotics right away.

Sudden testicular pain. If it's not because you got a knee in the groin playing basketball, take action fast. If you're an adult, you might have a hernia or an inflammation of the ducts that carry sperm from the testicles to the penis. These conditions need to be treated, but they're not dangerous.

More serious is testicular torsion. "The cord suspending the testicle becomes twisted, cutting off the blood supply," explains Dudley Seth Danoff, M.D., senior attending urologic surgeon at Cedars-Sinai Medical Center in Los Angeles and author of *Superpotency.* "If this isn't corrected within a few hours, you will likely lose the testicle. This is most common in prepubertal boys and rarely happens to anyone over age 20, but it always needs immediate attention."

on the immune system, see page 200.)

2. Do something yourself. If you feel a need to take some action, you can take a couple of painkillers, put on an elastic bandage, take an antacid, jump in the Jacuzzi or just get into bed for some extra rest. You can treat the symptom, says Dr. Zamarra, or you can make an educated guess at the underlying cause and go after that.

The vast majority of minor health symptoms fall into these first two categories. Only the more serious health problems go beyond the stage of self-diagnosis and self-treatment, says Dr. Zamarra. If you have a headache, athlete's foot or a sore knee from a fall in a basketball game, it's unlikely that you'll go to the doctor. You'll take care of it yourself.

But here's the catch: Although the list of symptoms that we can handle ourselves is very long, all of them can require a physician's attention if they go on long enough or are intense enough. It is important to keep a record and monitor your symptoms without denial or exaggeration, says Dr. Zamarra.

3. Consult a professional. Certain symptoms are just beyond our understanding or ability to handle. If you suddenly find blood in your urine, or you get dizzy when you stand up, or you become out of breath walking up a flight of stairs, you need to see a doctor. Confounding, life-affecting symptoms mustn't be ignored, notes Dr. Zamarra.

4. Race to the emergency room. When a symptom strikes that completely debilitates

many instances. Most mild symptoms are probably best left untreated if the body is in balance and healthy, says Dr. Zamarra. The body's magnificent healing mechanism will often take care of things without any interference. (For more

you or is terrifyingly strong, such as sudden blindness or an inability to breathe, there is no question what to do, says Dr. Zamarra. Life is too valuable not to get to a doctor immediately.

How do you know which of these four categories you're dealing with? Here are a few ways to improve your reading of the signals that your body sends you.

Be prepared. If you have some knowledge of the language of symptoms, you'll have a better idea of whether your symptom needs attention from a health care professional, suggests Dr. Zamarra. You'll know whether you can use the wait-and-see strategy or whether there's something you might be able to do yourself. A little reading, some analytic thought and objectivity will go a long way toward figuring out what a symptom is saying. At the very least, we should all be ready to recognize the kind of symptom that shouts "Take me to the emergency room!"

Learn to read yourself. "Most people are not aware of their bodies—or are not aware enough of their bodies," says Dr. Zamarra. "So they don't tune in on a regular basis to see how they are."

Dr. Grossman concurs. "Listening to your body is a complex thing," he says. "It takes time to do it and to learn to do it. But it's very, very important."

Quiet the noise. "I'll give you an example of tuning in," says Dr. Zamarra. "People who meditate, who can quiet their minds enough to feel what's going on in their bodies, are much more likely to be aware of when they're not feeling well and of what's going on to create the imbalance.

"On the other hand, people who don't take the time to meditate, whose attention is always outward, may be walking around with a lot of stress and may think it's normal to feel tight, tense and nervous all of the time. They may not even know they're tense! So I think meditation can be a crucial key—it's a neglected key—to a healthier lifestyle."

Know what you can't know. Many of the more insidious diseases are completely symptomless. High blood pressure, clogged arteries, liver disease, cancer, diabetes: Often it is impossible to know you have these in their early stages. That's one more compelling reason not to play the mule and to align yourself with a doctor who can test for things every few years, says Dr. Zamarra. (For what you need to get checked and when, see "Routine Medical Tests for Men" on page 49.)

Getting to the Underlying Cause

Western medicine has a genius for symptom relief. Go to any pharmacy, and the shelves will be filled with over-the-counter painkillers, antacids and other symptom alleviators. But think about this: Virtually all of these deal with the symptom, not with the underlying cause. Taking a cough lozenge to stop your hacking may work, but it does absolutely nothing to get rid of the irritant that is causing the cough.

"Treating the symptom is fine up to a point," Dr. Grossman explains. "But in many illnesses, the symptom is a manifestation of an underlying imbalance. If you have a stomachache, you can treat it with tablets and eliminate the symptom temporarily, but the symptom will keep recurring until you change something in your lifestyle, or your thinking, or your manner of dealing with the stress in your life."

It's the same message with headaches, infections, even heart attacks. The symptoms may be unique and clear, but the underlying cause of all could be stress, for example, says Dr. Grossman. It takes clear thinking to identify that.

"If something is wrong and you really want to be healthy, not just temporarily symptom-free, you need to treat the underlying imbalance in your life, the underlying patterns that don't work—patterns of dealing with stress, with upset," Dr. Grossman concludes. "You may have to change your patterns of rest, activity, exercise. It may be necessary to reprogram your thinking and your attitude. All of these things are crucial if you want to be healthy."

☺Medical Tests

- **Know what tests you need.**
- **Know when you need tests taken.**
- **Consider home screening kits.**

Cancer. Heart disease. Diabetes. Cirrhosis. High blood pressure. AIDS. They have many things in common, most of which you know: They are bad diseases. They kill lots of people. You don't want them.

But they have something else in common that you probably haven't realized, and it's perhaps the most important commonality of all.

"Many illnesses, including quite a few serious ones, have absolutely no symptoms, particularly in the early stages," says Michael Grossman, M.D., a family physician in El Toro, California, who specializes in preventive medicine. "You don't know you have a problem until it's too late."

Think about that. It's feasible that you have a serious medical problem but no idea that it's there. Now we don't like to use scare tactics to goad you into action. But there is no more compelling argument for getting yourself tested regularly than the knowledge that testing is the only way to discover many diseases before they do serious harm to your life.

High blood pressure, for example, causes no pain and no noticeable symptoms. "There's no correlation whatsoever between what people think their blood pressure is and what it actually is," Dr. Grossman points out. "That's why it has been called the silent killer."

Elevated cholesterol is another example. Judging by how you feel, you have no clue as to what your cholesterol level may be. Yet if it's high, you are again setting yourself up for possibly serious health problems.

The thing is, medical tests are cheaper and easier to conduct than ever before. Many tests that once required a costly visit to the doctor can now be done at home. And with a growing emphasis in the Western health establishment on preventive medicine, regular testing is becoming part of most health routines, says Dr. Grossman.

Test Types

Medical tests come in three varieties.

- Screening tests are given when you feel healthy and have no complaints to see if you might have any hidden problems. These tests, such as a standard blood test, urinalysis and a vision test, are relatively low-cost, comfortable and risk-free, says Dr. Grossman.
- Diagnostic tests explore more deeply the condition of someone who does have symptoms and complaints to help the physician pinpoint the problem and choose the most effective course of action for healing.
- Monitoring tests are used to evaluate a patient's progress once treatment has begun.

In this chapter, we will concern ourselves with screening tests. We'll review the different types that you should get and when you should get them. But before diving in, we need to make two important points.

Medical tests are not a substitute for a good relationship with a doctor. Medical tests, as valuable as they are, can't compare in value with a good relationship with a careful, caring physician, says Dr. Grossman. He believes that a physician can accurately diagnose the vast majority of a patient's problems without the help of medical tests, simply through the routine complete physical exam and complete personal history. As that great medical expert Yogi Berra commented, "You can observe a lot by watching."

Medical tests are not a substitute for true prevention. Medical testing sometimes goes under the name "prevention." This is something of a misnomer. It's certainly true that appropriate tests can detect signs of disease you may not have known about and that this early warning gives you a better shot at healing. But tests do not prevent disease; they only uncover it. "Early detection, which is what the medical tests do for you, is not the same as prevention," says John W. Zamarra, M.D., founder and director of the cardiac rehabilitation program at Placentia-Linda Community Hospital in Placentia, California. "Real prevention is more comprehensive. If you just take some tests and think you're doing okay, you're fooling yourself, because you can have lifestyle habits that are wrong for you and that are going to cause you problems later."

Real prevention, says Dr. Zamarra, "is to avert the danger that hasn't come. For that, you have to know how to live properly." All of the tests in the world could never substitute for not smoking, using alcohol moderately (or not drinking at all), eating fresh, healthy foods, practicing safe sex and managing stress. "Health is more comprehensive than just passing a test or a group of tests," says Dr. Zamarra. "It's a state of consciousness and a way of life."

The Tests You Need

There are roughly 19 routine medical tests to screen a man's health, says Dr. Grossman. Several of them are easily done at home; the rest require a visit to a doctor. Dr. Grossman notes that most need to be done every three years before age 40 and every two years once you hit that age. (See "Routine Medical Tests for Men" for a timetable.) What follows are brief explanations of what each test does and why each is important.

History and physical. Doctors used to advocate getting a complete physical every year, but many now feel a longer interval is acceptable, especially if you're young and healthy, says Dr. Grossman. However you and your doctor decide to space them, these visits are important for several reasons.

- To discuss strategies for health

> ## How to Do a Testicular Self-Exam
>
> "If you're under the age of 40, the only genital examination you need is a testicular examination, and you can do that yourself," says Dudley Seth Danoff, M.D., senior attending urologic surgeon at Cedars-Sinai Medical Center in Los Angeles and author of *Superpotency.*
>
> Gently examine each testicle with both hands. Place your index and middle fingers underneath and your thumbs on top of a testicle. Roll the testicle between your fingers.
>
> "Your testicles should feel like two peeled hard-boiled eggs," says Dr. Danoff. "They should have that rubbery, smooth consistency, and if you feel any lumps, bumps, tenderness or hardness, you should consult a physician." Dr. Danoff recommends that you do this self-exam at least once a month, while you're in bed or in a warm shower. This avoids the reflex "that makes the testicles squish up into your abdomen, like when you jump into a cold swimming pool. It's very hard to examine the testicles if the scrotum is contracted."

---

maintenance (exercise, stress management, diet and so on)
- For early detection of disorders and illnesses
- To build a relationship with the doctor, so he learns how you function when you're well and can more easily spot problems if they arise

Complete blood count. Blood is unique in that it's the only liquid tissue found in the body. And while it appears to be a homogenous solution, it contains a number of components with entirely different functions. The complete blood count measures the quantities of the three types of blood cells that you need to be healthy.

- Red blood cells, which transport oxygen from the lungs to the entire body. These make up about 45 percent of total blood volume.
- White blood cells, which fight infection. These, along with platelets (below), make up less than 1 percent of blood volume.

Routine Medical Tests for Men

Below is a rough timetable for 19 medical tests every health-savvy male should be getting, based on studies, books and interviews with several doctors. Two caveats: First, there is no agreement whatsoever among medical professionals that this is the correct list or timetable. Any doctor—or insurer—would likely say some of the tests are too frequent, or too infrequent, or downright unnecessary. But the doctors we talked to, with a few exceptions, feel this is a good consensus list. Second, your particular health situation and family history might suggest a different schedule, so be sure to discuss these with your doctor.

Twenties

History and physical	Every 3 years; at 40, switch to every 2 years
Complete blood count	Every 3 years; at 40, switch to every 2 years
Blood glucose	As needed to monitor diabetes; otherwise, every 3 years; at 40, switch to every 2 years
Blood pressure	Every 3 years; at 40, switch to every 2 years
Cholesterol	Every 3 years; at 40, switch to every 2 years
Tuberculin skin test	Every 3 years, or more often depending on social circumstances (if you are a teacher or health care worker, for example)
Urinalysis	Every 3 years; at 40, switch to every 2 years
Vision	Every 3 years; at 40, switch to every 2 years
Testicular self-exam	Every month; at 40, switch to every few months
EKG	Baseline once per decade throughout life
HIV	Regularly depending on sexual activity

Thirties
Add to the above . . .

Glaucoma	Start if family history; at 40, switch to every 2 years
Hearing	Only if difficulties emerge
Stress EKG	Every 3 years starting at 35
Chest x-ray	Only if there are symptoms or family history of disease or if you are a smoker

Forties
Add to the above . . .

Blood in stool	Every 2 years
Digital/rectal prostate exam	Every 2 years
Sigmoidoscopy	Every 2–3 years if family history of colon cancer; every 2–3 years after 50 if no history

Fifties and Above
Add to the above . . .

PSA screening	Every 2 years; after 60, every year

- Platelets, which help the blood clot and so prevent excessive bleeding.

Blood glucose. Glucose, a sugar manufactured by our bodies from the carbohydrates we eat, is our primary energy source. High levels of glucose in the blood may indicate diabetes (although other disorders are also possible), while low levels indicate hypoglycemia (low blood sugar). Diabetes often has no symptoms in its early stages, making screening very important. Untreated, it can cause blindness, heart and kidney disease and problems with the nervous system. Your blood glucose level is usually checked as part of a comprehensive blood test. Pharmacies may also carry a screening kit for home use.

Blood pressure. Because high blood pressure has no symptoms you can feel, you may walk around with it for years unless it's detected by the simple blood pressure cuff. Detected, it can be treated; undetected, it can lead to heart attack, stroke, blindness, cardiac failure or kidney failure. Blood pressure monitoring is normally part of the complete physical but can also be done at home.

To check your own blood pressure, you have to understand what the numbers mean.

- Systolic pressure, the top number, measures the force of blood flow at its peak. A normal systolic pressure is about 120. Keep in mind that this is a high-pressure system. If the aorta were open during the systolic period, blood could spurt

Medical Tests You Can Do at Home

Accurate home screening kits for blood glucose, blood pressure, urinalysis, vision, cholesterol and blood in stool are available in your pharmacy at relatively little expense, says Michael Grossman, M.D., a family physician in El Toro, California, who specializes in preventive medicine. And a home test for AIDS (HIV) will soon be available, according to Ernst J. Schaefer, M.D., director of the lipid clinic at New England Medical Center in Boston and the lipid metabolism laboratory at Tufts University in Medford, Massachusetts, and an expert on home screening tests.

"These tests are convenient, can save you money and give you more of a sense of control over your own health care," says Dr. Schaefer. And some home tests can be more accurate than tests done at the doctor's office. "Monitoring your blood pressure when you're relaxed and in more normal circumstances at home, rather then when you're tense because you're in a doctor's office, can give you a truer reading," suggests Dr. Grossman.

"But," he cautions, "if you have symptoms that suggest a potentially serious condition, such as blood in your stool, that's the time not for a home test but for a visit to a doctor."

Here are the main tests you can do at home, according to Dr. Grossman.

Testicular self-exam. No expense at all for this one. Do this test regularly between the ages of 15 and 40. (See "How to Do a Testicular Self-Exam" on page 48 for instructions.)

Blood glucose monitoring. If you have diabetes, your doctor may tell you to periodically monitor your blood sugar level at home. This home test involves sticking your finger to obtain some blood and letting a machine analyze the blood for sugar content. Most pharmacies carry good selections of home monitoring systems, with prices ranging from less than $40 to more than $100. Talk to your doctor about which make and model would be best for you.

Blood pressure monitoring. "Almost every hypertensive person would do well to have a blood pressure cuff at home," says Dr. Grossman. "You can buy a good one for about $80. I usually have a patient check his cuff against mine at the office in the beginning, to make sure he's reading it right and using it right."

Urinalysis. Several types of home kits are available for easy performance of a urine analysis. Most involve a plastic dipstick with chemically treated pads that change color in the presence of various substances in your urine. You then compare the color on the test pad with a master chart to determine the levels of substances in your urine. Most pharmacies carry home kits to test for sugar and protein in your urine. Expect to pay $10 for 100 sugar test strips and around $40 for 100 protein test strips.

Vision test. You can easily check your vision periodically by putting an eye chart up on your wall and reading it from the designated distance, says Dr. Grossman. Just follow the directions that come with the chart and be sure you have enough light. Eye charts are available through most medical supply stores for about $15.

Cholesterol test. A finger-stick self-test for total cholesterol is on the market and available in most pharmacies, and "a home test for HDL cholesterol (the good cholesterol) will be available soon," says Dr. Schaefer. "Then people will be able to calculate the ratio of total cholesterol to HDL, which is a very powerful predictor of heart disease." Test kits for total cholesterol cost around $15 for a single test and $20 for two (so you can recheck your level later).

Blood in stool test. "A lot of people don't do this test because they don't like dealing with stool," says Dr. Schaefer. "But it's very worthwhile to do in terms of screening oneself for colon cancer and other colon problems." The kits are available in most pharmacies for around $5.

HIV test. Home test kits for HIV, using urine rather than a blood sample, are being developed by several pharmaceutical companies and might already be available to you, says Dr. Schaefer.

Some final tips from Dr. Grossman regarding home medical testing: First, follow the manufacturer's directions carefully. Second, consider doing a trial run with your doctor the first time you use the test to be sure you're doing the procedure properly and interpreting the results correctly. Finally, remember that no test is perfect. There is always a chance that you are getting a false-positive reading (the test shows a problem but you are actually okay), so don't panic. If you're surprised by a result, repeat the test yourself or consult your doctor.

upward as far as five feet.

• Diastolic pressure, the bottom number, measures blood pressure at its lowest point. A normal diastolic pressure is about 70 to 80.

Tuberculin skin test. Tuberculosis is not extinct; in fact, it's on the rise, even in the United States. This test is especially important for people living in crowded conditions as well as for teachers and health care professionals. Men are about twice as likely as women to have tuberculosis, and non-Whites are about four times more vulnerable than Whites. This is a simple skin test administered in your doctor's office. You must return to the office in two or three days, so your skin can be examined for a reaction.

Urinalysis. Requiring no needles and no high-tech equipment, a test of your urine yields a wealth of information about the overall state of your body. It screens for diabetes, kidney stones, urinary tract infections, the health of your liver and gallbladder, high blood pressure, hormone imbalances and more. Home urinalysis kits are available in most pharmacies.

Vision. The routine vision test simply uses an eye chart to measure your visual acuity. You'll probably notice if you're not seeing as well as you should, but since we depend so much on our eyes, an occasional test won't hurt just to make sure you're seeing as well as possible. Eye charts are available so that you can test your vision at home. But it's usually best to see a doctor for an accurate exam.

Glaucoma. Glaucoma is a serious eye disease that can lead to blindness. It can't be cured, but if it's detected and treated, its progress can be stopped. The test, called tonometry, is quick, simple and painless.

Cholesterol/triglycerides. These tests measure the amounts of HDL (the good cholesterol), LDL (the bad cholesterol) and triglycerides in your blood. High levels of cholesterol, especially LDL, may contribute to the buildup of plaque in the lining of the arteries, leading to increased danger of high blood pressure, heart disease and stroke. An at-home finger-stick test for total cholesterol is now widely available.

Testicular self-exam. This self-exam detects possible testicular cancer, which often has no symptoms other than a lump you can feel with your fingers. At least once a month, follow the procedure.

Hearing. "There's no possibility of prevention by testing here," says Dr. Grossman. "The only treatment we have so far is a hearing aid, and that doesn't reverse the condition." For this reason, most doctors will test you only if you're having difficulty hearing. The test uses a special machine that emits tones, which you hear through headphones, and is performed by your doctor or audiologist.

Blood in stool. This test screens for colon cancer by detecting minute amounts of blood in your stool. You provide a stool sample; a small amount is placed on a slide and tested. Home kits are also available for initial screening, but you should always see a doctor if you suspect a problem.

Digital/rectal prostate exam. This

When the Doctor Wants to Probe

So far we've been talking about routine medical tests when you're symptom-free. It's a different story when you're sick, when you have some symptoms or when a screening test turns up evidence of a hidden disorder. Then your doctor may want you to have some of the literally hundreds of tests available in today's sophisticated health care system.

Many of these tests are expensive and may be covered by insurance only if your symptoms and diagnosis warrant their use. Not all are pain-free or risk-free. Play an active role in deciding which tests, if any, you want to have performed. According to Michael Grossman, M.D., a family physician in El Toro, California, who specializes in preventive medicine, here are some of the questions you need to ask.

Do I really need this test? Be sure to get a satisfactory answer before proceeding. Ask how the recommended test would change your unique situation. If either your diagnosis or your treatment would be improved by the results, you probably want to do it.

How should I prepare for the test? Do you need to fast or to avoid certain foods? Certain medications may interfere with the test and may need to be temporarily curtailed. Will you need someone to drive you home?

How is the procedure performed? Knowing exactly what will be done to you and how long the test will take can ease your state of mind and help you cooperate with the person performing the test.

What will I feel? You have a right to know whether

may have spawned more jokes than any other medical test. But even though some men are uncomfortable with it, it's important in the detection of prostate problems, says Dudley Seth Danoff, M.D., senior attending urologic surgeon at Cedars-Sinai Medical Center in Los Angeles and author of *Superpotency*. Here the doctor inserts a gloved finger into the rectum to examine the prostate gland for swelling or other abnormalities. Both benign enlargement and inflammation of the prostate, as well as prostate cancer, affect a huge number of men.

Prostate-specific antigen screening. This test of blood taken from a vein in your arm measures the level of prostate-specific antigen, or PSA, in your blood. The PSA test detects

the test will hurt or be otherwise uncomfortable or unpleasant. Most of us would rather know it's going to hurt and then prepare ourselves for it than have the anxiety of not knowing what's going to happen.

What are the risks? When the body is penetrated by a needle or a tube, the risk of infection is always present, as is the possibility of bleeding or other damage to your internal structures. There may be significant exposure to radioactive materials or possible reaction to drugs. Be sure you know the complete story and weigh the risks against what can be learned that may help you.

What do the results mean? Be sure you understand exactly what the test can tell about your health problem. You'll want to know both the numbers by which the results are measured and how to interpret them. You need to fully understand such results so that you can participate in the decisions about your treatment that will be based on them.

How much will it cost? You'll certainly want to know this if you're paying for it yourself. But the fact is that every test performed pushes up the price of insurance or HMO membership fees for you and everyone else in order to cover those costs. You may want to take this into consideration when making your decision (though it's a secondary matter if the test is crucial to your diagnosis or treatment).

Finally, you may want to read up on the procedure or procedures in a medical reference book. Numerous nontechnical books now exist describing medical tests in detail.

of your heart. You lie quietly on a table while the readings are made. Almost all kinds of heart disease will cause some abnormal readings and alert the doctor that further diagnosis is required.

Stress EKG. Also known as the treadmill or exercise tolerance test, this monitors your heart's response to the demands of exercise. In addition to providing EKG readings, the test measures blood pressure and heart rate as you walk on a treadmill or pedal a stationary bike. If your coronary arteries, which carry blood to your heart, are narrowed or blocked by cholesterol plaque, the heart is likely to produce abnormal electrical activity, which gets picked up by the EKG.

Chest x-ray. Until a few years ago, this test was part of the routine physical. Now doctors believe that zapping us with radiation every few years may not be wise. Chest x-rays are recommended only if there are symptoms indicating lung cancer, tuberculosis or other problems requiring Superman's view of your lungs, says Dr. Zamarra. But some doctors feel that if you're a smoker, you need one each year.

HIV. The blood test for HIV, the virus that causes AIDS, is recommended for all sexually active people. "If somebody tests positive," says Ernst J. Schaefer, M.D., director of the lipid clinic at New England Medical Center in Boston and the lipid metabolism laboratory at Tufts University in Medford, Massachusetts, "it's unconscionable to have unprotected sex. The only way to treat an epidemic like this, in the absence of any kind of a cure, is to contain the disease. I think that every person in the United States who is sexually active and who is likely to be engaging in sex with more than one partner ought to be tested."

noncancerous problems with the prostate (inflammation and infection, for example) as well as cancer. "As a man gets older and his prostate gets larger, the PSA level will go up," explains Dr. Danoff. "Mere elevation of PSA does not indicate cancer; it just indicates that we have to look further."

Sigmoidoscopy. This test involves insertion of a flexible fiber-optic tube known as a sigmoidoscope into the anus and up into the colon. It primarily screens for colon cancer but can detect other disorders as well, including ulcerative colitis.

Electrocardiogram. The electrocardiogram (EKG) uses electrodes on your wrists, ankles and chest to pick up the electrical activity

✚ Pain

- **Identify the cause accurately.**
- **Treat the condition smartly.**
- **Keep your attitude positive.**

Pain stings, burns, grips, grabs, sears, stabs, jolts, shoots, aches, throbs, grates, prickles. It is sharp or dull, specific or general, hot or cold, jagged or straight. It varies in intensity from barely noticeable to unbearable. When pain becomes too unbearable, we often lose consciousness.

Pain does more than tell us that something hurts; it tells us what's doing the hurting—and what we should do to make it stop. Don't touch the hot stove. Don't put weight on the injured foot. Race to the emergency room before the appendix bursts. (To determine if a particular pain is screaming "Get me to the hospital now!" refer to "Knowing an Emergency" on page 44.)

Thank goodness, most pain does not last long. It has an identifiable cause and a predictable duration, and most of the time it can be dulled. This type of pain is called acute pain, says Margaret A. Caudill, M.D., Ph.D., assistant clinical professor of medicine at Harvard Medical School and author of *Managing Pain before It Manages You*.

By contrast, there's the constant, nagging and often disabling pain known as chronic pain. This type of pain may be severe or merely bothersome. But it can last for a long, long time, undermining our productivity and interfering with our enjoyment of life.

What Is Pain?

Our tissues and organs are densely packed with millions of sensory nerve endings that constantly report to the brain what they're feeling. One sensor may say, "Hey, it's getting hot over here." Another may report, "I feel something vibrating." And a third might say, "Something is touching me."

Consider what happens when you bang your funny bone, says Dr. Caudill. First, you immediately feel a sharp, tingling sensation. That is your brain's response to pain sensors, which zap their signals to the top guy at about 40 miles an hour. This, in turn, is followed by a dull ache that spreads along the inside of your arm. This results from pain messages that crawl along at a more sluggish 3 miles an hour.

Finally, instinctively, you grab your elbow and rub vigorously. This is soothing because rubbing stimulates still other nerves, ones that carry touch and pressure messages at speeds of up to 200 miles an hour and can override or block the pain messages.

Most pain we experience is the result of a particular blend of nerve responses, says Dr. Caudill. That's why, for instance, an inflamed kidney, a skinned knee, a bruised arm and a cramping leg all hurt differently. Different combinations of nerve sensors are at work.

As hard as it is to believe when we're experiencing it, acute pain is our friend, says Norman J. Marcus, M.D., medical director of the New York Pain Treatment Program at Lenox Hill Hospital in New York City and president of the International Foundation for Pain Relief. If we didn't feel pain, we wouldn't act to protect ourselves from further injury. We wouldn't jerk away from the hot stove or rush to the hospital when the appendix swells.

Distant Warnings

Pain isn't always as straightforward as a bang on the elbow or a gashed hand. Sometimes what you're feeling in one place actually originated somewhere else. Often pain is caused not directly by the injury itself but by your body's response to the injury.

Consider inflammation. When you cut yourself, cells in the damaged area release chemicals that cause swelling and also irritate pain-sending nerves. It hurts, but it's an important type of short-term damage control: The body uses pain to remind us to treat the area with care.

Perhaps the most unusual pain of all is referred pain—that is, damage in one part of the body that causes pain somewhere else in the body. An example: When our testicles are hit sharply, we don't sense two clearly defined sore spots within the scrotum. The whole groin lights up, and we feel paralyzed. That's referred pain.

Another type of referred pain is a trigger point. Tender spots or "knots" in tense muscles, trigger points occur even when the actual problem area is far away, says Jane Cowles, Ph.D., in her book *Pain Relief*. Some therapists successfully relieve pain by locating and firmly pressing on a trigger point for a moment or so until the knot seems to dissolve. Shiatsu massage therapists treat pain by pressing on acupuncture points related to, but often far from, the area where the pain is felt. Western doctors sometimes inject anesthetics or cortisone into trigger points to relieve pain both locally and at distant points.

What causes an injury in one place to be felt somewhere else? Pain signals from different regions may travel along the same pathways, and the messages sometimes get mixed up, confusing exactly where the pain is, says Durwood Neal, Jr., M.D., associate professor of urology at the University of Texas Medical Branch at Galveston.

One last thing to consider in this discussion of the general nature of pain: We're all individuals. Identical injuries in different men will not cause identical experiences of pain. How we feel pain depends on genetics, stress levels and cultures. Some of us may experience pain more than others. And most of us sense pain more acutely when we're tense than when we're relaxed.

Quick Relief for Sudden Pain

In order to ease pain, you need to cut off, alter or overpower pain messages being sent to your brain. Rubbing works when you bang an elbow. Quickly icing an injury (which reduces circulation and hence swelling) is common sense and good medicine. So is taking an over-the-counter painkiller such as aspirin, ibu-profen or naproxen sodium (Aleve), says Dr. Caudill. If you're having surgery, you'll be given local or general anesthesia to deaden the nerves during the procedure and maybe some prescription-strength painkillers to numb pain while you heal.

Most sudden aches and pains are muscular, particularly in muscles that are tense, weak or in spasm, says Dr. Marcus. Sore muscles crowd and irritate neighboring nerves. Even headaches are often the result of muscle tension in the neck and shoulders, says Dale L. Anderson, M.D., coordinator of the Minnesota Act Now Project and author of *Muscle Pain Relief in 90 Seconds*.

Here are some smart ways to beat acute muscle pain, according to doctors.

Put it on ice. If the pain is the result of an obvious injury, such as a twisted ankle, and the area is starting to swell, wrap or cover it with an ice pack. Leave the pack on for 20 minutes, then remove it for 20 minutes, continuing this cycle for the first two hours after the injury. Then for the next day or so, apply the pack for 8 to 10 minutes of every hour. If you don't have a ready-made ice pack, put ice cubes in a plastic bag, recommends Dr. Marcus. Whichever cold treatment you use, don't apply it directly to the skin; it could cause tissue damage. Wrap it in a towel instead.

In addition, William S. Warren, Jr., M.D., a pain specialist in Hot Springs, Arkansas, advises that you stop using the ice if your circulation becomes sluggish. To check your circulation, pinch the area and watch how quickly blood returns to the area.

Get it high. You can reduce pulsing pain by elevating the injured area, says Dr. Marcus. Stack pillows if that helps.

Bring on the heat. If a sore, overworked muscle is in spasm or otherwise complaining, soothe it with a heat pack. A hot-water bottle works well; more sophisticated packs are available in medical supply stores. Drape the heat pack around the painful area or lay it on the sore spot, according to Dr. Warren.

Take a pill. Ever since Bayer introduced

Pain-Relieving Pills

Type	As Treatment for . . .	Dosage	Warnings
Acetaminophen (Tylenol)	Headaches, minor muscle aches and pains; not much anti-inflammatory action.	1–2 325-mg. tablets every 4–6 hours or 2 500-mg. tablets every 6 hours, not exceeding 4,000 mg. in any 24-hour period.	Chronic use can cause kidney and liver damage.
Aspirin (Anacin, Bayer)	General aches and pains, swelling and inflammation	325–650 mg. every 4 hours, not exceeding 4,000 mg. in 24 hours. Take with milk or food to avoid stomach irritation. Coated aspirin is available for people with weak stomachs.	Thins blood; can cause stomach bleeding. Don't take aspirin if you have ulcers or are taking blood-thinning drugs. Consult your doctor before taking aspirin if you have asthma or allergic rhinitis.
Ibuprofen (Advil, Nuprin)	Pain and inflammation; good for overworked-muscle injuries	1–2 200-mg. tablets every 4–6 hours, not exceeding 1,200 mg. in 24 hours. Take with milk or food to avoid stomach irritation. The dose may be higher if approved by your doctor.	Don't take ibuprofen with alcohol or if you have a history of kidney failure, high blood pressure or heart disease. Regular use can lead to kidney and liver damage.
Naproxen sodium (Aleve)	Pain and swelling; is long-lasting	Take 1 220-mg. tablet every 8 hours, not exceeding 660 mg. in 24 hours. Take with milk or food to avoid stomach irritation.	Don't take naproxen sodium with alcohol or if you have a history of kidney failure, high blood pressure or heart disease. Regular use may damage kidneys and liver.

aspirin in 1899, the world has been a less painful place. Aspirin helps block the body's production of prostaglandins, specialized chemicals that cause pain and inflammation. Because of its tendency to cause side effects such as stomach upset and bleeding, aspirin isn't always the pain reliever of choice, says Dr. Marcus. Coated aspirin is available to prevent stomach upset, adds Dr. Warren. (To see which medication is best for you, consult "Pain-Relieving Pills.")

Work it out. Strained and spasming muscles may need to be massaged and stretched before they will relax. You can do a lot with your fingers, your palm and the heel of your hand, though certainly, a sore back is out of reach. Beg a friend or lover to work on your back, or make an appointment with a professional massage therapist. Or grab a product called the Thera Cane and massage yourself according to the instructions in the accompanying videotape, recommends Dr. Warren. (For a description of the Thera Cane, see the tip "Work your trigger points" on page 60.)

Don't be afraid to move. Most muscle tightness will work itself out with movement, particularly controlled stretching, says Dr. Anderson. The opposite is true, too: Tightness could worsen with immobilization.

Note: If pain gets substantially worse with continued movement, self-treatment may not help. Something could be broken, and you should probably see a doctor.

In his book, Dr. Anderson recommends a "fold and hold" technique for relieving muscle pain. He suggests trying this first before attempting any stretches. The essence of fold and hold is to probe the painful site for the most tender spot, then find a position that folds the muscle over itself at that point and releases the tension (you are actually shortening the muscle rather than folding it). Be ready to get into poses that look awkward, he says. You've found the right position if the pain eases up by at least 75 percent and the area feels comfortable.

Hold the fold position for 90 seconds. This is the treatment phase, allowing the muscle to relax. Then slowly and gently return to your normal position. There are many possible fold positions; Dr. Anderson illustrates a number of these in his book.

Using the Fold and Hold Technique

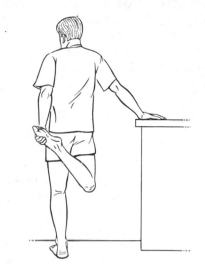

For a shinsplint or an achy Achilles tendon:
1. Locate the tender spot. It will likely be in the mid- to lower inner leg, immediately behind the leg bone, or tibia.
2. Stand near a table or chair or another support. For pain in the right shin, bend your right knee and grab the toe of your right foot with your left hand. Let your right heel rest against your left buttock. Point your toes toward the ceiling.
3. Fine-tune the position until the tender spot is 75 percent improved. Hold for 90 seconds, then gently let your leg down.

Chronic Pain

Imagine being in constant pain. Sometimes it roars; often it's just there, nagging, hurting. It never leaves for more than a few minutes or hours—maybe a day, if you're really lucky. Then it comes back, screaming in your face like a bitter witch. You can't shake it.

Chronic pain: It's a disease, not a symptom, says Dr. Caudill. It saps your vitality and distorts your mind, body and spirit. It changes your behavior, your outlook and your relationships.

Chronic pain often starts with an injury but then does not get better as expected. It may be that the pain-sending system goes haywire and starts misfiring. Doctors aren't sure how or why this occurs. Once it does, though, a lot of things can go wrong.

Pain increases stress, and stress forces the brain to release chemicals that increase sensitivity to pain. It's a vicious circle, notes Larry J.

Feldman, Ph.D., director of the Pain and Stress Rehabilitation Center in Newark, Delaware, and author of *Feeling Good Again: The Most Powerful Medicine Is What You Can Do for Yourself.* Many people with chronic pain spiral downward into feelings of helplessness, hopelessness, depression and isolation, which only compound the crippling power of chronic pain.

In most cases, there isn't a readily identifiable cause of, or a simple solution to, chronic pain. A relatively new test called provocative discometry, which consists of injecting saline directly into a spinal disk, can help identify the nerves and disks involved in excruciating pain, says Nelson Hendler, M.D., director of the Mensana Clinic in Stevenson, Maryland, one of the nation's first pain clinics. In some cases, doctors inject anesthetic into specific nerves to stop the pain. They may recommend having the nerves decompressed—that is, having scar tissue removed from them.

In the past, people with chronic pain were often advised to avoid physical activity altogether. Yet pain experts now believe that prolonged inactivity makes matters worse, says Dr. Marcus in his book *Freedom from Chronic Pain.* Muscles degenerate, bones lose calcium, and the body weakens and may put on substantial weight. All of this, in turn, brings on secondary aches and pains.

Here's the bottom line: You can't drug away chronic pain. You can't ignore it. And your doctor probably can't cure it. It's your pain. Get the upper hand with a multifaceted approach that enlists and actively involves your mind, your body and your spirit, says Dr. Caudill. Let's look at each one in turn.

The Mind

We know that sensations of pain are the result of the mind processing different signals and giving orders. And we know that we can change the orders the mind gives, for better or for worse, with our actions and reactions. Rubbing a banged elbow soothes the pain; feeling helpless and stressed increases it.

Clearly, one key to reducing the effects of chronic pain is to change how we think about it and respond to it. We'll deal with ways to develop an overall pain-conquering attitude in the section on the spirit below. Here we'll deal with actively putting our minds to work in the fight against pain. Here are strategies from some of the country's finest pain specialists.

Record your pain. Maintain a daily pain diary. Document your pain; track its ebbs and flows. We tend to develop such fear of and respect for our pain that we come to believe that it is omnipresent, says Dr. Caudill. In truth, it constantly varies in intensity and in response to factors such as the weather, what we're doing, how much we've slept and how we feel.

To understand your pain, make notations three times a day in a daily log. Note both the intensity of your pain (the physical sensations) and the intensity of your distress (how you feel). Use a scale of 0 to 10, with 0 being no pain or distress and 10 being the worst. Alongside each entry, note what you are doing at the time: watching television, eating dinner, driving, whatever. Keep the diary for three months. Over time—consciously or not—you will gradually modify the behaviors that make you hurt more and increase those that make you hurt less, says Dr. Caudill.

Control tension. Learning to drop your stress level by just 5 to 10 percent is enough to lower pain sensitivity and give you more control over chronic pain, says Dr. Feldman.

"The goal is not to eliminate tension or to achieve deep relaxation but to gain control over tension," he says. "Deep relaxation will just naturally happen as you become more aware of the importance of being less tense and as you learn that you can control surplus tension."

Dr. Feldman suggests this exercise: Four or five times a day, sit in a quiet place where you will not be interrupted. Silently count backward from 40 to 0, saying the word "relax" after each number. This should take three to four minutes. The goal is to gain control over your tension and stress.

Transform Pain with Hypnosis

Close your eyes, breathe slowly and deeply and count your breaths, counting backward from 40 to 1. With each breath, silently tell yourself to relax. When you reach 1, try this simple exercise, says Margaret A. Caudill, M.D., Ph.D., assistant clinical professor of medicine at Harvard Medical School and author of *Managing Pain before It Manages You*. Remember, she cautions, if you have any problems trying this, don't hesitate to seek professional assistance.

With your eyes still closed and your breathing deep, slow and steady, imagine your right hand becoming warm, pleasantly warm, and heavy. Each time you exhale, the warmth and heaviness increase a notch until your hand is so heavy that you cannot move it.

Feel a pleasing numbness beginning in your right thumb. When your thumb is numb, feel the numbness spread to your index finger as you exhale. With each breath, the numbness spreads to the next finger until all of the fingers of your right hand are warm, heavy and numb. Then let the numbness fill your palm and spread to the back of your hand, stopping at your wrist. Now your whole hand is warm, heavy and numb.

Place your right hand on the painful area or imagine the numbness moving from your right hand to the painful area. Let the painful area absorb all of the numbness. Once it has, resume focusing on your breathing and the word "relax." When you're ready to stop, transfer the numbness back to your right hand. Then feel normal sensations return first to the back of your hand, then to your palm, pinkie, fourth finger and so on in reverse order. Gradually, with each breath, your hand feels more and more normal. Count to three and open your eyes.

It is best not to practice this technique more than once daily. But the more days you do it, the more adept you will become at developing the sensation of numbness quickly and transferring it to any area of pain, says Dr. Caudill.

That's it. The key elements are the word "relax" and adopting a passive attitude toward other thoughts that pass through, says Dr. Feldman. Studies show that after a month of daily practice of this and similar exercises, people become substantially calmer, more chipper and less likely to tense up in stressful situations.

The hardest part for most people, says Dr. Feldman, is remembering to do the exercise. Dr. Caudill suggests posting a sign that says "Please do not disturb. I'm relaxing, per my doctor's orders."

After a month, notes Dr. Feldman, you'll find yourself often shortcutting the exercise, counting only a few numbers or just saying the word "relax" in tense situations and immediately feeling more at peace and more in control.

Learn to breathe. Another simple tension-fighter that offers long-term benefits is breathing deeply, says Dr. Feldman. Every few minutes or so, remind yourself to take a slow, deep breath and to exhale completely. Mentally say the word "relax" as you exhale, and you will actually relax even more, Dr. Feldman says. "Just saying the word 'relax' causes you to," he explains. "Your brain starts sending out the neurochemical message that says 'Relax.' "

The Body

Much of the physical therapy that works in reducing chronic pain involves relaxing, stretching and toning muscles. That's because muscle tension is present in most cases of

Other thoughts will crowd in again and again; that's okay. Acknowledge them, then let them go and gently return your focus to counting, breathing and the word "relax." When another thought appears, recognize that it is there, then let it go and return to counting. If you lose count, pick up at 20.

chronic pain, says Dr. Marcus. It can come from overworking muscles, particularly weak or weakened ones.

This is why rest is not the treatment of choice for chronic pain. The less we tone and work our muscles, the weaker they get, and the more likely we are to experience increasing pain, says Dr. Caudill.

Pain therapy involves physical therapy, actually working the muscles to relax, stretch and strengthen them. If you exercise carefully and slowly, you are not likely to make your condition worse, says Dr. Caudill.

Try tai chi. Or yoga. These Eastern systems of stretching, posturing, moving and breathing offer excellent stretching exercises and mind-body awareness and concentration, says Dr. Caudill. If you have movement limitations, ask the instructor to modify the positions so that they will work for you.

Work out in water. Most colleges and community pools offer low-impact water aerobics classes. About 70 percent of the effect of gravity is lost in water, so movement is easier, says Dr. Caudill. And you still get the benefit of the workout.

Check the attitude at the door. Your body's attitude, that is. Look at your posture, your facial expression, the timbre and tone of your voice, says Dr. Marcus. People with histories of pain often slump, frown and appear demoralized, all of which discourage the brain from releasing painkilling, feel-good chemicals called endorphins, notes Dr. Feldman.

Enjoy healing waters. Many people find relief and relaxation in hot tubs, whirlpools and saunas, says Dr. Caudill.

Apply heat. Or cold. Either one, applied during a pain flare-up, can help make you feel better fast, says Dr. Caudill. Use whichever you prefer. Ice is better for reducing swelling, while heat relaxes muscles.

Work your trigger points. Use firm thumb or fingertip pressure for a few seconds on a point of pain that feels knotted, if you can reach it comfortably. This often offers lasting relief, says Joan Johnson, massage therapist to sports superstars and author of *The Healing Art of Sports Massage.*

If you can't reach a point on your back, lie on your back on the floor, put a tennis ball under the point and shift your weight onto the ball, she suggests. Or buy a Thera Cane. A Thera Cane is a curved fiberglass stick issued to patients in many pain clinics as well as to players in some major sports clubs, including the Los Angeles Dodgers, says inventor Daniel Hennessey, a longtime chronic pain sufferer. It has handles and knobs that can reach just about any knotted, sore spot on your body.

"You apply the pressure yourself, exactly where it's needed and at the right angle of attack to relieve the spasm," says Dr. Warren. With proper pressure, you relieve the spasm and, with a couple of months' regular use, break even the most severe pain syndrome, says Dr. Warren. The tool is found in medical supply stores. It comes with instructions and a helpful video for about $50. If you can't find a Thera Cane locally, you can get one by mail order from Stretching (1-800-333-1307).

Lose weight. Extra weight not only robs you of energy but also can increase your pain, particularly if you have arthritis or back pain, say doctors at the Tampa (Florida) Medical Group, which treats chronic pain. Extra pounds put more weight on your back and joints. If you are overweight, talk to your doctor about starting a sensible weight-loss plan.

Get comfortable. Be sure that any chair you sit in, or any desk you sit at, for long periods of time gives you proper support. When standing, maintain a comfortable, straight-up-and-down alignment, says Dr. Caudill.

Massage those muscles. Massage offers temporary pain relief and relaxes tense and spasming muscles, says Dr. Caudill. It can cost anywhere from $40 to about $60 an hour, however, and is rarely covered by medical insurance. Many schools that train massage therapists operate low-cost clinics in which advanced students offer treatment to get the required number of hours of experience necessary for graduation and licensing. Call your

How to Pick a Pain Clinic

Of all of the pain treatment centers in the United States, only 184 are accredited by the Commission on Accreditation of Rehabilitation Facilities (CARF). To receive information about accredited centers near you, send your request, along with a self-addressed, stamped envelope, to CARF at 4891 East Grant Road, Tucson, AZ 85712.

Before selecting a clinic, consider the following, advises Nelson Hendler, M.D., director of the Mensana Clinic in Stevenson, Maryland.

• What portion of the clinic's services will your insurance cover?

• Is the clinic affiliated with a medical school? Some of the best are.

• Does the clinic use a multidisciplinary approach and offer different types of programs for different types of pain? Avoid clinics that use only one type of therapy.

• Does the clinic advocate the use of narcotic, sedative, analgesic or hypnotic drugs? If so, it's not for you.

state licensing board to find out which schools offer massage therapy. Then call the schools to see if they have low-cost clinics or sliding scales for payment, Dr. Caudill adds.

The Spirit

We all know that when we look for things to complain about, we find them. And the more we complain, the worse we feel.

Pain compounds the effect. Its every twinge reminds us that we're not our carefree selves anymore. And we begin perceiving disaster. And we express it.

"There's no use trying."

"Why me?"

"God is so unfair."

"I'll never get back to work."

This is what Dr. Marcus calls catastrophizing. It's the "poor, pitiful me" syndrome that nearly every chronic pain sufferer experiences sooner or later. To get control of your pain, he says, you must get control of your attitude. You must rebuke despair, because it compounds pain. Of course, that's easier said than done.

Building tolerance and lessening pain with the mind-body exercises we've suggested make it easier. Here are ways to develop a winning attitude.

Think about your thoughts. Examine each despairing thought. Write it down on paper immediately after it pops into your mind or out of your mouth. Many of the thoughts are distorted, hasty conclusions, says Dr. Caudill. That's revealed when you write one down and ask "Is this 100 percent true? What is true here?"

Monitor your self-talk. A lot of bad stuff gets said in the running dialogue you have with yourself in your brain, says Dr. Caudill. Don't be defeatist, even with yourself. Make a conscious effort to replace negative thoughts with positive ones.

Distract yourself. Develop a list of activities that you utterly enjoy, that you can immerse yourself in. Then incorporate some into your daily life despite your pain, says Dr. Caudill. You'll find that when you're immersed in an enjoyable activity, you feel much less distressed about your pain. Use your pain diary to identify activities that seem to lessen pain and do those things more often.

The Last Resort

If all else fails, check in to an accredited pain clinic, advises Dr. Caudill. They combine all of the techniques we've talked about—and more. Contact the American Pain Society at 4700 West Lake Avenue, Glenview, IL 60025, to locate the facility nearest you.

The services provided by accredited pain clinics are comprehensive and are usually covered by insurance. They involve physical therapy, psychological therapy, occupational therapy (learning to work around your pain), biofeedback and more.

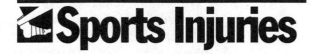

Sports Injuries

- **Always warm up before and cool down after a workout.**
- **Lift weights for a sturdier body.**
- **Constantly monitor your body.**

You are a smart man. We truly believe so. And we have no intention of talking down to you, as if you were some wild kid in need of a stern parental lecture. You've gotten pretty far in life without us, and we respect that.

But you know, you hardly ever see people stretching at the first tee on a golf course. Or at the tennis courts. Definitely not at the gym, either. Lots of lifting, but not much warming up or cooling down.

Not coincidently, go by a sports doctor's office, or a back or joint specialist's office, and the parking lot is full; business is good. There's a correlation: Many active men just don't take the simple steps necessary to prevent injury. We're going to tell you what those steps are here. And they are simple; for some of them, you'll slap your head and say "I paid money for this?" We hope you'll then ask yourself "So why aren't I doing these things?" Our message: Wise men rarely suffer sports injuries.

The Basics of Prevention

Your first line of defense against injury is actually a double line: strengthening the muscles you use most in your sport through weight lifting, and making your muscles and joints as flexible as possible through stretching, says Lyle J. Micheli, M.D., former president of the American College of Sports Medicine, associate clinical professor of orthopedic surgery at Harvard Medical School and author of *The Sports Medicine Bible*.

It's true for running, for swimming, for throwing a baseball, for riding a bike. Weight lifting and stretching help prevent injury for every physical activity, says Wayne Westcott, Ph.D., strength-training consultant for the YMCA and other national organizations. With increased strength and flexibility, you'll move better and more efficiently. And after you play or work out, your level of soreness will be minimal—if there's any soreness at all. As a bonus, you may even look better.

Stretching you probably knew about. But there still is a bias out there against weight lifting as a training tool for sports. So let's deflate some myths. Weight lifting will not make you muscle-bound, it won't reduce your flexibility and range of motion, and it will not slow you down, states Dr. Micheli. Nor will your muscles turn to fat if you stop weight lifting.

And assuming you are a healthy guy who isn't restricted from any activity by your doctor, weight lifting is perfectly safe and healthy for your heart and circulatory system, notes Dr. Micheli.

The stronger your muscles, the less you'll feel the effects of physical activity on them as well as on your tendons, ligaments, joints and bones—the body parts most prone to sports injuries. And here's another weight-lifting bonus: It may help fight osteoporosis.

Part 3 of this book provides exercises and programs for each major muscle group of the body. But we'll cover a few important points here.

Train all of your muscles. Weight lifting is muscle-specific. Do a biceps exercise, and the only muscles that benefit are your biceps. Picking out specific muscles that relate to your sport and training only them is called sport-specific exercise. Although some doctors recommend this method of training, Dr. Westcott does not. He believes that focusing on the same muscles you use in your sport can put excess stress on them, making them susceptible to overuse injuries. Instead, Dr. Westcott recommends strengthening all of the major muscle groups. Once you build all-over muscular strength, then you may want to emphasize some of the specific muscles that are more important to your sport.

Try three a week. Most authorities agree

that three workouts weekly, with a day off between sessions, produces the best results. Don't work out on back-to-back days under the belief that you'll speed up the strengthening process, says Dr. Micheli. Muscle strength and size both increase on the off days.

Be smart about how much you lift. A muscle increases in strength when demands are placed on it beyond its normal ability. In weight-lifting jargon, this is called overload. But too much overload may cause injury. The right amount of weight and the proper number of repetitions—together, these two factors are known as intensity—are essential to the success of your workout program, states Dr. Micheli.

The weight should be from 50 to 80 percent of your maximum lift capability. Use closer to 80 percent and do fewer repetitions when you want to develop the capacity for short bursts of intense power (say, to sprint a short distance). Use less weight and more repetitions to train muscles for stamina (to run a ten-kilometer race, for example), advises Dr. Micheli.

Be smart about how you lift. Use the two-four method: Take two seconds to lift, four seconds to lower. When you feel it's time to increase the weight you're lifting, do so gradually—say, by no more than 10 percent, says Dr. Micheli.

The Right Routine

Many sports injuries are caused by body parts bending beyond their capacity. Well, as one of its many benefits, stretching gives you the capacity to bend more without breaking, states Dr. Westcott.

In part 3, we provide stretches for each major muscle group. Unlike weight lifting, stretching can be done daily to increase range of motion, says Dr. Westcott.

The Golden Rules

In a rush? We've boiled down the most important steps in injury prevention to the following must-do's:

1. Warm up correctly.
2. Stretch slowly and thoroughly.
3. Wear the right shoes.
4. Wear clothes appropriate to the weather.
5. Start slowly.
6. Stop immediately if you feel dizzy, get very short of breath, feel pain or break into a cold sweat.
7. Cool down gradually after your workout or sport.
8. Stretch again.
9. Be mentally tough. Always be alert to your body and your surroundings.

A couple of general tips: Don't tug or bounce during a stretch, warns Dr. Westcott. Instead, slowly stretch until you feel a healthy tension in the muscle or joint, then hold still for the recommended amount of time. And remember to bring your entire body to the party, which means don't neglect any of the major joint-muscle connections. Start at the top and work your way down: shoulders, elbows, wrists, waist area, lower back, hips, knees and, finally, ankles.

There are two more pieces to the injury prevention routine: warming up and cooling down, says Dr. Micheli. The former starts the blood flowing to your muscles so that they, along with your heart and lungs, are prepared for the action soon to follow. Warming up also helps you mentally prepare for your activity, sharpens your focus and helps you relax. A warm-up can be almost any slow-going, easy-does-it repetitive activity—walking or jogging, for example.

Cooling down lets your body slowly return to a relaxed, stable exertion level, which is healthier for your heart and lungs. When cooling down, do what you did when warming up: easy, gentle movements until your heart rate returns to normal. Runners, joggers, walkers, swimmers and cyclists can just gradually move slower while the heart settles into its regular rhythm. Men who play racquetball, handball and similar sports can either jog slowly, then walk, or hit the treadmill or stationary cycle at an easy pace. Taper off and stop when your ticker is ticking at its usual rate, says Dr. Micheli.

After cooldown, end your session with five final minutes of stretching. This will help keep your muscles from tightening and aching and help you stay flexible, says Dr. Micheli. Remember the stretches you did before you began your workout? Do them again, but briefly this time, with emphasis on the areas of your body used in your sport or activity.

So we have all of the components of the perfect exercise or sports routine, one that will go a long way toward preventing injury.

1. Warm up.
2. Stretch.
3. Work out.
4. Cool down.
5. Stretch.

But that adds four steps to what you normally do, you say? Relax: Ten minutes for the first two and ten minutes for the last two is not a lot of time to keep yourself injury-free, says Dr. Micheli.

The Right Shoe

It's bad enough if you overextend yourself. But to get hurt because of ill-fitting, improper gear—that's adding insult to injury.

In particular, the right shoes with the right fit are essential protection against injury. Your feet take a brutal beating during most

The Most Common Injuries

What travails await the unprepared athlete? Here are the most common injuries in eight popular activities, according to H. Winter Griffith, M.D., former team physician at Florida State University in Tallahassee and author of *Complete Guide to Sports Injuries.*

Aerobic dance. All of that bouncing is tough on joints and limbs. Sprains and strains are particularly common in the feet, ankles, legs, pelvis and abdominal wall. Also common are runner's knee and shinsplints.

Baseball. Most injuries are to the arm. What's common: tennis elbow (or as it's known in baseball, pitcher's elbow), upper-arm muscle strain, elbow fractures, elbow joint strain, shoulder dislocations, shoulder sprains, shoulder bursitis and finger fractures and dislocations.

Basketball. Fingers get it worst (dislocations, fractures and sprains). But the limbs are also susceptible to ankle sprains, shinsplints, runner's knee, groin pulls, shoulder dislocations and shoulder bursitis.

Football. This is a rough sport; injuries can occur almost anywhere. Among the most common sites are the head, neck, pelvis, legs, knees and ankles.

Handball. Finger and hand injuries are particularly common. Also be prepared for ankle sprains, shinsplints, runner's knee, groin pulls and shoulder dislocations.

Running. Protect those legs! Muscle sprains and strains in the legs, ankles and feet are typical. So are runner's knee, shinsplints and hamstring injuries. It's not so unusual to get muscle injuries in the shoulders, arms and abdomen as well.

Racquetball/squash. The eyes get hit often in these sports. Also common: sprains and strains in the neck, shoulder area, back, arms, wrists, hips, legs, knees and ankles, as well as shinsplints, shoulder bursitis and tennis elbow.

Tennis. All of that multidirectional sprinting means high potential for muscle sprains and strains in the neck, shoulders, back, arms, wrists, hips, legs, knees and ankles. Also common are eye injuries, shoulder bursitis, tennis elbow and shinsplints.

sports. And the impact from running, jumping, twisting and turning can ripple through your feet all the way up your legs: ankles, knees, pelvis, hips and back.

But walk into a shoe store, and bam! Instant shoe store blues. You have only two feet and too many shoe categories to choose from. Footwear made specifically for physical activity includes shoes for running, walking, cross-training, tennis, racquet sports, bicycling, football, baseball, basketball, weight lifting and golf.

A right-fitting athletic shoe should be about one-quarter inch wider than your foot. There should be enough room in front for your toes to wiggle comfortably, according to Morton Walker, D.P.M., co-author of *The Complete Foot Book*. The shoe should fit snugly at the heel and instep. Keep in mind that shoe sizes are not uniform from manufacturer to manufacturer, so always try on shoes rather than relying on the size.

Also, when you're shopping for footwear, wear the socks that you intend to use with your shoes. As for the best sports socks, Dr. Westcott recommends 100 percent cotton. Socks absorb shocks and moisture and protect the feet from shoe abrasion. Wear socks that are one-half inch longer than your feet. Put on a freshly laundered pair of good athletic socks whenever you work out or do your physical thing.

Other Gear

Now that your feet are covered, let's work our way up. As many as 90 percent of eye

How to Be Prepared

In California, they drive around with cases of bottled water and canned chili in their trunks in case an earthquake suddenly hits. Why not? A trunk is a big space. Why be sorry?

Active guys have a far greater chance of getting injured while exercising than of getting hit by an earthquake. So out-cool those wacky Californians: Make up a simple first-aid kit in a toolbox or tackle box, stash it in your car trunk and take it with you whenever you work out or get physical. According to the American Red Cross, here are the supplies you'll need for a truly complete kit.

- Adhesive bandages (assorted sizes)
- Adhesive tape
- Antibiotic ointment
- Antiseptic/anesthetic spray
- Antiseptic ointment
- Antiseptic wipes
- Bulb syringe
- Butterfly bandages
- Calamine/antihistamine lotion
- Candle and matches
- Change (for a pay phone)
- Chemical cold "snap packs"
- Cotton balls
- Cotton-tip applicators
- Disinfecting soap
- Disposable gloves
- Elastic bandages/wraps (three-inch width)
- Emergency telephone numbers
- Eyecup or small plastic cup
- Eye patches
- Flashlight and extra batteries
- Ipecac syrup
- Paper drinking cups
- Pencil and paper
- Plastic bags (handy for ice packs)
- Safety pins
- Scissors (blunt-tipped)
- Space blanket
- Sterile eyewash
- Sterile gauze pads (two- and four-inch)
- Sterile nonstick pads
- Sterile self-adhering gauze roller bandages (two-, three- and four-inch)
- Thermometer
- Triangular bandages
- Tweezers

injuries are preventable. So don't worry about how you look (ugliness scares competitors anyway). Wear plastic safety glasses when you play sports with a high incidence of eye injuries, such as football, soccer, racquetball, squash, badminton and hockey.

As for the rest of your body, the big issue is temperature. In hot, humid weather, the goal is to wear clothes that wick away or absorb sweat. There's a whole science to fabrics that we won't get into here. Dr. Westcott is happy with cotton. Make sure you wear loose, light, white clothing that breathes and absorbs moisture. Keep your head covered, too. Excess sun on your noggin can make you do strange and unhealthy things, like overheat and pass out.

While on the topic of hot weather, Dr. Westcott offers a hardy dose of the obvious: Drink lots of water to keep your innards cool and to replace all of that sweat. The water should be cool but not iced. Drink before, during and after your activity. You can also drink Gatorade or a similar beverage to replace lost electrolytes (minerals important to muscle function), says Dr. Westcott; dilute every two parts sports drink with one part water to help absorption.

As for cold weather, the message again is pretty plain: Keep your skin covered, states Dr. Westcott. Exposed skin—on your face (especially your nose), ears and fingers—is susceptible to frostbite, particularly when wet. Dress in layers; the air between garments is an excellent insulator against cold. Wear a polypropylene garment next to your skin to carry away sweat and to prevent rapid cooling. The outer layer should protect against the wind. Runners and cross-country skiers, however,

Shoe Characteristics

Which shoes for which sport? Here are the characteristics to look for when shopping for shoes for various activities, as described in the *The Complete Foot Book* by Donald S. Pritt, D.P.M., and Morton Walker, D.P.M.

Baseball
- General: cleats of hard rubber or plastic.
- Upper: either nylon and leather or just leather.
- Sole: sharp-edged to provide the necessary traction.

Basketball
- General: heavy, sturdy high-tops to provide lateral support and stability. Extra cushioning at the ankle and midsole.
- Sole: hard rubber; cupped for dependable traction.

Biking
- General: snug fit.
- Sole: stiff for pedaling, particularly for racing; slightly more flexible for touring. Should fit tightly in pedal toehold.

Football
- General: sturdy; made of thick leather for protection.
- Heel: strong.
- Sole: spiked rubber. Hard artificial surfaces such as

need venting in their outer garments to release heat. A hat will prevent heat loss through your head. Mittens will keep your hands warmer than gloves. Instead of mittens, Dr. Westcott suggests wearing gym socks on your hands when you run. "I find they work as well as mittens and are more convenient, because I can easily throw them in the washer," notes Dr. Westcott.

Small Fixes

Accidents do happen. So remember this simple acronymn: RICE. It'll remind you what to do for your sprains, strains, pulls and pops, states Dr. Micheli. RICE stands for rest, ice, compression and elevation—four effective techniques that are used together to treat an injury.

Rest. Rest the injured area for at least 24 hours to prevent further damage.

AstroTurf require soles with small cleats for traction. Replace cleats with hard plastic studs for playing on soft grass.

Racquetball, Handball and Squash

• Sole: round-edged; tacky for a good grip on wooden floors. Insole should be well-cushioned to give comfort for rapid moves.

Running

• Flexibility: should bend easily.
• Upper: light, soft, breathable, flexible.
• Heel: somewhat raised; firm, with sharp edges for stability.
• Sole: turned up fore and aft, like a gentle crescent; grooved, studded or waffled for traction, with cushioning at the midpoint.

Tennis

• General: heavy and strong, with cushioning, especially at the midsole, for shock absorption.
• Upper: breathable material.
• Heel: firm.
• Sole: flat, hard and square-edged, with patterns for on-dime turning.

Ice. Quickly apply ice to limit internal bleeding and reduce swelling. Don't apply ice directly to your skin; wrap it in cloth or apply it over an elastic bandage. Apply the ice for 20 minutes, then remove it for 20 minutes. Continue this cycle for the first two hours following the injury. Then for the next day or so, apply the ice for 8 to 10 minutes of every hour.

Compression. Compressing the injured area with an elastic bandage immediately after the trauma limits fluid leakage into nearby areas and so helps reduce swelling. Make sure the bandage is not too tight. Loosen the bandage if you experience pins and needles, pain or numbness or if your skin turns blue below the bandaged area.

Elevation. Raise the injured area to decrease swelling and improve fluid drainage. Serious injuries, of course, require medi-cal attention. But use RICE until the injury can be evaluated by a physician.

Some Final Notes

A few other suggestions for staying on your feet and in the game:

Eat at the right times. Never eat just before a workout or game. Allow from 2 to 4½ hours for your system to digest food before starting strenuous physical activity. Also, don't eat high-fat foods and protein before your activity, says Allan M. Levy, M.D., director of the Department of Sports Medicine at Pascack Valley Hospital in Westwood, New Jersey, and author of *Sports Injury Handbook.* They take longer to leave your stomach, which could hurt your performance. Instead, Dr. Levy recommends high-carbohydrate, low-fat foods, such as breads, cereals, pastas, fruits and fruit juices and low-fat dairy products, for pre-activity eating.

Also, no alcohol for at least six hours before your activity. Lay off the candy as well. It won't give you a quick energy boost; it just temporarily spikes up your blood sugar level. The result: Insulin is released, blood sugar reserves are burned up, and energy is sapped.

Stay alert. Any good competitor knows that mental training is almost as important as physical training. Alert, upbeat, thinking athletes are the ones who excel. They also have fewer self-caused injuries, says Dr. Westcott. So when you are engaged in a physical activity, always think, think, think: "Is that a bump I'm about to ride over?" "Is my calf tightening up too much?" "Am I breathing deeply?" "Am I executing properly?" By constantly monitoring your body and your surroundings, you stand to not only prevent injury but also improve your performance, states Dr. Westcott.

ᙂSleep

- **Men who sleep alone have more sleep problems than those who sleep with a partner.**
- **Percent decrease in immune function that results from losing three or more hours of sleep: 50**
- **Number of Americans who regularly watch television between midnight and 3:00 A.M.: 20 million**
- **Ratio of men with sleep problems to women with sleep problems: 1:2**

Strange States

When you sleep, your mind doesn't lose consciousness so much as redirect it. Brain waves speed up and slow down. Electricity surges, then diminishes to a murmur. The unreal becomes real.

Experts have identified four different states of consciousness.

Deep sleep. You regain most of your energy and your sense of restfulness during this phase. Men who sleepwalk usually do it during deep sleep.

Dream state. Also called rapid eye movement sleep or REM sleep, this is the phase in which dreams occur. The eyes shudder beneath closed lids (hence the name). The brain is remarkably alert, perhaps even more so than when you're awake. Not only must it respond to the environment of your dreams but it must also create that environment in the first place. Paradoxically, the muscles in your body are profoundly relaxed; physical movement is nearly impossible. Perhaps this is a protective mechanism to prevent you from "acting out" your brain's otherworldly commands.

Light sleep. You spend most of your night in light sleep, which hovers near the border between sleeping and waking. While that may seem wasteful, it's far from it, says Patricia Murphy, Ph.D., postdoctoral research associate at the Institute of Chronobiology of the New York Hospital–Cornell Medical Center in New York City. It's during light sleep that your body performs most biological functions, such as protein synthesis and the release of hormones. But the balance of sleep will shift in favor of deep sleep if you've experienced a great deal of emotional strain or physical exertion, on the scale of running a marathon.

Waking state. You open your eyes and regain consciousness. You probably don't remember your dreams. You're in a different world—until the next time you sleep.■

How to Maximize Sleep

If the bags beneath your eyes are starting to look like suitcases, you know you're not getting enough sleep. Here are a few ways to log some extra Zzzs, courtesy of Deepak Chopra, M.D., in his book *Restful Sleep.*

Eat early and light. Late-night chow is great for poker games and midnight movies, but it's lousy for your sleep. You need to give your metabolism some quiet time. You'll further enhance digestion and feel more relaxed if you take a 5- to 15-minute walk after dinner.

Start winding down. Late night is for rest, not for jamming on the guitar. Or cleaning the house. Or calling in for messages. Basically, you want to be bored and sleepy by the time you hit the sack. Wind down with an amusing magazine, mellow music or a conversation with your wife or girlfriend. And go easy on the hot brew; caffeine stays in the bloodstream for up to six hours and can keep you awake half of the night.

Do your body good. It's not just an old wives' tale that drinking warm milk before bedtime will help you fall asleep. Milk contains tryptophan, a natural amino acid that aids in sleep. ***Drink easy.*** Although alcohol can knock you out, it doesn't provide restful sleep at all. In fact, drinking can inhibit dream sleep, which is why having even a few drinks can make you feel more fatigued the next day.

Be a day owl. Being busy and active during the day will help you sleep better at night. The body demands good sleep to replenish energy and keep you feeling good.

Appreciate atmosphere. Studies show that looking at pleasing things is relaxing and may help you sleep. Make your bedroom pleasant. If you have a room with a view, position the bed to face out the window. Or consider hanging a picture or putting a bowl of fish on the bureau.

Set the clock. If you're often tossing and turning an hour or more after going to bed, try turning back the clock. Simply set the alarm to go off a few minutes earlier each day for a total of 15 to 30 minutes per week. Getting up earlier will naturally cause you to feel more tired in the evening, so you'll fall asleep more quickly.

It's important, however, to stick to the new schedule, even on weekends. Otherwise, your body won't be able to acclimate to the new hours.∎

The Sleep You Need . . .

How much sleep you need varies with age. You began life requiring 16 hours a night; by the time you're in your thirties or forties, you need only about 7 hours a night.

Some men do fine on less than seven hours of sleep a night. Studies show, however, that cutting your sleep time short can prematurely cut you short. An American Cancer Society study found that men who sleep less than four hours a night have a 300 percent higher mortality rate than those getting between seven and nine hours of sleep each night.∎

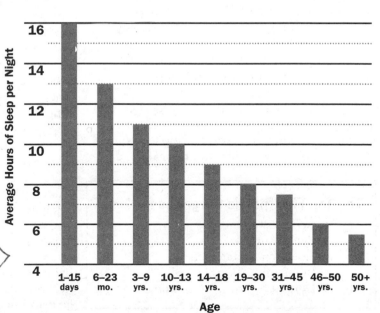

Chart: Average Hours of Sleep per Night vs. Age

Age	Average Hours of Sleep per Night
1–15 days	16
6–23 mo.	13
3–9 yrs.	11
10–13 yrs.	10
14–18 yrs.	9
19–30 yrs.	8
31–45 yrs.	7.5
46–50 yrs.	6
50+ yrs.	5.5

Plastic Surgery

- Be realistic about the outcome.
- Shop carefully.

Like all tourists, ancient warriors liked to collect mementos commemorating their exploits. But since there weren't a lot of roadside souvenir stands selling "I Conquered Rome" T-shirts in those days, these jolly fellows would simply lop off the noses of their captured enemies.

To repair those wounds, ancient doctors began performing the first crude plastic surgery in the seventh century B.C., fashioning new noses out of skin grafted from the forehead.

That operation is still performed, but plastic surgery—the term is derived from a Greek word meaning to mold or give form—has evolved into a sophisticated medical art. Every year, nearly 55,000 American men undergo some form of plastic or reconstructive surgery, including face-lifts, nose reshaping, penis enlargement, scalp reduction, pec implants and wrinkle removal. Overall, men account for about 14 percent of all plastic surgery in the United States.

"A lot of men seek plastic surgery to get a competitive edge over younger men in the job market. Others just want to look as young as they feel," says Patricia Rooney, M.D., a plastic surgeon at the Cleveland Clinic Florida in Fort Lauderdale.

The Tools of the Trade

Plastic surgeons have mastered an impressive array of techniques to enhance a man's appearance.

- Dermabrasion, for instance, removes fine wrinkles and acne scars. Basically, it involves sanding the face with a tool that looks a lot like a dentist's drill. Essentially, dermabrasion sands down the high spots on the face, making the skin look more regular. The procedure isn't particularly painful, but there is significant post-procedure crusting and oozing.
- During a chemical peel, doctors apply acid and other chemicals that strip away the outer layers of the skin and remove wrinkles and age spots.
- In addition to removing wrinkles, the focused energy of a laser can eradicate birthmarks, tattoos and scars. A new laser can resurface aged skin by vaporizing tissues.
- Injections of collagen, a fibrous protein that holds the skin together, also are an effective way to eliminate wrinkles and scars. While collagen improves the appearance of wrinkles and scars, it is eventually reabsorbed by the body, meaning that the benefits gradually fade.
- Liposuction, another popular technique, can help eliminate beer bellies, flabby legs and other areas of fatty tissue. The surgeon makes a small incision, frequently less than a half-inch long, and inserts a cannula, a hollow, blunt-tipped instrument that works like a vacuum cleaner wand, to suck out excessive fat.
- Nose reshaping is the most common cosmetic surgery performed on men. An incision is made inside the nostril, and the surgeon separates the skin from the underlying bone. The bone is then remolded into a more appealing shape.
- For a face-lift, incisions are made at the hairline and around the ears. Fatty tissue is removed, and loose skin and muscle around the face and neck are tightened. Like the face,

---

The Top Five Plastic Surgeries for Men

1. Nose reshaping
2. Eyelid surgery
3. Liposuction (fat suction)
4. Breast reduction
5. Dermabrasion (skin sanding)

baggy eyes can be tightened with an eyelid lift.

• About 5,000 men a year opt for breast reduction surgery. It is particularly common among overweight men and former weight lifters, who develop flab in the chest as shrinking muscle is replaced by fat.

Is It Right for You?

Many of these procedures can be done on an outpatient basis in less than two hours and cause only minimal discomfort. As with all surgeries, however, they involve some risk, including infection, nerve damage, excessive blood loss and permanent skin discoloration—not to mention severe bleeding from the wallet, since insurance usually won't pick up the tab if there is no compelling medical reason for the surgery.

Also, keep in mind that while the result can be spectacular, it often isn't permanent, and the procedure may need to be repeated every five to ten years. Here are a couple of other things to consider.

Be real. If you want plastic surgery because you think it will transform your life or make women flock to your side, you may be disappointed. "The 40-year-old guy who just went through a divorce and wants plastic surgery so that he can attract a 20-year-old woman, or the man who comes in and says he wants to look like his favorite actor, isn't the best candidate for plastic surgery," says Alan Matarasso, M.D., a plastic surgeon and clinical assistant professor of plastic surgery at Albert Einstein College of Medicine in New York City. Before you see a plastic surgeon, ask yourself what really bothers you about your appearance. Then write down three reasons why you

Makeup and Men

Plastic surgery can do wonders, but restoring the skin's luster can be expensive and painful.

There is a low-cost, pain-free alternative that can mask many scars, burns, birthmarks and other skin imperfections. The catch is: It's makeup.

"Guys are leery of corrective cosmetics because the term conjures images of lipstick and blush. They think that these products are going to make them look effeminate. But corrective makeup is something entirely different that can make a dramatic difference in a man's life," says David Nicholas, a licensed makeup artist in Boston who specializes in reconstructive and corrective makeup.

Corrective cosmetics are specialized makeup; they are waterproof and resistant to perspiration, and they won't rub off. The result is a natural-looking, durable shield that covers the skin problem and protects you from the sun's damaging rays for up to 24 hours. With practice, most men can learn to apply this makeup in a matter of minutes.

"Corrective cosmetics are wonderful. In truth, they may be as effective a solution as surgery if you're dealing with a small spot," says Alan Matarasso, M.D., a plastic surgeon and clinical assistant professor of plastic surgery at Albert Einstein College of Medicine in New York City.

Ask your doctor if corrective cosmetics may help you. Several brands, including Dermablend and Covermark, are available at many department store cosmetics counters.

want the surgery. It will help you and your doctor determine if you should go through with it.

Find the right surgeon. Take your time, advises Dr. Matarasso. Find a plastic surgeon who listens to your concerns, answers all of your questions and doesn't push you into having the procedure. Be sure to ask about specifics, including cost, risk, healing time, pain and what you can realistically expect to look like after the procedure is done. Find out how many times he has done this surgery and try to get telephone numbers of former patients who have had the procedure you're contemplating. Ask if he is certified by the American Society of Plastic and Reconstructive Surgeons with a specialization in aesthetic surgery.

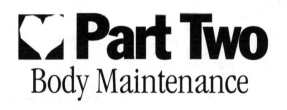

Part Two
Body Maintenance

Achilles Tendons

- **Stretch them before exercise.**
- **Stretch them after exercise.**
- **Stretch them some more.**

As superheroes go, Achilles was kind of a cut-rate Man of Steel. Sure, he was powerful. Resourceful. Feared by no-goods from Athens to Olympia. Your basic ancient Greek warrior-god, capable of leaping a Trojan horse in a single bound.

But once his enemies found out they could pierce his heel with an arrow, Achilles was so much mythological meat.

That's why the Achilles tendon is so aptly named. It's the strongest, toughest tendon in your body. The Achilles connects your calf muscle to your heel bone and, when healthy, lets you walk, run and leap, say, a fire hydrant in a single bound.

But when things go wrong, they can go really wrong. Tendinitis in the Achilles tendon makes it tough to even walk, let alone fight off columns of charging Romans. And if you're unlucky enough to rupture the tendon, you're looking at months of rehabilitation and possibly surgery.

The best way to avoid Achilles tendon trouble is to stretch it thoroughly before exercise. This goes double if you're over age 30, when you start to lose elasticity in the tendon, says Suzanne M. Levine, D.P.M., clinical podiatrist at the New York Hospital–Cornell Medical Center in New York City.

Here are a couple of suggested stretches. If your Achilles tendon is sore after exercise, Dr. Levine suggests elevating your foot and applying ice for 15 to 20 minutes. It's best to wear a sock while icing down the tendon to protect your skin. You can also take a pain reliever such as aspirin, acetaminophen or ibuprofen. If pain continues for more than a couple of days, see your doctor. You may be developing tendinitis.

Wall Leans. Stand facing a wall, with your feet about 12 inches apart. You should be about two feet from the wall. Place the palms of your hands on the wall at shoulder height. Lean forward, keeping your legs straight and bending your arms at the elbows. You should feel a stretch in your calves and the backs of your heels. Keep your heels flat on the floor and hold for 15 to 20 seconds. Repeat several times.

Wall Leans

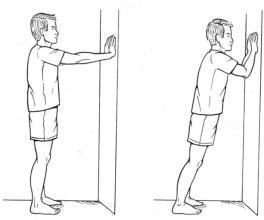

Heel Drops. You can do this stretch standing on the edge of a step or curb. Stand flat and slowly slide your right heel over the edge of the step or curb. Bend your left knee and lower your right heel until you feel a comfortable stretch in your right calf and heel. Hold for 15 seconds, then switch feet. Repeat several times with each foot.

Heel Drops

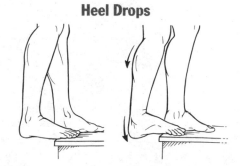

⌂ Adam's Apple

Adam and Eve were sitting around that fateful day, just tossing around the apple. Adam snatched the forbidden fruit, chomped and gulped. And gulped. His neck resembled a snake just after it swallows a mouse whole. Only the bump wouldn't move lower than the middle of his neck. The apple got stuck. And, so the legend from the 1700s goes, that bulge became known as Adam's apple.

Today we know that we're not walking around with apples lodged in our throats. And despite what the legend would have you believe, women have Adam's apples, too. But much smaller ones.

Doctors refer to the Adam's apple as thyroid cartilage. It consists of two plates that form a shield at the front of the throat, partially encasing the vocal cords. And as the name suggests, it sits just above the thyroid gland.

In young boys and girls, the Adam's apple is the same size. But once boys hit puberty, the apple grows, as do other parts of the throat. That is one reason why the male voice deepens.

For some people, the apple grows too much. The solution: an apple job. "You can actually have it shaved down. It's just a piece of cartilage," says Frederick Godley, M.D., an otolaryngologist at Harvard Community Health Plan in Providence, Rhode Island.

Because it's cartilage, about the only thing you can do to your Adam's apple is fracture it. And that is a rare occurrence. It's possible that an elbow to the throat during a basketball game could do the trick.

While the cartilage is low-maintenance, what's behind it is a different story. "There's rarely any bacterial infection of the larynx, though vocal abuse and viral infections regularly affect the voice," says Charles J. Krause, M.D., chief of clinical affairs and senior associate dean at the University of Michigan Medical School in Ann Arbor.

☀ Adrenal Glands

You are about to be attacked!

Did that get your heart beating? If it did, it means you just got a rush of the hormone adrenaline. Adrenaline is shot into your system whenever you become angry, scared or surprised. Adrenaline causes your heart to beat faster and your metabolism to rev up. It instantly prepares you for sudden challenges.

The adrenal glands make adrenaline. These two small glands, one located at the top of each kidney, also churn out hormones that regulate your blood sugar level, keep your blood volume where it should be and contribute to normal sexual development.

There isn't much you can do to keep your adrenal glands in good condition besides control your stress level, says Mitchell Harman, M.D., Ph.D., chief of endocrinology at the Gerontology Research Center of the National Institute on Aging in Baltimore. Chronic stress causes the adrenal glands to secrete too many hormones. Under extreme chronic stress, such as refugee conditions, the adrenal glands may even become enlarged from overuse.

"Relax. Get enough sleep. Keep things in perspective. Get away from it all once in a while," suggests Dr. Harman.

Adrenal gland diseases are rare. One is Cushing's syndrome, in which the glands produce too much of the steroid hormone cortisol. This causes unexplained weight gain, along with dark purplish stripes on the abdomen and buttocks. The disease can be treated with surgery or medication.

The flip side is when the glands stop producing hormones. This can cause Addison's disease, which is lethal if undetected but easily treated by taking replacement hormones two times a day.

▶◀ Ankles

- **Keep them stretched.**
- **Strengthen your calves.**
- **Work on your balance.**

The Achilles' heel of many men is the ankle. Consider: The average person takes between 5,000 and 10,000 steps a day. Every time that person's foot hits the ground, it sends a micro-jolt of stress through the ankle. Running is even tougher: Runners hit the ground with about 500 pounds of pressure. All of which helps explain why so many guys walk around with limps and with miles of mummy tape wrapped around their ankles.

Ankles are simply hinges—highly complex and mobile, but hinges nonetheless—that connect your feet to your legs. Those big bumps on the sides of each foot are where the leg bones, the tibia and the fibula, lock into the heel bone. In between those bones, of course, is a web of ligaments, tendons and muscles.

There's not a lot of support in there. Although the ankle is a powerful joint, capable of shifting your entire weight or reversing direction almost instantaneously, it's built more for speed and flexibility than for endurance. As a result, it's surprisingly delicate and prone to injury.

A sprain results when you wrench your foot to one side, stretching or tearing one of the ligaments that connect bone to bone. This is the most common type of ankle injury, and it happens easily. Stepping off a curb wrong can do it.

Nature never intended the ankle to be indestructible. But there are ways to maximize its flexibility while at the same time keeping strains and pain under rein.

Stand like a stork. "One of the reasons we trip and fall is that our sense of balance isn't good," says Steven I. Subotnick, D.P.M., a sports podiatrist in Hayward, California. To improve your balance while strengthening the ankle joint, "take off your shoes and stand on one leg, like a stork," he advises. Bend your other leg up behind you.

"Close your eyes while you do the exercise. Hold the pose for up to a minute," Dr. Subotnick advises. Then switch legs. He recommends repeating this several times a day.

Make your calves bullish. The calf muscles are critical for supporting and controlling the ankles, says Reba Schecter, director of exercise physiology at the Canyon Ranch health spa in Lenox, Massachusetts. To make them stronger, she recommends heel raises.

Stand facing up a flight of stairs, with the balls of your feet on one step. Your feet should be parallel and a few inches apart. Holding the railing for balance, slowly rise up on your toes. Then gently lower your heels as far as you can, always keeping the motion under control. Then rise all the way up again. Repeat eight to ten times. (For a slightly harder version involving weights, see the workout for the calves and lower legs on page 372.)

Heel Raises

Do this exercise three times a week, with a day or two between sessions, Schecter advises. You want your calf muscles to feel pleasantly, not painfully, fatigued after each set. If they don't, increase the number of repetitions until they do. For most guys, it's best to stick with a maximum of 12, she says.

Go for flexibility. One of the best ways to reduce your chances of ankle injury is to keep your muscles flexible. This is another exercise you can do with your toes on a step. This time, though, you don't raise your heels, and you hold your position rather than doing lots of repetitions.

To do it, simply lower your heels until you feel a good stretch. Hold the stretch for 10 to 30 seconds, then relax. Repeat three or four times. It is best to do the stretch while your muscles are warm, such as after walking, says Schecter.

Step Away from Ankle Pain

Ligaments have to be strong enough to hold bones together while at the same time sufficiently elastic to permit movement. Sometimes they're a little too stretchable; the ligaments that lash ankle to leg have the unfortunate habit of stretching and then staying that way, like taffy. It can take ten or more days for the ligaments to shrink and become normal-acting fibers again. In the meantime, your ankle hurts like hell.

To speed healing and ease pain, here's what experts advise.

Let it rest. You can't expect an injured joint to heal if you keep banging on it. At the same time, you want to do everything you can to prevent swelling and keep pain under control. For maximum relief, experts recommend the tried-and-true procedure known as RICE—rest, ice, compression and elevation. We cover this treatment in the chapter on sports injuries (page 62). But here's how it works, specifically for the ankles.

Proper Ankle-Wrapping Technique

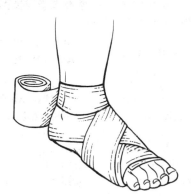

Start at the base of the toes and use a figure-eight pattern around the ankle and the arch, overlapping three-quarters of the bandage with each pass.

Rest. An injured ankle needs time to heal. Your job is to provide it. Staying off a sprained ankle as much as possible for at least 24 hours, even using crutches if necessary, is the best way to help it heal.

Ice. Applying cold, with either a cold pack or ice wrapped in a washcloth or towel, can help prevent swelling while helping to ease the pain. Apply cold where it hurts the most or where swelling is greatest. Leave it on for 20 minutes, remove it for 20 minutes, then repeat. After a few applications, you can cut back to once every hour or so, says physical therapist William Case, owner of Case Physical Therapy in Houston.

Compression. Wrapping your ankle with an elastic bandage will also help keep swelling under control. Starting at the base of your toes (leaving your toes exposed), wrap the bandage upward toward your ankle. Use a figure-eight

The Lowdown on High-Tops

Despite conventional wisdom and the relentless marketing efforts of athletic-shoe manufacturers, high-top basketball shoes don't protect your ankles from sprains any better than low-tops do. That's the conclusion reached by physicians at the University of Oklahoma in Norman who spent one season recording ankle injuries among 622 intramural basketball players.

In the study, each participant was given a pair of low-tops, a pair of standard high-tops or a pair of high-tops with pump-up chambers to wear during each game.

Ankle injuries were dispersed among the shoe types: seven in high-tops, four in low-tops and four in pump-up high-tops. "It's probably better for people to wear whatever shoes they are comfortable in rather than feeling they have to wear high-tops," says researcher James R. Barrett, M.D., lead author of the study.

pattern around your ankle and the arch of your foot, overlapping three-quarters of the width of the bandage with each wrap around your foot. You want the bandage to be firm but not so tight that it interferes with circulation.

Elevation. This is the fun part. Raising your foot—on pillows, the arm of a couch or anything else—will help keep swelling down. Make sure your ankle is higher than your heart. Keep the remote control within reach. And a good book.

Experts advise following these steps until the swelling goes down and the pain diminishes, up to two days. If there's no improvement by then, check with your doctor.

Other tips:

Pedal to strength. It's not smart to run right after an ankle injury, but you can strengthen the joint by using a stationary bike. "The bike is a good way to strengthen your ankle without putting a lot of weight on it," Case says.

Set the tension between minimum and medium. Pedal for 5 minutes, twice a day. After a few days, start working up to 10 minutes, three times a day. Eventually, you can be doing 15 to 20 minutes at a stretch. Bicycling not only strengthens the ankle but also provides a decent aerobic workout.

Take some relief. One of the most effective ways to reduce inflammation and ease pain is to take aspirin or ibuprofen, says Scott Haldeman, M.D., Ph.D., D.C., associate clinical professor of neurology at the University of California, Irvine, and adjunct professor in the research department at the Los Angeles Chiropractic College. To reduce stomach upset, experts often advise taking buffered or coated aspirin. Or your doctor may recommend a prescription anti-inflammatory drug instead.

Anus

- **Keep your stool soft through diet and drink.**
- **Keep it clean and dry.**

It's the butt of a lot of wisecracks. Yet in the end, the anus often has the last laugh.

Because no matter if it's swollen, sore, bleeding or itching, an irritated anus can disrupt your sleep, dampen your social life and generally demoralize you.

"You have to be nice to your anus; otherwise, it will bring you down. It will start to itch and could cause an unpleasant odor or pain. So there are a lot of reasons to keep your anus happy," says gastroenterologist Robert Charm, M.D., assistant clinical professor of medicine at the University of California, Davis, School of Medicine.

Keeping It Happy

When you defecate, your abdominal walls contract and push feces out of the rectum, a solid waste storage tank at the end of the colon, and into a 1½-inch-long canal called the anus. Here rings of muscle called the anal sphincters relax and allow the excrement to pass out of your body. Then the sphincters clamp shut until you need to defecate again. How long that will be varies from man to man. For some, it will be a matter of hours. Others may not feel the urge for three or four days.

Because the anus is such a simple structure, it seldom causes problems if it is kept clean and dry. "The anus will generally take care of itself if it isn't abused by overstraining, overstretching or excessive wiping," says Eugene S. Sullivan, M.D., a colon and rectal surgeon in Portland, Oregon.

But those are the exact things that many American men do. Why? The typical American diet is one big reason. A lot of us still eat highly refined, low-fiber foods that form small, dry, hard stools. These stonelike feces are difficult to expel and require an extra amount of straining that can stretch or even tear the sphincter walls as they pass through. And because the residue of a hard stool is harder to remove from your bottom, you might wipe too vigorously and further irritate the anus.

"The perfect stool is big, bulky and soft. It comes out easily, so the area isn't overworked and you don't have to do a lot of wiping," Dr. Charm says. "The key is diet. If you put the right products in your mouth, you'll get the right waste products on the other end. It's that

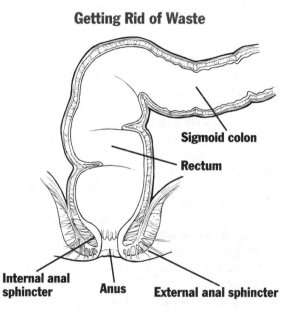

Getting Rid of Waste

Internal anal sphincter

Sigmoid colon

Rectum

Anus

External anal sphincter

Drinking lots of water and eating plenty of fiber makes defecating easier and puts less wear and tear on your plumbing.

simple." Here are a few dietary changes that can help you form Dr. Charm's vision of the perfect stool.

Drink, drink, drink. Water and fruit juices help soften your stool so that it can slip out of your body without a lot of straining. Drink the equivalent of six to eight eight-ounce glasses of water a day, Dr. Charm suggests.

Have a fiber feast. Your anus is less likely to become a troublemaker if you eat

plenty of fiber, an undigestible substance found in fruits, vegetables and plant foods that helps keep your stool soft and fluffy. Doctors recommend eating about 25 grams of fiber a day, but most American men consume between 15 and 20 grams a day. Try to eat at least six servings of grains, such as breads, rice and pastas, and at least five servings of fruits, vegetables and beans a day, Dr. Charm says.

Grind it up. Large chunks of hard, fibrous foods such as seeds and nuts that aren't fully digested can cut and tear the anus as they leave the body. So chew your foods well, Dr. Sullivan says.

What Can Go Wrong

See your doctor if you have tarlike, black or rust-colored stools, if you bleed between bowel movements or if you feel a lump around your anus. If your bottom does revolt, it's more than likely that one of a couple of minor culprits is to blame.

Hemorrhoids: A Swell Scourge

Hemorrhoids aren't subtle. They don't just swell, they balloon. They don't just itch, they grate. They don't just ache, they torture.

"All patients worry about hemorrhoids. It seems like every complaint they have about their anuses they attribute to hemorrhoids," says David E. Beck, M.D., chairman of the Department of Colon and Rectal Surgery at the Ochsner Medical Clinic in New Orleans.

Although plenty of other ailments, including fissures (cracks in the skin surrounding the anus), cysts, abscesses, polyps and sexually transmitted diseases, can cause discomfort, hemorrhoids are one of the most common anal problems.

Located just inside the anus, hemorrhoids are a group of blood vessels that normally form a tight seal and help prevent stool, gas and mucus from leaking out of the rectum. If one of these vessels becomes swollen or slumps out of its normal position—often from intense straining to pass a hard stool during a bowel movement—it can begin to itch, hurt or bleed.

Here are some things you can do to prevent or treat hemorrhoids.

Don't make the bathroom your library. The toilet is great for disposing of waste, but it isn't the best seat for reading books, magazines or newspapers. Prolonged stretches on an open toilet seat can strain anal muscles and make you more vulnerable to hemorrhoids, Dr. Beck says. If you insist on reading, put the toilet lid down, so your rear end has more support.

Pacify it with a potion. Soak a cloth with equal parts glycerin and witch hazel, then apply it to the hemorrhoids for about an hour, Dr. Sullivan suggests. He cautions that this is for external use only. The glycerin will absorb water and reduce swelling, and the witch hazel, a mild antiseptic and astringent, will soothe the surrounding skin. Both products are available over the counter in most drugstores. "For acute hemorrhoids, this glycerin–witch hazel pack is certainly as good as anything you can get over the counter," Dr. Sullivan says.

Chill out. If your hemorrhoid symptoms are severe, ice can sometimes relieve them, Dr. Beck says. Put some crushed ice into a plastic freezer bag, wrap the bag in a towel and apply it to the area for 10 to 15 minutes.

Dunk it. Fill a tub with just enough warm water to cover your buttocks (about three to four inches), then soak in it for 10 to 15 minutes. This should help thoroughly clean your bottom and soothe any hemorrhoids, says Gerard Guillory, M.D., a Denver internist and author of *IBS: A Doctor's Plan for Chronic Digestive Troubles.* If possible, do this two or three times a day in water that is very warm but not painfully hot to your hand.

Pruritus Ani:
An Itch That's Hard to Scratch

No itch is harder or more embarrassing to scratch. But for many men, an itchy bottom is an all-too-frequent nemesis.

Men are four times more likely than women to have *pruritus ani*, the medical term for an itchy anus, according to Dr. Sullivan. The underlying cause can often be elusive. Hemor-

rhoids, pinworms, fissures, anal warts and fungal infections are likely suspects. But improving your toilet habits and cutting back on certain foods and beverages might be all that is necessary to eliminate the problem, says Dr. Sullivan. Here's how.

Hit the head first. If you feel the urge to have a bowel movement in the morning, don't hold it in until after you've bathed. Instead, go to the bathroom first, then carefully rinse your anal area with warm water as you shower, Dr. Guillory suggests.

Rinse but don't lather. When showering or bathing, avoid rubbing soap in the anal canal, Dr. Sullivan says. Soap is highly alkaline, and its residues can get trapped in the folds of the skin and cause irritation.

Avoid the fancy stuff. Scented or perfumed toilet paper can irritate the skin and cause itching. Stick to soft, plain two-ply rolls, Dr. Charm says.

Use a wet wipe. After a bowel movement, use a wet cotton ball or facial tissue to thoroughly clean the area, Dr. Sullivan says. Then pat, don't rub, the area dry with a piece of toilet paper. Rubbing will only irritate the skin and make the itching worse.

If the itching is worse just after a bowel movement, try using a bulb syringe to cleanse the area with three to four ounces of warm water, Dr. Sullivan says. Again, be sure to pat the area dry.

Try absorbing trouble. Sticking a thin piece of gauze or cotton against the anus can help absorb irritating sweat and mucus, Dr. Sullivan says. The gauze can be lightly dusted with cornstarch or baby powder to improve its absorbency.

Watch what you eat. Spicy foods such as salsa and curry, citrus fruits such as oranges and tangerines and beverages such as milk, coffee, beer and other alcoholic drinks can all cause secretions from the anus that trigger itching, Dr. Sullivan says. If you suspect that one of these foods is causing you trouble, eliminate it from your diet, and your scratching may quickly end.

▼Appendix

- **Know where it is.**
- **Don't be in denial if abdominal pain hits.**

Jutting off the end of your large intestine like an overfed worm, the appendix—at least in adults—serves about as much purpose as a lawn mower in the desert.

"The appendix seems to be a totally purposeless organ," says John Schaffner, M.D., director of clinical gastroenterology at Chicago's Rush-Presbyterian-St. Luke's Medical Center. "Why it's there we still have no clue."

Some doctors, however, aren't as quick to write off this curious appendage. They speculate that the appendix might have an important role in developing protection against disease. According to this theory, the appendix slowly loses its role in the immune system as we mature so that by early adulthood, it is just an insignificant cul-de-sac along the digestive highway.

When Trouble Strikes

A narrow tube usually three to six inches long, the appendix can easily get clogged with hardened bits of fecal matter. Once it is clogged, fluids no longer have an escape route. Pressure builds up, bacteria invade, and the appendix becomes infected. Left untreated, it can eventually swell up and burst.

Some rare cases of appendicitis have been triggered by accidental swallowings of coins, nails and other objects, but the cause is usually untraceable and unstoppable. "There really is nothing that can be done to prevent appendicitis,"

says Alex Aslan, M.D., a staff physician with Northbay Health Care Services and Fairfield Medical Group in Fairfield, California. "It simply appears to strike out of the blue."

So managing appendicitis boils down to recognizing its onset, getting to the doctor and having your appendix surgically removed before it bursts.

While an infected appendix is little more than painful, a ruptured appendix can cause all sorts of trouble. When the appendix bursts, you instantly become a candidate for peritonitis, an inflammation of the membrane that lines the abdominal cavity.

As a general rule, you have roughly 12 to 48 hours between the onset of appendicitis and rupture. But this time frame can vary dramatically depending on how bad the infection is, so it behooves you to see a doctor as soon as you begin experiencing symptoms.

In almost all appendicitis cases, there's pain. At first, it may be vague and mild and spread across the abdomen. But typically, the pain increases and localizes above your appendix, on the lower right side between your navel and hipbone. Other symptoms may include fever, nausea, vomiting and diarrhea.

When pain localizes, it's time to see your doctor. If the pain suddenly lessens, you need to see a doctor even faster. This can be a sign that the appendix has ruptured. You have several hours, according to Dr. Aslan, before your condition becomes critical.

In most cases, treatment of appendicitis is a routine procedure. Doctors remove the offending culprit via surgery, and you go about your business good as new, minus a few inches of faulty plumbing. A standard appendectomy will have you in the hospital for one to two days and back to work within ten days.

Where Appendix Pain Might Be Felt

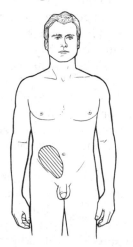

📺 Arteries

- **Check your cholesterol.**
- **Reduce saturated fat.**
- **Stay in shape.**

We often think of New York City's subway system as a model of bustling, complex efficiency, if not exactly the best in sanitation. Compared to your circulatory system, however, it's about as intricate as a driveway. Consider: The subway has about 230 miles of track. In contrast, your blood vessels cover about 60,000 miles. That's the equivalent of about 24 round-trip train rides between New York City and Los Angeles.

Despite its astonishing complexity, your circulatory system has a simple task: moving blood. It does this very well. In one minute, more than 5 quarts of blood flow through your various vessels, from the vast interstates near your heart to the tiny lanes that lead to each cell. If you happen to be exercising, the volume of blood flow can increase to more than 25 quarts. Per minute.

There's a reason for this high-power efficiency. Blood is responsible for moving various molecules—hormones, oxygen, nutrients, antibodies and so forth—from one part of your body to another. (For more on blood, see page 104.) That's why anything that interferes with blood flow, such as cholesterol buildup in the arteries or a drifting blood clot, can be so dire.

In fact, if you were a gambling man wagering on what will trigger your death, you'd be wise to put most of your chips on damaged arteries, particularly if you are over age 40. Heart disease is by far the number one killer of men, with stroke close behind at number three (cancer is in between). Either is caused by damaged or clogged arteries in many cases.

This is why doctors are so hung up on how much fat you eat and how much exercise

you get: Both are directly related to the health of your arteries. We'll be looking at a few of the ways you can keep your arteries clear and flowing. In the meantime, here's a quick look at what goes on beneath the surface—and what can go wrong.

Straight from the Heart

It's no exaggeration: Your arteries are your lifeline. Powered by the heart and the pulsing of their own muscular walls, they propel blood away from the heart (after it has been enriched with oxygen in the lungs) to tissues in every part of your body, from the tip of your toes to the farthest corner of your cranium. In case you have to get through a biology class someday, here's a tip: The *A* in artery stands for "away."

We often think of arteries as being enormous conduits, like water mains. Indeed, arteries near the heart are nearly large enough that you could slip a small finger into them. As you move farther away from the heart and closer to the individual cells, the arteries get progressively smaller. By the time blood reaches the arterioles, the tiny vessels leading to the capillaries that feed the cells, the inside diameter is less than 0.3 millimeter.

Once blood is used by the cells, it's returned to the heart and lungs via the veins for restocking. Then the whole cycle starts again.

Given the critical importance of reliable blood flow, it's not surprising that arteries are designed to maximize movement and minimize friction. The inside surface of an artery is glazed with a slick lining called the tunica intima, which enables blood to slide smoothly past.

Over time, however, this pearl-like lining begins to roughen. Experts aren't always sure what causes this to occur. A high level of cholesterol almost certainly plays a role, says Malcolm Perry, M.D., professor of surgery at the University of Texas Southwestern Medical Center at Dallas Southwestern Medical School. Circulating toxins, such as compounds in cigarette smoke, may also cause damage. So can the pounding turbulence caused by high blood pressure. For some men, it's simply that a roll of the genetic dice came up craps and passed on the tendency to develop arterial disease.

"Once a break in the lining happens, a whole cascade of events occurs," explains Edward S. Cooper, M.D., professor emeritus of medicine at the University of Pennsylvania School of Medicine in Philadelphia. For example:

- As soon as damage occurs inside an artery, disklike blood components called platelets rush to make repairs.
- A roughened lining becomes a natural magnet for drifting fat molecules. Like lint, they hang up on the coarse surface. As more and more fat accumulates, it gradually compresses into a dense goo called plaque, which begins to block the inside of the artery. This is what doctors refer to as atherosclerosis.
- As more and more plaque accumulates, it becomes harder for blood to pass through the increasingly narrow channel. At the same time, it's difficult for nutrients to penetrate the thick layer of goo. Artery muscle cells die, and inelastic scar tissue takes their place. This is called hardening of the arteries, or arteriosclerosis.

When atherosclerosis becomes this severe, you'll want to make sure your life insurance policy is paid up. It's a life-threatening situation. Not only is the artery clogged, but it doesn't have the flexibility to expand when it needs to. And as if that weren't enough to worry about, a blood clot may be just around the corner, says Dr. Cooper.

- Eventually, the artery gets so congested that blood can scarcely move. Stagnant blood tends to clot, and a clot tends to drift downstream and jam its way into a narrower artery. This can happen anywhere but is most likely to occur in the coronary arteries that

Cholesterol: The Good, the Bad and the Not So Ugly

A couple of years back, many of us got the message that cholesterol is bad. So we cut down on it. Then we found out that some of it is okay. So we got confused. Here's a quick primer.

Our bodies produce many types of fat, including cholesterol. This waxy goo is needed to make cell membranes, vitamin D and certain hormones. Some cholesterol is produced by the liver, and some comes from the foods we eat, such as meats and dairy products. Too much cholesterol can lead to heart disease.

Being a fat, cholesterol floats, like oil on water. In order for it to float through your bloodstream, it needs a coating of protein. This coating is called lipoprotein.

One type of lipoprotein, called high-density lipoprotein, or HDL, is good for you. Like dental floss for the arteries, it helps remove plaque. Getting exercise and plenty of vitamin C–rich fruits and vegetables, such as oranges and broccoli, will help boost your level of HDL.

The other kind of coating, low-density lipoprotein, or LDL, is bad for you. Eating foods high in saturated fat increases your body's production of LDL.

To remember which is which, here's another primer: H (as in HDL) is for healthy; L (as in LDL) is for lethal.

The American Heart Association and the National Cholesterol Education Program recommend keeping your total cholesterol level below 200 milligrams per deciliter of blood. More specifically, your HDL level should be above 45 milligrams per deciliter, and your LDL level should be below 130 milligrams per deciliter.

If you haven't already done so, ask your doctor to check your total and HDL cholesterol levels. You should get this test done every three years up to age 40 and every two years after that. More frequent tests may be needed if your total cholesterol is too high. A test of your LDL level can give an even better picture of your risk of heart disease and requires fasting for about 12 hours. The results could put you on the right track—for life.

serve the heart, the carotid arteries to the brain or the femoral arteries to the lower legs, says Dr. Perry.

   • A clot that stops blood flow to the heart causes coronary artery disease and perhaps a heart attack. A clogged carotid artery can lead to a stroke. Even if blood isn't stopped entirely, the reduced flow can cause problems, says Dr. Perry. Angina pectoris, a recurring pain in the chest, occurs when the heart muscle gets some, but not quite enough, blood and oxygen. Angina is not a heart attack. But it certainly is a wake-up call of the highest order.

Restoring Flow

   We tend to think of heart attacks and blocked arteries as happening mainly to beer-guzzling, stogie-sucking, out-of-shape guys who have had remote controls surgically attached to their thumbs. There's no question that lifestyle factors play a huge role. But we're all at risk.

   "The process begins in childhood. Even adolescents have fatty streaks forming on their arteries," says JoAnn E. Manson, M.D., associate professor of medicine at Harvard Medical School and co-director of women's health at Brigham and Women's Hospital in Boston.

   Yet there is increasing evidence that the damage can be prevented or even reversed by making relatively simple changes in diet and lifestyle. "Heart attack and stroke are the most common causes of sudden death, next to trauma," says Dr. Perry. So the changes are well worth making. Here's what experts advise.

   Cut back on fat. This is the big one. The average American gets about 35 percent of calories from fat, and about one-third of that amount is the saturated kind—the kind most likely to raise your cholesterol. In addition, a high-fat diet causes men to put on weight, which is another leading risk factor for heart disease. (For a full discussion of the different types of fat and how they affect you, see page 2.)

   The American Heart Association recommends a diet limited to 30 percent (or less) of calories from fat. That's not hard to accomplish, says Dr. Cooper, but it does

require some simple changes. For example: Have no more than one six-ounce serving (or two three-ounce servings) of meat, fish or poultry a day. Limit red meat to two or three servings a week. Eat plenty of fiber-rich foods, such as vegetables, fruits and whole grains. Chances are that after a few months of following this regimen, your blood cholesterol level will drop substantially, says Dr. Cooper.

   Be a teetotaler. Whether black, green or an Asian strain called oolong, tea can help

The Stages of Artery Disease

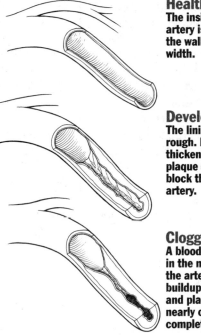

Healthy
The inside surface of the artery is smooth, and the walls are a normal width.

Developing
The lining of the artery is rough. Deposits of fat thicken the walls, turn to plaque and start to block the inside of the artery.

Clogged
A blood clot is jammed in the narrow opening of the artery. Increased buildup of fatty deposits and plaque on the walls nearly closes the artery completely.

keep your arteries unclogged. "Tea, though not the herbal variety, can play a role in protecting the body against damage to the arteries," says A. Venket Rao, Ph.D., professor in the Department of Nutritional Sciences at the University of Toronto.

   Green and black teas contain antioxidant compounds also found in fruits and vegetables. What these antioxidants do is help neutralize free radicals, harmful active oxygen molecules that can damage and cause buildup on blood vessel walls. Dr. Rao found that men who drank six cups of tea a day for two weeks had significant reductions in these harmful molecules. That may be a lot of tea for most of us, but, says Dr. Rao, "every little sip helps."

Take a hard line. Although most men can control cholesterol with simple changes in diet, others need more help. A few experts—among them Dean Ornish, M.D., president and director of the Preventive Medicine Research Institute in Sausalito, California—recommend a strict vegetarian diet with very little fat.

In fact, studies by Dr. Ornish have shown that a super low fat diet, when combined with exercise, giving up cigarettes and reducing stress, not only lowers cholesterol but also may reverse existing blockages in the arteries.

Eat well. A huge amount of research has shown that a diet high in antioxidant nutrients—vitamins C and E and beta-carotene—can help keep arteries healthy.

"There have been decades of studies showing the protective effects that eating vegetables has on the arteries," says Dr. Perry. Most experts agree that there's nothing wrong with taking supplements. But whenever possible, he adds, it's best to get nutrients in their "natural" state from fresh fruits and vegetables.

Citrus fruits such as oranges and grapefruit and vegetables such as broccoli are great sources of vitamin C. You can get vitamin E from wheat germ, hazelnuts and whole-grain cereals as well as from corn oil, soybean oil and other oils. Fruits, dark green, leafy vegetables such as spinach and kale and yellow and orange vegetables such as sweet potatoes, carrots and squash are high in beta-carotene.

Here's another benefit of dark, leafy greens: They contain a B vitamin called folate (the supplement form is called folic acid), which lowers the level of an amino acid called homocysteine. "People with high homocysteine levels can sometimes have as much as an eight-fold increase in the risk of coronary disease," says Paul N. Hopkins, M.D., associate professor of internal medicine at the University of Utah School of Medicine in Salt Lake City.

Cook some protection. For years, natural healers and folklorists have sworn by

the healing powers of garlic. Scientists are starting to agree. Research led by Yu-Yan Yeh, Ph.D., professor of nutrition at Pennsylvania State University in University Park, has shown that taking garlic—either as a deodorized capsule or fresh, in its most odoriferous form—can help keep cholesterol levels down. In his study, Dr. Yeh found that men who took nine garlic capsules a day were able to lower their LDL cholesterol (the bad kind) by 10 percent. Fresh garlic will produce the same results, although your social life may suffer.

Quit smoking. Now. Smoking accelerates hardening of the arteries, adds to the likelihood that you'll have high blood pressure and lowers your level of HDL cholesterol (the good kind). In addition, there may be particles in smoke that cause the blood to clot more readily. "Smoking is turning out to be even more important in causing heart disease than we thought 20 or 30 years ago," says Dr. Cooper.

Almost as soon as you quit smoking, you'll start to see the benefits, adds Dr. Manson. Your blood pressure, for example, will drop almost immediately. And after three to five years without smoking, your risk of arterial disease will be reduced to the level of a person who has never smoked, she says.

Tone up your arteries. Exercise is good for your heart, your head, your lungs, your muscles, your skeleton—and your arteries. "The good effects of exercise go even beyond the factors we can measure, such as blood pressure, LDL, body weight and diabetes," says Dr. Cooper. "Exactly how it improves the health of arteries, beyond the control of risk factors, is still being studied, but improved anticlotting factors and greater elasticity of artery walls are some possibilities."

You don't have to be a gym rat to get the benefits of exercise. Even taking a quick walk 20 minutes a day can make a major difference, experts say.

Go ahead—have an egg. Eggs have long gotten clobbered because of their high cholesterol content. There's now a crack in the research, and a sunny side has emerged for egg-lovers. Some experts say that for healthy men who have normal cholesterol and are eating low-fat diets, having an egg daily isn't going to send their arteries into coronary care. If your cholesterol is elevated, however, limit eggs to no more than three per week, says Dr. Cooper.

Beyond Home Care

It would be nice to report that every man can keep his arteries healthy by eating well and getting regular exercise. To be sure, all men can benefit from these things. But sometimes more is needed.

Some men, for example, have a genetic tendency to manufacture huge amounts of cholesterol, and diet and exercise won't stop it. Their arteries would quickly clog up without cholesterol-lowering medication. But prescription drugs such as lovastatin (Mevacor), cholestyramine (Questran) and niacin (Nicolar) can lower cholesterol—and with it, coronary artery disease—to a more manageable level, says Dr. Cooper.

The same is true of conditions such as high blood pressure and angina pectoris. Exercise and diet help, but often the only real "cure" is medication, says Dr. Perry. In fact, he adds, blood pressure drugs are among the most prescribed medications in the country today. Surgical procedures such as coronary bypass and angioplasty are options when the other steps are not enough, says Dr. Cooper.

Another condition that can be tricky to treat is intermittent claudication. *Claudication* comes from a Latin word meaning "to limp"; people who have intermittent claudication often stop to rest their aching calves. The pain comes from narrowed, clogged-up arteries in the legs, and surgery is sometimes the treatment of choice.

Here's the good news. "There have been several good studies showing that people with this condition get better with exercise therapy than they do with procedures to clean out their arteries," says Dr. Perry. More often, a good diet, exercise and no tobacco will eliminate the need for any procedure, he says. "If only we could get people to do these things."

Back

- **Stretch it.**
- **Strengthen it.**
- **Watch your posture.**
- **Be realistic; pain is all but inevitable.**

Have bad backs changed the course of history? Maybe. There are those who believe that the murderous disposition of Russia's Ivan the Terrible may have had something to do with his twisted spine. Likewise, intense back pain may or may not have affected the way John F. Kennedy made presidential decisions; we can only speculate. (Marilyn Monroe, following a private meeting with the president at the White House, was reported to have remarked, "I think I made his back feel better.") And who can predict how life as we know it would be different if back trouble hadn't forced basketball great Larry Bird into early retirement in 1992.

Back pain is one of life's most common ailments. Virtually every man will have it at some point. Besides colds and sore throats, back pain is the single most common condition that doctors treat. It's estimated that on any given day, between 15 and 20 percent of the U.S. population is suffering from back problems.

With odds like these, you might think that anyone with a backache may as well look for a bell tower to hide out in. But the opposite is the case. There's plenty of reason for back pain sufferers to be optimistic. A comprehensive study of back pain conducted for the Public Health Service by the Agency for Health Care Policy and Research in Rockville, Maryland, revealed an extraordinary statistic: Nine in ten people with lower back problems, which are by far the most common type, recover within one month or less. The same study found that only 1 in 200 cases of back pain has a serious cause, such as an infection or a tumor. We now know, too, that the chronic, debilitating back pain so many of us fear affects only about 5 percent of all of those who experience back pain and that many of the most common and debilitating treatments for back pain—extended bed rest, painkilling drugs, surgery—can actually make patients worse rather than better.

New Thinking about Backs

Not surprisingly, doctors have begun to conclude that when it comes to back pain, perhaps they've overreacted. "If you look at it historically, back pain wasn't considered a major medical problem until after World War II," says David Imrie, M.D., who designed a back pain prevention program used by the National Safety Council. "The reason for this may be that the surgical procedure for ruptured disks wasn't developed until 1932. So how did people manage for thousands of years before that? You start to look at this and say 'Hey, maybe we have to rethink the whole problem.'"

And that's just what is occurring now. Doctors are realizing that less is more when it comes to back pain treatment: less bed rest, less medication, less surgery. Whether you're suffering already or hoping not to suffer, doctors now believe the same rule applies: Take care of your back, and your back will take care of you. We'll get to just how that's done in a minute. But first, it will help to have a basic understanding of the remarkable system we're talking about when we talk about the back.

Strong and Flexible

"A stack of tin cans separated by jelly doughnuts." That's how Augustus A. White

III, M.D., professor of orthopaedic surgery at Harvard Medical School and director of the Spine Fellowship Program at Beth Israel Hospital in Boston, describes the basic structure of the back.

The tin cans he's talking about are the vertebrae that make up what we think of as the backbone. There are 24 of these hollow, cylindrical bones stacked one on top of the other, each attached to the one above it and the one below it by little joints. (The sacrum and the coccyx, or tailbone, are also made up of vertebrae, but these are fused together rather than connected by joints.) Each vertebra has an opening behind its body to allow the spinal cord to run through it. Major nerves branch off

---

Backbreaking Labor

What jobs are most often associated with back pain? Here are the top four contenders, according to Augustus A. White III, M.D., professor of orthopaedic surgery at Harvard Medical School and director of the Spine Fellowship Program at Beth Israel Hospital in Boston.

1. Drivers. Trucks, vans, buses, cabs: They all vibrate, and they all require that the driver be seated. That's a double whammy for back pain. A person who spends at least half of his job time driving a motor vehicle is three times more likely than the average worker to suffer a herniated disk, Dr. White says. Any other job that subjects a worker to constant vibration (jackhammer operators, listen up) also puts him on the endangered species list.

2. Heavy lifters. Any job that requires lifting, pulling or carrying can lead to back pain. And that doesn't apply only to you guys who drive moving vans and delivery trucks. Nurses, nurse's aides and farm workers tote their share of barges and lift their share of bales, too.

3. Firemen, policemen and emergency medical technicians. They don't necessarily lift things as often as deliverymen, but they are sometimes called upon to lift things quickly and in awkward positions. That's a prescription for back injury.

4. Desk jockeys. You guys who sit at word processors or who talk on the phone all day are putting pressure on the disks between your vertebrae. *Sitting* is one of the operative words here; *all day* are the others.

the spinal cord through openings in the vertebrae and out into the limbs. (For more on the spinal cord, see page 307.)

The jelly doughnuts separating the vertebrae are the disks. Each disk is a tough little bundle of fibers and cartilage, with a jellylike center. The disks are shock absorbers. They keep the vertebrae from grinding against one another, and they help cushion the spine against the pounding forces of a body in motion. Another way the body cushions itself is with the spine's curves, which give the back a springlike resilience.

The miracle of the back is that it serves two vital yet contradictory purposes so well. It has to be strong to protect the spinal cord from injury yet flexible so that the body can turn, bend, sit and lean at will. A complex set of muscles, tendons and ligaments makes that myriad combination of movements possible. Those same muscles, tendons and ligaments also help hold up the spine, much as guy wires hold up a radio tower.

Understanding Back Pain

With such a complicated tangle of tissue and bone wrapped around something as sensitive as nerves, it's hardly surprising that things go wrong in the back system. Spinal joints are as subject to wear and tear as the joints in your knees, hips and shoulders. Back muscles can cramp; back ligaments can get inflamed; back tendons can get strained. Disks can dry out and rupture or swell up and get pinched between vertebrae.

According to Scott Haldeman, M.D., Ph.D., D.C., associate clinical professor of neurology at the University of California, Irvine, and adjunct professor in the research department at the Los Angeles Chiropractic College, back pain appears most often in the lower back because as the body's halfway point, the lower back is a sort of fulcrum for a lot of the pressures that can lead to pain. Contrary to popular belief, ruptured (or herniated) disks probably aren't responsible for more than a small proportion of back pain. Muscle strain

may be the most likely culprit, although exactly what is producing back pain at any given moment is usually a mystery. In fact, doctors are unable to pinpoint the specific cause of back pain in as many as 85 percent of the cases they treat, says Richard Deyo, M.D., an internist at the University of Washington in Seattle and one of the chief investigators for the Public Health Service study.

One unusual study showed just how tricky back pain diagnosis can be. Researchers performed magnetic resonance imaging scans on 98 people. Two-thirds of those people were found to have some type of disk abnormality, and more than one-third had abnormalities in two or more disks. The twist? None of the people tested had reported having any back pain whatsoever.

Dr. Haldeman believes that the mistake we may have been making with back pain all of these years is assuming that there's something abnormal about having it. "It seems that we have back pain simply because we live on this earth," he says. "The longer you're alive, the more strenuously you work, the more bumps, bruises and injuries you sustain, the more likely you are to have back pain. For about 90 percent of the population, back pain appears to be just part of the aches and pains of living."

You may not be able to eliminate those pains from your life entirely, but there are plenty of steps you can take to minimize them. Read on.

How to Avoid Back Pain

Maybe we don't think about keeping our backs in shape because when we look in the mirror, we don't see them—you know, out of sight, out of mind. Or perhaps we think they're just bones. But our backs need the same sort of overall toning and maintenance that we regularly devote to other key parts of our bodies. "The back is a stepchild," says David Lehrman, M.D., co-director of the Spine Center at Miami Heart Institute in Miami Beach. "We're aware of our knees, our lungs, our hearts; we tend to address exercises to those parts of our bodies quite readily. We assume our backs will come along for the ride."

Without question, taking care of your back before you develop back pain is worth the effort. Statistics show that once you've had an episode of back pain, you're seven to eight times more likely to have a repeat episode than people who haven't had back pain. Here are some basic principles to think about when it comes to keeping your back healthy and happy.

Make conditioning critical. Staying in good overall shape is the first step in avoiding back pain. The various muscles, ligaments and joints in the back benefit enormously from good aerobic exercise, according to Dr. White. Low-impact activities such as swimming, cycling and walking improve circulation and build overall muscle strength and flexibility.

If you're not already in the habit of working out, Dr. White recommends gradually building up to a point where you're working out at your own pace for 30 to 45 minutes, three to five times a week. For walking, a brisk pace would be four miles per hour. That means you'll cover two to three miles per session.

Support your support systems. When it comes to your back, good overall conditioning is a start, but it's not the whole story. "Good fitness by itself does not

Mind over Back

It's remarkable how often people who work on back for a living end up talking about heads. Doctors are convinced that stress and attitude play big roles in lots of health problems, but in back pain more than most.

"Research shows that people with negative mental attitudes or social situations demonstrate markedly diminished tolerance for the aches and pains of everyday life," says Scott Haldeman, M.D., Ph.D., D.C., associate clinical professor of neurology at the University of California, Irvine, and adjunct professor in the research department at the Los Angeles Chiropractic College. "People who are happy tolerate back pain. People who are unhappy don't."

This doesn't mean that back pain is all in our heads. It does mean that our mental attitudes can affect how we experience the pain and perhaps even contribute to it. Dr. Haldeman points out that people who are under stress have tense muscles, which makes those muscles more vulnerable to strain. Research also indicates that stress causes the disks to absorb moisture, thus putting pressure on other structures of the spine.

Stress has a tendency to go to different parts of the body in different people, says Roger Nelson, Ph.D., professor of physical therapy in the College of Allied Health Sciences at Thomas Jefferson University in Philadelphia. "Not everyone gets ulcers," he explains. "Some people get heart trouble, some get headaches, and some get backaches. Stress can express itself in the back."

Given this head-back relationship, it stands to reason that a little work on the former might help the latter. Lauren Schwartz, Ph.D., a clinical psychologist at the University of Washington in Seattle, works in a pain clinic where stress management is a major part of the treatment. "We try to help our patients figure out what they can and can't control in their lives," she says. "You can learn how to change the way you think: Sometimes we can change the amount of stress we experience by changing how we interpret situations."

A positive mental attitude is also important in learning to believe that back pain can be overcome, according to Ted Wernimont, rehabilitation coordinator for the Spine Diagnostic and Treatment Center at the University of Iowa Hospitals and Clinics in Iowa City. "The people who tend to get better aren't the ones who sit back and say 'Fix me,'" Wernimont says. "The people who get better are the ones who say 'I'm going to beat this thing.'"

necessarily confer good fitness for the spine," says Jeffrey Young, M.D., assistant professor of physical medicine and rehabilitation at Northwestern University Medical School and an attending physician at the Center for Spine, Sports and Occupational Rehabilitation, both in Chicago. "We see plenty of people with back pain who can bench-press 300 pounds or run five-minute miles."

The problem, Dr. Young says, is that as well-conditioned as these athletes are, they have neglected the muscles that provide crucial support for the spine. The most important of these, he says, are in the abdomen and the butt. Paying special attention to keeping these muscles fit will help your back hold up under the load it carries every day. (See page 364 for abdominal exercises and page 368 for butt exercises.)

Watch your technique. Some sports that are great exercise when done right can hurt your back when done wrong. Take swimming, which is generally considered one of the most back-friendly sports there is. Dr. Young warns that a faulty breathing technique can create back problems. To breathe the right way, logroll your entire body to reach the water's surface with your mouth rather than craning your neck or lifting your entire head out of the water for air. Back problems can also result from bad form on golf swings, bowling approaches and tennis serves. Ask a coach to watch your style or take a few refresher lessons.

Alternative Back Treatments

A smorgasbord of alternatives is available for the treatment of lower back pain. Some sound exotic, even strange; others are ancient, natural, intuitively appealing.

As with ice and heat, there's no solid proof that any of these treatments actually works. Nonetheless, many physicians don't object to their patients trying them, especially when more conventional treatments aren't working.

"These therapies aren't the first line of thinking for us," says Jeffrey Young, M.D., assistant professor of physical medicine and rehabilitation at Northwestern University Medical School and an attending physician at the Center for Spine, Sports and Occupational Rehabilitation, both in Chicago. "But for pain modification for some patients, they definitely have benefits. What you have to remember is that the farther you go from the medical mainstream, the more your treatment will be hit or miss. That's why it's best to have a referral rather than just going someplace in a mall that has a sign out saying 'Massage Here.'"

One way to gauge a prospective therapist's credibility, Dr. Young adds, is to ask if he is willing to discuss your treatment with your regular doctor. If you're told that won't be necessary, consider another option.

Here are snapshots of a few alternative remedies for backache, from the book *New Choices in Natural Healing.* If you're interested in any, you'll need to search out experts or manuals in the particular healing method.

Acupressure. Pressing a few particular points behind your knees is said to open energy pathways in the back, so the pain can flow out.

Aromatherapy. A massage oil of blue chamomile, birch, lavender and other ingredients is said to ease the pain.

Hydrotherapy. Alternating hot and cold showers (one to four minutes of hot spray on the back followed by a cold spray for 5 to 30 seconds), repeated as often as hourly, could ease back pain.

Juice therapy. Drinking a cup of room-temperature fresh grape juice daily, apart from meals, supposedly is effective in reducing back pain.

Stay limber. The more limber you are, the less likely you are to strain your back. "If you don't have a great deal of flexibility and you try to move to another position, you'll put a lot of strain on the soft tissues of your back, such as the ligaments, and that's what leads to back pain," says Malcolm Pope, Dr.Med.Sc., Ph.D., director of the Spine Research Center at the University of Iowa in Iowa City.

Generally, men are less limber than women, says Judith Lasater, Ph.D., a physical therapist in San Francisco and author of *Relax and Renew: Restful Yoga for Stressful Times.* This is because men tend to favor exercise that develops muscle mass rather than flexibility. One way to increase flexibility is to do yoga. Dr. Lasater says that yoga and other stretching exercises can help you literally reset the length of your muscle fibers so that you can stretch them farther without injury.

Warm up. Sudden activity can cause sudden back pain. That's a warning to weekend warriors in particular: Sitting at a desk all week long and then rushing out onto the tennis court first thing Saturday morning is a setup for back strain. The same goes for guys who are active at work, says Dr. Pope. He recommends that any man whose job is physically demanding start the day with some stretching exercises. "You wouldn't dream of going out to play sports without stretching," he says. "So why would you go to work in a warehouse without stretching?"

Warm up gently with three to five minutes of easygoing exercise, such as walking. You'll know you're ready to stretch when you begin to sweat. Dr. Young suggests you concentrate in particular on stretching the hamstring muscles in your upper thighs. Strong, tight hamstrings can pull on the pelvis and fight the muscle systems that support the back, possibly to the point where these muscle systems irritate low-level back pain problems that you might not have noticed otherwise.

Snub cigarettes. A number of studies show what Dr. Haldeman calls "a clear and definite statistical correlation between smoking and back pain." Why exactly that is, we don't know, he says. It may be that smoking reduces circulation to the disks and other parts of the back, or it could be that people who smoke tend to be out of shape in general. In any event, if you have a cigarette in your mouth, the odds say you're courting back trouble.

Stay trim. Carrying a lot of extra weight in your belly puts stress on your spine. Over the course of a day, that stress adds up. "Take two ten-pound bags of sugar, put them under your shirt and walk around with them for an hour. Then see how your back feels," says Roger Nelson, Ph.D., professor of physical therapy in the College of Allied Health Sciences at Thomas Jefferson University in Philadelphia.

Stand Tall, Sit Pretty

As Merle Haggard says, Mama tried. When we were kids, every so often in the supermarket or at the dinner table Mom would all of a sudden give us a whack between the shoulder blades. "Stand up straight!" she'd say. "Your posture is atrocious!"

Well, many of us didn't listen, and it'll be hard to change now. There's little evidence that adults will change postural habits acquired over a lifetime, says Dr. Haldeman. Once a sloucher, always a sloucher, apparently. But don't despair. Slumping at the dinner table doesn't necessarily mean you'll get a backache.

"The position of the body is more of an aesthetic consideration than anything else," says Dr. White. "Drooping shoulders and a slouch may look bad, but there are no data to support the contention that posture has anything to do with back pain."

Nonetheless, many doctors still believe that you can help keep back trouble at bay by

How to Sit

To minimize back strain, sit so that your buttocks point to where the seat and backrest meet. Consider a pillow for the small of your back if you're on a straight-back chair. Sit comfortably erect. Feet should be flat on the floor.

watching the way you sit, stand and move, especially on the job. "You can reduce the fatigability of your back during your work activities," Dr. Haldeman says. Since fatigued muscles are more prone to injury, he explains, one way to prevent back pain is to avoid the sort of strain that tires out your muscles. Here are some good ways to accomplish this goal.

Sit right. If you're a computer jockey who spends your day roaming the Internet, sitting is serious business. In his book *Sitting on the Job: A Practical Survival Guide for People Who Earn Their Living while Sitting*, Scott Donkin, D.C., a chiropractor in Lincoln, Nebraska, explains how to develop a healthy relationship with your chair.

If you don't have a chair that's adjustable, consider investing in one, Dr. Donkin says. The seat and the backrest should fit the specific contours of your back and hips. You should sit so that your buttocks are aimed at the point where the seat and backrest meet. If you must sit in a straight-back chair, a back support pillow that fits between the small of your back and the chair can help provide support for your lower spine. The goal is to sit comfortably erect. Armrests help decrease the load on your back and shoulders.

The height of the seat should allow you to plant your feet firmly on the floor or on a footrest. Position your chair so that you face your computer (or whatever you're looking at) square on, without keeping your neck crimped either up or down. If your chair can't be raised or lowered to fit your desk, perhaps your desk can be raised or lowered to fit your chair.

Also, try to avoid awkwardly reaching for things. Repeatedly twisting your back and shoulders increases back strain.

Drive right, fly right. You can apply many of the above suggestions for sitting at work to driving in a car or flying in an airplane. Your seat should give your lower back good support, Dr. White says. If it doesn't, put a small pillow or a rolled-up towel at the small of your back. Slightly shifting your weight around in your seat may help. And don't sit too long

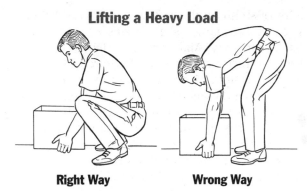

Lifting a Heavy Load

Right Way　　Wrong Way

without taking a stretch break.

If you're buying a new car, Dr. White recommends getting one with cruise control. It will give you more freedom to change positions on long drives.

Take a break. Many doctors believe back pain is the cumulative result of a lot of strains so minor that you don't notice them until it's too late. Relieving those tiny tensions with frequent breaks can prevent that accumulated strain, says Chris Grant, Ph.D., a research fellow with the Center for Ergonomics at the University of Michigan in Ann Arbor. Research has shown that short breaks of a minute or less can be as effective as longer ones, she says.

At the least, try not to sit for more than 20 minutes without standing and stretching. "Sitting in one place for a long time cuts off nutrition to your disks," says Dr. Pope. Breaking up your workday by mixing up the tasks you have to do is another effective way of avoiding the repetitive strain that can quietly undermine your back.

Stand tall. Taking frequent breaks is just as important if you work standing up. In addition, Dr. White recommends getting a stool about six inches high, so you can stand with one leg raised about six inches off the floor. Every so often, switch the stool to your other foot.

Lift right. There are at least three good ways to wreck your back while moving a box of stuff. The easiest is to bend from your waist to pick up the box. Always bend at your knees, keeping your back as vertical as possible, so

Carrying a Heavy Load

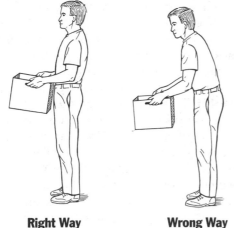

Right Way   **Wrong Way**

your leg muscles handle the heavy lifting, according to Dr. White.

The second easiest way is to hold the box out in front of you, away from your body. That puts a lot of strain right on the vulnerable muscles in your lower back. Always keep the load you're lifting as close to your body as possible, says Dr. White.

The third quickest route to back pain from lifting is to twist your torso while holding something heavy. Even empty-handed torso twisting has been known to hurt backs. According to Dr. White, orthopedists got plenty of extra business during the twist dance craze of the early 1960s.

Stay inside the beltway. There's no proof that those back support belts worn by movers, stockpeople and weight lifters do their backs any good, according to the National Institute for Occupational Safety and Health. Dr. Pope, however, believes the belts may have some benefit as a sort of early-warning device, reminding people who wear them to be conscious of the stress they're putting on their backs.

Pack right. The heaviest lifting a lot of guys do is slinging garment bags over their shoulders on the way into the airport. That is why it's worth thinking of your back when you buy luggage, according to Alfred Davis, Jr.,

D.C., a chiropractor in Montclair, New Jersey.

Dr. Davis says a rolling carry-on bag is better for your back than a garment bag, provided the handle is extendable, so you don't have to lean over as you pull. He also recommends a thin bag rather than a fat one. "A wide bag forces you to extend your arm out, away from your body," he says. "That's very bad for your lower spine."

Sleep right. As far as your spine is concerned, the best sleeping posture is on your back or on your side, according to Dr. Donkin. Sleeping on your stomach exaggerates the curve of your lower back and keeps your neck twisted. Use a pillow that keeps your neck in straight alignment with the rest of your spine.

When it comes to mattresses, Dr. Donkin says, go firm, young man, go firm. Remember, however, that the key to a good mattress is support, not hardness. It's the quality of the inner spring that really matters.

Beating Back Pain

If, despite your best efforts, you do get back pain, don't blame yourself. Although the preventive measures we've described can help, they can't guarantee you won't be among the millions who wake up one morning with a backache. "There's nothing that we know of,

Sleeping Posture

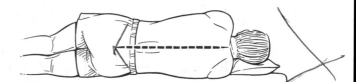

Right Way: Proper pillow height and a firm mattress help keep your spine straight while you sleep.

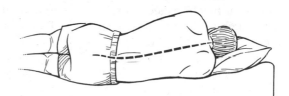

Wrong Way: Any mattress or sleeping position that has your spine curve can lead to back pain or injury.

other than death, that absolutely prevents back pain," says Stanley Bigos, M.D., an orthopedic surgeon at the University of Washington and chairman of the Public Health Service's back pain study.

The first step in treating acute (meaning temporary) back pain is to not panic. "Most backaches are like the common cold," says Dr. Deyo. "They don't require medical care. Except in unusual circumstances, they can be taken care of at home. The main problem is getting through the symptoms early on."

Here's how that is done.

Stop. If pain starts while you're in the midst of some activity, says Dr. Deyo, the first step is to stop what you're doing. Continuing the activity could further inflame the problem, he says, and exacerbate the pain.

Take aspirin. Aspirin, acetaminophen and ibuprofen are all effective tools for reducing moderate back pain, according to Dr. White. Follow the dosage suggested on the bottle by the manufacturer or take as your physician advises. In the past, doctors had often prescribed muscle relaxants, opiate-based painkillers and antidepressants for lower back pain. The Public Health Service's study of lower back pain discourages using any of them.

Take it easy, but not too easy. Something else that doctors had routinely prescribed for back pain was lots of bed rest. That has changed, too. According to Dr. Deyo, studies have found that bed rest for more than four days actually interferes with recovery. Why? Because the longer you stay in bed, the weaker your muscles become, including the muscles

that support your back. You're also more apt to get depressed, and studies have found that attitude can have a distinct impact on your recovery from pain.

Doctors now believe the best way to get over back pain is to return gradually but promptly to your normal activity. Two days of bed rest, Dr. Deyo says, is usually plenty.

Cool it, heat it. Although there's no proof that using ice or heat treatments actually works, many doctors think both can help ease pain. Ice is recommended for immediate relief, because cold reduces inflammation. Wrap some ice cubes or some frozen vegetables in a towel and apply the towel to the sore spot for 20 minutes, then break for at least 20 minutes. Continue this cycle for the first two hours after

Chiropractors: No More Great Debate

For many years, ranked high on the list of the world's great feuds—just below the Hatfields and McCoys—was the grudge match between chiropractors and medical doctors. Lately, though, their relationship has improved significantly. More and more doctors are referring patients with mild back pain to chiropractors, and some prestigious orthopedic clinics have even added chiropractors to their staffs.

Perhaps the biggest breakthrough for chiropractic credibility came when a major study conducted for the Public Health Service by the Agency for Health Care Policy and Research in Rockville, Maryland, concluded that spinal manipulation—which is what chiropractors mainly do—is an effective short-term treatment for lower back pain.

"That report was an acknowledgment that in the eyes of the medical and scientific communities, the research on spinal manipulation is now sufficient to justify use of this treatment," says Scott Haldeman, M.D., Ph.D., D.C., associate clinical professor of neurology at the University of California, Irvine, and adjunct professor in the research department at the Los Angeles Chiropractic College.

The Public Health Service panel defined short-term treatment as one month. According to Dr. Haldeman, who sat on the panel, that's not a hard and fast rule. Some people may see improvement within one or two visits, he says, at which point they can discontinue treatment. Others may be

the onset of pain. Then cut back the applications to 8 to 10 minutes of every hour for the next 24 to 48 hours. After 48 hours, an electric heating pad or a hot-water bottle may help reduce muscle pain and spasms, but be careful not to fall asleep on it and burn your skin.

Crack your back. Several studies have shown that spinal manipulation—having a vertebra or a joint realigned using a sharp thrust—can provide some short-term relief from lower back pain. Although most people get their backs cracked by chiropractors, osteopathic physicians and some physical therapists are trained to do it as well.

If you do decide to seek spinal manipulation, be aware that having numerous x-rays,

magnetic resonance imaging scans and other diagnostic tests isn't necessary. Dr. Haldeman feels a single set of x-rays prior to the start of spinal manipulation makes sense. Taking a new set every three to six months, he says, is excessive.

Also be leery of letting just anyone manipulate your neck. In the wrong hands, that can lead to serious injury, warns Dr. Haldeman.

What to Do about Chronic Pain

Chronic back pain has been defined as pain that interferes with your activities for more than three months. Not many of us would want to put up with it for nearly that long without seeing a doctor—nor should we, in the opinion of Dr. Lehrman. "Personally, I wouldn't wait longer than three to four weeks," he says.

"Use your judgment," recommends Willibald Nagler, M.D., physiatrist-in-chief (a physiatrist is a physician with special training in physical medicine and rehabilitation) at the New York Hospital–Cornell Medical Center in New York City. "If the pain is not from an obvious source, such as a basketball game you played the day before, you should think about seeing a doctor, at least the first time the pain occurs. Get a line on what's happening."

Back pain that goes away but keeps returning is one good reason to seek professional advice. "If you have a repetitive complaint, something has to be done," Dr. Lehrman says. "There's a pattern somewhere in your life that needs to be addressed; somebody has to do some detective work. Chronic pain is a loud signal that you're doing something wrong."

feeling better after a month and want to continue treatment slightly longer. "The point is to set a general boundary that amounts to short-term treatment, rather than indefinite treatment," he says.

Just what is spinal manipulation anyway? Basically, you lie or sit on a table while your chiropractor (or your osteopath or physical therapist) uses his hands to push on or apply a vigorous thrust to one joint or a group of related joints in your back. In layman's terms, you're getting your back cracked; the chiropractor calls it an adjustment. The idea is that joints and vertebrae can get out of line or locked in one position and that manipulation can restore them.

No one is sure just why spinal manipulation works, and some doctors believe its value is as much psychological as physical. Whatever the reason, the real goal, according to Roger Nelson, Ph.D., professor of physical therapy in the College of Allied Health Sciences at Thomas Jefferson University in Philadelphia, should be to get away from the need for spinal manipulation—or any other treatment. "Spinal manipulation is similar to an aspirin," he says. "You take an aspirin to get rid of a headache, but what's the source of the pain? Once you have spinal manipulation, you need to go to work to find what caused your pain in the first place. You want to avoid losing the flexibility you've just gained, so you don't have to go back."

The danger of ignoring such a signal, Dr. Lehrman adds, is that injuries to the back can build on themselves, causing a deconditioning that can lead to greater vulnerability as time goes on. "You have to find a way to intervene to keep this from continuously happening," he says. "If you don't step in and do something, then you will continue to have problems."

There are some danger signals that call for consultation with a doctor sooner rather than later. One such signal, says Dr. Haldeman, is pain so severe that you can't get out of bed. Dr. Haldeman also recommends promptly seeking professional care if you're having pain that radiates into your legs, especially if your legs are weak or numb. You should also call your doctor if your symptoms include fever, stomach cramps, weight loss, chest pain or difficulty breathing. Loss of bowel or bladder control requires immediate attention: This symptom could indicate nerve damage, a progressive infection or disease or even a severely herniated disk.

If you'd like to see a doctor about your back pain but you're not sure what sort of doctor to see, Dr. White suggests that you start with your primary care physician or internist (a physician who specializes in the diagnosis and treatment of diseases, particularly of the internal organs, in adults). Depending on the indications, he may refer you to a rheumatologist (a joint specialist), an orthopedist (a bone specialist), a physiatrist or a neurologist. If the problem is unrelated to severe disease or neurological injury, a chiropractor may be worth a try.

Beard

- **Soften it.**
- **Shave slowly.**
- **Go with the grain.**

If you were a lumberjack, you might be jealous of razors: A razor fells 16,000 stumps in just a couple of minutes.

But you probably aren't a lumberjack, and you probably have no great awe or respect for the razor. If you're like most of us, you dread it. Shaving is something most of us do on automatic pilot. Sometimes we hit a little turbulence.

There's not much science to the science of facial hair. It grows. The characteristics of your facial hair depend on your genetics. Some guys are hairy beasts; some guys can barely raise a shake of pepper. (For details on how hair grows, see the chapters on body hair, page 109, and hair, page 170.) What we are going to concentrate on here is what probably matters to you most: how to shave well, and how to make facial hair look good.

Does it matter what kind of razor you use? *Consumer Reports* says it does. The magazine found that cartridge razors outperform disposables across the board. But they are more expensive, and they're used by less than half of all shavers.

Five Steps to a Perfect Shave

Sure, in the old days, the barber did the job. But barbers are a dying breed, and you aren't going to wait at a barber shop every morning for a shave. We know you better than that.

So get with the program. Memorize these five steps, recommended by the experts at the Gillette Company, and you'll do as good a job as any barber—if not better.

Soften up. Soften your beard. A barber would wrap steaming towels around your face for a couple of minutes. Not necessary. Just take a steaming shower first. Wash your face in the shower to remove oil and dirt and sebum, which block pores and keep your beard from absorbing water. Then when you get out, splash your face with warm water and lather on a favorite shaving cream or gel to hold in the heat and moisture. Some men like to shave in the shower; steam-resistant shower mirrors are available for them (and for narcissists). If you're not showering first, soak your face in hot, soapy water for two minutes before lathering. Two minutes seems like too much time to spend? Compare that with three or four days of living with nicks, scratches and bloody blotches.

Wet hair offers much less resistance to the blade than dry stubble. Each of the 16,000 stubbly little hairs on your face would love to absorb up to one-third of its weight in water. Give it the opportunity. The warmer the water, the quicker it is absorbed. (Be sensible here; aim for a water temperature of about 125°F.)

A good reason to use a shaving gel or cream (instead of, say, bar soap) is that it contains lubricants to improve razor glide. We want the razor to glide rather than to grip and skip and skid.

Sharpen up. Start with a fresh blade and discard it at the first sign of pulling or tugging. The average guy can expect to get five shaves from a blade, but this varies with the thickness of the beard and how well it is prepared for shaving.

Get cheeky. Shave your cheeks first, then move to the sides of your face and neck. This gives tough areas, such as your chin and the area around your lips, more time to soften. Save them for last. Use slow, light, gentle strokes on your face, always going with the

An Ingrown Hair

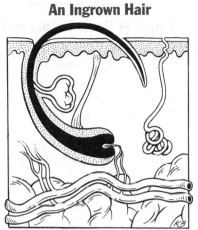

Some men with beards suffer from ingrown hairs. That's when the tip of a curly hair re-enters the skin. The result: pain, sometimes inflammation, sometimes infection.

grain of your beard. While your beard is dry, feel the direction that the hair on your neck grows; then shave in that direction. It varies some from man to man. Take your time and be particularly gentle around your Adam's apple.

Keep it clean. Rinse the blade frequently, flushing away beard and cream buildup on the cutting edge and in the cartridge.

Rinse off. When you're done, rinse your face and neck with cool water and pat dry. If you prefer a little fragrance, you can finish up with an aftershave, a balm or an alcohol-free shave splash. To avoid irritation, stay away from products that have a high alcohol content or are not formulated for use after shaving. Thoroughly rinse the blade and shake it dry. The experts at Gillette warn against wiping the blade, as this damages the shaving edge.

Cuts and Other Bad Strokes

Even the most experienced shaver slices himself now and then. It usually happens when we're in a hurry and is especially likely when using an old, clogged or rusty blade.

To stop bleeding immediately, use the old-fashioned styptic pencil, or firmly hold a small wad of tissue against the cut for a couple of minutes. It'll stick to the cut, so leave it there until you're ready to head out the door. Then moisten the paper with a few drops of water and slowly, gently peel it off your face, suggests Jerome Z. Litt, M.D., assistant clinical professor of dermatology at Case Western Reserve University School of Medicine in Cleveland.

A few bits of not-so-common wisdom from Dr. Litt:

• Skip shaving just before exercising. Sweat irritates freshly scraped skin.

• Don't loan or borrow a razor. Razors can spread herpes, warts and impetigo (a rather ugly skin disease).

Another common "side effect" of shaving is pseudo-folliculitis barbae—razor bumps to us. Generally, these sensitive bumps indicate inflammation caused by the razor-sharpened tips of curly whiskers arcing back into the skin and growing inward. (That's why this condition is especially common among African-American men and other men with curly hair.) Once the hairs grow back into the skin, they're attacked by the body's natural defenses just as any foreign body is, setting the stage for painful inflammation and possible infection, says Dr. Litt. To avoid ingrown hairs and razor bumps:

• Use the right razor. Dr. Litt suggests using a disposable single-track razor.
• Don't shave in more than one direction in any given area. If you do, Dr. Litt says, you're cutting it too close.
• Don't shave against the grain. True, cutting against the grain gives a closer shave, but it irritates the skin and encourages development of ingrown hairs.
• Don't stretch your skin taut while scraping it with the blade. That's likely to cut the beard hairs below the skin surface, increasing the likelihood of ingrown hairs.

If razor bumps develop, lay off shaving for at least a few days, advises Dr. Litt.

Which Is Best: Rotary or Foil?

Ouch. Some electric shavers grab hair and pull. Some buzz like floor sanders. Some are bulky and awkward. Some vibrate in your hand like massagers. But they all chop hair with one of two cutting patterns: circular or back and forth.

Circular cutters, which are found in rotary razors, feature spokelike blades on wheels that spin beneath round combs. Hairs captured in the combs are clipped by the spinning blades. Brands such as Norelco and Remington feature this design. You move a rotary razor in a circular motion on your face.

Shavers with back-and-forth cutters covered by screens of perforated foil are known as foil razors. Hairs are caught in the perforations and sliced off by the rapid movement of the blades rocking back and forth. A foil razor is used with up-and-down strokes.

Which works best? Back in 1989, *Consumer Reports* reported that the difference between the best of both types was a close shave—too close to call. It was strictly a matter of preference.

But competing manufacturers have continued to increase cutting power, hone designs and add features. And in the fall of 1995, the *Consumer Reports* panel of testers expressed a distinct fondness for two particular Norelco rotary models, though they also found one Braun foil model and one Panasonic foil model to be acceptable runners-up. We're sure that shaver technology will continue marching forward and that this is not the last word.

Buzz It Off

Some men—about one in four, according to *Consumer Reports*—prefer electric razors. The companies that manufacture them insist that you get your best electric shave if you forgo the wet shave altogether and use electric exclusively. "Beard hair growth adjusts to the method of shaving," says Ron Sinclair, product manager for Norelco shavers. "It takes about three weeks to adjust." Shave with an electric exclusively, he says, and your facial hair begins to stand up straighter and the shaver trims hair closer, so your face looks smoother.

For electric shaving, your face must be

A Guide to Beard Styles

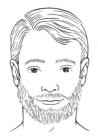

Full beard and mustache: best for narrow faces.

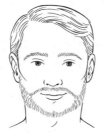

Lean beard and mustache (clean cheeks and lower lip): best for round faces.

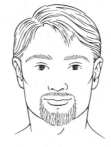

Goatee and mustache: best for round or square faces.

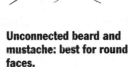

Unconnected beard and mustache: best for round faces.

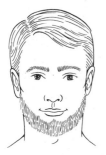

Full beard, no mustache: best for narrow faces.

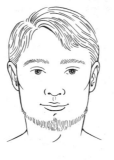

Lean beard, no mustache or sideburns: best for square faces.

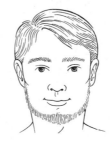

Lean beard, no mustache: best for square faces.

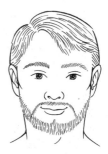

Standard beard and mustache: best for oval faces.

dry and your beard stiff. To set up your beard and improve razor glide, use a preshave lotion or liquid.

While experts are at odds on this, some recommend that you alternate with or switch to an electric razor if blade shaving irritates your skin. Some men find electric razors irritating, certain models more so than others.

And despite the manufacturers' recommendation that you do only one or the other, many men who blade-shave in the morning carry rechargeable electric razors in their cars or attachés for quick touch-ups before important encounters late in the day.

Norelco is the industry leader, but Remington, Braun and Panasonic are significant players. Periodically, *Consumer Reports* rates the various products. If you're considering a purchase, you might check for their latest assessments. Electric shavers aren't cheap: Expect to pay anywhere from $20 to more than $100 for cordless, rechargeable models. The shavers come in two styles: rotary and foil— that is, round head and rectangular head—and each works differently.

Sprout a Beard

Not everyone, of course, feels the need to shave. But ancient cave drawings tell us that even early man went clean-faced some 60,000 years ago, reports Jonathan Zizmor, M.D., in the book *The Complete Guide to Grooming Products for Men*. Ancient Egyptians shaved with bronze knives. Romans ground off their beards with pumice stones. Still, in many cultures, a beard is thought to impart an air of wisdom to its wearer.

Shaving became common among Anglo-

Saxons in the seventh century A.D., according to *The Columbia Encyclopedia*. The beard, though, makes a regular comeback and has been an acceptable American alternative since the 1960s.

A beard makes moot the many problems with shaving and can dramatically change a man's appearance. Plus it can have a cosmetic effect: Since a beard covers the bottom half of the face, it focuses more attention on the top half and on the eyes, notes Lia Schorr in her book *Lia Schorr's Skin Care Guide for Men*. A wide, short beard strengthens a thin, long face. An Abe Lincoln jawline beard overcomes a weak chin, she says.

Growing a beard isn't freedom from shaving and grooming; a beard needs daily cleaning and regular trimming and shaping. Even with a stylish full beard, you still need to shave your neck and perhaps portions of your cheeks.

Wash your beard daily while shampooing your scalp. Moisturize the skin beneath with a skin moisturizer or conditioner (such as Phyto 7, available in salons and specialty stores), suggests Christina Griffasi, head of the styling department at Minardi Salon in New York City.

Most beards and mustaches need twice-weekly trimming. A beard is trimmed dry; for best results, comb and untangle it first. Electric beard trimmers, such as those made by Wahl and other companies, make the job easy, says Griffasi. They look like barber clippers, but they are smaller and come with attachments that control the length of the cut. Home barber clippers can also be used, though they are somewhat bulky and thus more difficult to maneuver.

Wahl's instructions advise first redefining the lines at the edges of your beard. At the end of the trim, you'll need to clean up the lines by shaving along them. Beard trimmers don't cut close enough to give you a clean shave.

Then using the length attachment provided, mow the sides of your beard, holding the trimmer lightly and mowing a trimmer-width row at a time, from bottom to top. The instructions advise starting with a longer than desired length and working your way down.

Take It Off, Take It All Off

Removing a beard can be either a bloody mess or a smooth job done in minimal time. It's up to you. We'll tell you how to do it smoothly.

First, if you possibly can, do it on a Friday night. This gives your face a couple of days to recover before you have to shave again, suggests Griffassi. The skin is tender under there, brother; it does not welcome the blade.

Also, make sure you have a fresh razor or razor blade. Don't even attempt this with an old blade.

Start by mowing off all of the beard hair you can with a beard trimmer or barber clippers or cutting it off with scissors, suggests Griffassi. Next, hop in a steamy-hot shower and moisten your beard and face for at least five minutes. While your beard is still wet, coat it with lots of shaving gel or cream and let it soften up for a few minutes. Then with the fresh blade, shave slowly and carefully, rinsing the razor thoroughly between each stroke, says Larry Christman, owner of Larry Christman's Hair Center in Whitehall, Pennsylvania. If you need more cream or water, by all means apply it, says Christman. Don't shave any spot more than once. Shave only in the direction that your beard grows.

Finish by patting your face with a towel and applying a nonallergenic moisturizer, advises Dr. Litt. If you're heading outdoors, Dr. Litt offers a word of caution: Wait at least a half-hour after you shave to apply the moisturizer; otherwise, it could sting. Then give your face a few days' rest from the blade. By Monday, your face should be over its shock and ready to meet Mr. Razor again.

◼ Belly Button

It's an enduring reminder of where life begins. Yet few men think much about the belly button until that rare moment when a midwife hands over the scissors to cut a newborn child's umbilical cord.

For most of us, the navel is just a glorified lint trap. But the belly button—doctors call it the umbilicus—is actually a scar formed when the stub of the umbilical cord falls off, usually a couple of weeks after birth. A thick cord filled with lots of robust blood vessels is more likely than a thin cord to leave a small protrusion (an outie) when it falls off.

Newborn infants sometimes get belly button hernias; this rarely happens in adult men. Bacterial infection can be more of a problem when you get older. You can eliminate that risk if you scoop out any debris and wash your navel with soap and warm water every couple of days.

"The risk of infection isn't very great. But if you don't wash, material can get impacted there and form a smelly, disagreeable mass," says Albert M. Kligman, M.D., Ph.D., professor of dermatology at the University of Pennsylvania School of Medicine and an attending physician at the Hospital of the University of Pennsylvania, both in Philadelphia. This is especially true for disadvantaged individuals unable to care for themselves, says Dr. Kligman. And no, it's not a knot, so you can't untie it and peek at your stomach.

More commonly, men are getting their belly buttons pierced as a fashion statement. Piercing is particularly popular among men ages 18 to 25, but it is not as appealing to guys in their thirties or above, says Bill Krebs, owner of Pleasurable Piercings in Hawthorne, New Jersey. A dermatologist or cosmetic surgeon can eliminate a piercing hole if you tire of it, but the procedure gets more involved the longer the hole is in place.

◼ Birthmarks

He helped end the Cold War and oversaw the collapse of the Soviet empire. But what most of us remember about Mikhail Gorbachev is that weird purplish blotch on his forehead. Life, we all know, is not fair.

What Gorbachev, the last president of the Soviet Union, really has is a birthmark called a port-wine stain.

Many of us are born with some type of birthmark, such as a tiny spot of discolored skin. It usually isn't very noticeable and often fades early in childhood. No one is sure why we get birthmarks, but they may be inherited, says Paul Lazar, M.D., a Highland Park, Illinois, dermatologist and co-author of *The Look You Like: Medical Answers to 400 Questions on Skin and Hair Care.*

Some birthmarks such as café au lait, a light brownish spot, are caused by excessive skin pigment. Vascular birthmarks like port-wine stains and strawberry marks are caused by the overgrowth of small blood vessels in the skin.

Strawberry marks can appear on any part of the body and grow rapidly in the first few months of life. They are red and soft and protrude from the skin. Nine in ten of these birthmarks disappear by age nine.

Port-wine stains are most common on the face and neck. Usually flat at birth, they can thicken and develop small bumps and ridges as a man gets older. Unlike strawberry marks, port-wine stains seldom fade away on their own.

Special corrective cosmetics such as Dermablend, which is available in many department stores, can help some men camouflage prominent birthmarks. For a lasting solution, however, see a dermatologist or plastic surgeon, who can recommend a treatment.

The two typical removal choices are incisional and laser surgery. Be aware that a scar may be left behind, even with the laser surgery, says Dr. Lazar.

◨ Bladder

- **Drink lots of water.**
- **Urinate often; don't hold it in.**
- **Monitor for sudden changes in urine color, force or frequency.**

In *A League of Their Own*, a sentimental film about a women's baseball league during World War II, Tom Hanks, portraying the team's drunken manager, staggers into the locker room and urinates into a toilet for nearly a minute as his female ballplayers watch in astonishment.

"Boy," one of the shocked women finally says. "That's some good peeing."

Good, but hardly extraordinary. Some men claim they can maintain a steady urine stream for more than two minutes. In fact, a typical man urinates for 15 to 20 seconds five to seven times a day.

No matter what you call these torrents—taking a leak, draining the main, pointing Percy at the porcelain—the driving force behind them is the bladder, a muscular, punching bag–shaped holding tank that seldom causes men trouble.

"For most men, the bladder is just there. It's something that we take for granted. About the only time we think about it is when the urge to go to the bathroom hits us," says Raju Thomas, M.D., professor of urology at Tulane University School of Medicine in New Orleans.

When Nature Calls

Urine is constantly dripping into the bladder from the kidneys. The flexible bladder walls gradually expand until the reservoir is full, usually at 6 to 16 ounces.

When you urinate, a couple of things happen. Nerve signals relayed back and forth between the bladder and the spinal cord relax the urethral sphincter, the ring of muscle that holds the urine in the bladder. At the same time, the main bladder muscles squeeze like a

fist and push the fluid through the sphincter and into the urethra, the tube that carries urine out of the body.

How much you pee varies daily. The amount can range from a pint to about two quarts, depending on how much you sweat, eat and drink (alcohol and coffee are diuretics that increase urine production). Because the kidneys ease up at night, urine production usually drops by about 25 percent when you're asleep. Weather also affects urination: Colder temperatures trigger more pit stops.

Bladder problems are far more likely to affect women than men. Drinking at least six to eight eight-ounce glasses of water a day and urinating when you feel the urge are the best ways to prevent bladder irritation, Dr. Thomas says.

Men can get into trouble, however, if they get in the habit of holding fluid in for too long, says Dr. Thomas. That increases your risk of developing bladder stones, painful clumps of mineral deposits that can obstruct or completely block urine flow. And if you're a smoker, holding out for longer than normal may expose your bladder to high concentrations of cancer-causing tobacco residues that are normally flushed out of your body in urine, he says.

Pushing your bladder to the edge of its capacity also stretches its lining and makes it more difficult for muscles to expel all of the urine. Any residual urine becomes a cesspool that is a breeding ground for infection-causing bacteria. But more often than not, a man who gets a bladder infection has a more serious underlying problem, such as a tumor or an enlarged prostate gland, says E. David Crawford, M.D., chairman of the Division of Urology at the University of Colorado Health Sciences Center and director of the Colorado Prostate Center, both in Denver.

See your doctor if you notice blood in your urine, a change in the frequency of your urination or slowness of your urine stream; if urinating is painful; or if you frequently feel an urgent need to go that isn't relieved by urinating.

Finally, there's the issue of wet spots on

Bashful Bladder:
Learn to Go with the Flow

A chronic inability to use public rest rooms when nature calls is more than just a personality quirk of a few shy men. About one in ten men occasionally comes up dry when trying to urinate in a strange place, says Joseph A. Himle, Ph.D., a lecturer in the anxiety disorders program at the University of Michigan Medical Center in Ann Arbor. A few of those have a more severe form of social phobia known as bashful bladder syndrome.

The disorder, which seems to run in families, varies in severity, ranging from merely needing to use a stall instead of a urinal to being unable to urinate anywhere except in the privacy of your own home.

"It has nothing to do with faulty plumbing, because these folks can urinate at home quite easily with a good, full stream. It's just when they get out into social situations, where others are present, that it becomes difficult," Dr. Himle says.

What happens is that something— maybe your boss walking up to the next urinal—makes you uneasy, and as a result, you involuntarily tense up the muscles that control the flow of urine out of your bladder. Then you get into a vicious circle: Because you're worried, you tense up and can't urinate. Because you can't urinate, you get more worried, and so on.

"It's not as if these men were gripped by terrible fear standing over the urinal. It's just that their anxiety interferes to enough of a degree that it doesn't work," Dr. Himle says.

To overcome bashful bladder, Dr. Himle recommends this: Set aside an hour to practice in a public rest room with multiple stalls and urinals, such as in an office tower, an airport or a hospital. Then load up on water and other beverages, and allow your bladder to fill to the point that you can barely stand it. (You need all of that fluid because you'll be urinating up to ten times in the next hour.) Start by urinating a small amount in a stall with the door closed. Then try stopping the flow in midstream, so your bladder is still fairly full. Take a two-minute break. Then urinate again, this time with the stall door open. Once again, stop the flow and take another break. Try to move progressively from the stall to a urinal with no one in the room, to a urinal several feet away from other people and, finally, to a urinal right next to someone else.

If you're still having problems after six attempts at this self-treatment, seek professional help, Dr. Himle suggests.

your pants. Some men have the problem of a small amount of urine trickling out onto their trousers or shorts after they think they are done urinating. For the most part, urine dribbling is a result of poor urination habits and/or weak muscles, not a bladder that has lost control (a more serious problem called incontinence).

Bad habits? Well, yes—things like not pulling your shorts far enough away when you urinate, so there's pressure on the urethra, blocking flow. The solution: Pull your pants far away from your penis, and don't try to urinate by pulling your penis over the top of your underwear. Also, when you're done urinating, apply gentle pressure behind your scrotum to coax out any remaining urine. This is where the widest part of the urethra is located and where urine could pool.

As for weak muscles, we are talking about the pelvic floor muscles through which the urethra passes. Kegel exercises can help give you far greater urinary control. Slowly and tightly squeeze the muscles that you normally use to stop the flow of urine, then release. Do three sets of five each and every day. As you get better, add repetitions to each set.

Blood

- **Get enough iron.**
- **Take your vitamins.**
- **Limit your alcohol intake.**

In Hollywood, they call the stuff that splatters on movie and television screens reel blood. Made of corn syrup, red dye and paste, it comes in a variety of shades, including fresh, aged and dried. A typical horror film may use more than 30 gallons of the stuff.

Movie blood may be a nifty special effect. But real blood, the sticky serum that life depends on, is far more awesome.

Consider these facts: Of the 50 to 60 trillion cells in your body, more than half of them are blood. Every second, two million red blood corpuscles are destroyed, and two million new ones enter the bloodstream and join a massive transportation system that is responsible for nurturing every cell in your body.

Yet these corpuscles are so tiny that they can squeeze through a capillary thinner than a strand of hair. And they're packed together so tightly that an average guy could drain all five quarts of his blood into an oil pan.

"Blood is truly amazing. It really is the essence of life," says Mercedes Brenneisen, M.D., a hematologist at Good Samaritan Hospital in Los Angeles.

How It Works

With each heartbeat, blood rushes life-sustaining oxygen to your cells and sweeps toxic carbon dioxide back to your lungs. At the same time, it helps warm your body and distributes hormones and chemicals that regulate every bodily function, from heart rate to erection. In addition, white blood cells and other disease-fighters that comprise your immune system diligently circulate in your bloodstream, ready to pounce on any invading organism that might harm you.

Every hour, your body is producing up to ten billion new blood cells in your bone marrow and destroying an equal number of old ones in your spleen or liver. Early in life, the spleen, the liver and almost any bone can produce red blood cells. After age two or three, only the skull, breastbone, ribs, spine, pelvis and thighbones continue to create red blood cells and platelets. White blood cells are also manufactured by the bone marrow, but some types are produced in the lymph nodes as well.

Keeping It Healthy

Blood is fairly resilient and requires little care or maintenance to do its job. Eating a balanced diet that includes at least five servings of fruits and vegetables a day is the best way to ensure that your blood stays healthy, Dr. Brenneisen says. Here are some other important things you can do.

Stoke up on iron. Without iron, your body stops making red blood cells, and the red cells you do have have difficulty absorbing oxygen as they pass through your lungs. As a result, you can develop anemia, Dr. Brenneisen says. Anemia is rare in otherwise healthy men; it's more of a female problem because of the blood loss during menstruation.

Most men need about ten milligrams of iron daily, which you can easily get by eating a well-balanced meal. Good sources of iron include lean meats, poultry (dark meat is best), clams, oysters, dried apricots and dark green, leafy vegetables such as spinach and broccoli. Avoid taking iron supplements without your doctor's consent, since too much iron can lead to a condition known as hemochromatosis, which can hurt the liver.

Recharge with B_{12}. A low level of vitamin B_{12} disrupts the reproduction of red blood cells and increases your risk of heart disease. But B_{12} deficiency is rare, because the vitamin is easily stored in our bodies, Dr. Brenneisen says. Vitamin B_{12} is found almost exclusively in animal products: fish, beef,

A Blood Test Primer

Like any great detective, your doctor is always looking for clues. Your blood is often a good starting point. Although normal results vary depending on your age, your sex and the method a laboratory uses to conduct its tests, a typical blood screening can reveal a lot about you. Here's a look at the most common blood tests.

Complete blood count. This is the most basic test. It determines the number and appearance of red cells, white cells and other components present in the blood. A complete blood count will also tell your doctor how much oxygen your blood cells can carry and how well they can fight disease.

Blood glucose (blood sugar). A high level of blood sugar could be a warning sign of diabetes.

Bilirubin. A high level of this pigment, which is released when old blood cells are destroyed, may be an indication of liver disease or anemia. Jaundice, a yellowing of the skin and eyes, is also caused by an excessive amount of bilirubin in the blood.

Creatinine and blood urea nitrogen. An elevated blood level of either of these two waste products, which are normally excreted in urine, may be an indication of a kidney ailment.

Potassium. A high level may be a sign of kidney failure.

Sodium. An excessive amount in the blood could be a sign of dehydration or congestive heart failure.

Chloride. A low level of this important chemical, which helps keep body fluids in balance, may point toward infection, intestinal obstruction or severe diabetes.

Carbon dioxide. A high level suggests a lung problem, such as emphysema or pneumonia.

don't store folate, we need a daily dose of at least 200 micrograms. One-half cup of legumes, such as lentils, can deliver nearly all of your day's folate requirement. Wheat germ, oranges and green vegetables such as asparagus are other good sources.

Get an E grade. Vitamin E, an antioxidant, may help protect membranes and keep aging blood cells vigorous, according to Stephen Shohet, M.D., professor of laboratory medicine at the University of California, San Francisco, School of Medicine. Vitamin E is most abundant in oils, nuts and seeds. Unfortunately, these foods are also high in fat. But taking a multivitamin/mineral supplement daily will usually supply you with enough vitamin E to maintain your health.

Don't forget the C. Vitamin C, another antioxidant, might also help keep your blood cells healthy, says Joanne Curran-Celentano, R.D., Ph.D., associate professor of nutrition at the University of New Hampshire in Durham. It's abundant in the diet as long as you eat plenty of fruits and vegetables, such as oranges, strawberries, brussels sprouts and red bell peppers, every day. Although 60 milligrams is the Daily Value, Dr. Curran-Celentano recommends that you get 100 to 500 milligrams daily for healthy blood.

poultry and dairy foods such as cheeses and yogurt. If you are a vegetarian, you should talk to your doctor about whether to take a supplement. Men should aim for two micrograms of B_{12} daily.

Think folate. Folate is another B vitamin that is crucial to the development of healthy red blood cells, Dr. Brenneisen says. Deficiency can cause fatigue, weakness, cramps, depression and other symptoms of anemia. Since we

Take an aspirin. Aspirin can reduce the stickiness of blood platelets and reduce your risk of stroke and heart attack. Take one 325-milligram coated aspirin tablet every other day, suggests Dr. Brenneisen.

Ax the smokes. Smoking increases the carbon monoxide level in your bloodstream and destroys hemoglobin, a protein that helps transport oxygen in the blood. Smoking also stimulates the production of extra red blood cells, which can thicken the blood and make you more vulnerable to a stroke or heart attack triggered by a clot, says Arthur R. Thompson, M.D., Ph.D., hematologist and professor of medicine at the University of Washington in Seattle.

Limit booze. Overindulging in alcohol can interfere with the absorption of folate. Consume no more than one or two drinks a day, Dr. Brenneisen says.

What Can Go Wrong

If you get sick, your blood probably isn't the culprit. "What's amazing is how well blood works and how uncommon diseases of the blood really are," says John Harlan, M.D., a hematologist at the University of Washington School of Medicine in Seattle. Here are diseases you should be aware of.

Anemia, a lack of red blood cells, is one

Transfusions and Blood Parts

If you ever need to receive a transfusion, your doctor will likely choose to give you the single blood component, such as platelets, red cells or plasma, that is the most vital to your survival.

"When you donate blood, 98 percent of the time we're going to separate it into components. That allows us to use our resources more efficiently. So instead of giving someone a unit of whole blood, we can use that same blood, broken down into its components, to help several people," says Liz Hall, a spokeswoman for the American Red Cross in Washington, D.C.

Here's a look at the different parts of blood and when they get used in transfusions.

Platelets are the smallest of the blood cells and live only nine days. They clump together and form blood clots that quickly stop bleeding. Platelets are often needed following chemotherapy for leukemia and other types of cancer because the treatment destroys the bone marrow cells that make them.

Red blood cells are the most numerous. They are essentially supertankers, hauling oxygen and carbon dioxide into and out of your lungs. Hemoglobin, an iron-rich protein that gives these cells their distinct color, is what red blood cells use to efficiently carry gases such as oxygen through your body.

Without hemoglobin, you would need 75 times more blood to do the same job.

A typical red blood cell travels more than

The Key Components of Blood

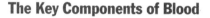

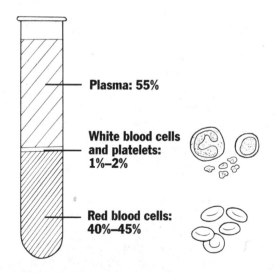

Plasma: 55%

White blood cells and platelets: 1%–2%

Red blood cells: 40%–45%

Your blood is primarily made up of four ingredients. Plasma is the main fluid and carries lots of essential chemicals. Red blood cells cart oxygen and carbon dioxide to and from your cells. Platelets form clots as needed for healing. White blood cells protect the body against infection.

of the most common blood diseases, affecting roughly 1 of every 500 American men. When you have it, your blood has trouble getting enough oxygen to your vital organs and removing carbon dioxide from your body. Symptoms include pale skin, fatigue, weakness, cramps, depression, fainting and heart palpitations. In extreme cases, an anemic man may eat or crave unusual things such as ice chips, newsprint or even clay. Anemia can be caused by deficiency of iron, vitamin B_{12} or folate.

Leukemia is a cancer of the blood-forming tissues—bone marrow, lymph nodes and spleen—that causes abnormal white blood cells to reproduce at an accelerated rate. These abnormal cells prevent the production of healthy red and white blood cells and platelets. As the disease progresses, it causes anemia, interferes with blood clotting and impairs the body's ability to fight off infection. Untreated, it can cause death. Leukemia afflicts about 1 of every 800 American men. Symptoms include chronic fatigue, bone pain, weight loss, easy

300 miles through your arteries and veins during its 120-day life. Red blood cells are needed by a person who is losing a lot of blood quickly because of trauma, such as a gunshot wound or an automobile accident.

Plasma is a straw-colored fluid containing water, sugars, proteins, vitamins, minerals and electrolytes such as sodium and potassium. (Electrolytes are important conduits for electrical and nerve impulses throughout your body.) Plasma makes up about 55 percent of blood.

Plasma helps people who have been burned or are in shock by increasing the amount of fluid and electrolytes in the bloodstream. Plasma also contains proteins that help in clotting, which is important for those who are losing large amounts of blood.

White blood cells protect the body against infection by destroying bacteria, viruses and other invading organisms. Some types of white blood cells can live for up to ten years. These cells are sometimes used in transfusions to boost the diminished infection-fighting capabilities of people with cancer.

Whole blood, like red blood cells, is transfused into people who have suffered traumatic injuries. It contains both red cells and plasma.

Donated blood is tested for infectious diseases such as hepatitis, syphilis and HIV, the virus that causes AIDS. If it tests positive for any, the donated blood is destroyed.

Healthy blood is usually separated into its components in a centrifuge. It's then refrigerated and stored in a hospital blood bank for up to 42 days. Despite rigorous safeguards, there is a minimal risk of getting a serious disease from an undetectable virus in donated blood.

"There is no such thing as sterilized blood. It can't be done, because if you sterilize it, it loses its life-giving capabilities," Hall says. "The Red Cross makes it as safe as possible by selecting healthy donors and testing them for disease."

Improved testing methods, however, have reduced the risk significantly. The odds of getting HIV from transfused blood, for example, have dropped from 1 in 2,500 to 1 in 420,000 in less than a decade.

If you will be undergoing surgery in the next six weeks and the type of surgery usually requires a limited number of blood transfusions, you can eliminate the risk of infection by receiving a transfusion of your own blood. Just arrange to donate blood prior to your surgery. The blood bank will reserve it for you, so it can be transfused back into you during the operation.

What Your Blood Type Really Means

In 1667, doctors attempted to transfuse sheep's blood into a young boy in an attempt to cure his sickness. The procedure didn't work, but fortunately, the patient lived.

Since that first miserable stab at a transfusion, doctors have learned that there are several types of blood and that if blood types aren't compatible, a person receiving a transfusion could have an immune reaction and die.

Blood is classified by the types of proteins that coat each red blood cell. Your blood type can be A, B, AB (meaning you have both A and B proteins) or O (meaning you have neither A nor B proteins). People develop antibodies to the proteins that their blood cells don't have. The following chart shows who can receive transfusions of what types of red blood cells:

If You Have ...	You Can Be Given ...			
	A	B	AB	O
A	√			√
B		√		√
AB	√	√	√	√
O				√

About 46 percent of people have type O blood, 42 percent have A, 8 percent have B, and 4 percent have AB.

Another blood grouping system, the rhesus (Rh) factor, divides people into Rh-positive and Rh-negative. About 85 percent of men are Rh-positive. Transfusion of Rh-positive blood into an Rh-negative person can cause a serious reaction if he has developed antibodies to Rh-positive blood from previous transfusions.

bruising and bleeding and fever.

Polycythemia is a condtion in which you have an unusually large number of red blood cells in your body. Sometimes, it's a good thing: When your tissues aren't getting enough oxygen because of a thin atmosphere, your body responds by creating more red blood cells. People who live in very high altitudes may always be polycythemic. However, in some cases, a genetic aberration can make a person polycythemic. Or, it could be a sign that an underlying ailment, such as lung or heart disease, is disrupting the flow of oxygen in your body. In response, the bone marrow produces more red blood cells than are needed. Because polycythemia thickens the blood, clots are more common, and that increases the risk of heart attack and stroke.

Malaria, caused by a parasite that's transmitted by a mosquito bite, is a common blood disease in tropical regions. The parasite attacks red blood cells, causing them to rupture. To prevent malaria, ask your doctor to prescribe an antimalarial drug before you travel to an area where the disease is prevalent. And while there, keep your skin covered with dull-colored clothing, wear insect repellent and use a bed net at night.

Hemophilia, a genetic bleeding disorder that prevents blood from clotting, afflicts 1 of every 10,000 men in the United States. It is almost exclusively a male disorder, passed on from women who carry the hemophilia gene to their sons. England's Queen Victoria was a famous carrier of the disease, and several of her royal descendants—including Alexis, the last crown prince of Russia—developed the affliction.

Sickle cell disease, an ailment that causes abnormal hemoglobin in 1 of every 1,000 African-Americans, is another rare but well-known inherited blood disorder. In this disease, sickle-shaped cells disrupt blood and oxygen flow to vital tissues.

Body Hair

- **Don't worry about it.**
- **Trim it yourself.**
- **Know your family history.**

Clark Gable, king of Hollywood tough guys and lady-killers, shaved more than just the area around his pencil-thin mustache. He took the blade to his chest and underarms, too. No little curly hair would mar his perfect bod, according to newspaper reports.

Some of today's silver-screen action heroes are following Gable's lead, though these days waxing—in which hot wax is put on hairy skin and then pulled off like a bandage after it solidifies, yanking out the hair—may be more popular than shaving. One Beverly Hills styling salon admits that it will mow a man's chest hair with electric clippers upon request. Competitive bodybuilders don't hide the fact that they remove all hair that might otherwise obscure hard-earned ripples.

Hair comes in two varieties: vellus hair, which is the thin, colorless fuzz; and terminal hair, which is the thicker, longer, colored hair. How much we have, how quickly it grows and where it grows are all determined by our individual genes, says Toby Mayer, M.D., co-director of the Beverly Hills Institute of Aesthetic and Reconstructive Surgery and clinical professor in the Division of Facial Plastic and Reconstructive Surgery at the University of Southern California in Los Angeles.

Most terminal hair follicles, other than those on the scalp and in the eyebrows, produce short, curly hairs. A hair rarely exceeds an inch or two in length before it falls out and is replaced by a new one. That's why, for instance, you can't grow your chest hair long and comb it back over your shoulders (as if you'd want to). That's also why doctors don't transplant hair follicles from your chest, back or groin to the scalp to replace hair lost to balding.

Grooming Your Body Hair

Most of us probably aren't so concerned about body hair, and that's fine. There's not a single medical problem related to the stuff, and women's opinions about it vary with the wind. But for aesthetic reasons, we usually don't want tufts sprouting from our noses and ears. Nor do we want a third eyebrow between the other two. Hair grows in those places, increasingly so as we hit midlife.

Feeling insecure about an abundance of body hair? Rent any Robin Williams movie in which he removes his shirt. You'll feel better. Still want to take action? In the good ol' days, a barber snipped away those offending hairs as part of a haircut. We may have to do it ourselves these days, says Christina Griffasi, head of the styling department at the Minardi Salon in New York City.

To do so, buy grooming scissors with blunt, rounded safety ends, electric nose-hair clippers and an electric beard trimmer, Griffasi advises. "They make these wonderful things you can now buy in the drugstore," she adds.

Use the electric nose-hair clippers or the blunt scissors to trim long nose hairs, Griffasi advises. The electric beard groomer, without any styling attachment installed, is good for buzzing away any tufts of hair protruding from the ear canals, she says.

For hairs growing from the ridges of the ears, take the advice of John Romano, M.D., assistant clinical professor of dermatology at the New York Hospital–Cornell Medical Center in New York City: Shave them. While you're shaving, moisten the ear and carefully work the razor around the edge of the lobe.

Permanent hair removal by electrolysis is painful, expensive and time-consuming. An electrologist uses a needle, attached to an electrical current, to damage the hair root. It requires multiple visits, at a cost of $60 to $100 per hour, to thoroughly kill the root.

Brain

- **Keep thinking. Thinking is brain exercise.**
- **Get your brain nutrients: B₆, boron and zinc.**
- **Exercise often to keep blood flowing strong.**

Back in those heady, science-will-save-the-world days of the industrial revolution of the 1800s, inquiring medical minds left little to chance. They studied germs and gerbils, bacteria and birds, mold spores and monkeys—anything they could slice into little pieces and slip under a microscope.

When the opportunity presented itself, they even studied each other's inquiring minds. Fun-loving groups such as the Mutual Autopsy Society of Paris scoured the Western hemisphere for the brains of eminent men. When they got hold of one, they weighed it, measured it and tried to determine whether brain size had anything to do with intelligence.

What they found was that old, eternal truth of manhood: Bigger doesn't always mean better. Napoléon III, the nondescript nephew of Napoléon Bonaparte, weighed in with a robust 1,500-gram brain, 17 percent larger than poet Walt Whitman's 1,282-gram offering (after the weigh-in, an apparently unimpressed member of the American Anthropometric Society dropped Whitman's brain on the floor, splattering it so badly that it was useless for further study). Crazy King Ludwig II housed a 1,349-gram brain inside his thick Bavarian skull, besting Albert Einstein, Mr. Theory of Relativity himself, by almost 10 percent.

And history fails to even record the size of Abraham Lincoln's brain—perhaps because, as some historians say, either records were lost during the assassination mayhem or scientists found it embarrassingly small for a man of such stature.

The moral of all of this skullduggery? Envy not thy neighbor's cranium. If you take care of your own brain by feeding it the right nutrients, giving it enough mental stimulation and getting enough physical exercise, it will probably serve you well for decades to come, no matter what its size.

"People used to think that there was nothing they could do to help their brains," says Douglas Herrmann, Ph.D., a memory researcher at the National Center for Health Statistics in Hyattsville, Maryland, and author of *Super Memory*. "But that's not true. Nutrition and other factors can improve memory and other brain functions. You can definitely make a difference."

The Main Parts of the Brain

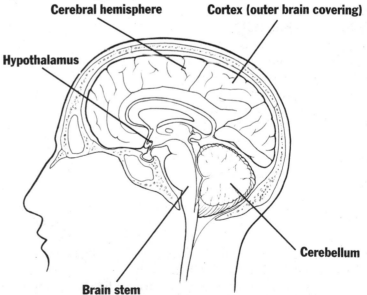

While the typical brain has some 100 billion nerve cells, age inevitably causes some deterioration in brain function. To combat it, exercise your brain (by thinking, reading, doing crossword puzzles), get sufficient vitamin B₆ and work out regularly.

Divvying Up the Duties

The brain is the business end of the body's central nervous system. It takes electrical impulses from nerve endings all over the body, sorts out what the body is trying to say and then transmits messages back through the nerve network, telling the body what to do: Flex a muscle. Sneeze. Sweat.

Of course, the brain does much more than that. It's responsible for higher functions such as language, creativity and logic. It stores memories. It interprets impulses from your eyes so that you can see. All of this in a three-pound package that fits neatly inside your skull.

The brain is divided into a number of interconnected parts, each of which controls different body functions. The cerebrum, the largest chunk of the brain, takes care of distinctly human traits such as reasoning and intellect. Most of this takes place in the part of the cerebrum called the cortex, the gray, folded layer of skin that covers the surface of the brain. The cortex takes information from nerves in the body and directs voluntary movements such as bending fingers and walking. It's also where you perceive the senses: The cortex sorts out impulses from your eyes, ears, nose, tongue and skin and figures out color, sound, smell, taste and touch. The cortex appears to house memories, too, storing many of them in the temporal lobes.

Deep under the cortex lies the thalamus. This area serves as a cerebral distribution center, routing information along sensory pathways to the proper part of the cortex. The thalamus, in fact, seems to be just a dumber version of the cortex. It can sense pain, for example, but it can't tell the difference between pain from a paper cut and pain from being cut in half by a ripsaw.

Even deeper in the brain is a cluster of structures that make up the limbic system, the ancient seat of our darkest, most secret emotions. Although *limbic* is derived from a Latin word for the peripheral limits of a system, this area controls many everyday functions such as digestion and heartbeat as well as

Locating the Thalamus

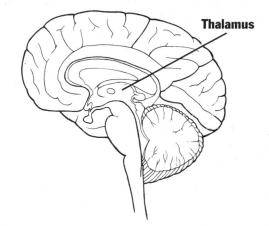

Thalamus

Located deep within the brain, the thalamus serves as a cerebral distribution center, routing information from the body's nerves.

many aspects of emotion and behavior.

The rest of your brain handles run-of-the-mill, any-mammal-can-do-it stuff. The brain stem controls activity in the heart, blood vessels and respiratory system. The tiny hypothalamus, located at the base of the cerebrum, controls body metabolism, temperature, blood sugar level, appetite and sexual arousal. The cerebellum orchestrates muscle action; when the cortex orders a movement, the cerebellum tells which muscles should move and how.

Brain Drain

The average human brain contains about 100 billion nerve cells. Each cell has several tiny branches of communication called dendrites that allow it to communicate with other cells. The point at which these dendrites meet is called a synapse. If you assume that each nerve cell can communicate with merely ten other cells—a very conservative guess—that means your brain can make more than a trillion separate connections with itself in a nearly infinite number of possible combinations.

While that may seem like more than enough for one lifetime, age and other factors can take their toll. As we reach late middle age,

MID-AGE

we start to lose a significant number of neurons. Neurons are the brain cells that send signals to each other; the other major type of brain cells, called glia, support and fix neurons.

The brain doesn't replace neurons, and that loss, over time, has a cumulative effect. We tend to lose lots of neurons from the brain stem, which, in time, can affect motor skills. That can mean slower movement, loss of flexibility and difficulty walking. Neurons also tend to break down or die in the cortex, which can affect learning, memory and other higher functions.

The brain apparently tries to compensate for its losses by rewiring itself, making new connections between existing neurons. Still, most people lose brain processing speed as they age. Their brains take longer to retrieve memories, and they have trouble doing other tasks as fast as they could when they were younger.

This doesn't mean you're doomed to senility. Dr. Herrmann says that unless you develop a brain disorder such as Alzheimer's disease or have a serious stroke, your brain can continue to function at a high level right through old age.

Dr. Herrmann uses a computer analogy to describe things. When you're young, he says, you have a Pentium-speed brain, capable of rapid calculations and instant recall. As you age, however, your brain becomes more of a 386 model: It can't process information as fast or store as much, but it can still get the job done.

When Memory Loss Gets Serious

Lost your car keys lately? You're hardly alone. More than half of Americans between ages 18 and 54 report misplacing items sometimes or frequently, according to the Charles A. Dana Foundation in New York City.

But when a person forgets what car keys are, it may signal a far more serious problem: Alzheimer's disease. Alzheimer's is a progressive, fatal disease that kills brain cells and leads to memory loss, dementia and loss of basic physical skills.

You're not likely to get Alzheimer's before age 65, although some cases have been reported in people in their forties and fifties. Still, according to Francis Pirozzolo, M.D., a neuropsychologist at Baylor College of Medicine in Houston, if you're worried about yourself or anyone else, look for these signs.

Inability to remember recent events. In the early stages of Alzheimer's, people forget seemingly innocent things, such as what they ate for breakfast. At this stage, the disease has not affected items stored in long-term memory, such as telephone numbers and Social Security numbers.

Difficulty understanding what people are saying. Alzheimer's can rob people of language skills. People with the disease can hear someone talking but can't figure out what the person is saying. They may also struggle to remember words.

Forgetting whole episodes. It's not unusual to forget details of a trip to the zoo. But Alzheimer's patients often forget they ever went to the zoo.

See a doctor immediately if you notice these symptoms. While Alzheimer's remains incurable, early detection and treatment can improve a patient's quality of life.

For more information on Alzheimer's, call the Alzheimer's Association at 1-800-272-3900. The association can answer your questions about the disease and refer you to a local chapter of the organization for information about support groups and other services in your community.

Like every supercomputer, your brain needs some ongoing, routine maintenance to stay sharp. Here are some tips to keep that gray matter strong.

B all that you can be. Vitamin B$_6$ helps

your body create neurotransmitters, chemicals that allow brain cells to fire off messages to one another, says Dr. Herrmann. One study of 38 elderly Dutchmen found that daily 20-milligram supplements of B$_6$ may improve long-term storage of memories. (The Daily Value for B$_6$ is just 2 milligrams, but 20 milligrams is well within the safe limit.) Your best bet, says Dr. Herrmann, is eating a balanced diet that contains lots of fruits and vegetables. Freezing and processing vegetables can rob them of 15 to 70 percent of their B$_6$ content, so favor fresh produce whenever possible. Other super sources of B$_6$ include chicken, fish and lean cuts of pork.

Let muscles go to your head. Working out your body can give your brain a boost. Studies have shown that regular aerobic exercise can, among other things, improve your ability to perform more than one task at a time and make you more creative. Doctors aren't entirely sure why this works, but they believe that since exercise improves your cardiovascular system, you may get more blood, oxygen and nutrients to your brain.

Use it or lose it. While you're at it, flex that cortex, too. Researchers have found that people with college educations who remain mentally active throughout their lives have 40 percent longer dendrites than less educated, less challenged people.

You don't really need a diploma to develop those dendrites. Most kinds of mental activity help keep the connections between your brain cells humming, so try continuing education courses at a local college, crossword puzzles or even playing along with television game shows, suggests K. Warner Schaie, Ph.D., professor of human development at Pennsylvania State University in University Park.

Mental activity may even help fight Alzheimer's disease. Research from Columbia University in New York City showed that people with high education levels and high achievement on the job have just one-third of the risk that others have of developing Alzheimer's. That may be because people who

use their brains build up reserves of synapses. That means there is less breakdown of communication between brain cells when Alzheimer's embarks on its path of destruction.

Keep the pressure down. High blood pressure is a three-pronged problem. It has been implicated in 40 percent of brain-busting strokes. It slows down your thought processes and appears to impair your short-term memory. Worst of all, a study of 35 men between ages 51 and 80 showed that high blood pressure appears to cause permanent structural changes and tissue loss in the brain. One of the authors of the study, Declan Murphy, M.D., senior lecturer and consultant psychiatrist at the Bethlem Royal Hospital in Kent, England, says that over time, this could cause problems with memory, language and sense of direction.

The standard recommendation is to have your blood pressure checked every three years, switching to every two years at age 40. But it's such a simple test, it's worth having it done every time you see a health professional.

Don't be a boron moron. A handful of peanuts may be the only thing standing between you and mental magnificence. According to James G. Penland, Ph.D., research psychologist at the U.S. Department of Agriculture Grand Forks Human Nutrition Research Center in North Dakota, the micronutrient boron appears to be good for memory, attention and motor skills. Research showed that men who consumed 3.25 milligrams of boron each day scored better on tests of all three of those traits than men who ate a low-boron diet. Peanuts are a great boron powerhouse, with 0.5 milligram per ounce. But be aware that peanuts are extremely high in calories and fat. Other foods that give you a boron boost: prunes, dates and raisins, each with 0.5 milligram per ounce, and honey, with 0.2 milligram per ounce.

And think about zinc. While you're minding your minerals, think zinc, too. This memory mineral may promote neuron function. Great zinc sources include oysters, with 8.2 milligrams per one-half cup; lean roast beef, with 5.3 milligrams per three-ounce serving;

lean pork, with 3.2 milligrams per three-ounce serving; cooked dried beans, with 1.8 milligrams per cup; and lima beans, with 1.7 milligrams per one-half cup. Experts don't recommend taking zinc supplements, since too much of this mineral can give you a serious case of the trots, nausea or vomiting and may even contribute to hardening of the arteries.

Save the starch for your collars. Carbohydrate loading may be great for marathon runners. But a Harvard University study showed that a meal consisting mainly of protein will keep your mind clearer in the short run. Men over age 40 who ate sherbet, made up of almost 100 percent carbohydrates, had up to twice as much trouble concentrating and doing other mental tasks as men who ate turkey. That may have been because high-carbohydrate foods elevate the brain's level of serotonin, a substance that makes us sleepy, according to Bonnie J. Spring, Ph.D., professor of psychology at the University of Health Sciences/Chicago Medical School. Conversely, high-protein foods such as turkey, fish and chicken contain tyrosine, an amino acid that has been linked to clear thinking and alertness.

Carbohydrates should be the primary source of calories in any diet. But when your head needs to be extra-clear for a few hours, protein is the prescription.

Drink to forget—it works. Alcohol kills brain cells randomly. Over time, alcohol can lead to long-term memory loss and crippling loss of muscle coordination. No one has set a "safe" dosage for alcohol, but a Finnish study found that drinking more than 32 ounces of beer, 2 ounces of wine or 0.5 ounce of spirits a day over a long period can have a damaging effect on brain cells. Dr. Herrmann says moderate drinking, maybe a couple of beers or mixed drinks a week, probably won't lead to serious problems.

Three-martini lunches can cause short-range problems, too, Dr. Herrmann says. Alcohol affects your concentration, so you are

Creativity: Where Man Beats Beast

It's the difference between Einstein and orangutan. Picasso and possum. You and yak. Thanks to our brains, we humans are creative. Thanks to their brains, animals stand around and grunt a lot.

You don't have to be some kind of beret-wearing, poem-writing, angst-riddled slacker to be creative, either. "Everyone has the ability," says William Shephard, director of programs for the Creative Education Foundation in Buffalo, New York. "In fact, creativity is becoming a survival skill. You have to come up with new and better ways to do things, or you and your company will get left behind."

Of course, you can't just sit down at your desk and say "Okay, brain, be creative." You have to know how to coax your mind into a creative state and learn how to take advantage of its ability to interpret information in new and unique ways. Shephard offers these tips.

Don't be so critical. A technique called brainstorming can help boost your creativity, either alone or in a group. First define the problem you want to solve, then start thinking up solutions. They don't have to make sense, be practical or even sound good; just keep kicking out ideas and writing them down. Don't make judgments about how good the ideas are until later. Go off in any direction the thoughts take you, as long as you keep the focus on the problem you're trying to solve.

After a set period of time, maybe 10 to 15 minutes, stop writing. If you can, put aside all of your notes for a day or so. Then go back and look at what you've written down. You'll probably find the solution to your problem right in front of you.

Change the subject. Sometimes we focus too hard on the task at hand, and our brains don't respond to the

less likely to focus on conversations or details when you feel a little buzz. That means you're also less likely to remember those conversations or details the next day.

Don't go pill-silly. You've seen those magazine ads for "brain cocktails"—pills or powders that are supposed to supercharge your brain. Be careful: Smart drugs may be a stupid idea. "The best advice I can give is not to fool around with them," Dr. Herrmann says.

"You may have an allergic reaction to them, or they may interfere with another medication you're taking." Besides, he says, we don't know enough about the roles of glucose, lecithin, selenium, amino acids and other ingredients in these pills to say whether they're going to help. "Maybe in a couple of years. But not yet," he says.

The Price We Pay

Complexity doesn't always come cheap. With billions of neurons buzzing in your brain, things sometimes go very, very wrong. Even a seemingly simple blow to the head can have you fluent in a language you haven't spoken in decades. It's possible, for example, for an 80-year-old man to suffer a severe brain trauma that erases 70 years' worth of English skills and leaves him speaking in the native Italian of his youth.

Other diseases are far more serious. Brain disorders range from infections such as meningitis to genetic breakdowns such as Down's syndrome to mental disturbances such as schizophrenia. "The brain is extremely complicated," says Francis Pirozzolo, M.D., a neuropsychologist at Baylor College of Medicine in Houston. "We're learning more about it every day, but it continues to puzzle us and frustrate us. Sometimes things go wrong that we just can't fix."

Alzheimer's disease is among the most feared of all brain diseases. About four

pressure. If you feel like you've hit a mental wall, take a break and do something entirely different. If you can't come up with the right phrase for a cover letter, for example, go pull some weeds. This gives your brain a chance to mull things over in a more relaxed setting.

Make a dream date—with yourself. Next time the boss catches you daydreaming, tell him you're actually doing some serious semiconscious creativity enhancement. Daydreaming for a few minutes lets you escape the pressure of the here and now and allows your brain to work its creative magic.

"Daydreaming should actually be encouraged," Shephard says. "You shouldn't drift away for hours at a time. But taking a little time to toy with an idea, to imagine its applications, can be tremendously helpful." Again, don't make judgments about what you're thinking. Just let the thoughts flow and worry about the details later.

Make new connections. Most of us think in preprogrammed ways. Table: chair. Salt: pepper. If you want to unleash creativity, compare things that seem to have nothing in common. French fry: B-52 bomber. Fence post: laptop computer. Take a few minutes to list all of the similarities you can think of between the items. "This helps you make new associations, see things in new ways," Shephard says. "It can break up the thought patterns that most of us always fall into."

Once you're done with that warm-up, move on to the real problem. If you're trying to think of new ways to market your company's candy bar, compare its attributes to those of the Eiffel Tower. Or Bigfoot. Or the paneling in the conference room. Make a list of the similarities, then see if any of them warrant further discussion.

(continued on page 118)

Memory

- **In May 1974, Bhandanta Vicittabi Vumsa recited 16,000 pages of Buddhist canonical text from memory.**
- **On May 29, 1992, Dominic O'Brien of Great Britain memorized a deck of shuffled playing cards in 55.62 seconds.**

Five Miraculous Methods for Magnifying Short-Term Memory

Yes, there are mental exercises that have been shown to help people remember things better. Here are some workouts recommended by Francis Pirozzolo, M.D., a neuropsychologist at Baylor College of Medicine in Houston.

1. WORK at it. To remember a short list of names or groceries, make a word out of the first letter of each item. Wanda, Omar, Rita and Ken become WORK. Soap, ham, oranges and pistachios become SHOP. These are known as mnemonics.

2. Distract yourself. Learn to concentrate amid chaos. Try reading a book with the radio turned up full blast. Or try watching two television sets at once. Then try remembering what you read, saw or heard. This will teach you to tune out what's not important, a key step in improving memory.

3. Gather in chunks. Your brain remembers items best when they're in groups of five to nine. So if you have to recall a long list of, say, 30 things, try dividing the items into six groups of five items each. The process is called chunking.

Group items with common themes. If you have a shopping list, for example, make a vegetable grouping, a canned goods grouping and so on.

4. Just imagine. If you have trouble remembering names, try visualization. Associate the person's name with an object or action, then make a mental picture of it. To remember Neil, for example, picture a man kneeling.

Rhyming can also solidify the connection. If Larry has a beard, try remembering him as Hairy Larry. Just don't call him Harry by accident.

5. Store in a drawer. If you're always losing your keys or misplacing your wallet, create a memory drawer. Make it a point to put easily lost items in this place every day. It doesn't have to be an actual drawer; a closet, countertop or nightstand will do fine. The process will quickly become a habit. And you'll never again have to run around the house checking the pockets of all of your pants and coats. ■

Where Your Brain Parks Memories

Scratch-pad memory. Your brain uses this to remember phone numbers, directions and the names of people you've just met. Good only for a few minutes before the memory disappears.

Mid-term. This is the temporary holding place for everyday memories: what clothes you wore today, what Dan Rather said on the news, what you had for dinner last night. This stuff hangs around for a couple of days, then gets jettisoned. You also use mid-term memory to memorize items for a test or presentation. If a memory is important enough, it gets transferred to long-term memory.

Long-term. Here's where all of the important memories end up: your wedding day (and, hopefully, your anniversary date), your Social Security number, your first kiss. It can be accessed directly by thinking about the event or item or indirectly by a cue such as a smell, a sound, a taste or a sight. ■

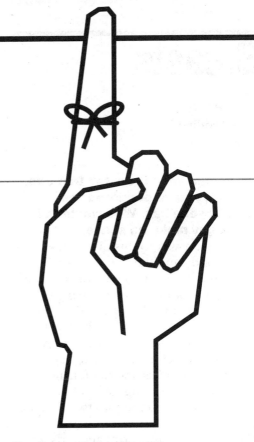

Brains and the Sexes

It's not just a stereotype: Men do think, react and speak differently than women. The proof is in the physiology. Here are some of the ways the male brain differs from the female brain.

• The fetal brain of the female develops faster than that of the male.

• The corpus callosum, which is the bridge connecting the right and left hemispheres of the brain, is bigger in women than it is in men.

• Brain scans that reveal "thinking" activities show that women tend to use both parts of their brains, while men weigh in more heavily on just one side.

• While men's brains are bigger by about 10 percent, women have 11 percent more neurons.

• Women seem better at verbal memory and fluency, but men do better at spatial tasks, such as reading maps.

• Men also do better at motor tasks, such as finger tapping. ■

Brain Busters: Six Sure Ways to Mangle Your Memory

1. Stress. So many memories, so little time. Stress decreases concentration and short-term memory in many men. If you need to remember something important, set aside a block of time to concentrate and allow no interruptions.

2. Lack of sleep. Your brain files memories while you sleep. And sleep makes you more alert during the day, so you concentrate better. So don't deprive yourself of your nightly sleep needs, or you may deprive yourself of memory.

3. High blood pressure. Impairs short-term memory, slows down mental processing and may also destroy brain tissues by depriving them of blood and nutrients. Get your blood pressure checked regularly.

4. Alcohol. Even a couple of beers will fog your concentration, so it's unlikely you'll retain details of an event where you've been drinking. Booze also kills brain cells. Over time, alcohol abuse impairs your ability to store and recall long-term memories.

5. Caffeine. Reduces concentration and can affect sleep patterns. One cup of coffee a day is probably okay, but anything more than that may hurt memory. Also avoid stimulant pills that contain caffeine. They'll keep you awake, but you won't remember much.

6. Cigarettes. Smoking impairs memory by constricting arteries and reducing blood flow to the brain. In one study, nonsmokers were able to recall a list of numbers more quickly than smokers, and nonsmokers also scored higher on standard memory tests. ■

million Americans have Alzheimer's disease, including one in ten people over the age of 65 and nearly half of everyone over age 85.

Simply put, Alzheimer's kills brain cells. Millions of them. As the cells die over the course of months and years, victims begin to suffer severe memory loss, loss of language and reasoning skills and physical deterioration, eventually leading to death. The disease can take from 3 to 20 years to run its course, and there's no known cure.

While Alzheimer's is the fourth leading cause of death among adults, its cause remains a mystery. People with the disease often show altered levels of neurotransmitters, which are needed for communication between brain cells. High levels of aluminum may be found in their brain tissues. Researchers are also studying factors such as genetics, head injuries, education and gender.

Parkinson's disease, unlike Alzheimer's, does not affect mental function. But it can lead to severe physical problems such as muscle tremors, slowed movements and difficulty walking. Parkinson's appears to be caused by a shortage of a neurotransmitter called dopamine. On the bright side: At least 90 percent of people with Parkinson's disease respond to drug therapy.

Stroke is one of the brain's deadliest enemies. The American Heart Association estimates that nearly 40 percent of men who have strokes die. That's more than 57,000 men each year.

Doctors say there are two basic kinds of stroke. The first is usually caused by a clot in one of the arteries leading from the heart to the brain. The clot blocks blood flow, cutting off oxygen and nutrients and killing brain cells. The second type of stroke, which is caused by a hemorrhage, happens when an artery in the head ruptures. This cuts off blood flow to the brain, and surrounding cells are deprived of blood. While hemorrhages account for one in five strokes, they are usually more deadly than strokes that are caused by blood clots.

Breasts

• **Check for lumps.**
• **Watch for swelling.**
• **Stay lean.**

Why do men have breasts? Don't lie: At some point, you've pondered the question. Everyone has. Who wouldn't? Nipples on a guy make no sense.

The simple answer to this question is that both the male body and the female body develop from the same template. You see, the physical structures of men and women aren't different initially (that is, during the first weeks in the womb). It's how hormones instruct the body to develop these structures that creates the differences between males and females. By this theory, the male penis and the female clitoris start as the same thing, but different hormones cause it to develop into two different organs.

In the case of breasts, boys and girls go until puberty being equal; the glands in the front of the chest remain inactive and undeveloped in both sexes. After the onset of puberty, however, testosterone causes the glands in a male's breasts to atrophy. For women, the female hormone estrogen causes a blossoming. Thank you, biology.

Health Issues

While the glands in the front of the chest may go unused in males, they are still there, and that means things can go wrong with them. Men account for 1,400 of the 183,400 new cases of breast cancer that are reported each year. While men are not nearly as susceptible to the disease as women, William Donegan, M.D., professor of surgery at the Medical College of Wisconsin in Milwaukee, believes that men should recognize the danger. "Just being aware of the possibility and being extra-conscious of your body while showering should be enough," he says.

Since the male breast never develops, there is less tissue to hide a cancerous lump that signals the disease. So the moment you detect an unexplainable lump, see your doctor. A study that tracked 335 males afflicted with breast cancer found that those who identified the cancer before it spread to their lymph nodes had an 84 percent survival rate over ten years. That's compared with only a 14 percent survival rate over ten years if the cancer spreads to four or more nodes.

The only other widespread problem of the male breast is called gynecomastia. With this, a mistaken jolt of the female hormone estrogen causes the glands in the breasts to swell. This most often happens around puberty, when a boy's body is flush with hormones (yes, the male body can manufacture estrogen as well as testosterone), and among men over age 50.

In one reported case of gynecomastia, a man returned from a vacation of heavy drinking with greatly enlarged breasts. The reasons: First, alcohol impairs the production of testosterone; and second, chicken in some foreign ports is shot full of female sex hormone to stimulate growth. Combined for a week, these factors turned this rooster into a hen for a short time.

Gynecomastia will hit 30 to 40 percent of men sometime in their lives, believes Dr. Donegan. Drugs are responsible for 18 percent of the cases, so if your breasts suddenly swell, talk to your doctor about your medication first. Liver disease can also cause breast swelling, since a defective liver can't break down the estrogen in your body.

A similar enlarged-breast condition called pseudogynecomastia can occur in men who are simply overweight. Fat can accumulate in the chest, causing men to look like they have breasts. The answer here is obvious: Lose weight. Some men opt for liposuction of the fatty area, says Dr. Donegan. Or if there's a lot of tissue, a doctor could remove it with traditional surgery.

Chin

Cary Grant's was a classic. Kirk Douglas has a nice one, if you're into dimples. Jay Leno wins points for sheer volume.

But the best chin of all time probably belonged to Edward Henry "Harry" Greb, an American boxer in the 1910s and 1920s. Greb went a record 178 consecutive fights without an official loss back in the days when men were men and knuckles were bare.

Unless you let ol' Harry pound on it, your chin probably will never give you too much trouble, either. After all, it's nothing more than a triangular piece of bone called the mentum that sits beneath your lower lip. (If your mentum has a couple of bumps on its front side, you'll end up with a dimpled chin.)

The only problem with chins, in fact, comes when you grow too many of them. As men get older, they're more prone to develop a double chin, sagging flesh that hangs under your jaw and gives you that stuffed sausage look. Men with low Adam's apples are more likely to develop double chins, according to Robert Kotler, M.D., a facial surgeon and clinical instructor in surgery at the University of California, Los Angeles.

For about $5,000, a plastic surgeon can trim away the excess fat and tighten things up for you. He can even drop in a silicone implant to give you a studly Dick Tracy jawline. But the easiest way to lose the double chin is to lose weight—as little as ten pounds, Dr. Kotler says.

Until you're done dropping the weight, wear loose collars, since buttons that are too tight force flesh up over the collar, suggests Massimo Iacoboni, fashion director for the Fashion Association in New York City. Buy shirts with pointed collars, which make the chin look longer and leaner. And never wear a V-neck sweater without a shirt underneath. Do you want to put those chins on display, or what?

⊙ Circulatory System

- **Number of red blood cells in an average adult: 35 trillion**
- **Number of new red blood cells produced every second in a healthy person: 2 million**
- **Miles of blood vessels in the body: 60,000**

How to Keep in Circulation

Here are five essentials for circulatory system health.

Eat less fat. Fat begets cholesterol. Cholesterol clogs arteries. The result: high blood pressure, heart attack, stroke. Forget bullets; cholesterol is the great man-killer of the United States. The best diet is rich in carbohydrates, low in protein and low in fat. Build your meals around fruits, vegetables and grains. Keep your intake of meat, poultry and seafood to six ounces a day. Avoid adding butter and oil.

Aerobicize. Your heart is a muscle, as are the walls of your arteries. Aerobic exercise makes them stronger. So get into a program of regular aerobic exercise, such as walking, swimming or bicycling. You don't have to exercise at a high intensity. As little as a brisk 30-minute walk three times a week can reduce blood pressure.

Watch your blood pressure. This is a measure of how hard your heart works. Persistent revving at a high rate can quadruple your risk of heart attack. Every one-point drop in diastolic blood pressure (the smaller number) lowers your risk of heart attack by 2 to 3 percent.

Reduce stress. If you can't easily name someone in whom you can confide, you may be at greater risk for fatal heart disease than other men. A Duke University study found that of the men with heart disease who weren't married and who had no friends or confidants, half died within five years of being diagnosed with the condition. Only 17 percent of similar patients with more social support died.

Drop the pounds. Being overweight makes your heart work harder and stresses your entire circulatory system. To determine your ideal weight, start with a base of 105 pounds, then add 6 pounds for each inch of your height above five feet. If you have a large frame, take 10 percent of the total and add on that amount.∎

The Numbers Game

Blood pressure. Your blood pressure reading consists of two numbers. The top one is systolic pressure; it measures how forcefully your heart pumps blood. When this number is too high, your heart is working harder than it should. The bottom number is diastolic pressure; it gauges the force of blood flowing through your fully relaxed arteries between heartbeats. A high number here could indicate clogged or constricted vessels. A reading of 120/80 or less is considered good. Repeated readings of 140/90 or more mean high blood pressure.

Pulse. When you take your pulse, you're measuring the rate at which your heart beats per minute by counting the shock waves that travel through your veins after your heart contracts.

To take your pulse, hold your left wrist in front of you, palm up. Place the first and second fingers of your right hand on your wrist, just below your thumb. Count the beats for 20 seconds. Then multiply that number by three for your baseline pulse. Rate your fitness according to the chart below.∎

50 or less	Excellent
51 to 65	Good
66 to 79	Bad
More than 80	Very bad

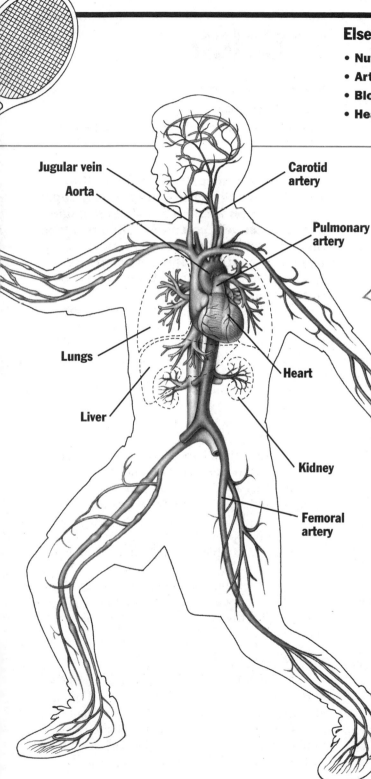

Jugular vein
Aorta
Carotid artery
Pulmonary artery
Lungs
Liver
Heart
Kidney
Femoral artery

Blood and Guts

Every cell in your body needs some nutrients to live: glucose, oxygen, minerals, water, whatever. Likewise, every live cell in your body creates garbage that needs to be carted away. The main job of the circulatory system is to deliver the good stuff and carry away the trash.

We'll start our tour of the circulatory system in the right side of the heart. This is where blood always returns. The right ventricle pumps the trash-filled blood to the lungs, where carbon dioxide gets dumped and oxygen gets picked up.

The blood returns to the left ventricle of the heart, which is the most muscular of the chambers. With a strong pump, the left ventricle sends the blood to the aorta, the body's main artery.

Some of the blood gets diverted to the kidneys, where it gets filtered for other wastes. Some blood goes to the intestines, where it absorbs nutrients. The blood also gets piped through an intricate web of smaller and smaller arteries, delivering needed materials to cells along the way and picking up waste.

After making its rounds, the blood travels through veins back to the right side of the heart, where it begins its cycle again. A typical drop of blood makes the complete loop in about 30 seconds. ∎

Collarbones

The collarbones are the main anchors for the muscles of your upper body. So every time you do a bench press or lift a box, muscles are pulling on your collarbones. That makes your collarbones stand out. It also strengthens your bones.

Your collarbones are located exactly where you'd expect: right where the collar of your shirt fastens. Each of these bones, also called the clavicles, extends in a long, S-shaped curve from the top of the breastbone, or sternum, to the top of the shoulder blade, or scapula. Making the connections between the bones are several ligaments.

People don't often dislocate a collarbone because the ligaments that connect it to the sternum and the scapula are so strong. Fractures are more common. If you fall and put out your arm to catch yourself, the jolt gets absorbed through your shoulder to your collarbone.

If you do get a fracture, you'll feel the pain, and your arm will feel like it has gone limp. If you suspect that you have a fracture, it's best to get an x-ray, says Bruce Janiak, M.D., director of the emergency center at Toledo Hospital.

In the past, a fractured collarbone was treated by immobilizing the upper arm and shoulder for several weeks. But this practice is changing, Dr. Janiak says. He believes that the collarbone can probably heal just as well on its own. So don't be surprised if the prescription is to just "take it easy."

If you want to strengthen your collarbones, you should work out the muscles of your upper body, states Scott Haldeman, M.D., Ph.D., D.C., associate clinical professor of neurology at the University of California, Irvine. And relax: Collarbone injuries during weight lifting are extremely rare. Most result from a direct blow or trauma, according to Dr. Haldeman.

Colon

- Drink lots of water.
- Eat lots of fiber.
- Exercise often to stimulate your digestive tract.

For a few disastrous years in the early twentieth century, surgeons thought that the colon was the body's bad neighborhood, an evil, poisonous slum to which ailments such as rheumatism, tuberculosis and even schizophrenia could be traced. Their simple solution: Wash it out or rip it out.

And so they did. Even when the ailment had nothing to do with the digestive tract, frequent enemas called high colonics, or washouts, were advised. As for surgery, one unfortunate boy who went to a clinic complaining of a sore throat lost his colon instead of his tonsils. And one man had his wife's colon removed with the hope that she would become a better-tempered companion.

These scalpel-happy doctors thought that once the colon was removed and the small intestine was attached directly to the rectum, aging would slow, illness would vanish and all would be well. They were wrong. In the 30 years that this procedure was in vogue, it permanently disabled many and killed more than a few.

When reason finally prevailed and the onslaught stopped, doctors found that the colon, rather than being a toxic dump, is a very practical organ after all.

The Body's Water Well

The colon, also known as the large intestine, begins in the lower right-hand side of the abdomen, where it connects with the small intestine. The colon bends in the shape of an M until it reaches the rectum, a five-inch-long tube that acts like a holding tank for solid waste.

By the time food reaches the colon, it has already been broken down, and most of its nutrients have been sucked out. In other words, it's barely food anymore; it's a semi-liquid sludge called chyme. All that remains for the colon to do is to absorb water and mineral salts, a process that can take anywhere from ten hours to several days. By the time the sludge reaches the end of the muscular five-foot-long, two-inch-wide colon, almost all of the water has been removed from it, and it has become what doctors politely call stool or feces.

The colon also serves as a breeding ground for harmless bacteria that devour digestive enzymes. Without these bacteria, the corrosive enzymes would literally eat through the anus and surrounding skin as they pass out of the body, says Eugene S. Sullivan, M.D., a colon and rectal surgeon in Portland, Oregon.

Keeping It Flowing

Lots of diseases can prey on the colon. In most cases, though, you can avoid them if you eat lots of fiber, drink plenty of water and follow other rules of colon maintenance.

Load up on fiber. Fiber, an undigestible component of fruits, vegetables and grains, speeds the movement of food through the colon, says Dr. Sullivan, which reduces the amount of time that the digestive tract is exposed to any cancer-causing substances that may be found in the food. Fiber also absorbs water and keeps your stool soft and pliable, so it can be expelled from your body without strain.

American men eat between 15 and 20 grams of fiber a day. Doctors say that we need at least 25 grams of fiber a day to keep the colon healthy. That's the equivalent of about ten apples; only Johnny Appleseed could happily gnaw on that many Granny Smiths every day. But if you eat a balanced daily diet that includes at least 6 to 11 servings of breads, cereals and other grains and 5 to 9 servings of fruits and vegetables such as straw-

berries, bananas, beans and peas, you should have no problem getting enough fiber into your gut.

"I tell my patients that if their stools are soft and fluffy (a consistency like heavy cottage cheese), they're doing great. If their stools are firm, like clay, they need to get more fiber into their diets," says David E. Beck, M.D., chairman of the Department of Colon and Rectal Surgery at the Ochsner Medical Clinic in New Orleans.

Go slowly. Suddenly increasing the amount of fiber in your diet can cause bloating, cramping and gas. So over a two-week period, add about three grams of fiber—the equivalent of an apple or one-half cup of chopped carrots—to your diet every day, so your digestive system has time to adjust, suggests Gerard Guillory, M.D., a Denver internist

"Pockets" in the Colon

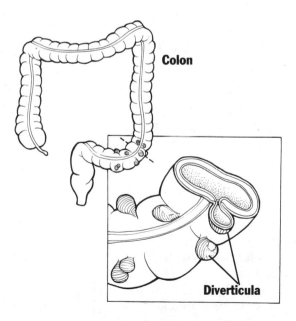

Colon

Diverticula

Diverticula are small saclike pouches that can form in the wall of the colon and protrude into the abdomen. Two-thirds of men develop them by the age of 85. Eating lots of fiber and drinking plenty of water will keep diverticula from becoming inflamed or painful, a condition known as diverticulitis.

and author of *IBS: A Doctor's Plan for Chronic Digestive Troubles.*

Keep the liquids flowing. Water, fruit juices and other liquids help fiber flush food through your colon. Drink at least six to eight eight-ounce glasses of fluids a day, suggests William B. Ruderman, M.D., a gastroenterologist on staff at the Orlando Regional Medical Center in Florida.

Clamp down on coffee. Coffee contains undigestible oils that can irritate the lining of your colon. Try to drink no more than two eight-ounce cups of java a day, Dr. Sullivan says.

Slash the fat. In addition to triggering cramping and diarrhea, an excessive amount of fat may increase your risk of some forms of cancer, Dr. Guillory says. Read food labels and try to limit your fat intake to no more than 30 percent of calories. As a start, eat no more than two three-ounce servings of red meat, poultry or fish a day.

Be wary of fat-free foods, too. Eating fat-free foods isn't necessarily good for your digestive health. Many of these products, particularly baked goods, are loaded with sugar, which is hard for some men to digest, Dr. Guillory says. Take a close look at the nutritional label before deciding whether to eat one of these foods, he suggests.

Take your colon for a walk. Regular exercise—even walking for just 20 minutes a day, three times a week—stimulates your digestive tract and keeps food moving through your colon, according to Dr. Ruderman.

Exercise may also reduce your risk of diverticulosis, according to researchers at the Harvard School of Public Health.

In a study of the physical activity of 47,678 men ages 40 to 75, the researchers found that the men who exercised the most were one-third less likely to develop diverticular disease than the least active men. A similar study by the same researchers found that men who exercise regularly have a significantly lower risk of colon cancer than men who don't.

Unwind. Stress can cause intestinal cramping and diarrhea or constipation. If stress upsets your digestive system, try a relaxation

---

Colon Cancer: It's Preventable, It's Curable

Of all of the ugly, screaming statistics that you may hear about colon cancer, this one is the most important for you to remember: Colon cancer is one of the most curable cancers if it is detected early. In fact, more than 90 percent of men who have colon cancer could still be alive five years after diagnosis.

But even this hopeful bit of news doesn't mean that you can relax your guard. About 75,000 new cases of colon cancer are detected in men each year, making it the third most common cancer (after cancers of the lung and prostate) among American men. About half of these men die of this disease annually, according to the American Cancer Society.

So it's important to be vigilant for the symptoms—rectal bleeding, blood in the stool, abdominal pain, unexplained weight loss and a change in bowel habits, such as constipation or diarrhea—and to seek prompt medical attention if you have any of them. It's crucial to get a digital/rectal exam as well as a stool test, to detect any hidden blood in your feces, every two years starting at age 40. You should also have an examination of your colon with a flexible hollow tube called a sigmoidoscope every two to three years starting at age 50 (men with family histories of colon cancer should begin this test at age 40).

You can further reduce your risk of colon cancer by eating plenty of grains, fruits and vegetables, which are

technique such as deep breathing, yoga or meditation, Dr. Guillory suggests.

A Glimpse at Your Colon's Enemies

Because diseases of the colon and rectum are often marked by similar symptoms, you should see your doctor for an evaluation of any persistent problem, particularly if you notice blood in your stool or you have a change in your bowel habits, such as chronic diarrhea or constipation.

While they're different in nature, many of these ailments can be prevented or controlled

high in fiber, says Sidney Winawer, M.D., chief of the gastroenterology and nutrition service at Memorial Sloan-Kettering Cancer Center in New York City. Doctors believe that fiber helps move food through the colon, so any cancer-causing substances are diluted and have less time to affect the cells along the colon wall.

Cutting back on the fat in your diet is also a good idea. Dr. Winawer says that a high amount of fat may indirectly increase the potency of any cancer-causing substances that are present.

Keep an eye on your weight, too. Overweight men are more prone to colon cancer than their leaner friends, says Dr. Winawer. So if you're carrying around a little extra bulk, try to shed it.

Also—and we know that this is starting to sound like a broken record—if you smoke cigarettes, quit. If you don't smoke, don't start. And go easy on the alcohol if you like to drink.

Finally, take a hike or get some other form of exercise regularly. In a six-year study of 47,723 men ages 40 to 75, researchers at Harvard School of Public Health found that the men who exercised the most had half of the risk of developing colon cancer compared with the sedentary guys. Like fiber, exercise probably speeds the movement of food through your colon and lessens your exposure to cancer-causing substances, Dr. Winawer says.

by the same three steps: adding more fiber to your diet, drinking more fluids and getting regular exercise, says Dr. Ruderman. Here's a rundown of some symptoms and disorders that commonly affect the lower digestive tract.

Diarrhea. A common symptom of many digestive ailments. When you get it, avoid eating solid foods and get plenty of clear liquids such as water, broth, juices and gelatin. Take an over-the-counter bulk laxative containing psyllium (such as Metamucil) as directed by the manufacturer, except mix it with half of the recommended amount of water. Instead of thinning your stool, that should help thicken it, Dr. Sullivan says. You might also want to try loperamide (Imodium), an over-the-counter antidiarrheal drug. Take one two-milligram tablet one to three times a day, Dr. Beck says. If diarrhea persists for more than 48 hours, see your doctor.

Constipation. Another common symptom of underlying digestive problems. For occasional bouts, drink more fluids, including prune, grape and grapefruit juices. Try taking a bulk laxative containing psyllium as directed by the manufacturer, except mix it with twice the recommended amount of water. That should quickly get things moving again, Dr. Sullivan says. If not, consult your physician.

Irritable bowel syndrome. The most common of all digestive disorders, irritable bowel syndrome affects about one in five Americans. This elusive syndrome has many names—nervous stomach, spastic colon—but it isn't considered a true disease. Instead,

Cutting Back on the Hot Air

A few years ago, perplexed museum officials in London couldn't quite figure out what was destroying their art. So they hired an atmospheric chemist, who quickly sniffed out the problem: bio-effluents, better known as farts.

According to the chemist, high levels of natural gases called sulfides, released in the galleries by patrons who passed wind, were the main culprit behind the blackened paintings, tarnished silverware and eroding photographs.

Fortunately, few men have priceless works of art hanging in their homes. But excessive gas, voiced at the wrong time, can be just as damaging to your social life.

The average man passes gas 10 to 20 times a day. Gas is formed in the colon by bacteria that feed on the unabsorbable portions of carbohydrate-rich foods such as beans and broccoli, says Michael D. Levitt, M.D., associate chief of staff for research at the Veterans Affairs Medical Center in Minneapolis. The result is a smelly concoction of nitrogen, hydrogen, carbon dioxide, sulfur and other gases.

Although the foods and beverages that cause gas vary from man to man, some common offenders are cheeses, onions, cabbage, apples, radishes, milk, carbonated beverages and alcohol. Swallowed air can add to the problem.

Here are a few ways to keep flatulence under control.

Eat slowly and chew well. The more food that gets into your colon undigested, the more gas you may form. Eating slowly allows the saliva in your mouth to thoroughly begin the digestive process, says Gerard Guillory, M.D., a Denver internist and author of *IBS: A Doctor's Plan for Chronic Digestive Troubles.*

Keep a gas diary. For a week, jot down when you pass gas and note everything that you eat and drink. If a particular food or beverage seems to cause gas, try eliminating it from your diet.

Soak your beans. Beans are terrific sources of fiber, but they also are notorious gas producers. Soaking them in a bowl of water overnight before you eat them might relieve that problem, says gastroenterologist Robert Charm, M.D., assistant clinical professor of medicine at the University of California, Davis, School of Medicine.

Reach for the enzymes. Over-the-counter products containing enzymes such as lactase (Dairy Ease) and alpha-galactosidase (Beano) can prevent gas by breaking down the sugars in milk, beans and other foods before bacteria in the colon have a chance to work on them, says Dr. Levitt.

it is a cluster of symptoms, including pain, cramping, bloating, constipation and diarrhea, caused by malfunctioning intestinal muscles that don't contract properly. In most cases, Dr. Guillory says, irritable bowel syndrome can be controlled with dietary changes and stress-management techniques.

Diverticular disease. Small saclike pouches called diverticula can form in the wall of the colon and protrude into the abdominal cavity, a condition known as diverticulosis. Often symptomless, these pouches occur in 33 percent of men by age 45 and in 66 percent of men by age 85. If a pouch becomes inflamed and painful, it's called diverticulitis.

Diverticulitis is easily confused with other things, even by experienced doctors. The periodic pain and diarrhea of relatively mild attacks can look like irritable bowel syndrome. Or it can be mistaken as ulcers or appendicitis if the pain is isolated to a particular spot. Once diagnosed, diverticulitis is usually treated with antibiotics. Usually, surgery is called for only to treat severe, complicated or recurrent episodes. After the infection has been remedied, it's time to boost the fiber in the diet to prevent reoccurrences.

Ulcerative colitis. A rare form of inflammatory bowel disease that attacks the lining of the colon. The cause of this chronic ailment is unknown. Diet usually has little impact on the disease, but drugs can control it in most instances. With persistent symptoms or long-standing disease causing permanent changes in the colon lining, surgical removal of the colon may offer the only cure. Chronic ulcerative colitis is often indistinguishable from Crohn's disease, which may also involve the colon.

Crohn's disease. Causes many of the same symptoms as ulcerative colitis, but Crohn's can occur anywhere along the digestive tract and is most common at the end of the small intestine. It attacks the entire wall of the digestive tract. Its cause is unknown, although it may run in families. Drugs can help control this disorder, but unlike ulcerative colitis, which is limited to the colon, surgery cannot remove the threat of further Crohn's disease. Crohn's is one of the few digestive diseases that may be helped by eating less fiber, says Dr. Sullivan.

Polyps. Benign growths on the colon wall that can cause bowel obstruction and that are considered to be a risk factor for colon cancer. Men are more likely to develop polyps than women. Often symptomless, they can be detected by a fecal blood test or by a thorough colon and rectal exam. They usually are surgically removed.

Diaphragm

- **Do belly-strengthening exercises.**
- **Avoid excessive bouncing.**

Some guys worry about their biceps. Others develop their chests. Then there's former Mr. Olympia Frank Zane. His most awesome muscle: his diaphragm.

From the tender age of 14, he'd lie back over the three-foot width of a downed tree trunk. Then he'd hoist 50 pounds up and down behind his head to expand his rib cage and strengthen his breathing muscle. Years later, he had such a strong diaphragm that he could flex it by sucking in his stomach almost to his spine. And he could stay in that pose, called the stomach vacuum in bodybuilding, for 30 seconds. The technique earned him the Mr. Olympia title three years in a row.

"It was the pose that brought the house down," says Zane, author of *Fabulously Fit Forever Expanded.*

No Time for a Break

Next to the heart, the diaphragm probably is your body's hardest-working muscle. The dome-shaped muscular sheet forms a wall between the chest and abdomen, with a few openings for tubes, nerves and blood vessels to pass through. The diaphragm's primary job: controlling your breathing.

The diaphragm is attached to the spine, the lower pairs of ribs and the lower end of the breastbone. When you breathe in, the diaphragm contracts downward into the abdomen. This causes the lungs to expand and air to get sucked in through the nose or mouth. When you breathe out, the diaphragm relaxes, expanding to its regular dome-shaped position just below the nipples. It compresses the lungs, pushing air out.

You can use your diaphragm for work besides breathing, too. It helps you bear down to get rid of urine and feces. And it helps you project your voice.

What Can Go Wrong

Generally, the diaphragm is a healthy, low-maintenance muscle. Its most common ailments are hiccups and side stitches. Less common and more serious are hernias.

• Hiccups are the result of your diaphragm having a temper tantrum. No one is exactly sure what causes them, though many fingers have been pointed at wolfing down food, slurping carbonated beverages and guzzling alcohol. When you get hiccups, your diaphragm contracts when you don't want it to. The action suddenly expands your lungs, sucking in air. But then the opening to your lungs quickly closes. So when the air hits that wall . . . *hic.*

Like a temper tantrum, hiccups usually go away by themselves within a few minutes. To stop them, you need to stop the spasm. Usually, swallowing something bitter such as a teaspoon of vinegar, drinking from the far side of a glass or being startled does the trick.

You can prevent hiccups by eating slowly, curbing carbonated beverages and alcohol and not letting creatures get in your ears. Seriously. The phrenic nerve, which gives the diaphragm its instructions, runs near the eardrum. One woman's case of hiccups was determined to have been caused by an ant in her ear.

• Hell's Angels, runners and camel riders all risk the same hazard: side stitches. Though no one knows for sure why we get these painful cramps of the diaphragm, exercise physiologist Owen Anderson, Ph.D., editor of *Running Research News*, has an idea: bouncing. Whenever you perform bouncy activities, your internal organs bounce, too. Many of these organs are attached to your diaphragm with ligaments. They pull and pull. And your diaphragm gets pooped out over the strain, says Dr. Anderson. Then you feel like you have a knife between your ribs.

Side stitches can be avoided. For one thing, don't mix eating with bouncing. Food makes your stomach heavier, increasing your chances of getting a stitch, Dr. Anderson says. Also, getting in shape usually helps ease their frequency.

For runners, breathing when the left foot hits the ground should help. Your liver, the heaviest organ, is on the right side of your body. When you breathe out on your right foot, your diaphragm is pulled up while your liver is plummeting down, creating strain. "Most of us are right-foot breathers. If you change over so that you breathe in and breathe out as your left foot strikes the ground, it will often relieve that right-side stitch," Dr. Anderson says.

Sorry, motorcyclists; we don't have much advice for you. About all you can do to avoid side stitches is search out smooth roads, Dr. Anderson says.

• Hiatal hernias occur in the diaphragm basically because the esophagus travels through, not around, the muscle on its way to the stomach. The hiatus is the opening in the diaphragm where the esophagus passes through. Sometimes the hiatus becomes enlarged, allowing stomach acid to creep upward to the esophagus and points north. This irritates the esophagus and causes a mean heartburn. Sometimes hiatal hernias need to be repaired with surgery.

You may be able to avoid surgery by losing weight and wearing nonconstrictive clothing, says Charles Itzig, M.D., staff surgeon at Schumpert Hospital in Shreveport, Louisiana. Having extra fat inside you allows your internal organs less room. This compresses your stomach and can force it up through your hiatus, which encourages food and acid to attempt to go north instead of south. Wearing tight pants and belts creates the same problem, says Dr. Itzig.

To Keep Huffing and Puffing . . .

Having a healthy, flexible and strong diaphragm improves your breathing. Starting with Frank Zane's two favorite exercises, here are some things you can do to accomplish that.

Pump iron. Lie back on a weight bench. Use both hands to lower a dumbbell behind your head as you inhale. Then lift the dumb-

The Pullover

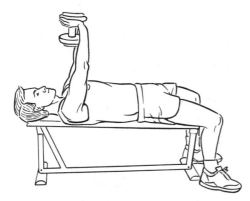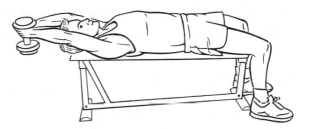

Inhale as you lower the dumbbell; exhale as you lift. This will help build up the diaphragm.

bell over your face as you exhale. Repeat. This exercise, called the pullover, is how Zane strengthened his diaphragm and expanded his rib cage.

Train it. Wait until your stomach is grumbling for food before you try this exercise. When you breathe out, use your diaphragm and abdominals to push out all of the air. Then instead of inhaling, suck in the diaphragm toward your spine. Visualize your abdominals touching your spine. You want to resemble the bodybuilding pose called the stomach vacuum, which looks just like the name sounds, Zane says. Hold the pose for as long as you can. Try to do this twice a day, gradually increasing the length of the workout. It will repress your hunger pangs for a short while, firm up your diaphragm and abdominals and make your waist look smaller, Zane says.

Do vocabulary resistance. Lie on your back and put a dictionary on your belly. When you breathe in, try to lift the dictionary. The exercise should strengthen your diaphragm, says Dr. Anderson.

Stop sucking it in. Washboard abs are glory. But what if you've never had 'em and never will? What if you have a stomach that hangs over your belt no matter how many sit-ups you do? Chances are that you compensate

by sucking in your stomach, suggests Jeffrey A. Migdow, M.D., a holistic physician and director of the Kripalu yoga teacher training program at the Kripalu Center for Yoga and Health in Lenox, Massachusetts. You may even breathe backward: Instead of pushing out your belly when you inhale, Dr. Migdow says, you may suck it in.

Look, your gut isn't like the space underneath your bed. You can't hide things there. If you can't get rid of it, the best advice we have for you is to get over it. Let it hang out. Because when you suck it in, it constricts your breathing muscle. And you won't get as much air, says Dr. Migdow.

Digestive System

- **Number of Americans who experience food poisoning each year: 24 million**
- **Percent of people who cite pizza as their favorite food to throw up: 6**
- **Distance the Guinness record holder can spit: 88 feet 5½ inches**
- **Volume of food the stomach can hold when fully distended: 1 gallon**

The Digestible Lifestyle

To keep your digestive system in top form, follow these seven suggestions.

Spread out your eating. Six small meals per day is far better than three big ones, not only for your digestive system but for your energy level as well. If that's just not possible, make your three meals smaller and eat healthy snack foods in between.

Don't get spoiled. Food poisoning is rampant in America. Usually, it's from bacteria on food. The answer? Do everything you can to keep your food free of cooties. Cook it thoroughly, wash it completely and don't leave it on the counter for more than a few minutes. Yes, put hot food directly into the fridge. The only thing at risk is your electric bill, which could go up a few pennies.

Fiberize! Fiber is undigestible plant matter. It's absolutely great for you because it cleans out your tubing and makes your stools softer. So eat plenty by filling up on lots of grains, fruits and vegetables.

Break the rules. Want spaghetti in the morning? Cereal and milk at night? Dessert before soup? Go ahead. Your body doesn't care what order food comes in; it's far more open-minded than your brain. What does matter is that you eat a good balance of food over a day's time and not too much in a single sitting.

Shut down early. Your digestive system secretes more acid at night, when your protective mechanisms are the least effective. Don't encourage it with food. The human body is designed to eat in the daytime.

Cut the fat. Not because it makes you gain weight, hurts your heart, helps cause cancer and otherwise ruins your life. From the digestive system's perspective, fat can cause the lower esophageal sphincter to relax. That can keep gastric juices bottled up in your tummy, and that hurts.

Mind your mint. Skip the after-dinner mint. Peppermint can weaken the esophageal muscles, causing heartburn.■

What Is a Stomachache?

You've just finished eating, and suddenly, your gut knots up. You spend the next 30 minutes on the toilet, sweating, cursing and hurting. A tummyache is no pleasure. But what is it?

There are three primary causes of sudden stomach pain, says Frank Lanza, M.D., gastroenterology professor at Baylor College of Medicine in Houston. The first is dyspepsia, or hyperactivity in the stomach. The second is colon cramps or spasms, which are often triggered by unwel-

come chemicals or secretions. The third is gastroesophageal reflux, a fancy name for stomach acid overflowing into your esophagus.

Often a combination of these factors is at work. If you eat an entire box of Twinkies, for example, the high fat content could stimulate your stomach to secrete more acid, causing dyspepsia. The increased stomach acid could lead your colon to spasm, or it could back up into your esophagus, causing painful heartburn.■

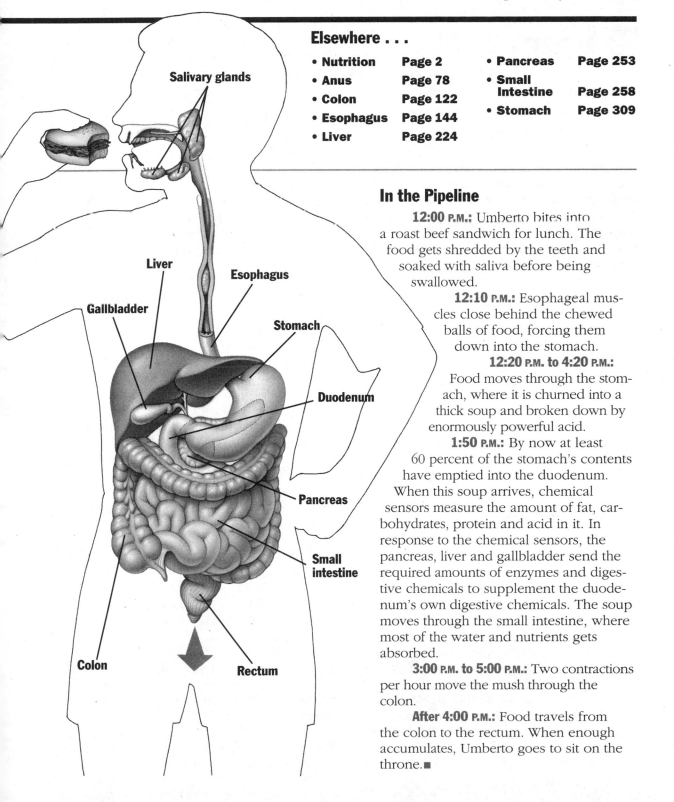

Salivary glands

Liver

Esophagus

Gallbladder

Stomach

Duodenum

Pancreas

Small intestine

Colon

Rectum

Elsewhere . . .

In the Pipeline

12:00 P.M.: Umberto bites into a roast beef sandwich for lunch. The food gets shredded by the teeth and soaked with saliva before being swallowed.

12:10 P.M.: Esophageal muscles close behind the chewed balls of food, forcing them down into the stomach.

12:20 P.M. to 4:20 P.M.: Food moves through the stomach, where it is churned into a thick soup and broken down by enormously powerful acid.

1:50 P.M.: By now at least 60 percent of the stomach's contents have emptied into the duodenum. When this soup arrives, chemical sensors measure the amount of fat, carbohydrates, protein and acid in it. In response to the chemical sensors, the pancreas, liver and gallbladder send the required amounts of enzymes and digestive chemicals to supplement the duodenum's own digestive chemicals. The soup moves through the small intestine, where most of the water and nutrients gets absorbed.

3:00 P.M. to 5:00 P.M.: Two contractions per hour move the mush through the colon.

After 4:00 P.M.: Food travels from the colon to the rectum. When enough accumulates, Umberto goes to sit on the throne.■

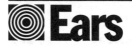 **Ears**

- **Turn down the volume.**
- **Don't poke or prod.**
- **Clean with great care.**

In the wild blue yonder of our lives, our ears are the radar system. They alert us to the approach of friends and enemies. They provide us with information—be it a half-whispered investment tip or a blaring car horn—that helps us chart a smooth flight path across our days.

The system's outer part is a pair of odd-shaped, fleshy dishes that pick up the telemetry of our noisy world and relay it to mission control. But we cannot see the truly wondrous part of the ears: the complex system of fluids, cilia and canals that not only allow hearing but help us keep our balance.

More than sensory devices, though, our ears are vessels of pleasure, allowing us to enjoy sound itself, whether it's the natural symphony of a pristine waterfall, the gut-level insistence of a favorite rock band or even the blessed sound of silence. Like sight, hearing is a sense that we should fight to keep healthy and strong.

Getting from There to Hear

Hearing starts when sound waves hit the outer ear, which collects sound and channels it to the eardrum, a fibrous circular membrane separating the outer ear from the twisting and turning caverns that form the middle ear. The eardrum vibrates in response to the sound waves and sends the signals on.

From there, the vibrations travel to three small bones called the malleus (hammer), the incus (anvil) and the stapes (stirrup), which form a chain across the middle ear. The vibrations continue on to the inner ear, where the cochlea, a snail-shaped organ that's lined with 20,000 groups of minute sensory hairs called cilia, transmits the vibrations to the brain.

In the big picture, your greatest ear worry is hearing loss. Alas, its most common cause is something you can't avoid: time. In fact, about 30 to 60 percent of people over age 60 have some kind of hearing loss, says Randy Oppenheimer, M.D., part-time clinical instructor of otolaryngology at the University of California, San Diego.

But the second most common cause of hearing loss is as obvious as a gunshot ringing through the air: loud noise. Going to rock concerts, hanging around pistol ranges, working with heavy machinery—all of these noisy activities take their toll on the cilia, says Steven D. Rauch, M.D., assistant professor of otolaryngology at Harvard Medical School. Assailing your ears with that kind of noise is like walking on the same grass over and over again, according to Dr. Rauch. For a while the grass bounces back, but constant wear eventually kills it. "Loud noise destroys the sensory cells of the inner ear," he explains. "They're brutalized by the intense vibrations, and they just wilt." So if you want to learn how to keep off the grass, get an earful of these hearing aids.

Know dangerous noise. If you're someplace so noisy that you have to shout to be heard—say, in a workshop where power tools are running, on a shooting range or even outside running a lawn mower—you're in the danger zone, says Clough Shelton, M.D., professor of otolaryngology at the University of Utah in Salt Lake City. "You should either move away from the noise or get some ear protection," says Dr. Shelton. Earplugs and earmuffs specially designed to baffle sound will work equally well. You'll find them in the gun section of most sporting goods stores.

Guidelines from the federal Occupational Safety and Health Administration say that you should wear ear protection if you're exposed to a noise level of around 80 decibels for eight hours a day. That's about what you'd hear at a symphony concert. According to the same guidelines, you should also wear ear protection if you're exposed to 85 decibels for four hours, 90 decibels for two hours or 95 decibels for one hour. These racket levels are the equivalent of a snowblower, a rock concert and a power saw, respectively.

Pick your protection. Although earmuffs are better at keeping out sound, you may not always find them practical. And in certain situations—at a concert, for instance—they completely defeat the purpose of being there. In these cases, think about wearing foam earplugs, which can at least provide some measure of protection.

"You know that old saying 'If it's too loud, you're too old?' Well, it's bull. At any concert where there's a sound system, you're going to hear the show just fine, even with earplugs in," says Roger Catlin, rock critic for the *Hartford Courant.* "I take my cue from the musicians; most of them are wearing earplugs up on stage."

Tone it down. Resist blasting your personal stereo, notes Dr. Rauch. "Keep the volume low enough that others can't hear sound coming from the headset," he says. "Otherwise, it is up too loud and could cause damage."

The Path to Healthy Ears

Although sound fairly easily finds its way through the labyrinthine depths of the ears, other items—such as foreign objects, water and harmful bacteria and viruses—don't fare as well. If you're not careful, they can stay trapped in the ears, causing all sorts of pain and discomfort and even hearing loss.

One of the most common ear problems is simple infection, the result of a virus or bacteria taking up residence in the warm, moist environment of your ear. You'll spot an infection pretty quickly: The main symptom is a head-splitting earache. You may also experience a feeling of fullness in your ear, some temporary hearing loss and even dizziness and nausea. An infection generally lasts from 24 to 48 hours, but if it persists, you may need to see your doctor for antibiotics. A bad infection can burst your eardrum, which causes the pain to stop completely but may also damage your hearing.

Other ear problems are a little more complex. Take tinnitus, a constant ringing in the ears. If you have it, you're likely to hear ringing, buzzing, whistling, hissing or clicking sounds whenever the background is quiet. Tinnitus is often caused by frequent exposure to loud noise. But it isn't just a problem in itself; it's a symptom, a possible side effect of a serious condition such as an auditory nerve tumor or Ménière's disease, an inner ear disorder. If your ears are ringing for more than a couple of days, think of it as an alarm and get yourself to your doctor.

Thankfully, the majority of ear problems are pretty temporary and pretty easy to solve. They range from earwax accumulation to air pressure buildup. Almost all ear problems can be avoided, though, with any number of simple steps.

Reach for alcohol. When water stays in your ear for too long, it can lead to an infection known as swimmer's ear. Rubbing alcohol is the perfect solution for wet ears, notes Thomas Pasic, M.D., assistant professor of otolaryngology at the University of Wisconsin–Madison. "After you swim, take an eardropper, drop the alcohol in your ears, then let it roll out. The alcohol dries up the water."

Blow it dry. Another surefire ear clearer is a blow dryer, notes Dr. Pasic. "Use a low setting—one that's comfortable. Aim the hair dryer at your ear until it's dry," he says.

Hop to it. If you get water in your ears while swimming or showering, tilt your head to one side and hop up and down on one leg as soon as you get out of the water. Then switch sides. "That's an old swimmer's trick for getting water out of the ears. It's very effective," says Charles P. Kimmelman, M.D., professor of otolaryngology at New York Medical College and attending physician at the Manhattan Eye, Ear and Throat Hospital, both in New York City.

Pass the vinegar. White vinegar is a surefire ear soother, says Dr. Oppenheimer. "White vinegar has acetic acid, which helps clear up outer ear infections," he explains. Squeeze a few drops into your ear using an eardropper, then put cotton in your ear to hold

(continued on page 136)

◎ Hearing

- **The smallest bone in your body: the stapes (stirrup), which conducts sound to the inner ear, at ⅒ inch long**
- **Number of men in every 1,000 who are hearing-impaired: 369**
- **Sound level of a whisper: about 20 decibels**
- **Sound level of a shout: about 90 decibels**
- **Sound level that could kill you: above 190 decibels**

Developing Super Hearing

To a certain extent, your ears—and your ability to hear—are like your family: You're stuck with them, no matter how much you might wish for better. But you can help keep your hearing from getting worse, and you can improve the way you listen, says Charles P. Kimmelman, M.D., professor of otolaryngology at New York Medical College and attending physician at the Manhattan Eye, Ear and Throat Hospital, both in New York City. Here are some examples to help you do just that.

Make life into a radio. At any one time, one sense tends to have your active attention while the other four fade into the background. And usually, it's your vision that has control. So to concentrate on your hearing, close your eyes. Try it the next time you're watching the tube. Pay attention to the voices; try to figure out what their inflections or the background sound effects are indicating. Next, close your eyes when you're listening to music or when you're sitting in your backyard. You'll find that you can hear far more when you concentrate on it.

Learn to isolate sounds. Rock critic Roger Catlin of the *Hartford Courant* is a proponent of closed-eye listening. He suggests trying to single out one instrument—the bass, for example—in a song and to follow only that instrument. Then you're really focusing your hearing, he says.

Give your ears a workout. Good fitness can keep your hearing strong and resilient. In a study of hearing loss, people who described themselves as highly or moderately fit suffered less hearing impairment than the least fit people. The reason? Regular exercise maintains the normal functioning of the circulatory system and ensures adequate blood flow to the inner ears, which are extremely dependent upon blood flow in order to function normally.

Take your B$_{12}$. Studies have shown that getting the Daily Value of six micrograms of vitamin B$_{12}$ might help ward off hearing loss. In one study of B vitamins, nearly half of the men who suffered hearing problems turned out to be deficient in B$_{12}$. Good sources of this vitamin include lean meats, poultry, fish, shellfish and low-fat dairy foods.

Avoid "too loud." Next time you are about to go into a concert or loud event, first tune your car radio to an all-talk station. Turn down the volume until you can just barely understand the words. Then after the event, turn on the radio to the same station and volume level. Chances are the voices that were understandable before aren't now. This is called a "temporary hearing threshold shift." Basically, it means the event's noise has overstimulated the hair cells in your inner ear, causing them to function less efficiently. Likely, your hearing will return to normal in 24 hours. But the effect can accumulate over time. The radio test is a good way to see if you are exposing yourself to noise thresholds that will hasten permanent hearing loss. ■

The Sound of Hearing

Your ears not only pick up sound, they generate it as well. This phenomenon is called spontaneous otoacoustic emission (SOAE), and your ears are doing it right now.

The noise starts when your ears first pick up sound. Delicate hair cells, called cilia, in your inner ears capture sound waves and con-vert them to nerve signals that the brain recognizes as sound. But the hair cells themselves vibrate in response to the sound they pick up, and that vibration, in turn, makes its own noise, a kind of inner ear echo. This is a good thing: Doctors say that by listening to the sound that these hair cells make, they can identify some of the hearing problems associated with these cells, which could, in turn, lead to better diagnosis of hearing loss.

But don't strain your ears trying to pick up the sound that these hair cells are making. Men give off fewer SOAEs than women; the reason why isn't clear. Also, the sound is too minute to be heard by conventional means.■

Coping with Airplane Ears

For some men, air travel is one of the perks of living in the modern world. For others, it's a fair approximation of hell, especially when their ears feel like they're about to ex-plode and all hearing becomes muffled, usually during descent of the aircraft.

This is called airplane ears, and it afflicts thousands of travelers. But the culprit isn't the airplane. It's the sudden change in air pressure and the havoc that it wreaks on your ears—or, more specifically, on your eustachian tubes, which connect the back of your throat to your middle ears, notes Anne Simons, M.D., assistant clinical professor of family and community medi-cine at the University of California, San Francisco, and co-author of *Before You Call the Doctor*.

The trick is to keep your eustachian tubes open despite the pressure change, says Dr. Simons. The best way? Yawn or chew gum.

But if those methods don't work and you don't have a sinus infection, try this for an ear-opener: Hold your nose closed, open the back of your throat as if you were yawning, bear down, then blow. That forces air into the back of your throat and through your eustachian tubes. You should feel blessed relief shortly.■

in the vinegar, instructs Dr. Oppenheimer. This treatment can be done several times a day.

Don't blow it. If you have a cold, blowing your nose too hard is a bad idea, says Anne Simons, M.D., assistant clinical professor of family and community medicine at the University of California, San Francisco, and co-author of *Before You Call the Doctor.* "You can drive bacteria-laden mucus into the middle ear," she notes.

Ease your pain. Take acetaminophen or aspirin for the discomfort of an ear infection, Dr. Simons suggests. She recommends 650 to 1,000 milligrams every four hours, but don't exceed 4,000 milligrams in 24 hours.

Deep-six the cotton swabs. These have done a lot of ear damage, and Dr. Simons doesn't advise using them. "The cotton swab is a common villain in outer ear ailments. Your ear canal is delicate; you can scrape off the skin deep enough to lose the canal's barrier to infection," she notes. "You can also push wax down inside, creating a plug in the canal that can trap water behind it."

Keeping Your Balance

As mentioned earlier, your ears are home to more than your own personal stereo system. They're also centers of balance. Deep in each inner ear you have a series of canals and fluid-coated hairs that are sensitive to gravity and acceleration as well as to the positions and movements of your head. This information is registered and sent via nerve fibers to your brain, so you always know which end is up. If your inner ears register conflicting information, such as when the cabin you're standing in is on a boat that your inner ears know is bobbing up and down, your sense of balance gets turned on its ear, and you may find yourself turning to the nearest bathroom for the old heave-ho.

Motion sickness isn't just the curse of the little kid who loses his lunch in the backseat of

---

Don't Pack the Wax

We poke, prod and probe our ears in an effort to keep them wax-free. But have you ever stopped to ask yourself why?

Earwax is actually a good thing, notes Steven D. Rauch, M.D., assistant professor of otolaryngology at Harvard Medical School. It serves as a moisturizing agent, has antibacterial properties and keeps out things such as dust, dirt and bugs, he notes.

In fact, the ear, which produces wax in glands located in the outer quarter of the inch-long ear canal, is a self-cleaning unit. So why do so many people use cotton swabs for wax control?

"The only safe thing to do with a cotton swab is clean the heads of your tape deck," Dr. Rauch says. "Using one in your ear is like muzzle-loading a cannon. You push all of the wax down inside."

But some folks' ears generate more wax or unusually hard wax. This is especially likely if your ear canals are narrow or if you're on the phone a lot. Still, you should skip the swab and try this method to prevent buildup: Fill an eyedropper with full-strength hydrogen peroxide (available in pharmacies) and put a few drops in each ear. Repeat about once a week, suggests David Zwillenberg, M.D., an otolaryngologist at Thomas Jefferson University Hospital in Philadelphia. "This keeps the wax soft, so the ears drain normally," he notes.

Or use this variation of the same method: Soak a small cotton ball in hydrogen peroxide and place it over the opening of your ear. Don't stick the cotton into your ear canal. Lie down on your side, with your other ear on a pillow. Let the liquid seep into your ear canal. Turn over and treat your other ear. Wait for five minutes, then take a shower, cupping your hand around each outer ear to guide the warm water in and rinse the peroxide out.

the car during a trip to the beach. It can happen to anyone, says Dr. Rauch. You'll recognize its onset from the classic symptoms: cold sweats, mild queasiness and light-headedness, moving right along to vomiting or dry heaves.

The more appealing alternative is to try to keep your balance system on the beam. The way to do it is to trick your inner ears into thinking you're living a balanced life, even when you're midway through the third loop on the Death Coaster. Here's how.

Get a front-row seat. When you're traveling, find a seat with a good view of what's happening, notes Dr. Rauch. In a bus or in a car, your best position is the front seat, where you can look forward out the window. If you're taking a train, be sure to take a seat that faces forward. Aboard ship, you may not be able to stay on deck the whole time, but the more you can, the better. Not only will the fresh air revive you, but it will give your brain a chance to register the rocking and swaying that your inner ears detect when you're below deck.

Make it a pressing matter. Try using an acupressure wristband, suggests Dr. Rauch. These devices, available in sporting goods stores and boating supply stores, have a plastic button that presses the inside surface of your wrist, short-circuiting motion sickness, says Dr. Rauch. If you don't have a band when you need it, you can put pressure on that point by pressing your thumb on the inside of your wrist, right about where your watchband lies.

Get ginger. Mom's old remedy of drinking ginger ale to settle a queasy stomach has some scientific basis. A number of studies have

---

Piercing Guidelines

We will not comment on whether men should or should not pierce their ears. We will not comment on whether they make a statement or what that statement may be. There are over 130 million men in America, and each has his own opinion. What you, we and everyone else must acknowledge is that plenty of men are doing it. If you're contemplating becoming one of the pierced, God-speed and more power—and these two tips—to you.

Stay south. The earlobe is fair game for piercing. But when you start adding holes farther along the outer edge of the ear, you get into cartilage territory. And you want to avoid that. "I say don't do it," says William Hendricks, M.D., a dermatologist in Asheboro, North Carolina. "There's a good chance that you can develop problems with the cartilage of your ear. You might get an infection that could become very severe." A serious infection of the cartilage can cause collapse of the ear at the infection site.

Stay light. Most men with pierced ears wear simple earrings, but there are the flamboyant among us who like to show off. Beware: A heavy wire earring can pull through the lobe and cause a split, notes Dr. Hendricks. A doctor can sew a split earlobe back together in his office in about 15 minutes, but why bother? Dr. Hendricks' advice: "You should wear lightweight earrings that don't put a lot of tension on your ears."

---

shown that powdered ginger can reduce nausea and vomiting—in some cases, even better than over-the-counter antinausea drugs. Although you'll find ginger in ginger ale and gingersnaps, if you want to fight motion sickness, you're better off buying ginger in capsules (you'll find them in most health food stores). Experts recommend taking about one gram of ginger when nausea hits.

Go over-the-counter. Your pharmacy should have any number of proven anti–motion sickness remedies. Look for the active ingredient meclizine hydrochloride on the product label, notes Dr. Oppenheimer. (One such product is Dramamine II.) "If you're going on a boat trip, take it about a half-hour to an hour beforehand," he says.

Elbows

- **Stretch surrounding muscles.**
- **Hold them near your body while working.**
- **Rest them often.**

After a grueling afternoon of twisting and turning, Anthony Foley's elbow rebelled and taught him a painful anatomy lesson that he hadn't learned in medical school.

"I was trying to put in a drain under my sidewalk. Instead of being smart and letting a professional do it, I was sticking my arm under the sidewalk and using a little hand trowel to burrow a hole in the clay. That's when it happened," says Dr. Foley, an M.D. who is assistant professor of family practice at Wright State University School of Medicine in Dayton, Ohio.

In an instant, he felt a dull ache and tenderness in his elbow that wouldn't go away. And for more than a year afterward, the joint would explode into excruciating pain whenever he lifted something even as light as a coffee cup.

That afternoon, Dr. Foley, like many weekend warriors, discovered that the elbow, which does a fine job when helping to perform routine tasks such as scratching a back and turning a doorknob, can transform into a wicked foe if it's abused.

Tennis Elbow, Anyone?

The elbow has the dual jobs of acting as a hinge (like the knee) and rotating, so you can turn your hand, wrist and forearm. If you hold your thumb and fingers on either side of one elbow and then slowly turn that arm from palm up to palm down, you might feel a portion of the joint rotating back and forth.

Although the bones of the elbow can be fractured, most injuries occur to the muscles, nerves, tendons and ligaments surrounding the joint. Most of us, for example, have experienced the shock of hitting a "funny bone." It

is neither funny nor a bone but actually a nerve that follows a groove right underneath your elbow. If you hit it just right, it sparks that strange pins-and-needles sensation in your hand and arm that jolts you like a power surge.

Occasionally, a hard blow to the elbow can cause bursitis, or swelling of the bursae, soft sacs that are filled with lubricating liquid. Bursae are located between the tendons and the bones in various joints.

Sprains, the tearing or stretching of ligaments that hold bones together, are fairly common in the elbow, particularly among children. Arthritis and tendinitis can also strike this joint. (For more information on joint problems, see page 209.)

But the most common elbow problem is the one that Dr. Foley had: tennis elbow, also known as epicondylitis. "Various conditions cause elbow pain, but basically, epicondylitis is the only problem that you see," says Pekka Mooar, M.D., assistant professor of orthopedic surgery at the Medical College of Pennsylvania and Hahnemann University School of Medicine, both in Philadelphia.

Tennis elbow causes swelling, pain and tenderness on the outside of the elbow where tendons anchor muscles to the joint. Tennis elbow is triggered by frequent and repetitive overuse of these tendons and muscles, whose full-time job is to straighten the fingers and the wrist. (A rarer form of epicondylitis known as golfer's elbow causes pain on the inside of the joint and affects the muscles and tendons that curl the fingers.)

Despite its name, tennis elbow can develop in men who have never touched a racket and who couldn't tell you the difference between Wimbledon and a Winnebago. Instead, it's usually an occupational hazard that can affect anyone from carpenters to librarians, Dr. Foley says. Hobbies such as gardening can also cause this condition.

"It doesn't have to be hard work to cause tennis elbow. It just has to be repetitive and done for a long period without a break," Dr.

Foley says. "Most household projects that we do on weekends are enough to cause tennis elbow."

Staying out of Trouble

Most elbow problems are minor, and most people who injure their elbows can treat themselves, says Richard L. Collins, M.D., an orthopedic surgeon in Scottsdale, Arizona. Here are some tips and exercises that may prevent injury or speed healing if your elbow is hurt.

Keep arm strength balanced. The best thing you can do for the elbows is to make sure that all the muscles that attach to it are not just strong but evenly balanced. Many men, for example, do lots of bicep exercises but neglect the triceps. Such muscle imbalances make you more susceptible to elbow injury.

If you're not doing so already, spend some time working on your triceps, biceps and forearms. Basic biceps curls and overhead triceps extensions, which are explained in the fitness section, ought to be enough to keep the muscles around your elbow strong and protected. Just be sure to pay attention to each muscle in equal measure.

Get closer. Whether you're tightening a screw, reaching for a book or digging in the yard, try to keep your elbows tucked in as close to your body as possible, Dr. Foley suggests. Overextending your arms while working on projects puts unwanted strain on your elbows.

Slow down. Take your time on home improvement projects such as remodeling the basement. "Basically, you can spend a year doing a project on nights and weekends, or

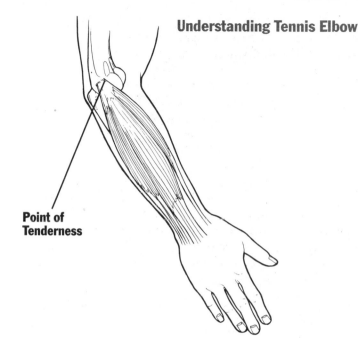

Understanding Tennis Elbow

Point of Tenderness

Tennis elbow is caused by frequent, repetitive overuse of the joint. It can be caused by most any motion—tennis is just one example. Symptoms are swelling, pain and tenderness on the outside of the elbow, where tendons connect muscles to the joint. To avoid it, take lots of breaks when doing repetitive tasks, keep good posture while typing, and strengthen the muscles that connect to the elbow.

you can do it in a week and then spend a year recovering from tennis elbow. The choice is yours," Dr. Foley says.

Take five. While working, take a 5-minute break every 30 minutes to stretch and relax your arms and elbows, Dr. Foley advises.

Sit tall in the saddle. Poor posture, particularly when sitting, increases stress on your joints and can cause elbow injuries, says William Loomis, D.O., an orthopedic physician in Spokane, Washington. Adjust your chair so that you can sit with both feet on the floor and your back straight up against the back of the chair. At work, be sure that your chair is at the proper height for your desk. You should be able to reach out and comfortably place your hands on a computer keyboard so that your wrists are flat and straight and your elbows are bent at 90-degree angles.

Reassess your game plan. If you play tennis, consider having an instructor evaluate your backhand, says Morris B. Mellion, M.D., clinical associate professor of family practice and orthopedic surgery at the University of Nebraska Medical Center and medical director of the Sports Medicine Center, both in Omaha. An improperly performed backhand, with the elbow bent instead of straight, is the stroke most likely to cause tennis elbow. At the same time, ask the instructor to check out your racket. If the racket is strung too tightly or the grip is too small for your hand, it can cause stress in your arm and eventually lead to tiny tears in elbow tendons.

Do a good turn. You can prevent a lot of elbow injuries simply by stretching the muscles surrounding the joint, Dr. Collins says. Here's one stretch to try: Make a fist and hold out your arm, with your elbow straight and your palm facing downward. Start rotating your fist through a full circle. Keeping the rotations

Hammer Turn

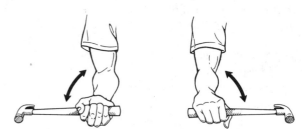

Slowly swing the hammer in an arc from one side of the wrist to the other. Do with each arm.

going, slowly bend your elbow until your fist is making circles above your shoulder. Still rotating your fist, return your arm to a full extension. You don't have to rotate your fist in any specific direction; just do what feels most comfortable to you.

Do five to ten repetitions, two or three times a day. If you feel any tightness, repeat the exercise only as often as you feel comfortable, says Dr. Collins.

Hammer it. Grasp a hammer as close to the end of the handle as possible. If you find the hammer to be too heavy this way, try moving your hand closer to the head of the hammer until you find a weight that you're comfortable with. Then slowly swing the hammer in an arc, turning your hand from palm up to palm down. Do this five to ten times with each arm, once or twice a day. This isometric exercise will not only strengthen your elbow muscles but also tone your forearm and wrist, says Thomas Rizzo, Jr., M.D., a consultant in physical medicine and rehabilitation at the Mayo Clinic Jacksonville in Florida.

Be a rubber-band man. To build elbow strength, securely fasten one end of a three-foot-

Moving Wrist Stretch

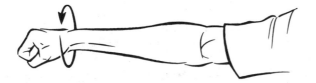

A. With your elbow straight out and palm down, start rotating your fist through a full circle.

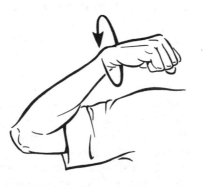

B. With the wrist still rotating, slowly bend your elbow until your fist is above your shoulder. Slowly return your arm to the starting position, rotating your wrist the whole time.

long piece of sports tubing (available in many sporting good stores) to the doorknob of a closed door, then sit in a chair facing away from the door. With the other end wrapped around your fist, bend your elbow and hold it at eye level. Then straighten your elbow as shown.

Rubber-Band Stretches

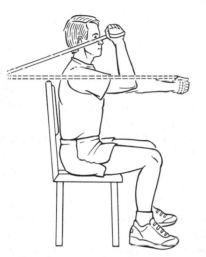

A. Fasten a three-foot piece of sports tubing to a doorknob and sit in a chair facing away from the door. Wrap the free end of the tubing around your fist, then bend and straighten your elbow at eye level.

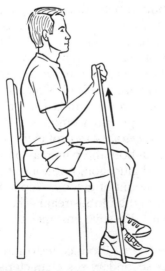

B. Place one end of the tubing under your foot and wrap the other end around your fist. Curl up your arm as far as possible.

Next, place the tubing under your foot and wrap the other end around your fist. Curl up your arm as far as possible, then lower slowly.

Once a day, do 25 repetitions of each exercise with each arm. Rest for a couple of minutes, then repeat the sequence two more times, says Mary Ann Towne, licensed physical therapist and director of rehabilitation and wellness services at the Cleveland Clinic Florida in Fort Lauderdale.

Take away the pain. If your elbow is sore but you haven't received a hard blow or fallen on the joint, loosely wrap it with an elastic bandage. Put several ice cubes into a plastic sandwich bag and apply the bag to the sore area for 25 minutes three times a day, Dr. Mellion says. (Be sure to lay the ice over the bandage or a towel to prevent skin damage.) For pain, take one 220-milligram tablet of naproxen sodium (Aleve) or two 200-milligram tablets of ibuprofen. Also, be sure to rest and to avoid the activity that you suspect caused the problem until your elbow feels better. If the soreness or swelling does not subside in a week, see your doctor.

If your injury is caused by a fall or hard blow and your elbow is swollen and painful, see your doctor immediately, Dr. Loomis advises.

Roll with the blow. Most people tend to stick their arms straight out when they fall. But that's a terrific way to injure your elbows and wrists. There's a better way, but it takes practice. The idea is to tuck your chin in to your chest and as you fall, to roll over your shoulder. It's how professional cyclists teach themselves to fall. If you cycle or skate a lot, or do any activity in which you fall regularly, practice somersaults and tumbling drills to break yourself of the stiff-arm-out falling instinct.

Don't lock yourself out. When lifting weights, it's tempting to lock your elbows at the apex of the lift, offering your muscles a brief rest. But it's a rest you're enjoying at the expense of your elbows. They're not designed like a deck chair—built to unfold, lock out and bear heavy weights. Extend your arms while lifting, but don't lock your elbows.

Endocrine System

- **Number of adults needed to make a pound of endocrine tissue: 4**
- **Number of hormone receptors on each receiving cell: up to 100,000**
- **Concentration of hormones in your blood: about 1 picogram of hormones per milliliter of blood (a picogram is one-trillionth of a gram)**

It's a Hormone Thing

Compared with the heart, liver or brain, the organs that produce hormones are rather small and nondescript. Yet these organs, collectively called the endocrine system, control virtually every response in your body's repertoire, from telling your heart to beat faster to putting more tension in a blood vessel.

The word *endocrine* gives a clue to the system's functions: *Endo-* means "within," and *-crine* means "secrete." The organs of the endocrine system, called glands, secrete hormones into the bloodstream. (In contrast, exocrine glands secrete substances into the gastrointestinal tract or urinary tract or to the outside of the body, as sweat glands do.)

Hormones are chemical messengers that tell individual cells what to do. Every second of every day, there's a veritable blizzard of hormones in your bloodstream, each targeting a certain organ and facilitating or inhibiting a certain response.

Thyroid hormones, for example, speed your body's metabolism. Growth hormone stimulates bone growth and muscle mass. A surge of insulin allows your cells to burn sugar. It's a never-ending process. Without hormones, your cells couldn't function, and you would die.

Hormones are extraordinarily potent. Because of a process called amplification, a single molecule of hormone can affect a number of processes and cells, and the receptor on a cell is capable of inciting multiple reactions. A little hormone goes a very long way.

Among the major endocrine glands in the body:

Pituitary. Called the master gland, it produces hormones that act directly on other glands, which, in turn, release hormones of their own to get things done.

Pineal. A tiny gland in the head, it releases melatonin and other hormones. It helps control the body's natural rhythms, including sleep cycles.

Hypothalamus. Regulates the body's water balance and plays a key role in body temperature.

Thyroid. Plays a key role in regulating the body's metabolism. Affects body temperature, oxygen consumption, blood pressure and more.

Parathyroid. Consisting of four tiny glands buried behind the thyroid gland, the parathyroid controls calcium balance.

Adrenal. Perched atop the kidneys, this pair of glands produces a variety of steroid hormones that regulate growth and metabolism and the body's response to stress. The adrenal glands also produce certain sex-specific hormones.

Pancreas. Islands of cells scattered throughout the pancreas produce insulin and glucagon, hormones that regulate the amount of glucose (blood sugar) in cells and in the bloodstream. The pancreas also contributes digestive enzymes to the intestinal tract.

Testicles. Produce testosterone, which regulates secondary sex characteristics such as facial hair and muscle growth and helps fuel the sex drive. ■

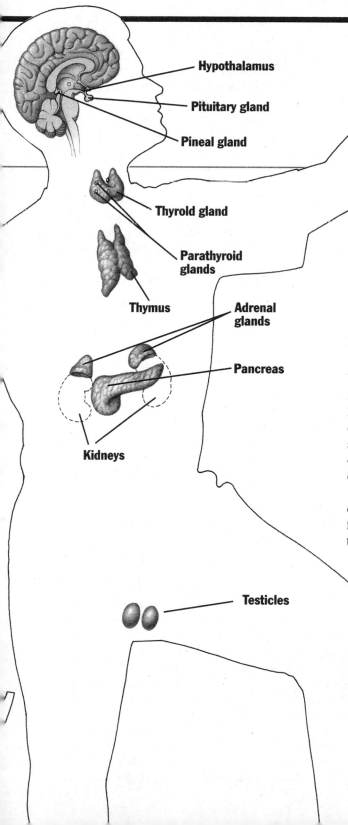

Hypothalamus

Pituitary gland

Pineal gland

Thyroid gland

Parathyroid glands

Thymus

Adrenal glands

Pancreas

Kidneys

Testicles

Elsewhere . . .

- **Adrenal Glands   Page 75**
- **Pancreas   Page 253**
- **Testicles   Page 323**
- **Thyroid   Page 328**

Inside Protection

Since the endocrine system regulates nearly every vital body process, you want to keep it healthy. Here's what Lila A. Wallis, M.D., clinical professor of medicine at Cornell University Medical College in New York City, advises.

Drink lightly. Alcohol in large amounts can affect the adrenal glands, impairing the production of testosterone.

Keep your weight down. There's a direct link between obesity and the onset of Type II (non-insulin-dependent) diabetes, in which the body has a reduced ability to utilize insulin, a pancreatic hormone. Obesity also disturbs the balance of androgenic (male) hormones, which can probably increase the risk of prostate and other hormone-related cancers.

Stay fit. Getting regular exercise has beneficial effects on a variety of endocrine system functions. Exercise also helps lower LDL cholesterol (the bad kind), the level of which is partly controlled by the action of testosterone. Finally, regular exercise can help keep your weight down, which, in turn, can help keep insulin working well.

Get plenty of sleep. Interrupted or inadequate sleep impairs your hormonal variations. Getting a steady amount of sleep should be your goal.

Keep stress under control. It can disrupt the hypothalamus, pituitary and adrenal glands, causing increased hormone production which can, in turn, have a direct negative impact on your health.■

⬇ Esophagus

- **Eat slowly and moderately.**
- **Don't lie down right after eating.**

Compared with the sophisticated feats that other body parts accomplish, the job that the esophagus has is simple: It transports everything you eat and drink from your throat to your stomach. Period. No digestive activities take place here. The esophagus is merely the digestive system's shipping department, a 10- to 12-inch corridor that can expand to up to 4 inches in diameter to accommodate bites of Herculean proportions—though the truly wise man will not test its limits.

Contrary to logic, gravity does not aid the flow of food through the esophagus. You could hang from your feet, and that whole enchilada would still make its way down. The esophagus is—don't choke on this term—musculomembranous, meaning that it's lined with muscles that undulate like a series of waves, enabling solids and liquids to surf their way through.

Don't Take It Lying Down

There are a few do's and don'ts that will help you and your esophagus maintain a long-term, healthy relationship.

One don't: Don't swallow javelins. Besides the fact that they don't taste that good, even the flexible esophagus has its limits. Sharp objects may leave scars in the lining of your esophagus, which could cause complications down the road. One such complication is globus hystericus, an injury whose very name suggests how annoying a persistent lump or lesion in the esophagus can feel.

One do: Do become friendly with a fellow nicknamed LES. That's the medical acronym for lower esophageal sphincter, the ring of muscle at the lower end of the esophagus that guards the passageway to the stomach.

The efficiency of this muscle is critical because the pressure in the stomach is normally higher than the pressure in the esophagus. When food reaches LES on the way to the stomach, the sphincter pops open, lets the food pass and then squeezes closed. But if LES loosens or relaxes, the acidic contents of the stomach back up into the esophagus. The sensitive mucous membrane that lines the walls of the esophagus does not like this stuff and lets you know as much by giving you what doctors call gastro-esophageal reflux, or acid indigestion. We know it most commonly as heartburn.

Heartburn is, in fact, a misnomer. It happens not in the heart or stomach but in the esophagus. The pain is felt in the chest, near the breastbone, because the esophagus passes that region en route to the stomach. Here's how to avoid the problem.

Don't overeat. If your stomach were a tank of gas, you wouldn't be surprised if you topped it off and some spilled out. Same principle here. Allow your stomach to do its thing before refueling. "Consider eating less but more often," suggests William B. Ruderman, M.D., a gastroenterologist on staff at the Orlando Regional Medical Center in Florida.

Don't lie down right after eating. In this case, gravity does take its toll. If you were to turn a full bottle of milk on its side, you would expect some spillage. Again, same idea. Wait a couple of hours to let the food settle and to let digestion begin to help move the food from your stomach to other parts of your body. Better yet, says William Ravich, M.D., clinical director in the Division of Gastroenterology at Johns Hopkins Hospital in Baltimore, "let gravity help things move south. If you lie down too soon, south becomes east, and that's not the direction you want the food to go."

Heads up. If nighttime reflux is a problem, consider putting six-inch blocks under the legs at the head of your bed. It's better than elevating your head with pillows, a strategy that Dr. Ruderman says actually makes leakage into your esophagus worse by bending you at the waist and compressing your stomach.

Don't eat too fast. That overworked LES

may not be able to keep up with the food you're scarfing down. Slow down and let those bites enjoy the scenery. "The faster you eat, the more you eat, and the more air you swallow," according to Dr. Ravich, "all of which increases the propensity to reflux."

Respect the offenders. Each body reacts differently to different foods, so don't think that there's something wrong if your friend can dive into a spicy Thai dish without repercussions while it repulses your digestive system. But doctors tell people prone to heartburn to avoid caffeine, cigarettes, fatty and fried foods, foods high in citrus (such as tomatoes, oranges and lemons), chocolate and mint.

Avoid other instigators. Watch out for especially hot foods, such as boiling water and hot potatoes. Also watch out for stress, which can trigger a bout. "Some medications, such as aspirin and ibuprofen, instigate it, especially if they get caught in the esophagus," says Malcolm Robinson, M.D., gastroenterologist at the University of Oklahoma Health Sciences Center and medical director of the Oklahoma Foundation for Digestive Research, both in Oklahoma City.

Weight lifters who put too much strain on the abdominal region also suffer symptoms. So do pregnant women, of whom we suspect you're not one.

Chew gum. The extra saliva created by the jaw action produces additional bicarbonate (one of the active ingredients in antacids), which neutralizes acid, suggests C. James Scheurich, M.D., a gastroenterologist at Pacific Communities Hospital in Newport, Oregon. Saliva also produces other proteins that provide a protective lining for the esophagus.

How Do You Spell Relief?

Ever wonder why they show so many antacid commercials during football games? The answer should come to you faster than you can spell *r-e-l-i-e-f*. You and your sedentary friends are an antacid ad agency's dream focus group, heartburns waiting to happen.

Most over-the-counter remedies for heartburn, acid indigestion, sour stomach and gas—household names such as Mylanta, Maalox, Di-Gel, Riopan, Gaviscon, Tums and Rolaids—contain basically the same acid-neutralizing agents. These are simple compounds that you learned about in high school chemistry: sodium bicarbonate, calcium carbonate, aluminum hydroxide and magnesium hydroxide (also called milk of magnesia). All of these products promote fast relief, but the relief is only temporary.

Dr. Robinson recommends antacids with both calcium and magnesium as active ingredients. He discourages sodium, including plain baking soda, especially for those who shouldn't have salt in their diets. He is also skeptical of aluminum, which can cause diarrhea. He recommends chewing tablets over taking capsules or liquids. "Chewing mixes saliva with the medicine, which keeps it in the esophagus longer, and that's where you want it," adds Dr. Robinson.

While the labels on most of these products suggest that you don't take more than eight doses a day for more than two weeks, "there's no risk in taking more," advises Dr. Robinson. "But if you feel you need these products that much, it's an indication that your condition is sufficiently acute that you should see your doctor."

Location of Heartburn Pain

Heartburn pain is a burning sensation that originates in the esophagus and can radiate to the upper chest, neck and arms. Because these symptoms are so similar to those of a heart attack, you should see a doctor if your chest pain is sudden and severe or if you consistently suffer from heartburn pain.

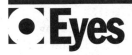Eyes

- **Don't blast them with too much light.**
- **Keep them moist and moving.**
- **Quit rubbing.**

Superman has it made. He never has to worry about making his connecting flight; he doesn't have to set foot in a gym; he can jump Lois Lane in a single bound.

But what you really have to envy is that super vision of his. Think about it: If you had telescopic vision, you could see trouble coming miles away. With the sharp glare of heat vision, you could burn your enemies and melt the hearts of women everywhere. And let's face it: What red-blooded American male couldn't make at least some use of x-ray vision?

Meanwhile, back in reality, we full-time Clark Kents would all be grateful if we could just read the newspaper without squinting, or have good-enough peripheral vision to see the idiot driver who's about to cut in from the next lane, or be able to put off buying those bifocals for one more year. Well, the way to do it is to keep our eyes clear and sharp. We get almost 90 percent of all sensory input through sight. That's a big responsibility, and the eyes have it. But they can also lose it if we don't follow a few simple steps.

Now that's not to say you can cure nearsightedness or exercise your eyeballs to the point where the women's locker room door becomes transparent. To a certain degree, much of your visual ability is genetically predetermined. If you're innately near- or farsighted, you probably needed corrective lenses by the time you reached puberty and are now reading this through a pair of glasses or contact lenses. Those of you who escaped into adulthood with 20/20 vision didn't make a clean getaway, however. As you get older, your eyeballs lose some of their focusing ability, meaning that you'll be seeing less and less. But no matter how good or how bad your eyesight is right now, you can still do things to make your eyesight better or, at minimum, to keep it stable. It won't take a heroic effort, either.

A Look behind the Lens

One of the great ironies of the eyes is that they can look at just about everything except themselves. Even when you look in a mirror, you're glimpsing a mere fraction of the highly technical equipment that allows you to open your windows on the world.

"People tend to think of the eyes as a static camera. You look at something and—click—take a picture. But there's much more to vision than that," says Paul M. Planer, O.D., president of the International Academy of Sports Vision in Harrisburg, Pennsylvania, and communications chairman of the National Eye Research Foundation in Chicago.

It all begins with muscles—a set of really strong muscles, in fact. They're attached to the outer layer of each eyeball and to the bone that forms each eye socket. When something draws your attention—say, a pop fly or a swishing skirt—these super-strong, super-fast muscles instantly steer your orbs in that direction. Coordination of these mighty eyeball rollers is entirely controlled by your brain. You're constantly moving these muscles, and your eyes, even when you think you're focusing intently on one spot.

Once you've locked onto an object, light waves bounce off that object and hit you right in your eyes. In each eye, the light passes through the cornea, the transparent membrane that curves around the front of the eyeball. The light then continues through the pupil, which is the black circle at the center of the iris. Here the eye muscles act like a tiny corps of press photographers, constantly making minute adjustments in the shape of the lens. With these adjustments, the light carrying the image is projected against the curved back wall of the eye (the retina) like a movie. Meanwhile, the pupil reacts to light intensity by expanding or contracting, adjusted by the iris that surrounds it.

The retina is the big-screen television in this multimedia system. It's a light-sensitive layer of membrane with two kinds of specialized nerve cells: rods and cones. Rods are sensitive to the dimmest light, picking up all of the dashes of color from the world around you. In bright light, the cones come into play, helping the rods do their image-processing work. Both rods and cones convert light energy into nerve impulses, which are conveyed back along the optic nerve, the cable hookup that leads to your brain.

This whole process occurs at a speed that makes the blink of an eye seem like slow motion. When light hits the rods and cones, the visual impulse, in the form of nerve energy, zooms from the eye into the brain at a speed of 423 miles per hour. That impulse first reaches the back part of the brain, where the shapes of objects and the spatial organization of a scene are interpreted. Then other parts of the brain do some further visual processing, and voilà! What you get is what you see.

The Villains of Vision

With something as sophisticated as vision rolling around in our imperfect heads, it's a wonder that our eyesight doesn't go on the blink more often. But in fact, our bodies are quite proficient at protecting our eyes. Tears wash out foreign objects and harmful bacteria. That powerful system of muscles and sockets protects our delicate orbs from impact and injury. And our bodies are constantly adjusting internal pressure on our eyeballs, keeping our vision at the best possible level.

But as with any other bodily system, all of the aspects of sight are subject to the ravages of time and abuse. As you get older, for example, the lenses of your eyes naturally get harder, which, in turn, makes it harder for you to focus on close objects. This all-too-common condition is known as presbyopia. But like most men, you won't think anything has happened to your eyes. "Patients come in and say 'Doctor, my arms aren't long enough anymore,' " says Mary Gilbert Lawrence, M.D., a Robert Wood Johnson clinical scholar at Yale University School of Medicine.

You may also begin to notice that your visual acuity just isn't what it used to be. You lose sight of the golf ball just seconds after you hit it. It's not so easy to pick your way down the hall to the refrigerator in the middle of the night. Worst of all, you're finding it harder to react to traffic on the
(continued on page 150)

The Parts of the Eye

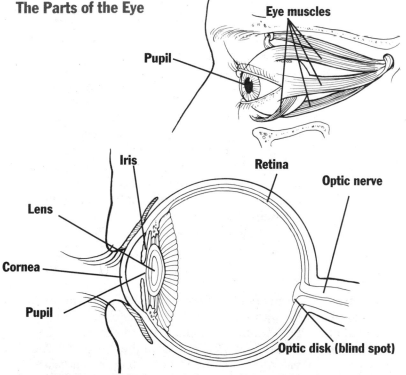

The eyeball is a mechanical wonder, the way it focuses light and converts images to nerve impulses. But just as vital are the many small but strong muscles that constantly and near instantly focus and direct the eyeball. Proper eye care focuses on both parts of the vision system.

◉Sight

- **Number of colors that the human eye is capable of distinguishing: 10 million**
- **First contact lenses: designed by Leonardo da Vinci in 1508**
- **Percent of total sensory input that we get from our eyes: 90**

Setting Your Sights Higher

Want to snag that pop fly, read road signs more quickly, catch the expression of the person beside you? To do these things, says Paul M. Planer, O.D., president of the International Academy of Sports Vision in Harrisburg, Pennsylvania, and communications chairman of the National Eye Research Foundation in Chicago, you need to practice, practice, practice at developing all of your visual abilities. Here's how.

Bob and weave. If you're trying to focus on a moving target, be it a pop fly that's coming at you or a clay pigeon that's moving away, take a moment to look at it from more than one angle. "Bob your head around; look at the target from a couple of different perspectives. Think of the owl. He's a great hunter because he's constantly moving his head, looking from every angle to get a precise fix on his prey," says Merrill Allen, O.D., Ph.D., professor of optometry at Indiana University in Bloomington.

Do focus drills. Try to focus on ten different objects in ten seconds by scanning around the room, says Dr. Planer. Then try to name the objects in the order you saw them. This will improve your eyes' ability to work together and to shift more rapidly. This skill will help you better remember that there's someone on second base or that two linemen are to your right.

Run a fine-print sprint. For another great focusing exercise, tack a page of newsprint to a wall at work, about eight feet from where you sit. Stop what you're doing every five to ten minutes and look at the newspaper. Bring the headline into focus, then look back at your work. Do this drill about five times, then get back to work, says Dr. Allen.

Be a better batter. You can improve your night vision in the blink of an eye—literally, says Dr. Allen. Simply bat your eyelids as many times as you can in a few seconds. "This stimulates your eyes and helps them adjust to darkness more quickly," he explains.

Get on track. To sharpen your ability to track a moving object, play catch with a friend, using a ball or beanbag marked with letters and numbers. As it comes toward you, call out the last letter or number you see before you catch it. Just toss the ball or beanbag slowly enough, without too much spin, so your friend has time to see the writing, says Dr. Allen.■

Warning Sights

Your eyes can do more than help you appreciate a beautiful woman, admire a sunset or put the wood to a baseball. They have their own built-in warning system, too. Here's what it means if you notice any of the following.

Seeing spots. Has your vision suddenly been invaded by what look like tiny black gnats or squiggly lines that others can't see? Usually, they're nothing to worry about—just harmless bits of your eyeball's inner fluid floating into view, says Merrill Allen, O.D., Ph.D., professor of optometry at Indiana University in Bloomington. Doctors call them floaters. The older you get, the more common floaters are. Nearsighted guys also get them more often. The spots go away on their own in time, but you can try moving your eyes up and down rapidly. That stirs up the eyeball fluid, causing the floaters to settle outside your line of vision.

Discharge. Sometimes when you wake up, your eyes have this yellow crust that practically seals them shut. In most cases, awakening with oozy, red-rimmed eyes means that they have been invaded by bacteria, sometimes due to oily skin. It is usually not serious. Degunk your eyes with a warm washcloth, then dip a cotton ball in a solution of one-half teaspoon of salt dissolved in one teaspoon of warm water and rub it along your lash lines, says Dr. Allen.

Another type of discharge—thinner, clear, noncrusty—indicates a cold, an allergy, a virus, dryness or an eyelash touching your eyeball. Again, clean your eyes and take care of the underlying cause.

Slightly blurred vision accompanied by a scratching sensation. If you can't see any obvious foreign object, chances are that you have a small scratch on the surface of your eyeball. If your own tears aren't soothing enough, use a couple of drops of an over-the-counter eye lubricant such as Refresh. Do not rub your eye or stick your finger in it; that will only make the problem worse. If the discomfort lasts for more than a couple of days, or if it's so severe you can't keep your eye open, see a doctor.

Double vision. Unless you've been drinking to excess, take blurred or double vision very seriously. Either could be a warning sign of cataracts, a concussion, a stroke or even certain types of cancer. Consult your physician.

Blind spots or flashes of light. If you develop any blind spots in your vision or notice streaky flashes of light, see your doctor immediately. These are common symptoms of a detached retina, the part of the eye that is sensitive to light. If the problem is caught early, the retina, which is usually damaged by an injury, can be reattached, and there's a good chance that your vision will return to normal. ∎

Great Moments in Sports Vision

- Baseball legend Ted Williams claimed that he could see the spin a pitcher put on a ball, which helped him determine exactly where to aim his bat. To prove it to a skeptical umpire, Williams, then 54 years old and managing the Washington Senators, coated his bat with pine tar and stepped up to the plate. With each pitch, he called out where he had hit the ball: along one seam, one-quarter inch above one seam and so on. When fielders recovered the balls, they checked to see where the bat had left its pine-tar marks. In five of seven hits, Williams called each one exactly right.

- When writer John McPhee was profiling basketball star Bill Bradley for his book *A Sense of Where You Are*, McPhee was so impressed with Bradley's peripheral vision that he coaxed Bradley to get it measured by an ophthalmologist. According to conventional measurements, the most anyone should be able to see while looking straight ahead is 180 degrees on the horizontal plane. Bradley's peripheral vision measured at 195 degrees. ∎

roads. You're becoming one of those trawling old guys you used to blow past at 80 miles an hour.

There are other conditions to keep an eye out for, too.

Pinkeye. One of the most common but least harmful eye troubles is conjunctivitis, or pinkeye. You can get it a few different ways: bacteria from dirty contact lenses (keep 'em clean with plenty of saline, boys), a viral infection from someone else or severe allergies. If you have it, you'll notice redness, discharge and a gritty feeling in your eye. Pinkeye won't blind you; it just feels that way. With the help of antibiotic eyedrops (your doctor can prescribe them), you can ditch the infection in about 72 hours.

Glaucoma. This is far more insidious and dangerous to your vision, and yet half of the three million Americans who have it don't even know it. Glaucoma often is an inherited disease, usually striking people over age 40. It results when too much fluid builds up in the eye, putting excessive pressure on the optic nerve. Because this buildup of pressure rarely causes symptoms at first, it's usually detected only through an eye exam. Your doctor will check your eye pressure; if it's high, he'll probably recommend regular treatment with eyedrops to lower it.

Cataracts. A cataract is a partial or complete clouding of the lens of the eye, the result of an eye injury, exposure to too much sunlight or one of a number of other factors. About 23 percent of the population will develop cataracts between the ages of 65 and 74;

nearly half of us will have cataracts after age 74. Like glaucoma, a cataract is hard to spot without a doctor's help. You'll first notice a cataract when your vision starts to get blurry around the edges; those edges will start closing in over time. Luckily, most cataracts can be removed, and vision can be restored, with a fairly routine surgical procedure that involves cutting open the eye and essentially removing the cataract.

Achieving the Vision Thing

If all of this makes it seem like you have nothing good to look forward to, think again.

Shady Dealings

It is rare for a health aid to make a strong fashion statement as well. Then there are sunglasses.

"It is absolutely a good idea to wear them. Never mind that they help you see better in bright light; they can also help prevent eye problems such as cataracts," says Mitchell Friedlaender, M.D., an eye surgeon at Scripps Clinic and Research Foundation in La Jolla, California.

But which shades give your eyes the most protection—the Wayfarers or the wraparounds that make you look like the Terminator? We got our experts to compose a quick checklist, so you can have it made in your shades.

• UV coating: The whole point of sunglasses as a form of eye protection is to screen out ultraviolet (UV) radiation from the sun. That's what causes blinding problems such as cataracts, says Dr. Friedlaender. So look for sunglasses with a label that says the lenses have UV coating or protection.

• Color: Although the tint of the lenses has little to do with preventing cataracts, certain colored lenses can distort colors, which puts a strain on the eyes. Stick with gray lenses, since they distort colors the least, says Mary Gilbert Lawrence, M.D., a Robert Wood Johnson clinical scholar at Yale University School of Medicine.

• Eye coverage: UV radiation doesn't just come down; it can come in at the sides, too. So to ensure that your eyes have the best possible protection, choose a pair of sunglasses that wrap around the sides of your eyes a little bit. "Not everyone likes the way this style looks, but it does offer the best protection," says Dr. Friedlander.

"So many people think that good vision, and all of its benefits and privileges, is just one of those things that they're going to have to give up as they get older. It doesn't have to be," says Merrill Allen, O.D., Ph.D., professor of optometry at Indiana University in Bloomington, who has studied the effects of aging on eyesight. "There are so many things you can do to keep your vision strong and clear. And the sooner you start doing them, the longer you'll have your good eyesight." Get an eyeful of these tips.

Pull down the shades. Because years of unprotected exposure to ultraviolet light has been shown to cause cataracts, it's a good idea to wear sunglasses outside, says Dr. Lawrence. Plus wearing sunglasses during the day will improve your night vision. "If you don't wear sunglasses, you'll expose your eyes to too much glare, which will blur your vision and keep your eyes from performing better in low-light situations," says Dr. Allen.

Don't let smoke get in your eyes. The pernicious leaf that's behind so many other health problems also contributes to cataract development, notes William Christen, M.D., instructor in the Division of Preventative Medicine of Harvard Medical School at Brigham and Women's Hospital in Boston. "It's not clear exactly why, but one possibility is that cigarettes decrease blood levels of nutrients that maintain lens transparency," he says.

Dr. Christen points to the results of one study that involved 371 participants. The study showed that people who smoked 20 or more cigarettes per day had about twice the risk of cataracts of people who had never smoked.

Peel an orange. Eating fruits and vegetables containing antioxidants such as vitamins C and E and beta-carotene may help slow cataract development, says Dr. Christen. Fruits such as strawberries and cantaloupe are rich in vitamin C, while yellow and orange fruits and vegetables are good sources of beta-carotene. Almonds, peanut butter and shrimp are high in vitamin E.

Blink more. When you blink, you're squeezing tears across the surface of your eyeballs, keeping them clear and moist. And although you already blink involuntarily several thousand times a day, you could benefit from doing it even more. "Blinking rapidly stimulates the eyes and helps them focus faster and adjust to darkness more quickly," says Dr. Allen. "So if you want to see better when you go into a dark room, for example, first blink as many times as you can in the space of a couple of seconds."

Don't rub 'em out. When allergy season or an errant speck of dust strikes, it feels as if you were walking around with splinters sticking in your eyeballs. They're sore and they itch. And as with any itch, you want to scratch it, in this case by rubbing your eyes.

But the rub of rubbing is that you could cause more of the problem that you're trying to relieve. "If you rub your eye when you have a foreign object in it—pollen or an eyelash, for example—you could scratch the lens," says Mitchell Friedlaender, M.D., an eye surgeon at Scripps Clinic and Research Foundation in La Jolla, California. You think a foreign object is painful? A scratch is ten times worse.

Should you scratch your eye, take comfort in the fact that it will heal quickly. Meanwhile, you can soothe the savage eye by using an over-the-counter eye lubricant such as Refresh and by applying a hot, wet washcloth. The heat speeds healing, says Dr. Allen.

Avoid squint stints. In your effort to avoid finally buying those bifocals so that you can read the paper, you may have noticed that squinting helps you focus on the fine print, especially in dim light. Contrary to what Mom might have told you, squinting—and reading in dim light, for that matter—won't really hurt your vision. But it can certainly wear you out.

"Squinting once in a while is fine, and it's certainly a natural protective reaction to bright light. But you don't want to do it for hours at a time," says Dr. Allen. "It's not so much that it damages your eyesight, but you can suffer temporary eyestrain. Your eyes feel sore and bleary, and you give yourself a good headache."

Make a safety play. If you play any contact sport regularly—yes, even a pickup game of basketball in the driveway with your kid—get yourself a good pair of safety glasses, the kind that fit snugly around your head and cover the front and sides of your eyes.

"It's one of the most common sports injuries: getting your cornea scratched by someone else as he's diving for the ball," says Dr. Planer. Although most of these injuries are minor, they're mighty painful. And some blows to the eye can cause permanent loss of vision.

If you don't normally wear eyeglasses, you can usually pick up a good pair of clear sports goggles in any sporting goods store. "And if you do wear glasses, it's worth the extra money to get a pair of prescription goggles," says Dr. Planer. And don't give us the excuse that they look stupid. "They're not stupid; they're the mark of a serious athlete. Look at Kareem and Horace Grant. No one says that they look dumb in their goggles," points out Dr. Planer.

Expand your horizons. Dr. Planer adds that 90 percent of having super vision depends on seeing as much as possible as well as possible. With this in mind, you can concentrate on improving your peripheral vision. "When he played basketball, Bill Bradley used to walk down the street, looking straight ahead, and ask himself what he could see on either side of him. You can do that, too. And the more you concentrate on exactly what it is that your eyes are taking in, the more you'll see, even at the periphery of your sight," Dr. Planer says.

Get your eyes checked. Finally, if you have good vision and no history of eye prob-

lems, one of the simplest ways to stay bright-eyed is to get an eye examination at least every three years, reminds Dr. Friedlaender.

On-the-Job Straining

If you're among the men who do the 9-to-5-or-longer daily grind, you may have noticed that most eye problems seem to flare up right there in the office, while you're staring at the computer screen. Computers may be the wonder of the age, but they're hell on the eyeballs. If you're suffering from watery, red eyes and blurry vision either at a distance or up close, chances are that you're feeling blinded by technology.

Experts say that computer-related eyestrain may lead to duller vision after years of

---

Toss Out Your Glasses for Good

Thanks to a revolutionary operation called radial keratotomy, contact lenses and glasses aren't the only answer for folks with faltering eyesight.

Since nearsightedness occurs when the eye is too long, the cornea is too steep or the lens can't relax enough to focus distant images, glasses and contacts won't correct the underlying cause of nearsightedness. But surgery can actually correct the shape of the eye. A surgeon cuts into the periphery of the cornea, which changes the focus by flattening the cornea out a bit.

Ninety percent of those who have the surgery don't need glasses anymore, says Herbert Kaufman, M.D., chief of the Louisiana State University Eye Center in New Orleans. "There might be some glare at night, but it's a very satisfactory procedure," he says. Some 200,000 radial keratotomies have been performed in the United States.

This operation can also be done with an excimer laser, which is so precise that it can cut a cell in half. "In 20 seconds, you'll never need glasses again," notes Dr. Kaufman. "It removes a little tissue from the top of the dome of the cornea and changes the shape, like grinding a lens in the front of the eye."

Though radial keratotomy is still considered experimental in the United States, it's widely used in Europe and Canada.

exposure. But you can screen out your computer screen's harmful effects right now by following these simple steps.

Dim the lights. Bright fluorescent light bounces off the computer screen in the form of glare, says Jeffrey Anshel, O.D., an optometrist in Del Mar, California, and author of *Healthy Eyes, Better Vision*. To see if the lighting in your office is too harsh, try this test: Shade your eyes with your hand as if you were looking over the horizon, then look at your screen. If your eyes feel better being shielded, the light is too bright.

Remember that paperwork reflects light, so you need brighter illumination for that than for computer work, which emits light. For paperwork, Dr. Anshel recommends a task light—

Sighting Up Your Computer

Your eyes should be 20 to 28 inches from your computer screen. The center of your screen should be 4 to 9 inches below your eyes, so you look slightly downward at the monitor.

that is, an ordinary desk lamp with an incandescent bulb—on your desk.

Keep your distance. The best distance from a computer screen is between 20 and 28 inches, says James Sheedy, O.D., Ph.D., clinical professor of optometry at the University of California, Berkeley.

Peer down. "Your eyes work most efficiently looking downward," notes Dr. Sheedy. The center of the screen should be four to nine inches below your eyes, so there's a 10- to 15-degree downward viewing angle when you're looking at the screen. "Anything higher than that is too high," says Dr. Sheedy.

Take a quick vacation. Perhaps the best way to prevent eyestrain is to simply look away from the screen every five to ten minutes, says Dr. Lawrence. "Hang a picture on your wall of something with an ocean or a lake and look at it every now and then," she says. "This helps relax your eyes when they're doing a lot of prolonged close-up work."

Be color-conscious. It's better to have black print on a white background than vice versa, notes Dr. Sheedy. "You want fairly equal brightness. With white on black, you're looking into a black hole that doesn't blend," he says. And be sure to adjust the screen for brightness, so there's plenty of contrast with the background.

Feet

- **Wash them.**
- **Pamper them.**
- **Buy good shoes.**

Think you're under a lot of pressure? Try walking a mile in your feet's shoes.

- With every step, the foot of a 150-pound man absorbs 570 pounds of pressure.

- In an average day, your feet face 5.7 million pounds of pressure. That's like letting every man, woman and child in Euless, Texas (population: 38,149), step on your toes.

- Every month, your feet must handle about 171 million pounds of pressure. That's the weight of the battleship U.S.S. Iowa—with every man, woman and child in St. Louis, Missouri, aboard.

- After 65 years of walking, your feet will have been asked to deal with more than 136 billion pounds of pressure. That's like dropping the Great Pyramid of Cheops on your penny loafers. Five times. For each foot. And then letting every man, woman and child in Brazil do the samba across your aching arches.

Should it surprise you, then, that 87 percent of us suffer from foot pain during our lives? With that much pressure, it's a wonder that we can stand up at all.

"Feet are remarkably good at taking stress and strain," says William L. Van Pelt, D.P.M., a Houston podiatrist and past president of the American Academy of Podiatric Sports Medicine. "But there's a limit. You have to take good care of your feet, or a lot can go wrong with them."

The list of foot ailments is enough to make you wish that man still swung from trees. But if you follow some simple advice—and stop buying shoes that don't fit—you may be able to lift some of the weight of the world off your soles.

Fast Foot Facts

Feet exist for two reasons: to bear the weight of our bodies when we stand and to propel us forward when we walk. As we've just learned, these are not simple tasks. Any body part that can take so much pressure has to be built to rigid specifications.

The key design feature of the foot is a flexible arch. While arches can vary greatly in height from human to human, they all perform the same function. As you stride forward and put weight on your foot, the arch flattens out slightly to absorb the pressure. It then springs back to its original shape as you shift your weight to your other foot. While you may have been told for years that "flat" arches—arches that almost touch the floor when you're not putting weight on them—are bad, that's not necessarily the case. In fact, "high" arches, which can be as much as an inch off the floor when they're not bearing weight, can flatten out too much during walking, causing far more problems, as we'll see later.

The foot is a complex network of 26 bones, 56 ligaments and 38 muscles. The bones of the foot are divided into three subgroups. The 7 bones around the ankle are known as tarsal bones. These join the foot to the tibia, which is the large bone in your lower leg. They're arranged so that you can rotate your ankle (if you've ever tried to walk in ski boots, you can appreciate how useful a flexible ankle can be). Then come the metatarsals, a collection of 5 long bones that form the middle portion of the foot, or the instep. Finally come the phalanges, which are made up of a disputed number of bones (about 14, depending on how you count them). These, scientifically speaking, are your toes.

In addition to providing endless amusement—what would childhood be without 5,000 rousing choruses of "This Little Piggie"?—toes perform two key functions. First, they help you keep your balance. Applying pressure or bending them just so keeps you from blowing over in a stiff breeze. And second, they help you walk. This role was more important before the advent of shoes, when toes gripped the ground and pushed the body forward. But even today, if you want to see how important toes are, just curl them up tightly and try to walk. Talk about your basic stumblebum.

Foot Pain: Don't Be So "Callus"

Your feet also have a vast collection of nerve endings, giving them a keen sense of touch rivaled only by your hands. Nerve endings are good when you're walking barefoot through a patch of clover on a dewy spring morning. But they're not so welcome when you develop a problem such as a corn, callus or heel spur, all of which can cause debilitating pain.

And even though women are more likely to complain about foot pain, men are at equal risk of developing it. In fact, Dr. Van Pelt says, we make things harder on ourselves by refusing to seek help.

"Men tend to neglect their feet. It's something in the culture," Dr. Van Pelt says. "Society says we're supposed to live with pain. The problem is that when men finally come in for help, their feet are much worse off. And we usually have to do something radical just to salvage their feet."

The first and best thing that you can do to avoid foot problems is to buy good shoes, says Dr. Van Pelt. But if you already have foot problems, our experts offer some suggestions for dealing with them.

Calluses are buildups of dead, yellowish skin that usually form where there's lots of friction. They often occur on the bottom of your feet, or the soles, which already have the thickest layer of skin anywhere on your body. If your shoes are too tight, or if you walk or stand improperly, you put extra stress on parts

Are You Overpronated?

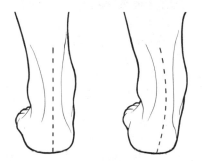

With bare legs, stand up straight. Have someone observe the structure of your Achilles tendon, ankle and heel from the back. Your Achilles tendon should run straight up and down the back of your leg. If it curves outward when it gets to heel level, you probably overpronate.

of your feet that aren't designed to handle it. Calluses are your body's attempt to shield your feet from extra damage, says Suzanne M. Levine, D.P.M., clinical podiatrist at the New York Hospital–Cornell Medical Center in New York City.

Normally, a callus isn't a big problem. To remove one, try soaking your foot in warm water for 10 to 15 minutes, then lightly rubbing the callus with a pumice stone, which you can buy in most drugstores. Try to take off a thin layer of the callus every day, Dr. Levine says, but stop if the callus gets sore or inflamed. When you're done with the stone, rub moisturizing cream onto the callus to keep it soft. Until the callus disappears, you can cover it with a piece of moleskin, available in drugstores, to help reduce the friction.

See your doctor if a callus becomes painful. It could be a sign that your foot has a structural problem that needs to be addressed, says Dr. Levine.

Corns are similar to calluses, except they form only on your toes. They're hard, yellow masses of skin that form in response to friction—again, usually from ill-fitting shoes.

To get temporary relief from a corn, Dr. Levine suggests soaking your foot in warm water and Epsom salts. After 15 minutes, take your foot out of the water and apply moisturizing cream to the corn. Cover your toes in plastic wrap and wait another 15 minutes. Then gently rub with a pumice stone, removing a thin layer each day until the corn is gone, says Dr. Levine.

Of course, unless you fix the underlying problem—your shoes—corns will never go away. If a corn becomes painful or red, see your doctor.

Heel spurs feel like sharp little thumbtacks piercing the bottom of your feet. A spur is a bony chunk of calcium that forms inside the heel and irritates the plantar fascia, a tough piece of tissue that stretches the length of the sole. Running and other activities that pound the heel are often the causes of heel spurs, Dr. Van Pelt says.

If you're feeling pain, take some aspirin or ibuprofen and apply ice, wrapped in a towel, for 15 to 20 minutes. For a couple of weeks, ease up on whatever activity is causing your heel pain. Dr. Van Pelt suggests using foam heel pad inserts in your shoes to help cushion the shock of running or walking. If heel pain persists, see your doctor. Sometimes surgery is the only way to fix a heel spur.

Other Manly Problems

Polls show that the vast majority of men are happy being men. Many of us have cool low voices and impressive chest hair. Unfortunately, many of us also have man-related foot problems, such as feet that smell like roadkill or big toes that throb after eating anchovies.

Here are three of the biggies.

Foot odor. Most times, Dr. Levine says, the problem is bromhidrosis. That's Greek for "stench sweat." Your feet smell because the sweat from your feet gets trapped in your shoes and socks, and odor-causing bacteria basically go nuts.

Dr. Levine's advice comes in four parts. First, wash and dry your feet often—at least twice a day. Second, change your socks at least once a day (do we

Buying Shoes: Don't Be a Heel

Forty percent of women admit that they've thrown a shoe at a man sometime in their lives. Small wonder. If you had to wobble around on five-inch spike heels because of the whims of some sandal-wearing European male fashion guru, you might get a little testy, too.

But women aren't the only ones feeling the pain. Most men are wearing shoes that are either the wrong size or the wrong style for their feet. And it's not doing them any good.

"It's amazing what we men will put up with when it comes to shoes," says William L. Van Pelt, D.P.M., a Houston podiatrist and past president of the American Academy of Podiatric Sports Medicine. "Men constantly buy the wrong shoes for the wrong reasons, and it's contributing to a lot of foot problems out there."

We're talking everything from blisters to bunions to heel spurs. So do yourself a favor. Save your soles with these simple shoe-shopping secrets from Dr. Van Pelt.

Find last-ing comfort. Shoes are made on three basic shapes, or lasts. People with flat arches should wear shoes made on a straight last; those with high arches should look for shoes made on a curved last. People with normal or "neutral" arches should buy shoes patterned on a standard last.

To determine which last works for you, sit in a chair, with your bare right foot on the floor. Place a piece of paper on the floor and trace the outline of your foot. Be careful not to put too much weight on your foot as you trace. Then consult the illustrations below to see which last you need.

Unfortunately, shoes, shoeboxes and shoe salesmen can rarely tell you what kind of last a brand uses. So just flip the shoe over and look at the sole. Again, the illustrations below show which sole you should look for.

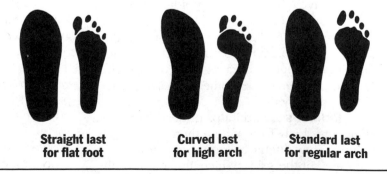

Straight last for flat foot   **Curved last for high arch**   **Standard last for regular arch**

really need to tell you that?). Third, give your shoes a rest. Try not to wear the same pair two

Measure up. Typically, a man's feet grow longer and wider as he ages, because they lose some of their elasticity. So just because you've been a size nine since high school doesn't mean you'll be a size nine next month. That's why you have to measure your foot every time you buy a new pair of shoes.

Always stand up when measuring your feet. When you stand, your feet spread and lengthen under the weight of your body. And measure both feet; chances are that one is bigger than the other. Always choose your size based on the larger foot.

Don't believe the label. Having implored you to measure your feet, we now need to add a caveat: Shoe sizes are as reliable as your average Middle Eastern peace treaty. Never buy a shoe just because the box says it's your size. If a shoe doesn't feel comfortable, try another size. If it's still not comfortable, try another style.

And never, ever buy shoes thinking that they'll stretch to fit your feet. They won't. Shoes that start small will always be small—and your feet will react to them with blisters and other problems.

Try to remember a little rule of thumb when picking shoes: There should always be a space at least as wide as your thumbnail between the tip of your big toe and the end of the shoe. Anything less than that, and the shoe is too small.

Take a wide berth. "Width" means different things to different shoemakers. That's because the width measurement—the most common for men is D—is figured by volume, not just by the distance across the shoe. So a man with a slightly wide foot may need a D in one style and an EE in another.

"You'll have to just try different styles to find the right one," Dr. Van Pelt says. In some shoes, the toe box is higher and shorter; in others, it's wider and lower. Unfortunately, nothing is standardized, and you're pretty much on your own. Once again, Dr. Van Pelt's recommendation: Keep trying on shoes until you find one that feels right.

Go late. Your feet are always their biggest late in the day, after you're done walking, running, standing and pounding on them. If possible, shop for shoes after work. That way, you'll be sure to pick shoes big enough to be comfortable 24 hours a day.

suggests looking for products that contain aluminum chlorohydrate. She especially recommends Dr. Scholl's Super Deodorant Foot Powder. Charcoal-activated insoles are also good, she says.

Athlete's foot. Sometimes foot odor is caused by a fungal infection, athlete's foot being one of them. Of course, athlete's foot also packs other problems, such as burning, cracking skin between your toes. To help you avoid athlete's foot, wear rubber sandals in the shower, especially in public locker rooms. And after showering, always dry and powder your feet thoroughly, says Dr. Van Pelt.

If you do get athlete's foot, try using antifungal foot powder or medication. Look for products that contain clotrimazole, such as Lotrimin AF and Mycelex OTC. Dr. Levine warns that over-the-counter treatments don't always work; sometimes a doctor needs to prescribe oral medication to clear up stubborn cases. In any event, don't let a case of athlete's foot get out of hand. It can lead to a nasty secondary bacterial infection.

Gout. A form of arthritis, gout usually strikes men, especially in the big toe. It's caused by a buildup of crystals of uric acid, a waste product of digestion that works its way down to your feet.

Foods high in purines can trigger a bout of gout. If you have trouble with gout, avoid beer and wine, organ meats and fish such as anchovies, sardines and herring. When gout

days in a row, so they have a chance to dry out. Finally, try a little foot powder. Dr. Levine

How to Walk

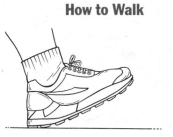

Your heel should gently but firmly make contact with the ground.

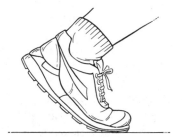

Then roll your foot forward toward your toe and allow your foot to press into the ground.

strikes, Dr. Van Pelt says, you should elevate your foot, take ibuprofen (not aspirin, which can decrease the uric acid level and lead to an inaccurate diagnosis) and apply ice, wrapped in a towel, for 15 to 20 minutes. Call your physician or podiatrist if the pain continues. Losing weight often helps control gout in the long term.

Ankle, knee or back pain. Is walking a pleasure or a pain? Well, it may depend on how you walk. Improper technique, especially when it comes to your feet, can cause everything from a blister to a bad back.

The most common walking malfunction is called overpronation. When you walk, the outside of your heel hits the ground first. As you stride forward, the weight is supposed to move forward and across your foot until you push off with your big toe. But if the weight stays on the outside of your foot, you

Leather and Laces: How to Fix the Ties That Bind

Nothing scuttles a workout like sore feet. You can't run. You can't jump. You can't hop, skip, walk, pedal, cross-country ski, climb stairs or slide on one of those stupid mats. You're left with two options: standing or crawling around, begging for Tylenol—neither of which is likely to get your heart rate within target range.

Obviously, the best way to deal with foot pain is to prevent it. One of the simplest ways is to customize your shoe-lacing style to your feet. You can help compensate for high arches, low arches, sore toes and other problems, says Carol Frey, M.D., associate clinical professor of orthopedic surgery at the University of Southern California School of Medicine in Los Angeles. She offers these suggestions.

Narrow foot. (A) Use the eyelets that are set wider apart on many running and cross-training shoes. This pulls up the sides of the shoe so that it's tighter across the tip of a narrow foot.

Wide foot. (B) Lace using the eyelets found closer to the tongue of the shoe to provide more width to the lacing area. It's like letting out a notch on your belt.

Foot pain. (C) If you have a bump on the top of your foot or pain from a tendon injury, leave a space in the lacing to alleviate pressure. Simply skip the eyelets at the point of the pain and lace through the next set of eyelets.

High arch. (D) Lace your shoe so that the shoelace travels in a straight line from eyelet to eyelet. Start by lacing the bottom two eyelets. Then with the left shoelace, skip an eyelet and poke the lace up through the next eyelet on the left side of the shoe. Then take the lace across the tongue and poke it down through the opposite eyelet. Now take the right lace, poke it up through the neighboring eyelet, take it across the tongue and push it down through the opposite eyelet. Repeat. By avoiding the crisscross effect, you eliminate the pressure points on the tongue of the shoe that cause pain on the top of your foot.

Ingrown toenail or corn. (E) Start by poking the shoelace through one of the top eyelets; leave enough of the

put extra stress on ligaments and muscles that aren't designed for the purpose. Then the rest of your body compensates, throwing other body parts out of alignment. The result is a throbbing mess of pain.

Much of overpronation is caused by flat-lace threaded through to tie the shoe when you're finished. Next, thread the longer section of lace through the opposite bottom eyelet. Lace across, then diagonally up, then across again and so on, always lacing over the section of lace running from the top of the shoe to the bottom.

Slipping heel. (F) Lace normally until you reach the second-to-last eyelets at the top. Instead of crisscrossing the shoelace, poke each end up through the eyelet and down through the eyelet above it. Thread each end across and under the loop you formed with the opposite lace, then tie the shoe.

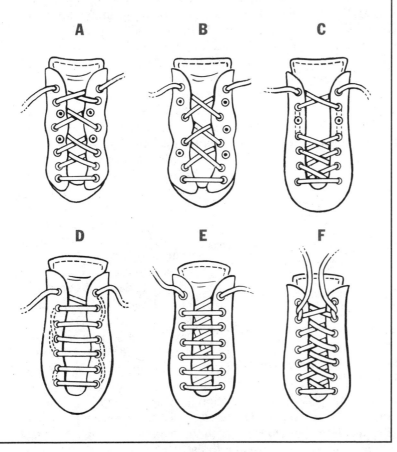

A   B   C

D   E   F

touching the ground, you're going to have problems. The entire weight will rapidly and excessively shift to the inside of the foot, and the whole foot will "roll over" on its side, says Dr. Van Pelt.

The telltale signs of over-pronation are excess wear on the outer edge and outside heel of your shoe. If this is a problem for you, ask a knowledgeable shoe salesman to point you toward athletic shoes that compensate for overpronation. And see your foot doctor about prescribing special insoles to keep your arches up and straighten out your stride, says Dr. Van Pelt.

One last note about walking: Yes, you've been doing it all of your life, but that doesn't mean you're doing it right. Think of your foot as the rocker on a chair. Your heel should land gently, hardly making a sound, according to Deena and David Balboa, directors of the Walking Center of New York City. Then your foot should roll forward easily, pushing off with your toes. The Balboas say that the soft heel landing brings more muscles into play than the typical hard heel strike. So be prepared for a few aching muscles at first, especially in your shins. The payoff: pain-free walking.

And one last note about feet: Be careful if you have diabetes. People with diabetes often lose sensation in their feet and can cause terrible damage without even feeling it. Avoid walking barefoot, Dr. Van Pelt says, since you could easily cut your foot and not notice a problem.

tening arches. We all grew up thinking that flat arches were bad (unless, of course, you wanted out of the Army). But the truth is, it doesn't matter how high your arches are when they're not bearing weight. If your arches flatten out when you walk, to the point of touching or almost

🔲 Fingernails

- **Keep them trimmed.**
- **Don't chew on them.**
- **Keep them moist but not wet.**

It's not one of life's great ponderables, but it may someday win you a bar bet: Which fingernail grows the fastest?

For most people, it's the nail on the middle finger of the dominant hand. Nobody is quite sure why. One possibility: "The middle finger is the longest, sticks out the most and gets bumped around all day," suggests Paul Kechijian, M.D., chief of the nail section at New York University Medical Center in Great Neck.

All nails, no matter how fast they grow, are made of keratin, the protein that also gives skin and hair their toughness. Nails serve three main purposes.

- To protect your fingertips from sharp and/or hard objects
- To increase the sense of touch in your fingertips
- To improve your ability to pick up and manipulate small objects

You really don't have to do much to keep your nails in decent shape. Just trim them and follow these simple tips.

Keep them out of your mouth. About 80 percent of all serious nail problems are caused by biting and picking, says Dr. Kechijian. Nail-biting can do several nasty things. It can leave sharp edges that catch on clothing and tear nails. It can injure the nail bed, which can cause a bacterial infection. Or it can cause your cuticle to tear. The cuticle, if you aren't clear, is that extremely narrow band of hardened skin that rings the bottom and sides of the nail where it meets your finger. Torn cuticles

can lead to a skin infection that could require a doctor's visit and an antibiotic prescription to clear up, says Dr. Kechijian.

Don't be a mushroom. Fungus infections give you thick, crusty, yellowish nails. "The fungus enters the small opening between the nail bed and nail plate of the finger," says Dr. Kechijian. "People come into contact with fungus all of the time."

For most guys, this is not a big issue; their bodies eradicate the fungus before it does harm. But some people can't help getting nail fungus; their immune systems don't fight it well. For these guys, battling fungus infections is an ongoing thing. As with bacterial infections, over-the-counter remedies don't work well. You'll likely need a dermatologist to prescribe something stronger.

Keep them dry . . . Too much moisture can lead to a bacterial infection, which causes dark spots on the nail. So wear gloves if your job has your hands perpetually in water.

To cure a bacterial infection, you'll need to see a dermatologist. He'll cut away the affected portion of nail and treat with iodine and alcohol. Some doctors say that you may also need oral medication. Again, over-the-counter remedies rarely work.

. . . But not too dry. Dry, chapped fingertips can lead to hangnails. Dr. Kechijian says that hangnails aren't really nails; they're pieces of dried skin along the edges of nails that can crack and stick out sideways. They often get caught on objects, tear and become infected. And only a hockey puck to the groin can match the pain of catching a hangnail on a sweater thread.

Avoid this problem by rubbing moisturizer on your fingertips and hands several times a day, especially after washing. If you do get a hangnail, use clippers or nail scissors to cut it at its base. Then apply moisturizer, cover it with a bandage and leave it alone. Don't bite it down, or you risk infection.

How to Trim

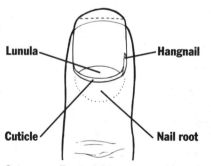

Lunula — Hangnail

Cuticle — Nail root

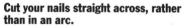

Cut your nails straight across, rather than in an arc.

Foreskin

- **If you don't have one, relax. You're not missing much.**
- **If you have one, clean it every shower.**

God, of course, knew that Abraham was a great salesman. So he assigned the 90-year-old leader the task of convincing his fellow Hebrews to take a sharpened flint and, without anesthesia, clip the tip off the skin covering the head of the penis.

Nowhere in the Bible is it recorded that even one man asked Abraham, "God said *what?*"

Circumcision has evolved since biblical times. Now the entire head of the penis, not just the tip, is denuded. And for most of a century, doctors in the United States advocated that all baby boys be circumcised for health reasons.

But today, doctors are again arguing the pros and cons of circumcision. Some cite studies showing that it lowers the incidence of rare diseases such as penile cancer. Others present contrasting studies and liken circumcision to mutilation—and argue that it robs men of sexual pleasure.

The Great Cover-Up

The foreskin is a flap of skin, or hood, that naturally covers the head of the penis. At birth, it is attached on the inside to the head of the penis, or glans. It slowly breaks its bonds and becomes fully retractable over the next 17 years.

The foreskin shelters the glans and keeps it soft, moist and sensitive. If the foreskin is removed, the glans hardens, toughens and loses sensitivity.

On its underside, the foreskin has a mucous membrane with a great number of small, sensitive, nerve-rich knobs and pleats. They are stimulated during sex as the foreskin glides back and forth over the glans and penis shaft.

Usually, the uncircumcised penis requires minimal maintenance. Men should pull back the foreskin when they shower and wash away any buildup of mucus or secretions, known as smegma. (Don't force back a baby's foreskin and wash it. That prematurely breaks bonds and can cause urinary tract infections.)

Occasionally in older men, the foreskin loses its ability to stretch and retract and must be treated with a topical steroid, slit open or cut off.

The Flap over Circumcision

For most American males, the issue of circumcision is . . . well, cut and dried. Approximately 80 to 90 percent of us have already been skinned. In contrast, only 7 percent of British men are circumcised. And the procedure is rare elsewhere in northern Europe, Central America, South America and Asia.

The American tradition of medical circumcision stems from nineteenth-century "cures" for masturbation, from concerns about cleanliness and from this century's emphasis on preventive medicine. In the past 25 years, the American Academy of Pediatricians has taken the position that circumcision is not medically necessary. The pediatricians do note, however, that circumcision may be beneficial. "It is a decision that should be left to the parents," says E. Maurice Wakeman, M.D., a pediatrician in Guilford, Connecticut, who served on the academy's most recent circumcision task force. While 90 percent of hospital-born boys were circumcised in the 1960s, only about 60 percent are today.

An intact foreskin can sometimes be linked to

Uncircumcised Penis

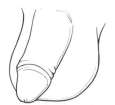

Circumcised Penis

certain diseases and conditions.

Penile cancer. This type of cancer is very rare, but in the United States, it seems more likely among uncircumcised men. The rate of penile cancer is lower in Denmark and Japan, where few men are circumcised. But the role of circumcision is unclear.

Urinary tract infections. Some data suggest that infection will strike 1 in 100 uncircumcised boys. That rate is ten times higher than for circumcised boys. While circumcision is preventive, urinary tract infections are routinely and easily treated with antibiotics.

Sexually transmitted diseases. Data regarding the role of circumcision in the transmission of sexually transmitted diseases are inconclusive, decided an American Academy of Pediatricians task force. Practice safe sex, and you needn't worry.

Stretching the Truth

Not only is circumcision less in vogue these days, but there's a small movement of men who are undoing their circumcisions—either quickly, through plastic surgery, or slowly, by tugging on the penis skin. At least 10,000 men have sought how-to instructions for reversing circumcision, claims Jim Bigelow, Ph.D., a psychologist in Pacific Grove, California, and author of *The Joy of Uncircumcising!*, the definitive work on methods of restoring the foreskin.

Dr. Bigelow is aware of hundreds of men who have undergone the process that he advocates, which is called skin expansion: stretching existing skin and ultimately growing new skin cells. Dr. Bigelow's do-it-yourself process involves pulling and taping skin from the penis shaft over the glans. With three to five years of stretching, taping and eventually attaching weights to the overhang, you develop a cosmetically acceptable foreskin.

The new model doesn't come with all of the original goodies under the hood. But it keeps the penis head warm and moist. And soon the mucosal covering reverts to a softer, more sensitive state, says Dr. Bigelow.

Freckles

Howdy Doody, the four-foot-tall puppet and television icon of millions of young baby boomers in the 1950s, had exactly 48 facial freckles—one for each state.

Howdy never complained about his spotted appearance, even after gaining another pair of freckles when Alaska and Hawaii joined the Union. But for flesh-and-blood men, freckles are a sometimes handsome, more often annoying reminder that they've spent too much time in the sun.

Freckles are harmless, tiny brown spots caused by excessive sun exposure. Normally, the sun's ultraviolet light triggers the production of pigments that darken the skin and evenly tan the body. But in some men, only small, scattered clusters of pigment cells respond to the sun's onslaught. Instead of tanning, these men freckle.

Freckles are often an inherited trait and are most common among fair-skinned, redheaded men. They vary in number from a few spots to hundreds dotting the face, back and arms. They are most prominent in the summer and usually fade in the winter. They are seldom found in the groin, the armpits and other areas that are shielded from the sun.

Minimizing sun exposure and regularly using a sunscreen that has a sun protection factor (SPF) of at least 15 will help avert new freckles and prevent the darkening of existing ones, says Paul Lazar, M.D., a Highland Park, Illinois, dermatologist and co-author of *The Look You Like: Medical Answers to 400 Questions on Skin and Hair Care.*

Over-the-counter bleaching creams rarely fade unwanted freckles. Tretinoin (Retin-A), a prescription acne medication, is effective in some cases. And for those desperate for monochromatic skin, dermabrasion, laser surgery and chemical peels can also eliminate the spots.

Gallbladder

- **Lose some weight, but do it slowly.**
- **Eat more often, but in smaller portions.**
- **Up your fiber intake.**

Lyndon Johnson, the earthy 36th U.S. president, was a fan of big things: big cars, big crowds, big election victories.

He was proud, too, of his big scar, the one he showed off to the world by pulling up his shirt for the press following gallbladder surgery in 1965. It was a priceless American moment, recorded photographically for all time.

But had he actually seen his gallbladder, the president might have been dismayed to find that such a small organ had caused his big pain.

Less than six inches long, the gallbladder is a pear-shaped reservoir that holds about one-quarter cup of pasty, yellowish green material called bile, which the body needs to digest fatty foods and absorb certain vitamins and minerals.

The gallbladder is connected to the liver, which produces bile, and to the small intestine, where the bile gets used, by tiny tubes called bile ducts. Bile flows from the liver to the gallbladder, where it accumulates and thickens. When you eat, the gallbladder contracts and spews bile into the small intestine to aid digestion.

Bile, which contains water, cholesterol, electrolytes and other chemicals, has a nasty tendency to crystallize—much like sugar at the bottom of a coffee cup—when it is stored in the gallbladder. These crystals can fuse together and form gallstones, lumps of solid cholesterol, calcium salts or bile pigments.

Stones with Gall

Gallstones are by far the most common problem affecting the gallbladder. Rare in childhood, gallstones become increasingly common as men reach middle age. By age 60, one in ten men will have at least one.

Gallstones vary in size, ranging from tiny specks to small balls. Most, however, are less than one inch long and seldom cause trouble. In fact, about 80 percent of all gallstones are "silent" and cause no symptoms at all. But if they do, you'll definitely know it.

"Gallstone pain is worse than a heart attack. It, and kidney stone pain, is supposedly the worst pain anybody can get," says Roger D. Soloway, M.D., a gastroenterologist and professor of medicine at the University of Texas Medical Branch at Galveston. In fact, the pain can be mistaken for a heart attack because it occasionally spreads into the back, chest and shoulders.

Typically, the agony begins when a small stone slips into the bile duct leading out of the gallbladder and gets trapped there. In most cases, the pain subsides only after the stone falls back into the gallbladder or the organ pushes it through the duct and into the small intestine. This intermittent but excruciating pain generally lasts for 30 to 60 minutes but may linger for more than three hours.

Other, more uncommon symptoms include fever and chills, vomiting and jaundice. In rare instances, gallstones can lead to liver damage or inflammation of the pancreas or can cause the gallbladder to burst, triggering a potentially fatal infection of the abdominal cavity.

Stopping 'Em before They Start

Doctors are still sorting out why some men get gallstones and others sail through life unhindered. Heredity may have a role; gallstones are almost unheard of in Africa and Asia, while 80 percent of Pima Indians in southern Arizona have them by age 35.

And although some evidence points to diet, most doctors say that the link between what we eat and gallstones is flimsy. What they do know is that men over age 60 and men who are overweight, who have recently experienced rapid weight loss or gain or who have diseases of the small intestine are at increased risk.

With all of that in mind, here are some ways you may be able to keep your gallbladder healthy.

Shed that jumbo look. If you're overweight, you're up to six times more likely to develop gallstones than someone who is slimmer, says Robert Charm, M.D., a gastroenterologist and assistant clinical professor of medicine at the University of California, Davis, School of Medicine.

To trim your waistline, graze, don't gorge, he suggests; eat several small meals each day instead of one or two large ones. Avoid junk foods such as potato chips, which are high in both fat and calories. Be sure to eat a balanced diet that includes eight to ten servings of fruits and vegetables, and exercise 20 minutes a day, every day, recommends Dr. Charm. "If you eat every day, you should exercise every day," he says.

But don't crash and burn. Rapid weight loss drastically increases the amount of cholesterol in bile, and cholesterol is the primary ingredient in 80 percent of all gallstones in the United States. As you lose weight, your body breaks down cells, and that process releases extra cholesterol into the bloodstream. The liver transforms that cholesterol into bile and sends it on to the gallbladder. But because the bile is suddenly saturated with cholesterol, it's more likely to form gallstones. To prevent that, Dr. Soloway suggests shedding no more than two pounds a week.

Eat small, eat often. Every time you eat, bile is expelled from the gallbladder. So the more often you eat, the less likely bile will pool in the organ and form stones, Dr. Soloway says. Eat four or five small meals, including breakfast and a small snack (such as half of a sandwich) just before bedtime, to cut down the amount of time you're fasting between meals.

Keep away from cholesterol. Most doctors consider dietary cholesterol an insignificant source of gallstones, since only 20 percent of the cholesterol in blood comes from what we eat. The rest is manufactured by our own bodies. But it may still be worthwhile to cut back on cholesterol-laden foods, says Henry Pitt, M.D., director of the Gallstone and Biliary Disease Center at Johns Hopkins University School of Medicine in Baltimore.

"If diet is a factor, following the same guidelines as you would to prevent heart disease will help prevent gallstones as well," Dr. Pitt says.

Cholesterol is found only in foods derived from animal sources, including beef, lamb, pork, poultry, fish, shellfish and dairy products such as milk, cheese and butter. Try to limit your consumption of dietary cholesterol to less than 300 milligrams a day (one egg yolk, for example, has about 213 milligrams of cholesterol, while a three-ounce piece of broiled chicken has about 73 milligrams). Eat no more than two three-ounce portions of meat, fish or poultry a day, and if you drink milk, you should switch from whole to skim. Doing these things will

Where Gallbladder Pain Might Be Felt

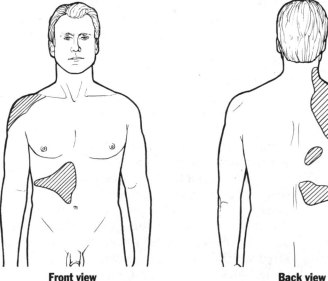

Front view   **Back view**

also slash the amount of saturated fat in your diet, which can also elevate blood cholesterol, adds Dr. Pitt.

Fill up on fiber. Men who eat more fiber seem to expel more bile from their gallbladders and have fewer gallstones, says Rajiv R. Varma, M.D., director of hepatology at the Medical College of Wisconsin in Milwaukee. It takes at least five servings of fruits and vegetables and six servings of grains such as breads and pastas each day to keep your fiber level appropriately high.

Take a swig. Drinking about two ounces of alcohol (the equivalent of three or four beers) each week may help prevent gallstones, says Gregory T. Everson, M.D., director of the Section of Hepatology at the University of Colorado School of Medicine in Denver.

You Can Live without It

If you do develop painful gallstones, doctors can try to destroy them either with drugs or, in Europe, by lithotripsy, a nonsurgical procedure that shatters the stones with shock waves. (Lithotripsy is being tested but has not yet been approved for use in the United States.) But neither of these options can prevent new stones from forming. The only way to ensure that is to surgically remove the organ.

"Most people can live comfortably without a gallbladder. Having it removed doesn't jeopardize your quality of life or your life expectancy," Dr. Varma says.

Nor does having it taken out mean that you'll end up with a Texas-size scar like Lyndon Johnson's. This once-complex surgery that required a three- to six-inch incision in the abdomen and weeks for recovery now is usually done with miniaturized instruments that are inserted through tiny cuts about the size of your belly button.

The procedure, called a laparoscopic cholecystectomy, takes about an hour and leaves few noticeable scars. In most instances, you'll be able to go home the next day and return to work within a week.

Λ Groin

- Keep stretched and strong.
- Monitor for lumps and bumps.

"A kick in the groin" is one of those guy phrases that doesn't need much explanation. The inference is pain, no more children, a higher voice, more pain.

Trouble is, these common notions are inaccurate. The testicles hurt. The penis is sacred. But they aren't the groin.

The groin is a complex of muscles and tendons where the abdomen meets the thighs. The groin muscles attach the upper legs to the pelvic region. These muscles control many important body movements: pulling the legs inward, kicking a soccer ball.

For those who are physically active, and particularly for someone who relies on leg power, it's not hard to injure a groin muscle. Like any other muscle group, groin muscles can be strained, overused and abused. Repeated stress over a long period can also hurt the groin. When you're jogging, for example, the repeated impact of your foot on the ground can ripple up your leg to your groin.

As for any other muscle group, the key to preventing a groin injury is to do exercises that strengthen and stretch the region.

Here are two good groin stretches, suggested by Bob Anderson in his book *Stretching*, to do before and after any physical activity. Sit on the ground and put the soles of your feet together. Hold on to your toes and gently pull yourself forward, bending from your hips, until you feel a good stretch in your groin. Hold for a long time—say, 20 to 30 seconds. Be sure not to bounce.

Another good stretch: Lie on the ground with your butt about three to five inches from a wall, your legs extended straight up and your heels against the wall. Your lower back should

Seated Groin Stretch   **Lying Wall Stretch**

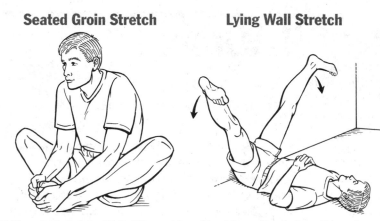

Hold each stretch for 20 to 30 seconds, without bouncing, to keep the groin muscles limber.

be flat on the floor. Slowly, carefully separate your legs, keeping your heels on the wall, until you feel a good stretch in your groin. Hold the position for 20 to 30 seconds.

Hernia Alert

You can have a ripped body (that's weight-lifting slang for well-defined muscles), but woe is he whose body accidentally rips. That's almost what a hernia is. More accurately, a hernia is when tissue or part of an organ protrudes through the thing that normally contains it. Of hernias occurring in the groin, inguinal hernias are the most common, accounting for about 97 percent of all cases. Hernias occur where the folds of abdominal flesh meet the thighs. With an inguinal hernia, intestinal or other abdominal tissue pushes through the abdominal wall or down toward the scrotum.

What causes a hernia? Some unlucky guys are born with a predisposition to have hernias. The transversalis fascia, a thin layer of tissue supporting the groin area, weakens. When it is weak enough, anything that increases pressure in the abdominal area, such as sneezing, lifting or bending, can cause the tissue to rupture, and presto! A hernia. Obesity can contribute to the pressure. And as you age, the chance of getting a hernia grows, in part because of an unstoppable deterioration of some of the tissue in the groin.

You don't want a hernia. It hurts. How can you prevent one? Since you can't change your genetic makeup, you should avoid doing things that trigger the rupture of the transversalis fascia, suggests Parviz K. Amid, M.D., director of the Lichtenstein Hernia Institute in Los Angeles. One thing you can do is lift properly. The right technique shifts pressure from your back and abdomen to your legs. (For tips on smart lifting, see page 92.)

And always watch for the signs. If you even think you have a hernia, get it checked by your doctor. You may be able to push the tissue back into place by yourself, but that won't fix the hole it came through, and you should not delay surgical repair, cautions Dr. Amid. Left alone, the hernia could become strangulated; that means the blood supply to the out-of-place tissue has been cut off. This is a serious situation, requiring emergency surgery. For a groin hernia, look for:

- A bulge or lump anywhere in your groin that is visible only when you're standing, straining or coughing. The protrusion may disappear when you lie down.
- Pain at the bulge or a lump when you're lifting
- Scrotal swelling
- Intense abdominal pain, indicating that the hernia is strangulated
- Pain, nausea, vomiting and loss of appetite, which may indicate a related intestinal obstruction

A hernia requires surgical repair, says Dr. Amid. With traditional surgery, which sutures together the edges of the tear, hernias have a recurrence rate of about 10 percent. A newer procedure uses a sheet of surgical mesh, which is stitched over the tear. This strengthens the entire area and reduces the probability of recurrence to virtually zero, Dr. Amid says.

Gums

- **Floss regularly.**
- **If it's not food, keep it out of your mouth.**
- **Let your dentist get in deep.**

War is hell. And hell is full of guys with really bad hygiene.

Imagine: It's the summer of 1918, and you've been stuck in some stinking, muddy Belgian foxhole for 17 weeks. You can't change your underwear. You can't shave your face. Your socks are permanently fused to your feet.

And now, after 119 straight days of canned meat—and 119 days of not brushing your teeth—you have an even bigger problem. The whole battalion has breath that could melt tank armor. You have trench mouth, the worst breath of the war.

Luckily, trench mouth is not a major concern during peacetime. But if you have bad breath, the cause is probably the very same thing that gave all of those GIs so much grief. Before you blame spicy food or dry mouth or Otto von Bismarck for your breath, take a look at your gums.

"Bad breath is one of the telltale signs of gum disease," states Howard S. Glazer, D.D.S., president of the Academy of General Dentistry. "When all of those bacteria get working inside your mouth, you can really get a bad case of it."

And halitosis, however unfashionable and socially awkward, can be just the beginning. If you don't control it, gum disease can lead directly to tooth loss. So if you want to hold on to your molars, you have to whip those gums into fighting shape.

Beware the Plaque Attack

Gums exist to protect your teeth. They're made of soft, pinkish tissue that wraps around the base of the teeth. They help anchor your teeth to your upper and lower jaws and also keep food and assorted junk away from the roots of your teeth.

The problem with gums is that they're fairly easy to damage. Brush too hard, and they'll erode. Poke at them with a toothpick, and they'll bleed. Neglect them by not brushing and flossing often enough, and they could develop diseases that may cost you that manly smile.

Now for something really scary: You probably already have some form of gum disease. The American Academy of Periodontology estimates that 75 percent of adults suffer from at least a mild strain of gum disease.

The first step toward a toothless future is called gingivitis. This disease is marked by swelling and puffiness of the gums. The gums also bleed easily when you brush and floss.

Gingivitis begins when bacteria collect around the teeth and gums. The bacteria feed on food particles that remain on and between the teeth and under the gums. The whole sticky bacteria-and-food mess is called plaque. Plaque can cause mild infections in the gums, making them sensitive and tender.

If you're not careful, gingivitis can be just a prelude to disaster. Left unchecked, the plaque forms rock-hard tartar (also called calculus) that sticks between the teeth and gums like concrete. Your gums start to erode, and little pockets form in the gaps next to the teeth. These pockets then become infected with bacteria, and you have periodontal disease.

This is serious stuff. The infection starts eating at your teeth. Then it turns to your jawbone. When your teeth and jaw lose their grips on each other, you lose your teeth. Hello, dentures or implants.

"Gingivitis can be reversible, but periodontal disease is much more difficult to control," Dr. Glazer says. "If you let your gums go that far, you might not be able to save your teeth."

While gingivitis and periodontitis (a more advanced form of gum disease) are the biggies, other factors can lead to gum damage. Scurvy, caused by a severe deficiency of vitamin C, can make gums bleed. Scurvy is very rare in the United States. In some cases, leukemia is to blame. Also, some drugs—most notably antihistamines, decongestants and medications for high blood pressure and heart disease—can lead to swollen or bleeding gums. If you're taking prescription drugs and notice gum trouble, talk to your doctor.

Don't Let Your Mouth Go South

Remember those disgusting mouth-from-hell photos that your dentist used to stick in your face every time he found a cavity? The ones that look like somebody ran gums-first into a concrete pillar, lost a knife fight with a ninja gum assassin and then flossed with razor wire?

Remember: *This doesn't have to be you.* Life may have dealt you bad genes (periodontal disease tends to run in families), but if you can open your mouth wide enough to stick a piece of pizza inside, you can also brush your teeth and floss your gums.

"That's the number one form of prevention," says Dr. Glazer. "If you start with good toothbrushing and flossing techniques, the odds of developing serious trouble diminish greatly."

We discuss proper brushing technique in the chapter on teeth (page 317). But here's a little refresher course. Choose a brush with soft, rounded bristles. Brush in an elliptical or circular pattern, not from side to side, so you don't wear away your gums. Turn the brush to a 45-degree angle, with the bristles pointing toward your gums, so the bristles can massage and clean your gums and work under the gumline a little. Brush three to five times a day, or at least after breakfast and before bedtime, for at least three minutes a session.

Now let's move to flossing. The concept is simple: You slide a piece of string between two teeth and gently work it under the gumline. This removes food particles and plaque that are hiding in places a toothbrush can't reach. (For a complete course on proper flossing, see "How to Floss Your Teeth" on page 320.)

Dr. Glazer recommends that you floss once a day. "It takes bacterial plaque about 24 hours to colonize," he says. "So if you break things up once a day, it'll never get a foothold." It's best to floss just before bed. That's because saliva flow diminishes at night, giving the bacteria a better chance to get established.

Here are some more tried-and-true tooth-saving tips recommended by Dr. Glazer.

Know the drill. Visit your dentist every six months for a routine exam and cleaning. He'll

---

Wax On, Wax Off?

You have your waxed and your unwaxed, your tape and your string, your thin and your thick, your mint and your regular. So which is the best kind of floss?

The kind you'll use.

"Floss doesn't do any good unless it gets inside your mouth," says Howard S. Glazer, D.D.S., president of the Academy of General Dentistry. "So if you're more comfortable with one kind than you are with another, by all means use it."

Dr. Glazer does, however, have a favorite kind: plain-Jane unwaxed floss. And he likes it for the reason that many of us don't. "When you slide it between your teeth, it breaks up into little strands," he says. "And those strands are more likely to catch and remove plaque than a single waxed string."

He also worries a little about the wider, tapelike floss. "It has an edge to it, and it can cut your gums. If you like to use the tape stuff, be gentle when you slide it under the gumline. The idea is to help your gums, not to injure them."

Flossing tools, such as those plastic spreaders that hold short pieces of floss between their tines, are fine. "Do anything you need to do to get the floss to those back teeth," Dr. Glazer says. "That's the only thing that's important here."

clean areas of your gumline in ways that you can't. He'll check for the onset of gingivitis or periodontitis. And he'll present you with a bill—but hey, that's the cost of keeping your teeth.

Don't be like Bela. As you age, your gums naturally recede a bit, exposing the roots of your teeth (thus the phrase "long in the tooth"). This has two immediate effects. First, your teeth become more sensitive to hot and cold foods, since your gums can no longer protect those squeamish roots from temperature changes. Second, your canine teeth, the pointed ones on your upper jaw, become more and more prominent, giving you that unmistakable Dracula look.

Unfortunately, that humble superhero of oral health, the toothbrush, can also turn on you and hasten the erosion process. If you brush too hard, or if you brush your gums from side to side instead of in an elliptical or circular motion, you'll wear away your gums. Usually, the only way to fix the problem is through surgery to graft tissue on the bare spots. While it's highly effective and almost always successful, it's still surgery. So it's best to go easy with the brush and avoid the problem altogether.

The way you grip your toothbrush is key to preventing erosion. (See the illustration on page 320 for the proper technique.)

Keep foreigners out . . . Toothpicks, straws, cherry pits, razor blades: Chew on any of them, and you're going to cause gum damage. Cuts in your gums are all the excuse that bacteria need to cause an infection. So if it's not food, keep it out of your mouth.

. . . Especially when they're on fire. If you're looking for another reason to stop smoking, here it is. The heat from cigarette, pipe and cigar smoke damages gums. And Dr. Glazer says that tar and nicotine create a sticky film in your mouth that offers sanctuary to those bacterial colonies we keep talking about.

Repeat after your dentist: Camels wreck enamels. Camels wreck enamels. . . .

C the difference. Vitamin C helps repair connective tissue such as gums. So Dr. Glazer suggests that people with gingivitis or other gum problems stock up on the stuff. The Daily Value, as set by the government, is just 60 milligrams, but you can safely take up to 1,200 milligrams a day. Also, eat high-C foods such as sweet red peppers, orange juice, citrus fruits and brussels sprouts.

If you're going to drink lots of fruit juice, be certain to swish a few ounces of water around your mouth afterward. Fruit juice is high in acid, which is hard on tooth enamel.

Forget swishing. Mouthwash really isn't a gum-saver. While it kills some bacteria, the effect is short-lived. "Mouthwash is pretty low on the totem pole of oral hygiene," Dr. Glazer says.

In fact, some mouth washes have stunningly high alcohol levels. And alcohol dehydrates your gums, which can cause damage in the long run. So if you're addicted to that minty-fresh breath, make sure you pick a mouthwash that's alcohol-free.

A Brush with Death?

Through the lips and over the gums—look out heart, here it comes.

For reasons that no one can yet explain, there seems to be a link between gum disease and heart disease, particularly in men under age 50. A study of 1,600 American men younger than 50 found that the guys with periodontitis, or advanced gum disease, were nearly twice as likely to develop coronary artery disease as those with healthy gums. These men also were at higher risk of dying from heart disease. In fact, men who had lost all of their teeth before age 50 were 2.6 times more likely to die before their time than those who hadn't.

Researchers say they doubt that plaque on your teeth leads directly to plaque in your arteries, however. Their explanation: Men with dental troubles may take poor care of their bodies altogether. So you'll need to do more than floss to keep your heart happy.

Hair

- **Wash it, perhaps daily.**
- **Condition it, too.**
- **Go ahead, make a statement.**

Your shiny shock. Your manly mane. Your crowning glory. Your proud pompadour. It's nothing but snake skin. That's right. Pick any hair on your head and magnify it 30 or 40 times, and you'll see "snake skin—bands of overlapping scales," says Toby Mayer, M.D., co-director of the Beverly Hills Institute of Aesthetic and Reconstructive Surgery and clinical professor in the Division of Facial Plastic and Reconstructive Surgery at the University of Southern California in Los Angeles.

P.S.: It's dead. Dead, dead, dead. The part of your hair that you see is as lifeless as the hair on a shriveled mummy at the American Museum of Natural History.

But at least it's unique. Commit a crime, and the cops are likely to vacuum up one or two of the hundred or so hairs that you shed each day and pin you to the scene. Because while most hairs on your own head are pretty much the same, to a trained eye they are not at all like hairs from another head.

Life and Death

The real life of hair takes place beneath the surface, in the follicles, says Dr. Mayer. Follicles produce one of two types of hair: vellus or terminal. Vellus is the colorless peach fuzz that covers much of your body. Terminal is the thicker,

longer, colored hair that you brush, comb, style, cut, spritz, spray, gel, dye and otherwise pamper—and whose almost certain eventual loss you either lament or learn to accept.

Each follicle is bulb-shaped. It is surrounded by blood vessels, which feed the bulb the nutrients it needs to manufacture the globs of keratin (a protein) and melanin (a pigment) that make up hair cells. As each new glob of hair cells is produced, it pushes the previous one up the bulb's stem. There it dries and dies and is glued by amino acid to the glob above it, becoming one more in a strand of hair. That's how hair grows, at a rate of about one-half to one inch per month, says Dr. Mayer.

"The very hairs of your head are all numbered," Jesus Christ said. Modern science seems to agree, after a fashion. Each hair carries a genetic code that regulates nearly everything about it.

Every hair on your body has a genetically predetermined length. Scalp follicles produce hairs up to 40 inches long. Chest-hair follicles produce short, curly hairs. Move a chest-hair follicle to your scalp, and you will grow a chest hair on your scalp, says Dr. Mayer.

Whether your scalp hair is straight or curly, wiry or soft, thick or fine is also genetic. And each follicle and each hair has a genetically predetermined life span. A scalp hair grows for a few months or years, up to six years, then falls out. Its follicle rests briefly, then—unless it receives a biochemical message to the contrary—develops a new hair.

At any given time, you are in the process of shedding about 10,000 of the 100,000 or so scalp hairs that you started with. The difference between men with full heads of hair and those who

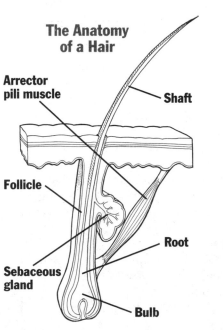

The Anatomy of a Hair

Arrector pili muscle

Shaft

Follicle

Root

Sebaceous gland

Bulb

are balding is that balding men don't always grow a new hair for each one that is shed.

If you are destined for baldness—and more men are than aren't—at some point your follicles get that message and quit producing new hairs. The process is well under way for half of us by the time we reach age 40. Chances are that if we're around to see snapshots of our 80th birthday parties, most of us will notice quite a bit of scalp shining through what once was a full, thick mop.

Just why we have hair is a matter of speculation. Writers of one edition of *The Encyclopedia Americana* thought it was to keep dust out of our eyes. In *The Bald Book: The Complete Book of Hair Loss and Regrowth*, science writer Walter Klenhard argues that hair—like a peacock's plumage—helps us attract mates. And in *Your Hair How to Keep It*, Neil S. Sadick, M.D., clinical assistant professor of dermatology at Cornell University Medical Center in New York City, suggests that early in evolution, when we had much more hair, its primary purpose was to protect us from the elements.

All of the above boils down to one thing: When it comes to your health, hair doesn't matter. At all. You can be bald, ponytailed, even dreadlocked—it has minimal effect on your physical health, unless someone pulls on it really hard.

Mental health is a completely different matter.

There is no denying that hair makes a huge personal and cultural statement. It helps identify an individual's personality, beliefs, income, attitudes. We want our hair to announce who we are, what we are. And so we spend a gazillion dollars to make this happen. We glance in every mirror and reflective window we pass to assess our appearance. We compulsively handle our hair to assure ourselves that all is well and in place.

Healthy, Shiny, Fluffy Hair

How do you keep hair healthy, shiny, fluffy and in place?

Remember, your hair is primarily made up of dead protein cells. When overly dried and bleached and oxidized by too much heat, sun, air pollution or chlorine or by overuse of styling products, the hair shafts become damaged. That leaves the hair looking dull, frayed, frizzy, even strawlike, says Gillian Shaw, senior barber at the Vidal Sassoon Salon in New York City.

Hair shines and is considered healthiest when the scales lie flat against the outside of the shaft, called the cuticle. Then the hair reflects light evenly instead of diffusing it at each scale. Hair shines even more when lots of healthy hairs lie together smoothly, reflecting light off one another, says Rebecca Caserio, M.D., clinical assistant professor of dermatology at the University of Pittsburgh.

Nature provides a sebaceous gland near the top of each follicle to secrete oil onto the scalp and hair shaft, keeping each hair soft, smooth and shiny. But nature never anticipated all of the stress and pollution that your hair is subjected to in modern times.

So now we have shampoos, conditioners, thickeners, gels and mousses that smooth scales and increase shine by coating the hair shafts with glossing agents or by infusing them with protein, notes Christina Griffasi, head of the styling department at the Minardi Salon in New York City. And we have special shampoos to wash away all of the product buildup that, over time, dulls hair. When this happens, you can use a clarifying shampoo, or after shampooing, you can wash away the buildup with one teaspoon of vinegar in a pint of warm water, worked through the hair and then rinsed out, says Griffasi.

Some products clog follicles and irritate the scalp, says Allison Vidimos, M.D., staff dermatologist for the Cleveland Clinic Foundation. Nearly all hair experts agree that each of us needs to experiment with shampoos, conditioners and other products until we find ones that work well. "Ask friends and your stylist for recommendations," says Shaw. "Don't be afraid to try different products."

Whether you have a thatch, mane or

fringe, here's how to keep your hair looking great with the least effort.

Keep it clean. Shampoo daily, unless your scalp is exceptionally dry. In that case, says Griffasi, rinse it well with water one day and shampoo it the next. Men tend to overuse dandruff shampoos, which overly dry hair and scalp, warns Shaw. Use a dandruff shampoo when you have a problem, then go back to a gentler shampoo. Use a shampoo for your scalp type: dry, normal or oily. If you're not sure of your scalp type, ask your stylist.

Condition, condition, condition. It takes only an extra minute or two in the shower, but it's a step that many men skip, says Griffasi. Shampoo first, then condition while soaping up the rest of your body.

Dry hair carefully. Towel-dry, then blow-dry. Use medium to high heat but low speed or airflow, says Griffasi. Keep the blow-dryer moving and at least six inches from your head to avoid overheating and damaging your hair. Don't overdry; stop while the top layer is still slightly damp.

Detangle gently. Use your fingers, a hair pick or a wide-tooth, vented plastic styling brush to desnarl. A bristle brush dragged through wet hair can do lasting damage, cautions Griffasi.

Avoid bleaching. Wear a cap or hat while golfing, gardening or sailing. If you swim in a pool regularly, rinse your hair thoroughly as soon as you get out, says Gregory Miller, head of the color department at the Vidal Sassoon Salon in New York City.

Why? The chlorine in pools is extremely rough on your hair. Think of it this way:

How would your jeans look if you washed them in bleach time after time after time? Chlorine has the same effect. It's not uncommon for chlorine to give hair a greenish tint, given enough exposure.

Keep your hair on the wagon. Skip products that list alcohol as an ingredient, advises Shaw. It dries and dulls hair.

Do a dab. To hold your hair in place and keep it out of your face, a dab of gel or mousse is great, according to Griffasi. If you have particularly dry hair, she recommends mixing three drops of silicone shiner, a styling product that you can buy in your salon, with a splat of gel and working it through lightly towel-dried hair like a pomade.

What It Is: A Man's Guide to Hair-Care Products

Looking for the right shampoo, conditioner, hair goop? You'll find only about 14 quadrillion different choices in the typical discount drugstore. Here's a quick rundown of various hair-care products, terms and ingredients.

Glosser, shiner, polisher, laminator, glass. Goop, usually loaded with silicone or oil, that you rub onto your hair to smooth it and make it gleam when it reflects light. Just two or three drops of silicone shiner worked throughout the hair brings especially dry hair to life, says Christina Griffasi, head of the styling department at the Minardi Salon in New York City. Skip these products if you have normal to oily hair, because they'll "weigh it down, make it look greasy and flat," advises Gillian Shaw, senior barber at the Vidal Sassoon Salon in New York City.

Thickeners, volumizers, body builders. Ingredients found in shampoos and conditioners; also stand-alone products. May infuse hair with proteins and actually expand the hair shaft from inside out or coat it with proteins, polymers and waxes to make it appear thicker. Some, Shaw warns, use alcohol to purposely dry out hair, because dry hair is fluffier. But the drying ones, she says, damage hair.

Clarifying shampoo. Use occasionally to cleanse away buildup from hair products such as from thickeners, says Griffasi.

Moisturizing. Term for shampoos, conditioners and

Skip the hair vitamins. Expensive nutritional supplements, taken orally, that claim to help your hair's health probably do little, says Dr. Mayer. "If you eat a normal, reasonably balanced diet, your hair will receive all of the nutrients it needs for growth," he explains. The type of severe malnutrition that does affect hair health is usually not found in the United States, he adds.

Switch often. "Don't get stuck with one shampoo; keep switching them often," says Diana Bihova, M.D., clinical assistant professor of dermatology at New York University Medical Center in New York City. "This is especially important for people with scalp problems like dandruff, psoriasis or dermatitis." You'll know that it's time to switch when the shampoo is less effective than it was when you first started using it. This doesn't mean that you have to buy a new brand every week. "Keep two main brands around and interchange them. For normal hair, switching gets rid of buildup."

Brush up your technique. To make your shampooing truly effective, first give your hair a good brushing. "This loosens excess grooming products, dirt and natural oil as well as stimulates your scalp," says Damien Miano, top hairstylist and co-owner of New York's Miano/Viél Salon and Spa. If you have long hair, begin by brushing just the ends of your hair to detangle it. Then gradually work your brush in toward your scalp. If you brush in one stroke from the scalp out to the ends, the force of brushing can damage the oldest part of your hair and cause the hair ends to split.

Don't brush too long or too strong. "You'll traumatize the hair if you brush it 100 times, like the old adage says," warns Dr. Bihova.

Neutralize static. Hair standing on end due to static electricity? It happens, particularly in winter. To get rid of it, wet a comb and run it slowly through your hair.

---

treatments that soften dry, brittle hair and hair exposed to environmental heat and dryness. Many contain glycerin, which helps hair grab and retain moisture. Some use oils to weigh hair and may give hair a flat, greasy look.

Conditioner. A treatment applied to wet hair after shampooing, then rinsed out. Often adds vitamins, moisturizer, shiner, proteins, detangler and more—sometimes even sunscreen—to your hair. Finding the right conditioner to leave your hair looking healthy and natural requires experimenting, says Shaw.

Leave-in conditioner. Applied and left in damp, towel-dried hair after shampooing. Some protein- and vitamin-infusing leave-in conditioners are great for men, says Griffasi. Some, warns Shaw, are gimmicks, causing too much buildup and irritating the scalp. Experiment.

Gel. When applied to dried hair, it "takes off the fluffy edge and holds hair in place," says Shaw. Use a dab or a lot. Especially good for styling short hair. Worked into wet hair, it dries hard, leaving a wet look.

Mousse. A foaming conditioner that helps hold hair in place. Good for curly and longer hair. Adds body and firmness.

Spritz, sprunch, spray gel. A lighter, liquefied gel, sprayed onto hair as a mist. "Good on all hair textures, applied wet or dry," says Shaw. Sprunching means shaping your hair with your hands as the spray dries.

How to Pick a Stylist

No matter how much hair you have, stylists agree, a good cut is the first step toward great-looking hair. And a good cut, says Shaw, is one that works with a person's natural features and hair—its natural part, texture, crown, cowlicks, curl, wave, lift and so on—to create an attractive, easy-to-maintain style.

Matching Hair to Face Shape

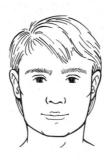

Square
Wider on top, flatter on the sides. Longer hair in back can create the illusion of a longer face.

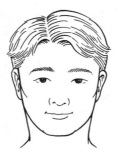

Round
Need to develop some angularity. A layered cut helps. Hairstyle should be wide on top and flat on the sides. Part off-center to slenderize the forehead.

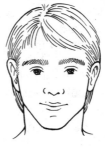

Diamond
Needs the illusion of a wider chin and forehead. Hair is fuller in back to offset the chin. Sides are close to the face. Off-center part hides a narrow forehead, creating the illusion of width. Bangs can work well.

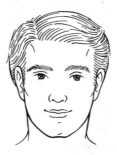

Oblong
Need to shorten face. Use a layered cut with full sides and a flat top.

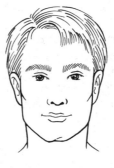

Sharp rectangle
Need to make the face appear wider and shorter. Styles that are flat on top help. Bangs are nice. Leave the sides full. Generally, hair should not be long in back.

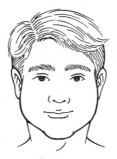

Pear
Similar to round. Fullness on top helps broaden the forehead. Bangs can create the illusion of width. Trim hair short on the sides.

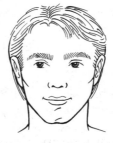

Triangle
Broad forehead and narrow chin. Hair should be full in back, adding weight around the chin area. Part off-center to trim the width of the forehead. Brush back the sides or keep them flat.

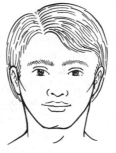

Heart
Need to narrow the forehead and widen the chin. Part off-center to cut the width of the forehead. Allow some fullness in the back to soften and draw the eye away from the chin-line.

A good short- to medium-length haircut lasts for about six weeks before "it starts to fuzz at the ends, lose its shape and look messy," says Griffasi. Regular sessions with the shears are a must to maintain a sharp, healthy look.

How do you find a good haircutter? Someone who'll make you look better than maybe God intended? Consider these tips from Barbara Bealer, Hair America artist and assistant education director at Allentown School of Cosmetology in Pennsylvania.

Watch the folks leaving. They shouldn't all have the same haircut. They should have styles that seem neat, natural, flattering and easy to maintain.

Look for someone who listens. Go for the stylist who asks questions about how you care for your hair, what you like and don't like about it and why you like various styles. A good stylist wants to know what kind of work you do and lets you know when trends that affect you change, so you can adjust.

Expect good instructions. Your stylist should advise you on shampooing, conditioning, drying, combing and so forth and should recommend products for your hair type and style that really do help. You should be able to ask "Which should I use: mousse, gel or axle grease?" and be able to then trust your stylist's answer.

Check the training. Is it up-to-date? Does the stylist have certificates posted showing that he attends continuing-education seminars to keep up with techniques and trends?

And finally, and perhaps most important:

Like your haircut, visit after visit. If this happens, you've hit gold. Most of us want a wash-and-wear cut that looks good every day with minimal maintenance. Let your stylist know if that's what you're after.

Types of Male-Pattern Baldness

Class 1
Frontal balding only, with or without a frontal tuft.

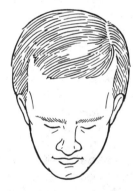

Class 2
Frontal and midscalp balding.

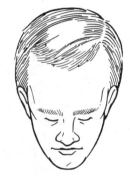

Class 3
Frontal to crown, or frontal and crown, balding.

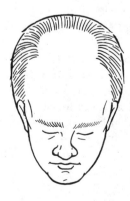

Class 4
Crown baldness without a frontal tuft.

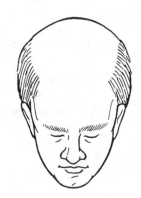

Great Styles

How you wear your hair affects how you look and the image you project to the world.

The "rebel farmer" look of the mid-1990s, a buzz cut on top and hair cascading down the shoulders in the back, may work fine for some country singers, welders and mechanics. But it isn't going to fly in most corporate boardrooms.

For most professionals, short- to medium-length styles are the right choice in the mid- to late 1990s, advises Shaw, though she notes that hairstyles can sometimes change almost overnight. A good stylist knows if you're edging obsolescence. Ask.

These days,

men's hairstyles are very much tied to the type of work we do. Creative, artistic types in all fields get away with longer, wilder hair than do executives, customer reps and spokesmen.

Besides fitting your role and image, your hairstyle can enhance your strongest facial features and de-emphasize less flattering ones. The drawings on page 174 (and accompanying text) show common facial shapes and how to best style hair for each, according to Bealer.

The Bald Truth

Not all of us will end up with a shiny dome and a horse-shoe-shaped fringe over the ears, but most of us will experience significant hair loss, says Dr. Mayer. We can do nothing to stop it. Even the so-called miracle of minoxidil (Rogaine) offers little hope. Only about 10 percent of males using the drug grow some cosmetically acceptable hair, doctors say.

A number of things can lead to hair loss: stress, chemotherapy, drugs, scalp infections, pulling hair. But by and large, the most common cause is genetically programmed male-pattern baldness.

This is classic baldness, where the hairline creeps backward toward the crown. Sometimes an ever-enlarging bald circle appears at the crown. Eventually, the open spaces merge.

Technically, what happens

Color to Dye For

We start life with a blend of up to eight different colors of hair on our heads. An example: Nature mixes together hairs that are blond, red and shades of light to dark brown to create a medium brown color that, in the sun, shimmers with blond and red highlights.

Over time, one by one, our follicles quit producing pigment, and we find less and less color and more and more transluscent, whiteish hairs in the mix. The less vivid combination of colors produces gray tones—tones that, as television wants us to believe, sap our vitality and consign us to obsolescence. We're taunted with images of restored youth, found in $7 bottles that "rinse away gray" and replace it with rich, natural color.

Don't believe it, says Gregory Miller, head of the color department for the Vidal Sassoon Salon in New York City. Dark, rich-colored home hair dyes turn all of your hair one solid color, which never looks natural, he says. And as your hair grows out, you have gray roots.

For natural hair coloring, Miller advises you to:

See a colorist. The best salons have people who specialize only in coloring hair. They'll advise you about what is and is not possible.

Blend in color. A professional colorist will blend in only a little color here and there, in areas that normally turn gray last. They'll "squeeze out very, very small wefts of hair and place them in aluminum packets with color," he says. "The foil keeps the color from going onto the other hairs."

Expect to invest real time and money. You'll spend a couple of hours in the salon every three months. It'll cost $200 in a famous-name salon, maybe as little as $50 in the heartland, says Miller.

Practice damage control. That means protecting your hair from the sun and chlorinated pools.

If you insist on hitting the bottle at home, take the advice of Angela McEntee, spokeswoman for Just for Men, which makes hair-coloring preparations for men.

• Follow all of the instructions on the package, including the color and skin tests.

• Pick a color that is a shade or two lighter than your natural hair color. A lighter-shade permanent dye will not lighten your existing dark hairs but will color your white hairs with the lighter shade for a more natural blending effect.

in men who are programmed for baldness is that chemical receptors in the hair follicles convert testosterone to dihydrotestosterone (DHT) at a genetically determined time. DHT in the follicles causes hair to grow thinner and weaker; eventually, all that is left is vellus hair. Even when abundant, this fuzz is of little consolation to the man losing his hair, according to Dominic A. Brandy, M.D., clinical instructor of dermatology at the University of Pittsburgh School of Medicine, in his book *A New Headstart! Doctor's Complete Guide to the Latest Advances in Hair Replacement.*

Heredity's precise role in balding has not been firmly established, but most of us seem to experience the hair-loss patterns of our fathers or maternal grandfathers, says Dr. Mayer. But there are always exceptions; heredity doesn't always mean destiny.

Scientific testing is underway on a number of chemical compounds that may someday slow or halt male-pattern baldness. Most interfere with how the scalp and follicles process testosterone. Many have nasty side effects. Minoxidil is the only drug available to the general public for dealing with hair loss. And, Dr. Mayer warns, no over-the-counter remedies advertised in magazines or on television have been proven to work. So for now, according to Dr. Mayer, those of us losing our hair can pick from the following menu of choices:

- Style around it.
- Accept it.
- Hide it under a rug.
- Surgically change it.

Style it. We all know someone who grows nine-inch-long strands just above one

Those Who Cut Their Own Hair

Not too long ago, the *Wall Street Journal* ran an article featuring some rather well-known men who insist on cutting their own hair. Most admitted that they have produced horrendous and laughable results at times. But they enjoy the element of danger, the potential for disaster. And besides, as graphic artist Chuck Beasley of Emmaus, Pennsylvania, says, "The difference between a good haircut and a bad haircut? A few weeks."

It's true. You can take the scissors to your own hair. Or you can buy a $79 Flowbee haircutting tool that connects to your vacuum cleaner and sucks your hair into whirring blades. Or try the $29 Wahl electric barber clippers.

If this idea appeals to you, we suggest that you stop at your local public library and check out a couple of books illustrating home haircutting techniques. You'll see that the logic, technique and art of haircutting can be mastered. You might even get good at it. We also suggest that you install a couple of great mirrors to leave your hands free and to allow you to see your head from all views, especially the sides and back.

ear, then combs them up and over his bald dome and cements them there. This is not a cover-up that stylists recommend.

Your haircutter, though, can help camouflage your thin spots and emphasize your strong features if you ask, says Dr. Mayer. If you don't bring up the subject, your stylist, out of politeness, probably won't, either.

Here are some general guidelines.

- Stick to a short style if you're obviously losing hair, says Shaw. Growing it long, or sweeping a few lonely wisps across the great divide, draws attention to a losing proposition, she says.
- Hide a small bald spot or disguise marginal recession by slightly altering your part and style and possibly by adding body and direction with a permanent wave or a spot perm, says Dr. Mayer.
- Comb hair forward a bit to disguise a receding hairline. An off-center part may hide

the deep V of scalp on each side, says Dr. Mayer.

Accept it. Sean Connery, the late Telly Savalas, John Malkovich, the late Yul Brynner, Michael Jordan, Charles Barkley, Patrick Stewart, George Foreman: All have capitalized on their baldness and are considered sex symbols. Savalas and Brynner shaved their heads, as do Jordan and Foreman, creating a bold, confident look—certainly an option for those who can carry it off.

Bury it. John Wayne, Humphrey Bogart, Paul Simon, Frank Sinatra: four men who wear wigs well, at least on film and videotape. Add Sean Connery (as James Bond) and now-you-see-it, now-you-don't Willard Scott.

A great hairpiece, properly cared for, works wonders. A bad hairpiece—well, you might as well wear a sign on your rear saying "Kick me."

A great hairpiece is custom-built to fit your skull and custom-matched to your hair color. It will probably have a slightly receding hairline and a hair density typical for men your age, so it looks real, says Dr. Mayer.

You can expect to spend $2,000 to $5,000 for two identical custom-made hairpieces. (You alternate between them, so you extend their wear and you don't go bare while one is in for cleaning and repair. Yes, hairpieces need regular maintenance.) If they're carefully maintained, you'll get two to three years of life out of them.

Replace it. A skilled, artistic, experienced surgeon can move flaps of hair from the sides of your head and rotate them into place across the front and top of your head, explains Dr. Mayer. By combining this procedure with tissue expansion techniques, scalp reduction surgery, individual hair transplants and some fancy styling, you can end up with a real and realistic-looking head of hair for somewhere between $10,000 and $40,000. Don't expect insurance to reimburse you.

And be very careful, warns Dr. Mayer. Any M.D. can set up shop as a hair-replacement surgeon, and too many have, he and Dr. Brandy agree. Insist on seeing tons of close-up, evenly lighted before-and-after photos and videos of their work. And even more important, "ask to see live patients who have your type of baldness and who have received the type of treatment that's being recommended for you," says Dr. Mayer. "See if you like what you see. That's the only way to judge. See live results."

National hair-replacement chains don't have great reputations, says Dr. Brandy. Both he and Dr. Mayer advise seeking a private physician who devotes his practice primarily to hair replacement.

The most realistic, effective and inexpensive way to surgically replace hair is a combination of the following techniques, Dr. Mayer says. All of these procedures are shown in detail in *The Everyman's Guide to Hair Replacement*, the book that Dr. Mayer co-authored with Richard Fleming, M.D.

Tissue expansion. A procedure borrowed from modern plastic surgery and modified. Balloons are implanted in the scalp beneath areas bearing dense hair and, over a period of two to three months, are inflated so that the areas grow up to one-third larger, resulting in the production of more hair.

Scalp reduction. Large sections of bald scalp are removed, and hairy areas on either side of the head are stretched over and sewn together. Sometimes the forehead is lifted slightly as well, removing wrinkles and excess loose, bare scalp.

Flap surgery. Long flaps, up to two inches wide, of hair-bearing scalp are cut from the sides of the head and grafted across the front and top to cover balding areas. Hairy areas above and below the donor sites are sewn together. The surgery involves several steps over two weeks.

Hair transplants. For the most natural results, flap hairlines can be further softened by moving and randomly placing single hairs along the flap hairline. In the early days of this surgery, plugs of hair were moved. Generally, the finished product looked like a bald scalp with plugs of hair transplanted.

Hands

- **Do exercises for finger dexterity and strength.**
- **Play a musical instrument.**
- **Give them regular breaks from typing and other intense work.**

Although they've been hardened by nearly 70 years of plucking the strings of his ancient bass, Milt Hinton's well-worn hands still gracefully weave his musical legacy.

"My feelings, my interpretation of life, my whole character comes out through my hands. They're like pencils that I use to draw what I feel in my soul," says Hinton, a jazz legend in his eighties who has performed with Louis Armstrong, Cab Calloway, Duke Ellington, Frank Sinatra and Paul McCartney.

In a sense, whether we're delicately stroking a lover's breast or throwing a haymaker into a drunken lout's ugly face, we all reveal a bit of our inner feelings through our hands.

"The hands are amazing parts of the body. Much of what we experience we interpret and express through our hands. So it's important to prize and value them," says Robert Markison, M.D., a hand surgeon and associate clinical professor of surgery at the University of California, San Francisco, School of Medicine.

The Brain in Your Fingers

The hands have 27 bones each, including 8 in the wrist, 5 in the palm, 3 in each finger and 2 in the thumb. These bones are interwoven by a complex series of muscles, tendons and ligaments. (Ligaments are the elastic cords that hold bones together, and tendons are the cords that connect muscle to bone.)

The most versatile body parts, the hands are extremely sensitive to pain, temperature and touch. The main muscles for controlling hand movement are in the forearms and are con-

nected to the fingers by strong tendons. When these muscles contract, the fingers open or close. The beauty of this system is that it gives your hands brute power from your arms to do many of the necessary tasks of life, such as hauling garbage out to the curb, shoveling snow in the wintertime and futilely hailing a taxi in a thunderstorm.

But your hands are also nimble enough to tie fishing flies and to deftly play a musical instrument. Dexterity comes from 20 small muscles within each hand. Hungarian pianist Franz Liszt was so dexterous that he sometimes played difficult compositions with two water glasses balanced on the back of his hands, never spilling a drop.

But as vital as your hands are for performing routine tasks—try turning a page, typing a letter or answering a telephone without them—they are also critical information gatherers for your brain. To get an idea of their importance, imagine that your brain's sensory centers are about the size of the United States. The space that your brain devotes solely to sensory input from your hands would equal Alaska, California and Texas combined.

Keeping Them Healthy

Most men have had their share of tumbles and accidents and have learned that the hands are among the most vulnerable parts of the body, particularly to cuts, burns and fractures. Tendinitis and arthritis are also common. (For more on these conditions, see pages 210 and 212.) Increasing hand dexterity and strength is often your best defense against all of these problems. Here are some simple exercises that can help.

Do a morning massage. Take a minute each morning to gently massage your fingers and hands. "During sleep, you don't move your hands very much. By taking a moment to massage them, you're waking them up and refreshing them," Dr. Markison says.

Begin with the fingertips of one hand and work your way down to your palm, gently squeezing and rolling the knuckles and joints
(continued on page 182)

Touch

- **Body part most sensitive to touch: tip of the tongue**
- **Body part least sensitive to touch: ball of the foot**
- **Number of nerve endings per square inch of the average fingertip: up to 50,000**

The Touch That Means So Much

There's nothing that a man respects more than a firm handshake, one that's not too tight or too limp. You often get only one shot at it, and that moment can determine if you get a job or continue scanning the want ads. How do you do know if it's just right?

It has a lot to do with your sense of touch.

Your skin contains thousands of touch receptors, specialized nerve endings that respond to particular sensations, such as pressure, heat, cold and pain. Other receptors keep your brain aware of the positions of your hands and feet. Some parts of the body have more of one type of receptor than another. The eyes, for example, are 100 times more sensitive to pain than the soles of the feet.

The fingertips are particularly sensitive to the slightest pressure and can detect objects that are millimeters apart. So when you shake someone's hand, nerves in your fingers relay signals up your spinal cord to the cerebral cortex in your brain, where they are interpreted. Your brain instantaneously sends signals back to your hand, so it can adjust the pressure to make the handshake perfect, says Yadollah Harati, M.D., professor of neurology at Baylor College of Medicine in Houston.

Touch often diminishes with age, as nerve receptors in the skin gradually die. Diabetes and alcoholism can also dull touch. But maintaining your overall health will help keep tissue alive longer. Like the rest of your body, nerves depend on nutrition, exercise and good circulation, Dr. Harati says. ■

How to Be a Sensitive Guy

As any safecracker can tell you, having a strong sense of touch is good. Sure, it helps you avoid pain and damage. But better, it allows you to enjoy the finer things in life: the smooth coat of a faithful hound, the warmth of a roaring fire, the delicious pressure of a partner's body against yours. Here are some simple ways to stay in touch with your world.

Make sex a science experiment. What better time to work on your sense of touch than during a feast of sensual touch? But be more selfish the next time you enter a sexual encounter.

Sensate focusing is a technique taught to men to control premature ejaculation. In it, you focus on your sensations when touching a partner. What do your fingers feel? Your lips? Your chest? Don't concentrate on your genitals; you already know how sensitive Mr. Happy is. By tuning in to total body sensations, you not only improve ejaculatory control but also enhance your general sensitivity.

Come in from the cold. When you're scraping your windshield this winter, be sure to protect your hands—and any other exposed patches of skin. "Frostbite may kill nerve endings in the skin and cause whole body parts to fall off," says John E. Wolf, Jr., M.D., chairman of the Department of Dermatology at Baylor College of Medicine in Houston. "But even occasional exposure to intense cold can cause blood flow to be directed away from skin surfaces." The result: loss of sensation over time. The remedy is simple: Wear gloves or mittens.

Screen out rays. You already know that too much exposure to the sun can cause skin cancer, which could really put a damper on your sense of touch. But basking too long in the sun's glow also causes your skin to harden and thicken over time. Even if you manage to avoid the ravages of cancer, your skin will be one big callus. So break out the sunscreen—and make sure it has a sun protection factor (SPF) of at least 15. ■

Moisturize. Men especially tend to suffer from dry, cracked skin, says Dr. Wolf. This makes your sense of touch overly sensitive. The elements, your clothing, even your very own body hair will constantly irritate your skin; your sense of touch will drive you crazy. But it doesn't have to.

"Men just don't believe in using moisturizing agents on their skin, and they should," says Dr. Wolf. Any over-the-counter moisturizing lotion, such as Purpose or Vaseline Intensive Care, will do. "Buy an unscented brand," says Dr. Wolf, since a perfume could further irritate your skin, not to mention that touchy male ego.

Get a rubdown. Besides stimulating your skin, massage is a wonderful stress reducer and sex enhancer rolled into one. Take turns with your partner giving and receiving massages. Keep the rubdown gentle; think light touching rather than deep kneading. ■

A Ticklish Situation

Why are we ticklish in some places but not in others? Why can't we tickle ourselves? Why are we ticklish at all? The answers to these ticklish questions lie in that nebulous link between the body and the mind. On one hand, tickling occurs when someone excites the delicate nerve endings just under your skin. That's clearly a physical response. But the tickler has to be the right someone, a person you're close to, in order for your mind to respond to the sensation as tickling. If a stranger tried to tickle you, you wouldn't respond to it as a playful attack. Your mind would interpret the sensations as some wacko messing with you.

Experts say that by sheer force of will, you can overcome the psychological urge to laugh when tickled. But your body may substitute a painful sensation instead. All we can say is good luck. It's hard to concentrate on anything when your wife or girlfriend has you backed into a corner, cackling madly as she plays your rib cage like a xylophone. ■

as you go. Keep working your way down into your wrist and upper forearm. Then massage your other hand.

Squeeze in a shower. Keep a palm-size sponge in the shower, so you can slowly squeeze the water out of it. Do this five to ten times with each hand every morning while you bathe, Dr. Markison says. It will help tone your hand muscles.

Name that tune. Playing an inexpensive and simple musical instrument, such as a recorder, for 10 to 15 minutes a day can improve your hand coordination and dexterity. "The recorder is perfectly designed for use by the hands. I play it every single morning to wake up my hands and brain," says Dr. Markison, who is also a professional clarinet and saxophone player.

Touch and go. To improve your finger dexterity and coordination, touch the tip of your thumb to the tip of each finger of your hand, moving from your index finger to your little finger and back again. Start slowly and increase your speed as you go. Do this five times with each hand, two or three times a day, says Mary Ann Towne, a licensed physical therapist and director of rehabilitation and wellness services at the Cleveland Clinic Florida in Fort Lauderdale.

Give yourself a break. Like your wrists, your fingers and hands need frequent rest stops, particularly if you're doing a repetitive-motion job such as typing or tightening bolts on an assembly line. Take a 5-minute break every 30 minutes to stretch and relax your hands, says Steven Bogard, hand therapy supervisor at the Mayo Clinic in Rochester, Minnesota.

Bend and stretch. Slowly bend your fingers at the knuckles farthest from the palm into a modified fist. You might feel a slight pulling sensation as the muscles in your fingers stretch. Hold this position for ten seconds. Do this five times with each hand,

Knuckle Stretch

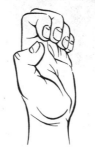

Hold the stretch for ten seconds, then relax. Do five sets with each hand, two or three times a day, to strengthen your fingers.

says. Do this five times per hand, two or three times a day.

Extend yourself. Loop a rubber band over the back of all of the fingers of one hand, positioning it between the middle and end joints. Hold this loop stable with your other hand and pull your fingers into a straightened position. Hold for three seconds. Do this five times with each hand, two or three times a day. This strengthening exercise can also be done with individual fingers, Bogard says.

Reach for it. Put a box of your favorite cereal on the highest kitchen shelf that you can reach, suggests Thomas Rizzo, Jr., M.D., a consultant in physical medicine and rehabilitation at the Mayo Clinic Jacksonville in Florida.

Rubber-Band Stretch

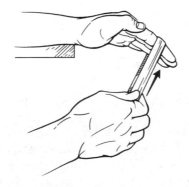

Do five sets with each hand, two or three times a day, to strengthen the muscles on the back of your hand.

two or three times a day, Towne says.

Spread out. Put your hand on a table and slowly spread out your fingers so that you're creating a fanlike effect. Hold for ten seconds, then relax and repeat, Bogard

Reaching for that box will not only stretch out your fingers but also limber up other important joint muscles in your wrist, elbow, shoulder and back.

Handy First-Aid

Of course, even the strongest hands can be injured. Here are a couple of first-aid tips.

Keep sprains under wraps. Immobilize a minor hand or finger sprain for three to four days, using a

Don't Be a Sucker If You Punch

The Marquis of Queensberry rules, boxing's sacrosanct version of the Ten Commandments, don't apply to street fights or barroom brawls. So when a jerk snarls in your face, he probably won't be gracious enough to let you dash off in search of a pair of boxing gloves before he swings at you.

If you're lucky, you'll be able to walk away from him without any fisticuffs. If not, beware: Doing battle bare-fisted can cause more harm to you than to your foe unless you know how and where to throw your punches.

"If you hit a person on a hard surface, such as the top of his head, you're likely to injure your own hand. If you're going to hit somebody, you'll incapacitate him quicker and protect your hands better if you hit him in the gut," says Flip Homansky, M.D., director of the emergency room of Valley Hospital in Las Vegas, who has been a ringside doctor for many world-championship bouts.

But if, like most men, you instinctively take a swing at your tormentor's head, avoid hitting him in his mouth. That's probably the worst place to hit someone, because the human mouth is awash with bacteria that can cause serious infection if you cut your hand on your opponent's teeth

To throw a punch that is safe but still packs a wallop, make a fist, but keep your thumb on the outside of your fingers and curled under-neath the bottom of the fist. Tilt your hand downward slightly and lock your wrist, says Michael Olajidé, Jr., former Canadian middleweight boxing champion. This ensures that the knuckles of your index and middle fingers, which are stronger and less susceptible to injury, make first contact.

Making a Fist

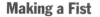

Keep your thumb outside and curled underneath your fingers. Tilt your hand downward slightly and lock your wrist.

Pick a target and throw as straight a punch as you can at it. Avoid swinging overhand; besides taking some of the steam of out of your punch, it will probably make you miss your target, says Olajidé.

On defense keep your hands close to your body and up toward your face to deflect punches. "Generally, guys will punch at the face first. Few think of going for the body," Olajidé says.

comfortable splint or a loosely wrapped elastic bandage, says David Lichtman, M.D., professor of orthopedics and head of the Division of Hand Surgery at Baylor College of Medicine in Houston. For pain, he recommends that you take one 500-milligram aspirin or two 200-milligram ibuprofen tablets every four hours.

To reduce swelling, Dr. Lichtman says, apply an ice pack wrapped in a towel to the injury. Leave it on for 20 minutes and then remove it for 20 minutes, continuing this pattern for the first 2 hours. Then apply it for 8 to 10 minutes of every waking hour during the next 24 to 48 hours. After a day or so, begin exercising the injured area to restore circulation. Elevate your hand as often as possible to drain away the fluid that causes swelling. If the injury is still sore after two days, apply a warm heating pad to the area for 10 to 15 minutes of every hour as needed. If the pain, swelling and discoloration persist for more than four days, see your doctor.

Don't be Ringo. Take off rings before working around machinery, because they can get caught in the inner workings of the device and rip off fingers, Dr. Lichtman says. If this happens, put the detached finger in a plastic bag, then put the bag into a chest of ice until you receive medical attention. You should never put the finger directly on the ice or use dry ice, because that will kill tissue. Gently rinse the finger in tepid

The Other Right Hand

Imagine being the first left-handed caveman, bumping elbows with everyone else in your tribe of right-handed mammoth slayers.

"You'd be treated as if you were cursed and either exiled from the tribe or killed," says right-handed Stanley Coren, Ph.D., professor of psychology at the University of British Columbia in Vancouver and author of the *The Left-Hander Syndrome.*

Although life has gotten somewhat better for lefties since man evolved from caves to cars, surviving in a world designed and built for righties still isn't easy. In his studies, Dr. Coren found that left-handers are 89 percent more likely to suffer injuries in accidents, and five times more likely to die from those injuries, than right-handers.

Here are some other leftover facts.

• Only 10 percent of humans are left-handed. Scientists aren't sure why. But based on cave drawings and other clues, researchers believe that man has been predominantly right-handed for at least 1.5 million years.

• In virtually every culture, "left" has unpleasant connotations. The Latin word for left is *sinister.* In German, *linkisch* means left, but it also means unhandy. The French word for left, *gauche,* also means clumsy. And the Old English word for left, *lyft,* also means weak or broken.

• The official handshake of the Boy Scouts is left-handed. The Scouts' founder, Lord Robert Baden-Powell, who was ambidextrous, apparently was impressed with a particular African tribe that greeted others with a left-handed shake. So he adapted it for his own organization.

• In Middle Eastern countries, the left hand is considered unclean because it has traditionally been used to wipe after defecating. In Saudi Arabia, it is against the law to use the left hand in public.

• Great left-handed dinner guests from history? Try Jack the Ripper, the Boston Strangler and Billy the Kid. For a more sedate evening, try Johann Sebastian Bach, Benjamin Franklin, Michelangelo and Leonardo da Vinci.

• Two dining rules for lefties to live by:

1. Let others sit first. It will almost guarantee you an outside seat, the best place for a lefty.

2. Don't be timid about rearranging your place setting to meet your needs.

tap water only if it is extremely dirty. To prevent unnecessary nerve damage, avoid using antiseptics and never wash or scrub a detached finger with soap, detergent or a washcloth.

The Rules of Handshaking

In a political campaign, there are two ironclad rules: Kiss every baby and shake all of the hands that you can.

"It's basic politics. Get out there, shake hands, be sincere and say hello. People relate to that," says Congressman John P. Murtha, a Pennsylvania Democrat who was first elected in 1974.

"During one campaign, I must have shaken hands with 5,000 people at a parade. Five years later, a guy came up to me and reminded me that I'd shaken his hand at that parade. That's the kind of impression that a good handshake can make."

So whether you're running for dogcatcher or interviewing for your dream job, your handshake counts. Here are some tips from Congressman Murtha.

• Look self-assured; don't be shy. Walk right up to the person you're meeting and offer your hand.

• Make sure that you tuck the inside of your thumb into the inside of the other person's thumb. It will prevent wear and tear on your hand and allow you to get a firm grip.

• Look the person in the eyes and smile. Then in one quick motion, squeeze his hand firmly, shake once and release.

◣ Heart

- **Exercise it regularly.**
- **Keep the plumbing clean by eating less fat.**
- **Reduce daily stress.**
- **Don't smoke.**

Leonardo da Vinci, who seemed to have words of wisdom on just about every subject, found himself almost speechless when describing the heart: "How in words can you describe this heart without filling a whole book? Yet the more detail you write concerning it, the more you will confuse the mind of the hearer."

He's right. So for clarity, forget everything that anyone has told you about the heart and know just this: It's a pump. Like any pump, it has tubes—tubes pumping stuff in and tubes pumping stuff out. And like most pumps, it's powered by electricity.

Really, there's not much else you need to understand, except what can go wrong with it. Fortunately, there's not much. The tubes can get clogged and gunky. They can crack, leak or bubble up. The electrical wiring can fray and short-circuit. A surge of electricity can overload it. Or more often, it simply stops working, usually from old age and when it's already many years past warranty.

It's a wonderful machine, this heart of man. Elegant in form and function. And yet it is so complex, so misunderstood, that every time you turn on the television or skim a newspaper or magazine, there's some new report telling you what to eat and what not to eat, what to do and what not to do to keep it pumping. We'll discuss these issues in just a bit, along with some bottom-line recommendations. In the meantime, here's a quick review.

- Lesson number one: The heart is made up of muscle. Flex it, and it gets stronger.
- Lesson number two: The heart has lots of plumbing. Keep the tubes clean, and it'll run more smoothly and for a long time.
- Lesson number three: Ignore the first two lessons, and all bets are off.

The entire machine metaphor can be taken only so far, but let's add one thing: Periodic checkups help keep things running. It works for your car and your water heater. It'll work for your heart, too.

Later on, we'll show you how to take heart readings, along with how to maintain heart health. But to start, let's take a closer look at the heart itself: where it's located, how it works and what can go wrong.

The Heartland

About the size of a clenched fist, your heart sits slightly to the left of the center of your chest, nicely sandwiched between your breastbone and spine and surrounded by your lungs. It consists of three layers of muscle: the endocardium, a moist, smooth inner layer that reduces friction for the stuff passing through; the myocardium, a thick, muscular wall that does the pumping; and the epicardium, a thin membrane that surrounds the whole thing and is part of a larger structure called the pericardium. The pericardium anchors the heart in place—a good thing, because nobody appreciates a wandering heart.

Imagine the heart as a four-room apartment, presumably one that's less messy than yours. Each room is one of the heart's four chambers. The top two rooms, the atria, are the collecting chambers; they collect "spent" blood from the veins as well as fresh, oxygenated blood from the lungs. The bottom two rooms, the ventricles, are the pumping chambers; they shove blood out of the heart, first to the lungs for oxygenation and then to the body's arteries for general circulation.

As you can see, the heart is a four-directional pump. Tubes lead to and from the body and to and from the lungs. To prevent blood from going in the wrong direction and from backwashing into the chamber it just emerged from, the heart also has a number of one-way valves. It's the opening and closing of these valves that make the sound of a heartbeat. That familiar *lub-dub* is caused by the two sets of synchronized contractions that make up the heart's cycle.

In the annals of folklore, history and art, the heart has long held an exalted position. Yet it's still a muscle, and like all muscles, it requires a constant supply of blood to keep its cells fed. Paradoxically, it can't drink from its own well; instead, it requires a number of arteries, called coronary arteries, to provide the necessary blood and nutrients.

From the top of the heart emerges the aorta, the big kahuna of arteries. Branching off the aorta are the coronary arteries. They trace along the surface of the heart, then circle the top and branch down like a crown.

There's a reason for all of this plumbing. Even at rest your heart works hard. It's a demanding muscle that requires a lot of blood. Consider this: Your heart represents less than 1 percent of your body weight, yet it uses about 5 percent of the total blood pumped. More than seven ounces of blood flow through your coronary arteries each minute.

Any damage to the coronary arteries—from accumulation of fatty, cholesterol-laden plaque, for example—threatens the heart muscle itself. Coronary artery disease causes more deaths than any other heart-related condition.

The Powers That Be

Your body does not come with an extension cord. There's no compartment for batteries. Nor is it solar-, wind- or water-powered—not yet, anyway. So it's natural to

ask: If the heart is a pump, what's powering it?

The heart comes equipped with a built-in generator. There's a bundle of cells called the sinoatrial node located in the upper part of the right atrium. It is the heart's natural pacemaker. Like the mechanical device of the same name, the pacemaker delivers the juice that makes the heart beat. It acts like a spark plug, sending a jolt of electricity that makes your heart contract, pump blood and relax, all in the space of about one second.

As you age, however, the impulses that drive your heart can misfire. "Damage to the heart muscle can block the electrical pathways," says cardiologist Geoffrey Tofler, M.D., assistant professor of medicine at Harvard Medical School and co-director of the Institute for Prevention of Cardiovascular Diseases at Deaconess Hospital in Boston. That can lead to abnormal heartbeats called arrhythmias. The

The Parts of the Heart

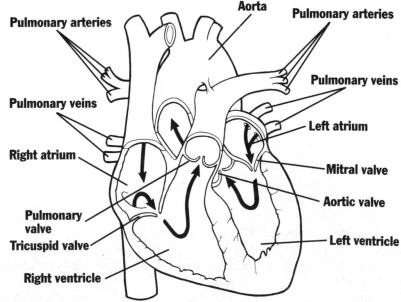

By eating less fat and keeping your cholesterol levels down, you greatly increase the chances that blood will flow smoothly through the tubes and chambers that make up your heart.

most dangerous type of arrhythmia, called ventricular fibrillation, causes the heart's beating to become very rapid and uncoordinated—entirely chaotic. When this happens, blood doesn't pump, and you can die.

Give It Air

Remember lesson number one above? The heart is a muscle and so needs regular exercise. The question is, how do you do that? If the technology of that classic sci-fi movie *Fantastic Voyage* ever comes to pass, someday you'll be able to shrink its star, Raquel Welch, to the size of a single cell and send her down to your heart with some barbells to lead it in a workout. But for now, there's one way to strengthen your heart: aerobic exercise.

Aerobic comes from the Greek word *aero*, which means air. According to our bedside medical encyclopedia (which we read occasionally as a cure for insomnia), an aerobe is "a microorganism that lives and grows in the presence of free oxygen." That would be all of us, bro.

Why is air so essential? Every cell in your body requires oxygen as part of the chemical reaction that creates energy. Without a steady flow of oxygen through your body, you would perish.

Aerobic exercise is any activity that requires a continuous heightened supply of oxygen, says Dr. Tofler. It could be swimming, walking, running, dancing or simply deep-breathing exercises, called pranayama in the yogic tradition.

How does aerobic exercise strengthen your heart? Say you're on a bicycle. Your leg muscles need more oxygen than usual to sustain the constant pedaling. So to get that oxygen to your legs, you breathe harder, and your heart pumps

more often. Sustain that heightened heart rate for a while, and your heart and lungs get stronger at delivering oxygen, Dr. Tofler says.

What's great about aerobic exercise is that it's not about brawn. Nor is it about accuracy, speed, hand-eye coordination or the competitive killer instinct. It's about making your body more efficient through steady activity. It trains your heart to go above and beyond the usual call of duty, to pump more blood in fewer beats. In the world of white coats, this is called stroke volume.

The real boon of a great stroke volume is that it can stretch the life of your heart. It works like this: If your heart was on a warranty, it would guarantee something like 2.5 billion beats in an average lifetime. If you improve your heart's efficiency so that each beat pumps more blood, you can save a beat here and there and then apply them to the other end of your life, when you'll probably be able to use a couple of extra beats. Consider aerobic

Understanding Blood Pressure

When your doctor (or, more likely, his assistant) wraps that little inflatable cuff around your arm and starts pumping, he is not acting out his sadistic side. His intention is to cut off circulation to your arm so that he can study how hard your blood pushes through your body.

There are two numbers to think about when looking at blood pressure. Consider a healthy reading of 110 over 60 (clinically written as 110/60 mm. Hg, since blood pressure is calculated as millimeters of mercury). The first or top number is the systolic pressure. It measures the pressure of blood when your heart is working hardest—when it beats. (If the aorta was opened at precisely that moment, blood would spurt about five feet.) The second or bottom number is the diastolic reading. It measures the strength of blood flow between beats.

When systolic pressure is too high (near 140 or above), your heart is probably pumping too hard. When diastolic pressure is too high (90 or above), the arteries are rarely getting a break or may be clogged. More than 50 million Americans have high blood pressure, many without knowing it. Untreated, high blood pressure can lead to heart problems, stroke and kidney disease.

exercise a long-term savings account in which heartbeats saved now offer a very good return on your investment later.

These are all very good incentives for choosing an aerobic activity that you enjoy and for doing it regularly. In part 3 of this book, where we discuss how to get in shape, fitness authorities suggest maintaining aerobic workouts for at least 30 minutes and doing three workouts a week. But here's a key point: There's nothing necessarily magic about these numbers. There's plenty of value in exerting yourself for 15 minutes. Even 10 minutes of fast walking has health benefits, says Dr. Tofler. And it certainly beats conning yourself into thinking that you're exercising by getting up to change the channel rather than using the remote.

Tubing and Heart Health

Gravity does not move blood around your body; pressure does. Pressure moves blood from your heart to the rest of your body and back again. The pressure, which is measured as the force of blood against the walls of the arteries, is determined by several factors: the pumping action of the heart, the resistance to the flow in the smaller arteries, the flexibility of the main arteries and blood volume and thickness. The numbers used to determine your personal blood pressure measure how well your arteries stretch and then relax to let

An Icon for the Ages

The next time she drops you a note with a tiny heart penciled next to her name, take that piece of paper and frame it. Bronze it. Or at least laminate it. Above all, cherish it. It says a lot more than you may think.

The heart does more than keep you vertical. In literature, religion and art, it's a universal symbol of love, intelligence, generosity—and more.

The image we're most familiar with, which shows up on everything from bumper stickers to heart-healthy menus, does bear a slight resemblance to the human heart. Historically, however, the connection wasn't quite so literal.

In the Middle Ages, the symbol that we use for the heart may have been more closely linked to the symbol for fire and flight. Another related notation represented union or togetherness.

In ancient Greece, the symbol for the heart was similar to the symbol for the lyre—a logical connection, since this was the instrument strummed by Eros, the god of sexual love.

In ancient Egypt and also among the Chinese, the heart was a symbol of life and the seat of emotion and intelligence. In our own culture, the heart has come to represent, above all, ardor, whether spiritual, sexual or romantic.

Meanwhile, what meaning can be derived from the fact that the biggest bank in the world, the Japanese Dai:Ichi Kangyo Bank, uses a heart-shaped silhouette as its corporate logo? Could it be the bank's attempt to win its way into the hearts, if not the wallets, of its countrymen?

Not all cultures are equally enthralled with the heart. In Sweden, for example, the heart symbol is used to denote public toilets; its meaning is the equivalent of derriere.

The lesson to be learned from all of this is that the heart is generally an enduring symbol of love and togetherness. But don't use it to punctuate a love note to a Swedish gal. The response might be more—or less—than you asked for.

The symbol used in the Middle Ages for fire and flight.

The ancient symbol for union or togetherness.

The modern symbol for sexual love; the arrow is from Cupid or Eros.

The ancient Greek symbol for the lyre, an attribute of Eros, the god of sexual love.

blood flow from your heart.

This should be the end of the story. Except that something like 50 million Americans of all ages—about one in four adults—have high blood pressure (readings of 140/90 or more), a condition also known as hypertension. Men are at greater risk for high blood pressure than women until age 55; after that, the risk evens out. And in about 90 percent of cases, the cause of high blood pressure is not known, though it doesn't take Sherlock Holmes to track down some clues.

For one, clogged and hardened arteries, which can come from eating too much fat and cholesterol, have less space for blood to flow through. For another, excessive salt draws fluid into the blood, increasing volume and therefore pressure in the limited artery space. A third cause might be the couple of extra pounds that a guy is carrying, since his heart must work harder to tote that excess baggage around.

Race plays a role as well. There's a higher incidence of high blood pressure among African-American men and men of Hispanic backgrounds than among Caucasians and Asians. And genes are a factor. If your father and your grandfather have had heart problems, you are more susceptible.

How does this discussion of blood pressure relate to the health of your heart? Well, think about that pump metaphor again. If it has to pump fluid through small or blocked tubes (clogged arteries), or if it's pumping more fluid than it's used to (too much salt), or if it's a small pump driving a big piece of machinery (overweight), that pump is going to poop out sooner rather than later. The extra wear and tear, the sheer additional effort, sets it up for breaking down in any number of ways.

The more your arteries are clogged, the higher your blood pressure, and the harder your heart has to work to get blood to where it needs to be. This weakens the heart and sets it up for a breakdown. This, again, is why the condition of your arteries is so critical to your heart's condition, says Gary James, Ph.D., associate professor of physiology at the New York

Hospital–Cornell Medical Center in New York City. That, you'll recall, is lesson number two above: Keep the tubes clean.

We explain how to keep your arteries clean and healthy in the chapters on nutrition (page 2) and the arteries (page 82). The message of both is to eat less fat and cholesterol. Trust us: Besides quitting smoking, there is just about nothing you can do that's better for your heart and your health than leaning down your diet. Be sure to read those sections thoroughly. Meanwhile, here are some additional tips that will hold off high blood pressure and other cardiovascular diseases.

Shake the salt habit. If you're like most people, you love salt—always have, always will. It's only human, since everyone needs a little salt to survive. But sodium, which makes up 40 percent of salt, draws fluid into your vascular system, increasing the amount flowing through your arteries and contributing to increased blood pressure. "If a healthy person periodically eats a lot of salt, it won't kill him," says Dr. James. "Your body is designed to handle big doses of salt occasionally. But people get in trouble when they eat a lot all of the time. And it catches up, probably beginning in your forties."

Be aware that table salt accounts for one-third of the sodium we consume. The rest is hidden in most processed, frozen and canned foods. And so-called softened water gets that way by adding many pounds of salt.

Dr. James suggests one way to eliminate salt from your body: Sweat it out. Another is to just cut down on sprinkling it on at the table. Use other seasonings and ingredients, such as lemon juice, hot spices, ginger and garlic.

Pray to your heart's content. The effects on the heart of praying "are profound, and they are good," says Larry Dossey, M.D., executive editor of the *Journal of Alternative Therapies in Health and Medicine*, author of *Healing Words: The Power of Prayer and the Practice of Medicine* and former chief of staff at Medical City Dallas Hospital. "When a person enters a state of prayer, meditation or relaxation, physical changes occur, characterized by lower blood pressure, a fall in heart rate, lower oxygen consumption, less carbon dioxide production and a heightened degree of wakefulness in the brain." Researchers such as Herbert Benson, M.D., Ph.D., of Harvard Medical School corroborated this in the 1970s, calling it the relaxation response.

Why this occurs remains somewhat of a mystery. While Dr. Dossey advocates praying, he also expresses a concern: "The danger is that people will use prayer as a pill and forget its primary purpose, which is to help them connect with something higher than themselves."

Take a yoga class. Doing those odd poses and stretches in the comfort of your living room can be an alternative to brisk walking as a way of exercising your heart and controlling high blood pressure, according to Linda DiCarlo, a researcher in the health and performance sciences department at the Georgia Institute of Technology in Atlanta. In one study, she and others found that heart rate and blood pressure readings were higher during a 32-minute session of hatha yoga than during 32 minutes of walking on a treadmill. (It's important to bear in mind that any exercise regimen that pumps up your heart rate and blood pressure is good, because those numbers will drop to below their normal rates when your body is at rest.)

Also, the researchers found that yoga utilized less oxygen than the treadmill walk. Translation: Yoga provides lower-intensity heart benefits than walking but is still considered beneficial.

Switch from red to white. Meat, that is. Ground beef is the biggest source of fat, particularly saturated fat, in our diets, according to Jayne Hurley, R.D., senior nutritionist for the Center for Science in the Public Interest in Washington, D.C. And that's the kind of fat that can send your blood pressure soaring.

While some men may consider cutting out meat altogether as a punishment worse than the crime, there is an alternative. Poultry and veal, the so-called white meats, are leaner than

red meats and will still satisfy your appetite for something substantial from the protein family to sink your teeth into without adding to your fat count. Hurley warns not to buy into the ads from the National Pork Producers Council that promote pork as "the other white meat." "They're bunk," she says. "Trimmed pork is one-third fattier than skinless chicken and twice as fatty as skinless turkey." Trimmed veal, however, is even leaner than skinless chicken.

Boost the big D. Researchers have found that men with higher levels of vitamin D in their blood tend to have lower blood pressure, while men with lower levels of D have higher blood pressure. Vitamin D is in milk and other dairy products (always choose low-fat versions). You also get it from exposure to the sun.

Vitamin D also helps the hormone insulin remove excessive sugar from your blood, notes Michael Weber, M.D., an editor of the *American Journal of Hypertension* and chair of the Department of Medicine at Brookdale Medical Center in Brooklyn, New York. Maintaining the right level of blood sugar can help control diabetes. (For more on diabetes, see page 253.)

Enjoy a little wine. Numerous studies have shown that there is reduced incidence of cardiovascular disease among moderate drinkers—that is, those who drink a glass or two of red wine on a daily basis. "We know that drinking wine in moderation causes a slight lowering of blood pressure as alcohol dilates blood vessels, which, in turn, reduces blood resistance," explains David Whitten, M.D., co-author of *To Your Health: Two Physicians Explore the Health Benefits of Wine*, assistant professor of physiology at the University of California, San Francisco, and chief of emergency services at Kaiser Foundation Hospital in Santa Rosa, California. Wine also has the effect of reducing the adhesiveness of platelets in the blood, helping to prevent them from gumming up the smaller arteries, he adds.

But, he warns, drink only in moderation: no more than two glasses of wine or bottles of beer a day (women should have only one a

Checking Your Pulse

Exercise buffs are always telling you to check your pulse, but they neglect to say exactly what the pulse is. Hint: It's not the beating of your heart. Not exactly.

The steady thrumming that you feel when you place your fingertips against your wrist is caused by the alternating expansion and recoil of arteries in response to surges of blood. Each throb is a wave of pressure caused by the beating of the heart.

The normal, healthy resting pulse slows as we age. In infants, it is about 140 beats per minute; in children, it clocks in at 100 to 120; in adults, it steadies at 60 to 100, with a truly healthy pulse being under 80. To check your pulse:

• Place the tips of your index and middle fingers on the underside of your wrist, about one to two inches below the bottom of your thumb.

• Press very gently. You should be able to feel blood pulsing through the artery.

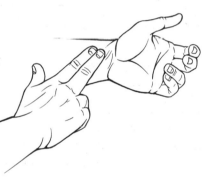

Where to feel for your pulse.

• Count the number of pulses in 20 seconds and multiply by three to get your pulse rate per minute.

day). Excessive alcohol consumption can raise blood pressure dangerously.

Give your lungs a lift. Once more, with feeling: Give up or cut down on cigarette smoking. "It's like running an exhaust pipe directly from your car into your mouth," says George Sopko, M.D., leader of the interventional cardiology scientific research group in the Division of Heart and Vascular Diseases of the National Heart, Lung and Blood Institute in Bethesda, Maryland. "Given the choice between oxygen and carbon monoxide, red blood cells go for the carbon monoxide," meaning that the blood delivered to your system is oxygen-deficient. That can injure your

blood vessels, leading to heart disease.

It's Got Rhythm

You may have as much rhythmic sensibility as Vice-President Al Gore dancing at the 1992 inaugural ball. But luckily, your heart has mastered the beat and would have no trouble sitting in with the Tito Puente Latin All-Stars.

The tempo of your heart is called the heart rate. This varies tremendously from man to man. But assuming that you are in pretty good health and happen to be resting at the time, your heart probably beats about 60 to 80 times a minute.

When you exercise or get excited, your heart speeds up in order to provide additional blood and oxygen to fuel the increase in metabolism. A 35-year-old man sprinting in the last leg of a 10-K race can generate a heart rate of about 185 beats a minute. In the throes of orgasm, your heart rate can reach 160 to 180 beats per minute.

A higher heart rate is natural and good when it's caused by physical exertion. But in general, a strong heart beats slowly. There are all types of unnatural triggers for an elevating heart rate. Tobacco, caffeine, alcohol and a variety of drugs can boost it. So can stress or any other emotion that increases your body's demand for oxygen.

As a man gets older, his heart rate naturally slows. At age 25, your maximum heart rate is about 200 beats a minute. By age 65, your top rate is about 155 beats a minute. The heart rate is also slower in a trained athlete, since the heart contracts more powerfully and is able to propel more blood with a single beat.

Following are the best ways to keep your

heartbeat slow and healthy.

Stay active. We discussed this above, but it bears repeating: Regular exercise strengthens your heart and helps it pump more blood with each contraction. Even light exercise will help make your heart more efficient and keep the rate from skyrocketing, says Gil Gleim, Ph.D., director of research for the Nicholas Institute of Sports Medicine and Athletic Trauma at Lenox Hill Hospital in New York City. "Even ten minutes of walking three times a day is better than nothing," he says.

Stay trim. When you're overweight, your heart has to work harder. After all, there's a lot more tissue that your blood has to reach, and you burn additional energy just hauling yourself around. The burden, directly or not, falls on your heart. "It's a function of physics," explains Dr. James. "It takes more energy to move something that weighs 250 pounds than something that weighs 175 pounds."

Laugh it off. Studies have shown that laughter, after the initial stimulation, can make your heart rate slower than it was before, says Dennis Swartout, M.D., a family physician at Lahey Hitchcock Clinic in Keene, New Hampshire. Researchers suspect that laughter and other positive feelings help trigger the release of chemicals called endorphins, which stimulate feelings of well-being and keep your body calm.

What Type Are You?

There are a lot of guys out there who can't stop checking their watches. Even when they're on vacation, they're always worried that there's something else—anything—they should be doing

this very minute. These men may well have what has been dubbed a type A personality.

Type A is a clinical term first coined by Meyer Friedman, M.D., director of the Meyer Friedman Institute in San Francisco. He and others have shown that those who exhibit type A tendencies develop heart disease at more than twice the rate of type B men, who are characterized as having a more easygoing approach to life. You may be type A if you are prone to being:

- Overly impatient
- Extremely aggressive
- Highly competitive

With a Song in My Heart

You will not understand cholesterol counts and high blood pressure by listening to the songs listed here. But you may glean a tip or two on how to handle a cardiovascular disease that even the most gifted surgeon won't touch. It's called broken heart, and for inexplicable reasons, it seems most prevalent among people living in the vicinity of Nashville.

Country, rock 'n' roll, the blues, popular music—hell, even Musak—all wax rhapsodic when it comes to the heart. The poor muscle works overtime in the music industry, playing the part of any old metaphor that lyricists can dream up: heart of gold, heart of stone, heart of soul—everything, it seems, but heart of artichoke.

And who can blame songwriters? Just mentioning the heart evokes images of moons and Junes, love and marriage, horse and carriage. We should praise the Goddess of Corn for these songs. Without them, torch singers, cabaret sirens and lounge lizards trying to be Barry Manilow would be out of work.

But the thing is, just skimming through this list might do your heart some good, especially if the songs evoke memories of some time when your own heart's desire inspired you to play Romeo to her Juliet and serenade her with a few bars of, say, "Heartbreak Hotel" (with apologies to Elvis). But mostly, remembering these songs may put you in touch with your own heart. And that always does you good.

- "Heartaches by the Number" (Guy Mitchell/1959; Johnny Tillotson/1965)

- Especially short-tempered
- Self-critical
- Hostile and angry

Type A's also tend to have frequent bouts with:

- Migraines
- High blood pressure
- Ulcers
- Irritable bowel syndrome

Dr. Friedman's label later evolved into one of those typical medical psychobabble terms: *coronary-prone behavior pattern*. In this case, however, it did clarify a vague term. It suggests that there are ways we behave, as opposed to ways we are, that affect our health. And it implies that if we can identify the behaviors that hurt our health, we can change them. The two that researchers found most related to heart disease are anger and hostility. These emotions cause the release of stress hormones, which increase blood pressure, heart rate, breathing and muscle tension. When combined with other factors—obesity, smoking, a family history of heart problems, lack of exercise, a diet high in fat and cholesterol—the additional work that you make your heart do when you act out type A behaviors can lead to a heart attack. (For more on anger and stress and their impact on your health, see page 21.)

Knowing this, you may want to consider small shifts in your personal style that will have a lasting impact on your heart, such as:

Do nothing wherever and whenever. As revolutionary as it may sound, you may need to learn to waste time. "Type A men need to get their minds off the tape loop that keeps telling them 'I gotta do more, I gotta do more,' " says Daniel Goleman, Ph.D., behavior writer for the *New York Times* and author of *Emotional Intelligence*. "They have to learn to break the cycle of continuously being frantic and harried." He suggests standing in line—at the bank, at the supermarket, at the airport—and forcing yourself to enjoy the mini-vacation from all of those pressing responsibilities. Miraculously, they'll all be waiting patiently for you at the end of the line.

Lose the watch. One sure way to stop watching the

- "Heartache Tonight" (The Eagles/1979)
- "Heart and Soul" (Larry Clinton and His Orchestra/1938; The Four Aces/1952)
- "Heartbeat" (Buddy Holly/1958)
- "Heartbreaker" (The Andrews Sisters/1947)
- "Heartbreaker" (Led Zeppelin/1969)
- "Heartbreaker" (Dolly Parton/1978)
- "Heartbreaker" (Pat Benatar/1979)
- "Heartbreaker" (Dionne Warwick/1982)
- "Heartbreak Hotel" (Elvis Presley/1956)
- "Heartbreak Hotel" (The Jacksons/1981)
- "Heart Full of Soul" (The Yardbirds/1965)
- "Heartless" (Heart/1978)
- "Heart Like a Wheel" (Steve Miller Band/1981)
- "Heart of Glass" (Blondie/1979)
- "Heart of Gold" (Neil Young/1971)
- "(The Gang That Sang) Heart of My Heart" (The Three D's/1954)
- "The Heart of Rock and Roll" (Huey Lewis and the News/1983)
- "Heart of Stone" (The Rolling Stones/1965)
- "Heart of the Country" (Paul McCartney and Wings/1971)
- "Heart of the Night" (Poco/1979; Juice Newton/1981)
- "Hearts" (Marty Balin/1981)
- "Hearts of Stone" (The Fontane Sisters/1955)
- "Hearts of Stone" (Bruce Springsteen/1986)
- "Heart to Heart" (Kenny Loggins/1982)

clock is to leave it at home. It may be a big adjustment at first. But after a while, you'll notice that checking the time is a compulsive habit that makes you more anxious, not less, says Dr. Goleman. You'll also notice that it's pretty easy to approximate the time without the aid of your Timex. You might even learn how to read the position of the sun.

Meditate on it. No longer the domain of mystics, yogis and gurus, meditation has entered the mainstream. It is being used in traditional medical settings as an effective strategy for reducing stress and for helping patients to deal with chronic pain. A pioneer in this approach, Jon Kabat-Zinn, Ph.D., director of the stress-reduction clinic at the University of Massachusetts Medical Center in Worcester and author of *Wherever You Go, There You Are: Mindfulness Meditation in Everyday Life*, recommends simple mindfulness exercises that involve paying attention to your breath, your body or your thoughts without getting attached to them. You will not necessarily feel less stress or pain, he notes, but you will develop an ability to cope and to live with it. And that in itself will ease tension.

What's a mindfulness exercise, you ask? Well, to help you get started, Dr. Kabat-Zinn suggests the following: Sit or lie in a comfortable place (your eyes can be open or closed). Feel your breath moving in and out without trying to change it in any way. Pay attention to all of the feelings associated with your breath moving, moment by moment. Every time your mind wanders, note where it has gone and gently bring it back to your breathing. Do this exercise every day for however long it feels comfortable, he advises.

Mellow out in the mornings. Sunday night the pressure begins to build: "Oh, no—not work again tomorrow!" It's not surprising that heart attacks most often occur during the early morning hours, especially on Monday mornings. The reason, according to Scott Sharkey, M.D., director of the coronary care unit of Hennepin County Medical Center in Minneapolis, is that your blood is more prone

to clotting in the morning. As your body tries to go from 0 to 60 in nothing flat, especially after lounging around all weekend, you may undergo hormonal changes that can ignite an attack.

Try reserving about 15 minutes on Monday mornings to indulge in some quiet time for yourself. A slow walk, deep breathing while looking out a window, some easy stretching, even a warm bath may be just the buffer you need to face the workweek and conquer the world.

Practice acts of kindness. If you're angry or hostile, "think charitable thoughts," says Dr. Goleman. "Research shows that thoughts and acts of kindness trigger physiological responses that alter your emotional state. It's a way of doing judo on your own negative thought processes."

Put matter over mind. Here's a switch on the familiar mind-over-matter model. Sometimes the best way to put unconstructive thoughts or feelings out of your mind is to divert your brain's attention to your body, says Dr. Goleman. Whether it's an athletic endeavor that requires your full attention—juggling beanbags rather than juggling appointments—or another activity that distracts you, nothing keeps your mind off your mind like your body.

A Heart Attack by Any Other Name

When you are man's number one killer, you can go by any name you choose. These are the major conditions related to the heart, with tips on how to recognize them. We could fill a volume with how they are treated, but we won't. We'll just say that if you feel any of these symptoms, get to a doctor fast. Your life could be at stake, says Dr. Sopko. Take the following seriously.

Myocardial infarction. Commonly called a heart attack, myocardial infarction occurs when a blocked artery keeps blood from getting to your heart muscle. This kills off critical tissue (*infarc-* means dead tissue in Latin; *myocardial* refers to your heart muscle). You'll know it's myocardial infarction when you feel like there's an elephant sitting on your chest and you can't breathe. You'll also experience a "feeling of impending doom," says Dr. Tofler. Other symptoms include sweating, nausea, discomfort and tingling in your left arm or your neck.

Unfortunately, these symptoms can be very mild in some people, so they don't recognize what's happening. Or they may think that they have a touch of indigestion, Dr. Tofler says. Since treatment that is given early enough can save your heart muscle or even your life, don't delay, he advises. Get to your doctor right away.

Cardiac arrest. This also is commonly called a heart attack. But in cardiac arrest, unlike myocardial infarction, the heart muscle doesn't necessarily die from a lack of blood supply. Instead, it just stops beating, usually because its natural electrical signals get disrupted.

There are two main types of electrical disturbance that can cause cardiac arrest. In the first, the rhythm of the heart gets so out of sync that the heart stops dead in its tracks. An electrocardiogram, which records the heart's electrical activity, would reveal a flat line, or no heartbeat. In the second type, called ventricular fibrillation, the heartbeat quickens and becomes chaotic, and the heart muscle goes into a shivering spasm, like when your eyelid spontaneously quivers. Usually, the only way to stop it is with an electric shock delivered in the emergency room or by a trained rescue team.

The most common symptom before cardiac arrest is feeling faint or dizzy. The feeling comes on quickly and is often over in less than a minute, says Dr. Tofler. You won't have a lot of time to think about what you've just experienced, however, because the faintness is followed by loss of consciousness.

Angina pectoris. This is a chest pain. It frequently shows up when you are exercising beyond your limit or you are under extreme stress. It's a sign that your heart is not getting enough oxygen. "It's your heart saying 'Back off,' " explains Dr. Sopko. It's also telling you to proceed directly to your doctor—do not pass go, do not collect anything. An angina attack is often a predecessor to a heart attack and can mean that your arteries are dangerously clogged. If you feel an unfamiliar new chest pain and you don't see your doctor, you are playing a deadly game of Russian roulette.

Aneurysm. This is a structural weakness of the blood vessel wall. "Vessels are like elastic pipes," explains Dr. Sopko. "If you damage the wall, the pipe starts to balloon out at the site of the weakness." The wall gets thinner and dangerously thinner. The common form of aneurysm, primarily related to hardening of the arteries, most frequently occurs in the segment of the aorta that runs through the abdomen. You can have a small aneurysm for years and not know it. But if it starts to balloon, it can affect blood flow and put pressure on surrounding organs. And if it ruptures, it can kill you quickly. Some people feel a pulsating sensation in the abdomen when the rupture occurs, but because there are very few other symptoms, "it can be a catastrophe waiting to happen," says Dr. Sopko. An aneurysm can be detected by x-rays and other tests during regular visits to your physician.

Stroke. The result of inadequate blood flow to the brain, a stroke can be caused by heart problems as well as by a clogged or ruptured blood vessel in the brain itself. What sometimes happens is that a blood clot will form in the carotid artery, a blood vessel that leads from the heart to the brain. This lack of blood flow can cause severe damage to the nervous system, says Dr. Sopko. Symptoms of a stroke are weakness, numbness, paralysis or another abnormality in a limb as well as speech, comprehension and vision defects.

↗Hips

- **Keep them stretched and strong.**
- **Eat for good bones.**

Today, broadcast television willingly shows naked buttocks. But there was a time, not long ago, when fully clothed hips were considered dangerous. Two hips in particular: Elvis Presley's.

When Elvis appeared on *The Ed Sullivan Show* on January 6, 1957, his third and final time, the CBS cameras showed him only from the waist up. This was necessary, network censors explained, because of the singer's "suggestive movements." In the words of biographer Dave Marsh, "Elvis made a mockery of the censorship, swiveling wildly, bumping and grinding with everything from his elbows to his eyebrows, using his shoulders as a metaphoric pelvis and grinning wildly at the undiminished screams."

Hidden in this rather quaint notion that a man's clothed hips could be offensive are two serious anatomical lessons. First, the rhyme: The word "pelvis," so often associated with Elvis, refers to the two conjoined hipbones as well as to the two attached bones at the base of the spine. Together these bones protect the internal organs and help provide a transition from torso to legs. Elvis could move his pelvis like Jell-O because the hipbones are connected to the thighbones by two of the body's strongest and most flexible joints. In a sense, it is the versatility of the hip joints that made Elvis Elvis.

Anatomy lesson number two: Like the shoulder, the hip is a type of ball-and-socket joint. The ball at the top of your thighbone fits into the socket at the side of your hip. When you move your leg (and sometimes your torso), the ball rotates within the socket. So unlike your knee, which essentially moves back and forth in one plane, your hip can move in an almost unlimited number of planes.

To accomplish the range of complex and difficult motions involved in a task such as running, each hip joint is attached to and surrounded by some of the most powerful muscles in the body, including the hamstrings, at the rear of each thigh, and the gluteus maximus, which makes up most of each buttock. These muscles also stabilize the joint when you move or stand in anything other than an upright position.

Problems That Affect the Hips

As joints go, your hips are fairly indestructible. Because of their flexibility and the powerful muscles surrounding them, they are

The Hip Joint

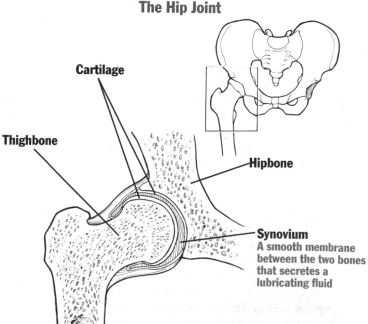

Cartilage

Thighbone

Hipbone

Synovium
A smooth membrane between the two bones that secretes a lubricating fluid

The hip joint is among the most injury-free joint in the body. If it starts hurting, stop what you are doing immediately. If the pain goes away in a few days, the problem likely was muscular. But if pain lingers, get it checked—it could be arthritis or bursitis.

far less prone to the myriad sprains and tears of ligaments and tendons that afflict joints such as the knees and ankles. In contrast to the shoulder, the hip is rarely dislocated. Tendinitis, the scourge of many an elbow, is rare in the hip. Hip fractures are rare, except in cases of extreme trauma (a car accident, for example) or among men with osteoporosis, a degenerative thinning of the bones seen in the elderly.

"It's the best of both worlds," says Gerald Eisenberg, M.D., a rheumatologist and director of the arthritis treatment program at Lutheran General Hospital in Chicago. "The joint itself is more flexible and moves in many different directions. It's also covered by a deep layer of muscle on all sides. Because the joint is inherently more stable and normally moves in more directions, it is inherently less prone to injury."

But things do go wrong. And because of your hips' strategic importance—it's impossible to walk without putting weight on them—when something goes wrong, it can be a tremendous inconvenience.

Muscle Trouble

In many cases, what's perceived as hip pain can be traced to an injured or overused muscle. Here's what to do if you suspect that the pain is muscular, says Thomas Rizzo, Jr., M.D., a consultant in physical medicine and rehabilitation at Mayo Clinic Jacksonville in Florida.

• If your hip hurts while you're exercising, temporarily eliminate the activity that's causing the problem. Ride a bike, for example, instead of running. Wait a week or two before resuming your regular workout, then see if you still feel pain. If not, it probably was a muscle, and it has healed. If pain is there, the problem might be something other than you think, and you should consider consulting a doctor. If the pain spreads to another part of your leg or keeps you up at night, consult your doctor.

• If your hip hurts after exercising, apply ice for 20 minutes. (Remember: Never put ice directly on your skin; wrap it in a towel instead.) If it still hurts a couple of hours later, reapply the ice.

• If your hip hurts and you haven't been working out, apply heat for 20 minutes. Moist heat—a towel soaked in hot water—works best, but you can also use a heating pad, with a dry towel on your skin to prevent burning. Massage and products such as Ben-Gay, Flex-all 454 and Eucalyptamint may help, too. Heat applied before exercise can also help by loosening the joint and muscles.

• When the pain stops, do exercises to make the joint and muscles stronger and more flexible.

Bursitis

Bursitis, or inflammation of the fluid-filled sacs called bursae that cushion and lubricate the hip joint, is another fairly common problem usually related to excessive use. Unlike more generalized muscle-related pain, you'll feel bursitis as very localized pain and tenderness—as, for example, a half-dollar-size pouch on the outside of your hip. Because your hip bears weight every time you walk, it's sometimes difficult to treat bursitis here. Cortisone shots, along with stretching, are the common treatment prescribed by doctors. For mild cases, rest, ice, over-the-counter analgesics and stretching exercises are all helpful, says Dr. Eisenberg.

There is a stretch that helps take the pressure off this joint, says Morris B. Mellion, M.D., clinical associate professor of family practice and orthopedic surgery at the University of Nebraska Medical Center and medical director of

Bursitis Stretch

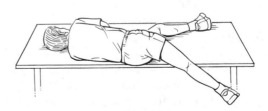

Using a sturdy table, lie down on your side on the hip not affected by bursitis. Drop your top leg behind your body so that your foot is about 12 inches below the tabletop. Hold the stretch for 20 to 30 seconds.

the Sports Medicine Center, both in Omaha. Try this: If you have bursitis in your right hip, lie on your left side on a sturdy table, with your back straight. You should be near but not on the edge of the table, facing the opposite edge. Bend your left leg at the knee and the hip, so your weight is firmly on the table. Then drop your right leg behind your body so that your right foot is about 12 inches below the tabletop. Hold this stretch for about 20 to 30 seconds. Do five to ten repetitions of this stretch three times a day. In mild cases, you can do the stretches without cortisone, but it's tough for more serious cases, says Dr. Mellion.

Joint Trouble

When physicians talk of hip pain, they usually mean pain in the hip joint, the place where the ball of your thighbone fits into the socket of your pelvis. Typically, hip pain is perceived not in the back but in the front. You'll feel this kind of a problem in your groin. To find out if you have a hip problem, lie on a table on your back, lift one leg ten inches and hold it. Then do the same with your other leg. If you feel pain within 10 to 20 seconds, you can be highly suspicious of a hip joint problem—namely, arthritis, says Dr. Mellion.

Arthritis is the most common source of hip joint pain. In fact, while our hips are relatively safe from the acute injuries that afflict other joints, often they simply wear out over time. Only our knees are more frequently affected by the most common form of arthritis: osteoarthritis, or degenerative joint disease.

Get Hip to These Exercises

Here are several exercises recommended by Thomas Rizzo, Jr., M.D., a consultant in physical medicine and rehabilitation at Mayo Clinic Jacksonville in Florida. For balance, stretch both legs equally. (For more stretches, see the workouts in part 3.)

Outer-Thigh Stretch

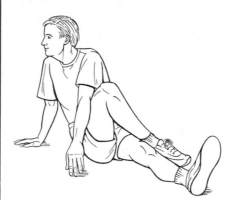

Butt Stretch

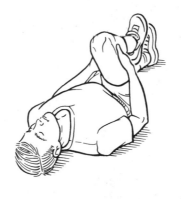

Outer-thigh stretch. Sit upright on the floor, with your left leg extended flat on the ground and your right knee bent and lifted. Place your right foot on the outside of your left knee. Lean back on your right arm and turn your upper body to the right about 90 degrees, using your left elbow to press the outside of your right knee. You should feel the muscles on the outside of your hip stretch gently. Hold for at least 20 to 30 seconds. Switch positions and do the other thigh.

Butt stretch. Lie on your back, with both legs resting on the floor. Grasp the back of one thigh and lift that knee toward your chest until you feel the muscles in your buttocks and lower back stretch. You

"Osteoarthritis is a disease of usage," says Dr. Eisenberg. "So those joints that we use more, whether to bear weight or otherwise, are more commonly affected." It's not a coincidence that arthritis affects our knees and hips most frequently; both joints routinely bear most of our weight.

At its most extreme, arthritis of the hip

can also pull the uplifted knee across your body. Hold the stretch for at least 20 to 30 seconds. Switch legs.

Elastic-band stretch. A large elastic band (available in some fitness equipment stores) or a piece of surgical tubing looped around a table leg can help you strengthen the muscles on the outside of your hip. Stand beside the table and place your outer foot inside the elastic band. Hold on to the table for balance. With your leg straight, stretch the elastic band away from the table by swinging your foot. Hold for ten seconds. Repeat 10 to 15 times with each leg.

For balance, work the inside of your thigh, too. Loop the leg that's closest to the table through the elastic band and swing your foot away from the table. Hold for ten seconds. Repeat 10 to 15 times with each leg.

Elastic-Band Stretches

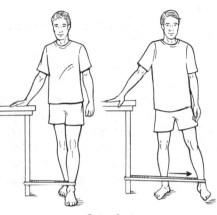

Outer foot

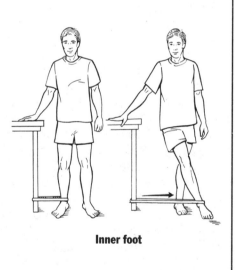

Inner foot

hip replacement don't even know the procedure is available. And many who need the procedure don't have insurance or access to good medical care. Many simply can't afford hip replacement surgery."

Referred Pain

What you experience as pain in your hip, however, may well be what doctors call referred pain, meaning that its true cause lies elsewhere. When there is pain in the buttocks or the back of the hip, the cause usually lies in your lower back or in the sacroiliac joint, where your spine and pelvis meet. Pain in this joint is occasionally caused by a progressive form of arthritis known as ankylosing spondylitis, which typically starts in men between ages 20 and 40. Pain in the hip area may even be caused by a hernia or a kidney stone.

Nerve Trouble

Sciatica pain is often perceived in the buttocks and sometimes shoots down the back of the thigh. This pain is caused by pressure on the sciatic nerve, the longest nerve in the human body, which originates in the spinal cord and branches throughout the legs. The pressure itself is usually caused by a problem with a disk in the lower back.

can necessitate total hip replacement surgery, in which a physician replaces the ball and socket of the joint with artificial ones. It is the most common type of joint replacement surgery; more than 45,000 men get new hips each year. "And we're not even beginning to replace all of the hips that need to be done," says Dr. Mellion. "Some people who need total

Hip Maintenance

No surprises here: Generally, what's healthy for your bones is healthy for your hips, says Dr. Mellion.

Lose weight. When you stand, walk or run, your hip joints support almost 70 percent of your body weight. The less weight your joints have to carry, the better off you'll be.

Stretch. Limber up your hip joints, especially before exercising.

Get your bone nutrients. Be sure to get enough calcium and vitamin D. Calcium is essential to strong, healthy bones, and your body can't absorb calcium without vitamin D. Select nonfat or low-fat dairy products such as skim or low-fat milk and yogurt and reduced-fat cheeses.

Bear weight. Lift weights or do an activity in which your body supports its own weight, such as brisk walking or running. Weight-bearing exercise stimulates the cells of your hips and back to build more bone. Running is not recommended if you have arthritis in your hips or knees, says Dr. Eisenberg.

Know when to seek help. Your hips might be sturdy, but hip pain can signal a serious problem. See a doctor if:

- The pain radiates to another part of your leg.
- The pain disrupts your sleep or interferes with everyday activities.
- The pain persists for several weeks, even after rest.

Follow these tips, and you will go a long way toward staving off osteoporosis, along with the disabling, even deadly hip fractures that sometimes come with it, says Dr. Eisenberg. Don't think you're immune just because you're a man. Our bones tend to be denser than women's, and we lose bone density more gradually as we grow older, but osteoporosis does affect us. In most cases, though, it affects us later in life than it does women. And smoking and drinking, among their many evils, significantly increase your chances of developing osteoporosis.

⊞ Immune System

- **Get all of your nutrients.**
- **Keep moving.**
- **Get happy.**

Among the many diseases that afflict humankind, chickenpox is neither glamorous nor usually debilitating. Usually, it's just a minor viral illness that you get when you're young and, in most cases, never get again.

Therein lies the magic of the immune system. Even though chickenpox is highly contagious—most people contract it by age ten—relapses are extremely rare. The same goes for colds, flus and pneumonia. It's unlikely you'll ever get the same bug twice.

The reason for this is simple: Your immune system is a very quick study. After one exposure, it knows the invader's secrets. It responds by churning out proteins, called antibodies, that help fight off that particular virus (or bacterium or fungus). Should the invader ever return—months, years or even decades after the initial exposure—the appropriate antibodies are already primed and ready for action. As long as your immune system is strong, there's a good chance that it will destroy microbes long before they have a chance to make you sick.

Scientists estimate that the immune system has the potential to create more than 100 million types of antibodies. Since the average person will encounter only a few thousand different invaders during his lifetime, it's obvious that the immune system is rather magnificently overbuilt. With a few frightening exceptions, such as HIV, the virus that causes AIDS, you're well-protected no matter what comes along.

A Whole-Body System

Unlike your heart, lungs and other organs, the immune system really isn't a "thing" at all. Nor can you find it gathered in a specific place. To some extent, virtually every part of your body plays a role in protecting you from outside onslaughts. For example:

Skin. Your body's first line of defense, it has a tough surface that prevents viruses, bacteria and fungi from getting in. In addition, the acidity of skin secretions such as sweat helps keep bacteria in check.

Respiratory tract. Your airways are densely covered with tiny mucus-coated hairs that trap bacteria and other particles. These invaders are then coughed, sneezed, blown or otherwise propelled out of your body before they cause harm.

Fluids. Both saliva in your mouth and fluid in your eyes contain lysozyme, an enzyme that kills bacteria.

Stomach lining. It secretes a highly concentrated solution of hydrochloric acid that's nearly as potent as battery acid. It kills microbes on contact.

While many parts of your body contribute to disease resistance as a sideline to their primary tasks, there are a handful of entities whose primary duty is to serve your immune system. Lymph glands, for example, help produce and store white blood cells. The spleen, which is actually a large lymph gland, stores white blood cells and returns fluids to the bloodstream. The thymus serves as a kind of incubator and schoolhouse; here T cells, a specific type of white blood

cell, mature and learn to function. (These crucial cells are destroyed by the virus that causes AIDS.) The system's foot soldiers are the trillions of white blood cells, which vary in structure and function but together serve a common purpose: Defeat the invader.

Ultimately, though, it all comes down to the trillions of specialized cells and molecules circulating throughout your body in lymphatic tissues and bodily fluids. Their job is to spot, identify and destroy foreign particles—not just

---

A Healing Blitz

Suppose you cut your hand and bacteria starts to pour into the wound. In the space of minutes or even seconds, dozens of mechanisms kick in to keep the damage under control.

Increased blood flow. Injured tissue cells release chemicals such as histamine, kinins and prostaglandins, which cause blood vessels to widen. More and more blood flows into the injured area, making it hot, red and swollen.

Swelling. As blood and protein-rich fluids flood the injured area, they bring in large quantities of oxygen and nutrients needed for repair. Swelling also helps keep the area immobile, aiding healing.

Pain. Swelling in the area presses on nearby nerves, causing pain. Also painful are the release of bacterial toxins and the presence of inflammatory chemicals.

Fever. When certain immune cells make contact with bacteria, they release pyrogens, chemicals that turn up your body's thermostat. The resulting fever helps inactivate invaders. At the same time, fever increases the metabolic rate of body cells, accelerating the process of healing.

Feeding. Specialized cells are chemically attracted to injured tissue; they arrive en masse to destroy bacteria and other microbes that have breached the surface.

Disposal. As the infection winds down, prodigiously hungry cells called macrophages arrive to clear the area of surviving microbes and to remove pus, an accretion of dead tissue cells and dead and dying immune cells.

Healing. To stop bleeding and keep the wound closed, a cascade of more than 30 substances causes clotting, usually within three to six minutes after the damage has occurred.

microbes such as bacteria and viruses but also things such as plant pollen, dust, chemicals and environmental toxins. Anything that isn't you may be perceived as fair game.

Silent Battles

Your body's response to invasion is exquisitely synchronized. Suppose, for example, a virus that made you sick once before returns for a rematch. Within minutes to hours of the virus entering your body, specialized immune cells and proteins mobilize in astonishing numbers. Some recognize the invader; others mark it for attack; still others go in for the kill. In short order, the thing, whatever it is, is surrounded, attacked and devoured for lunch. The remains are then disposed of, and the combatants return to their lairs, ready to fight another day. (Actually, some immune cells do die in the attack; that's what pus is.)

Unless you actually get sick, most immune system skirmishes occur in silence. You aren't aware that anything is going on. Once an infection takes hold, however, you may notice the lymph glands in your neck, armpits and groin getting swollen.

"A swollen lymph node is generally a sign of one of two things: either an infection or something more serious," says Ronald Glaser, Ph.D., professor of medical microbiology and immunology at Ohio State University Medical Center in Columbus. "The bottom line is that if you have unexplained lymph node swelling, go to your doctor."

Staying Strong

The immune system obviously isn't perfect; if it were, you'd never get sick. We'll

Understanding AIDS

Scientists have conducted vast amounts of research on HIV, the virus that causes AIDS, since it was first isolated in 1984. But the prognosis remains dire. Nearly a million Americans are infected with HIV. AIDS is the leading cause of death among men ages 25 to 44 (accidents are second). Among women in the same age bracket, it's the third leading cause of death.

The phrase "HIV-positive" means that your body is carrying the virus that causes AIDS. This virus multiplies in the lymph nodes. In time—and it could be a short or long time, even more than a decade—the lymph glands become destroyed, leaving your body defenseless against invaders. The slightest infection can rage unchecked; even minor infections, once easily conquered, can eventually prove fatal. When your body reaches the point where it cannot fight disease effectively, you have full-blown AIDS (that's short for acquired immune deficiency syndrome).

Although diagnostic tests to detect HIV are more effective than ever, a cure for AIDS has yet to be found, which is why it's so important to take precautions. Since the virus is spread exclusively by bodily fluids—semen, blood and vaginal secretions—there's a lot you can do to avoid contact with the virus.

• Abstinence is the surest protection against the AIDS virus. Given the power of the human sex drive, this isn't going to be a practical solution for most of us. Next best is to engage

talk in a bit about some serious problems that can leave your immune system reeling. Much more common, and correctable, are those everyday assaults that lower your defenses against colds, flus and other infections. To keep your immune system strong, here's what experts advise.

Blow off steam any way you can. A demanding boss. Sick children. Money woes. Stress is a multifaceted beast, and when it hits hard, the immune system goes down. In studies of students, for example, experts found that immune function took a nosedive during exam periods and bounced back when the stress of the tests had passed. One study found that highly stressed people who were exposed to a

only in monogamous sex with a partner who you know is HIV-free, says Terry Phillips, Ph.D., D.Sc., professor of medicine and director of the immunogenetics and immunochemistry laboratories at George Washington University Medical Center in Washington, D.C.

• Use latex condoms. When used with a spermicidal lubricant containing nonoxynol-9, these provide substantial protection, says Dr. Phillips. Don't carry condoms in your wallet, however, as this could damage the latex. Be wary of condoms made of natural animal products such as skin, he adds. The structure of latex is more tightly woven than that of lambskin and gives far better protection against disease and unwanted pregnancy.

• Understand the language of AIDS testing. You can get a blood test to check for the presence of HIV antibodies (proteins created by your body to fight the HIV virus). If these antibodies are found, you are HIV-positive and can infect others. If the test finds no antibodies, the virus is probably not living inside you; you're said to be HIV-negative.

But beware. The immune system can take as long as six months to develop HIV antibodies, which is what the test looks for. If you or your partner has recently been infected, it's possible to test HIV-negative and still be carrying the virus.

For the latest information about HIV, AIDS and their treatment, call the Centers for Disease Control and Prevention's National AIDS Hotline at 1-800-342-2437.

effects. "It sounds like witchcraft, but some patients respond to it, and we're slowly establishing the effectiveness of such methods with hard scientific data."

• Get happy. Years ago, Norman Cousins claimed that laughter could help you recover from illness. Research is confirming this theory. One study found that people who watched a 60-minute comedy video boosted their production of white blood cells by 39 percent and decreased their levels of a stress hormone by 46 percent. Researchers say that laughter can cut the immunity-dampening effects of everyday stress almost in half.

• Find a way to truly relax. Some people meditate, but you need not be so formal. Amid a hectic day, pause for five minutes, close your eyes and breathe deeply. Or take a walk. In tests, stress-busting techniques such as slow, deep breathing and even just relaxing with friends have been shown to boost levels of disease-fighting cells and antibodies.

Bone up on sleep. How often do you try to add a few hours to your life by cutting back on sleep, especially when the work is piling up on your desk? Problem is, your immune system needs that time in order to recover for another day. "Sleep is the repair shop for the immune system," Dr. Phillips notes. In one experiment, participants who missed three or more hours of sleep in a single night showed a 30 percent drop in some immune system activity.

How much sleep do men require? That varies from person to person. Most of us require about six to eight hours a night, but some energetic people may need nine, says Dr. Phillips.

cold virus were twice as likely to develop colds as less-stressed volunteers exposed to the same virus.

There's no way to avoid stress. But there are ways to keep it in check.

• Work on your attitude. Thinking yourself strong can make it so. Studies have shown that optimists have higher immune levels than pessimists. In his work with cancer patients, Terry Phillips, Ph.D., D.Sc., professor of medicine and director of the immunogenetics and immunochemistry laboratories at George Washington University Medical Center in Washington, D.C., found that those who "visualize armies of little white blood cells attacking their tumors" can experience positive

Keep up your workouts.
Numerous studies have shown that aerobic exercises such as walking, running and bicycling can boost immune function for a few hours after a workout. It also seems likely that regular workouts confer long-term benefits. One study found that people who walked 45 minutes a day, five days a week, ended up spending half as much time sick with colds and flus as those who were sedentary.

But don't overdo it. Regular workouts boost immune activity, but pushing too hard has been found to deplete it. Tests on marathoners have revealed that the activity of certain immune cells can be depressed for up to six hours after a run.

"The key is to control intensity," says David C. Nieman, D.H.Sc., of the Department of Health, Exercise and Leisure Science at Appalachian State University in Boone, North Carolina. "Going out at a moderate pace—anything from a brisk walk to an easy jog—for an hour won't do anything negative, but hammering hard for two to three hours will."

Eat wisely. The link between nutrition and immunity was first noted more than 40 years ago, when physicians in developing countries observed that malnourished children suffered more than their share of infections. What has only recently been understood is that even if you're apparently well-fed, your immune system may be running below its optimum level. "The role of diet in immunity is very direct," says Jeffrey Blumberg, Ph.D., professor of nutrition at the Jean Mayer USDA Human Nutrition Research

Allergies: False Alarms

It's comforting to imagine that like Father in the old television series, the human body knows best. Sometimes it does. But not when it comes to allergies. Then it's wrong every time.

An allergy is your body's misguided attempt to protect you from something that's generally harmless or even beneficial. Instead of reacting kindly to whatever you're allergic to, your immune system pounces. It treats the "stuff," be it pollen or pussycat dander, like an enemy invader.

Not surprisingly, your body's response to the allergen—blood vessels dilate, tissue swells, mucus secretes, muscles contract—is far more uncomfortable than anything caused by the stuff itself. If your allergy is severe, as are some people's allergies to certain foods or to insect stings, the reaction can be fatal.

To keep your allergy under control and your immune system calm, here's what experts advise.

Clear the house. By making relatively simple changes, such as using air-conditioning to filter air and replacing carpets with bare floors, many people can keep allergies to manageable levels. "If they're really diligent, most people can relieve 20 to 30 percent of their symptoms," says Gerald L. Klein, M.D., an allergist and professor of clinical medicine at the University of California, Irvine. "Others can virtually eliminate allergies, especially if they're allergic to dust mites or molds."

For information about how to allergy-proof your home, see an allergist or contact the Asthma and Allergy Foundation of America (1-800-7-ASTHMA) or the Allergy and Asthma Network/Mothers of Asthmatics (1-800-878-4403).

Flush out the molds. Having a vaporizer in the bedroom is good for keeping your nasal tissues moist, but don't forget to clean it every three days to prevent the buildup of allergy-causing molds, says David Zwillenberg,

Center on Aging at Tufts University in Boston.

"Specific nutrients play very particular roles in pushing immunity up and down," says Dr. Blumberg. You don't have to be a food scientist to know that eating less fat and more grains, fruits, vegetables and leafy greens will provide just about everything you need to keep your immune system strong.

Consider supplements. While many ex-

M.D., an otolaryngologist at Thomas Jefferson University Hospital in Philadelphia. Rinse it with a solution made of a teaspoon of bleach and a quart of water. Or you can use a 50-50 solution of vinegar and water.

Have a bleach party. Another way to avoid molds is by washing areas around sinks and bathtubs with bleach. You can use straight bleach or make a solution of bleach and water, says Terry Phillips, Ph.D., D.Sc., professor of medicine and director of the immunogenetics and immunochemistry laboratories at George Washington University Medical Center in Washington, D.C.

Get a dryer. If pollen is your poison, it's a good idea not to line-dry clothing, says Dr. Zwillenberg. "Clothes dried outside tend to trap pollen," he notes. "It's just one more irritant to deal with."

Seek chemical solutions. Various medical approaches treat the symptoms of allergies or make it harder for allergens to do their work. Here are the primary pharmaceutical tools.

Antihistamines. Available over the counter or by prescription, antihistamines such as diphenhydramine (Benadryl) and astemizole (Hismanal) work by blocking histamine, the chemical that fires up your body's allergic response. If antihistamines make you drowsy, ask your doctor or pharmacist about one of the nonsedating kinds.

Decongestants. Taken orally or by nasal spray, medications such as oxymetazoline (Afrin Nasal Spray) and pseudoephedrine (Sudafed) relieve nasal congestion by causing blood vessels in your nose to constrict. This helps reduce the swelling that can hinder breathing.

Allergy shots. Some people get permanent relief from allergies with desensitization therapy, in which your doctor injects minute amounts of the allergy-causing substance to help you build immunity to it.

John's and director of the World Health Organization Center for Nutritional Immunology, older men and women who took a daily supplement of vitamins and trace minerals suffered less than half of the infection-related illnesses of those taking a placebo. Nutrients that are particularly helpful include:

Vitamin A. Essential to microbe-catching membranes of the mouth and respiratory passages, it also fortifies the top layer of skin. This helps prevent cracks through which invaders can enter. Daily Value: 5,000 international units.

Beta-carotene. A study at the University of Arizona in Tuscon found that when older people raised their intakes of beta-carotene, they had increases in immune activity. While the government has not established how much beta-carotene you need in a day or whether the nutrient is entirely safe in supplement form, Dr. Michael Osband, M.D., adjunct professor at Boston University School of Medicine, suggests taking six to nine milligrams a day. That's the equivalent of 10,000 to 15,000 international units.

Vitamin B$_6$. Immune power fluctuates in direct response to your intake of this vitamin. "When older people were fed diets deficient in vitamin B$_6$, their immunity was lowered substantially," says Dr. Blumberg. Daily Value: two milligrams.

Vitamin C. This nutrient triggers the release of an important chemical that keeps viruses from multiplying. It also stimulates tumor-attacking cells. The Daily Value for

perts feel it's best to get the necessary vitamins and minerals from a healthy diet, some men simply aren't able or willing to eat the recommended five or more servings of fresh fruits and vegetables to meet their daily needs, says Dr. Phillips. Supplements can help fill the gaps. In a small preliminary study conducted by Ranjit Kumar Chandra, M.D., professor at Memorial University of Newfoundland in St.

vitamin C is 60 milligrams. Experts say it's safe to take up to 1,200 milligrams daily, although excessive amounts may cause diarrhea.

Vitamin E. In one study, people ages 60 and over who took vitamin E supplements raised their immune function to levels that matched those of people in their thirties and forties. Some researchers feel that the Daily Value of 30 international units is probably too low for optimum immune function. Dr. Blumberg says that taking supplementary doses of 100 to 400 international units daily is quite safe.

Magnesium. Some studies suggest that magnesium deficiency can cause the immune system to run amok, attack normal cells in the body and trigger autoimmune diseases such as rheumatoid arthritis. Taking a magnesium supplement may be a good idea for men on water pills or high blood pressure drugs. Both make you lose this mineral. So does drinking excessive amounts of alcohol. The rest of us can get the Daily Value of 400 milligrams without supplements by regularly eating leafy vegetables, potatoes, whole grains, milk and seafood.

Fighting Back

The immune system is a highly efficient machine, but it's a machine nonetheless. At the very least, it sometimes runs down or doesn't run very well. At worst, it can break down entirely or even turn against you, sometimes with disastrous results.

There are two ends of the spectrum when it comes to immune problems. At one end are immunodeficiency troubles, which occur when the body loses its ability to fight off invaders.

It's difficult to imagine the sheer chaos that ensues when the body becomes immunodeficient. Diseases such as cancer and AIDS can severely damage the immune system, leaving the body vulnerable to anything that comes along.

A number of prescription drugs—steroids, for example—can seriously weaken the immune system. While this often is an undesirable side effect, in some cases it's beneficial, as

when drugs are given to prevent organ rejection following transplant surgery.

Regardless of the cause, those with immunodeficiency typically suffer from frequent infections and recover slowly or incompletely from illness. They may be vulnerable to certain types of cancer as well.

At the other end of the spectrum, the body becomes overly sensitive to invaders. Allergies are probably the most common example. When you have an allergy, your immune system attacks a substance that poses no threat. This is called an autoimmune disorder.

In conditions such as lupus and rheumatoid arthritis, the immune system loses its ability to differentiate friend from foe, and the body stupidly begins attacking itself. Without treatment, an autoimmune disease can be quite serious, resulting in damaged skin, destroyed joints and wasted organs.

Perhaps the most common type of immune "disorder"—one you can't do anything about—is caused by getting older. The immune system tends to weaken with age, says Dr. Phillips. That's one reason older men often suffer more infections and illness, including cancer, than younger men.

But the fact that some men maintain healthy immune systems well beyond age 70 suggests that deterioration of the immune system is not inevitable. Some experts believe that at least part of this "inevitable" decline can actually be traced to poor nutrition. Eating a good diet and getting enough essential vitamins and minerals can help you stay strong well into old age.

"In the end," says Dr. Phillips, "it's how well we look after ourselves that decides how well our immune systems look after us."

Jaw

- **Relax your face.**
- **Exercise your jaw muscles.**
- **Maintain good posture.**

Kirk Douglas has a prominent one. Jay Leno's contains a miniature Grand Canyon.

But Tracy King, a truck driver from East Greenwich, Rhode Island, puts them both to shame. With a jutting jaw of Herculean strength, he balanced a 16½-foot, 70-pound canoe on his chin while appearing on *The Late Show with David Letterman.*

"I can balance anything up to 170 pounds and 40 feet high on my chin," states King, who is in his thirties. "In December 1994, I balanced a 12-foot Christmas tree during David Letterman's Christmas special. Your mandibular muscles are some of your body's strongest muscles."

Your jaw is made up of the mandible bone on the bottom, the maxilla above the teeth and the temporal bone in front of your ear. Together they form a powerful door to your mouth. The muscles that control your jaw can clamp down with more than 200 pounds of force.

Connecting two of the jawbones is the temporomandibular joint. This joint allows the jaw to open, close and move backward, forward and from side to side. This enables you to eat, speak, kiss and even balance canoes. By sliding a finger in front of each ear and moving your jaw, you can locate your temporomandibular joint and the dime-size disks that keep the jawbones from rubbing against each other.

Problems in Motion

Normally, your jaw just jaws on, a crucial, ever-in-motion cog in the machinery of your mouth. But as with any other machine, problems often arise in the moving parts. Your temporomandibular joint is no exception. It can get off track or break down, causing it to creak, pop, crack, grind and shoot pain through your neck, head and shoulders.

This problem is known as temporomandibular disorder, or TMD, and it afflicts one in ten men. TMD is often caused by a traumatic blow to the head, such as being hit in the jaw or having the neck jarred in a car accident. It can also result from a gradual deterioration of the joint brought on by a severe underbite, bad posture or tooth grinding.

Stress during the day can also contribute to the onset of TMD. Typical male reactions to stress—chewing on pens, gnawing on gum, clenching the teeth—can cause our muscles to tense, our jaws to ache and our jaw joints to cry out in pain.

It is easy to misdiagnose a malfunctioning mandible because the pain often shows up away from the joint. That's why TMD is often mistaken for a headache, a toothache or even a sore throat. "I'd say that fewer than one-quarter of my patients come in with complaints of aching jaws. They call TMD the great impostor because it mimics many

Locating the Jaw Joint

Temporal bone

Temporomandibular joint

Maxilla

Mandible

Opening and closing your jaw as you feel around in front of your ear will help you locate where your jaw joint is.

other symptoms," says Neil Gottehrer, D.D.S., director of the Craniofacial Pain Center in Abington, Pennsylvania.

The degree of pain that TMD sufferers experience can also vary enormously. "The pain can be so mild as to not be noticed or so severe as to render the patient suicidal," says Richard Goldman, D.D.S., director of the Institute for the Treatment and Study of Headaches and Facial Pain in Chicago.

Jaw Health

The goal of jaw maintenance is to keep the joint from malfunctioning. Here's how to keep your jaw in line.

Use your jaw less. Beavers must constantly chew to wear down their teeth, or their teeth will grow through their skulls and kill them. Luckily, guys don't have to worry about that, although you wouldn't know it from their behavior. Excessive mouth motion, such as chomping on gum or gnawing on a pencil or doing mouth gymnastics with a toothpick, is bad for you, says Gerald J. Murphy, D.D.S., president of the American Academy of Head, Neck and Facial Pain and a dentist in Grand Island, Nebraska. Give your mouth a break and quit overusing your jaw joint.

Battle bruxism. Bruxism, the medical name for grinding your teeth while you sleep, is murder on your jaw. It can be alleviated by a simple mouth guard from your dentist. "We put a hard plastic appliance over the upper teeth that keeps the teeth separated. So the lower teeth can glide over smooth plastic instead of biting into the uppers," says Charles Longenecker, D.M.D., a dentist in Emmaus, Pennsylvania.

Phone straight. Cradling the phone receiver between your shoulder and ear is a sure way to get TMD. It takes your jaw out of alignment and puts strain on your neck and shoulder, says Dr. Longenecker. Try a speakerphone or a headset instead. Either will let you gab all day without stressing your jaw joint.

Type like a man. Staring down at a computer screen or gazing down at a book all day puts extra stress on your neck and jaw muscles. "Changing your head posture changes your jaw position. Over the course of time, that relates to developing TMD," says Dr. Murphy. By raising your computer screen or book to eye level, you can eliminate this muscle stress.

Have soup instead of sirloin. If you're experiencing pain in your jaw joint, lay off foods that require you to tear and grind with your teeth, such as steak and taffy, says Dr. Murphy. Instead, feed on soft foods such as soup, Jell-O and well-cooked vegetables until the tension in your joint subsides.

Sleep facing the stars. Sleeping on your stomach, with your head twisted sideways, can aggravate your jaw joint and put undue stress on the muscles in your neck and jaw. "I recommend sleeping on your side or back if possible," says Dr. Gottehrer.

Try a pain pill. A nonprescription pain reliever that helps reduce inflammation, such as ibuprofen or aspirin, can help relieve the pain of a TMD flare-up, says Dr. Murphy. Be sure to read the product label for dosage recommendations.

Work in some heat. Locate your jaw joint using the method mentioned earlier. Then with a moist, warm washcloth, gently massage the joint in a circular motion for about 20 minutes. Dr. Murphy suggests that you try this technique in the morning and evening, when you are most likely to have jaw pain.

Pump up your jaw. Just like other muscles in your body, the muscles surrounding your jaw can be strengthened and toned to ward off those clicking and popping noises and prevent TMD. Dr. Gottehrer recommends light isometric exercises, such as putting your finger beneath your chin and trying to open your mouth against slight resistance. Repeat this exercise 10 to 15 times twice a day.

Do jaw exercises work? In one study of 44 TMD sufferers, half did jaw exercises while the rest did nothing. Researchers found that 18 of the 22 people who exercised eliminated the clicking, while none of the nonexercisers got better.

Joints

- **Keep surrounding muscles strong.**
- **Avoid excessive wear and tear and banging.**
- **Keep joints stretched, stretched, stretched.**

Consider the Tin Man's plight. Exposed to rain, his joints froze, forcing him to stand motionless alongside a yellow brick road. Finally, after he had waited for more than a year with an ax in his hand and his right arm uplifted, a young girl and a scarecrow wandered near enough to hear him mutter the word "oilcan" through his clenched jaw.

Heartlessness was the least of the Tin Man's problems. He needed working joints.

As the Tin Man might attest, life without functioning joints is not a moving experience. But not all joints move. You have a joint wherever two bones meet; joints are your body's seams as well as its pivots and hinges. Immovable, or fixed, joints are found, for example, in your skull, where the bones that protect your brain come together.

Depending on their structure and purpose, other joints allow you to move in different ways. Those in your back are relatively stiff, and each individual vertebra moves little. Your back is flexible because so many individual joints are aligned. So-called hinge joints—your fingers, knees and elbows, for example—move back and forth, primarily in one plane. Ball-and-socket joints in your shoulders and hips are the most versatile, capable of moving in many different directions. As a matter of necessity, they are also the most muscular. Muscles help hold your ball-and-socket joints together and provide the power to move in so many ways with stability. Also key are strong tendons (which connect muscle to bone) and ligaments (which connect bone to bone).

We've provided separate chapters in this book on the major joints such as the knees and wrists. But joints have much in common, in terms of both maintenance and problem resolution. So for limber, well-oiled joints from toes to nose, read on.

Use Them or Lose Them

There's no secret to keeping your joints healthy. Strong and supple joints are healthy joints. Here are ways that experts recommend to keep your joints jumping.

Keep your weight down. Extra weight puts added pressure on your leg joints, especially your knees, and wears them down.

Exercise. Physical activity makes muscles stronger, lessening the stress on your joints, and also strengthens your bones. For your joints, the best cardiovascular exercises are those that involve little or no impact, such as swimming, bicycling and walking, says Steven F. Habusta, D.O., an orthopedic surgeon in Toledo, Ohio.

Stretch. Loose joints are more likely to remain healthy. Among other things, stretching also increases your muscle strength. (To learn stretches for individual joints, see their respective chapters as well as the workouts in part 3 of this book.)

Don't become a ballet dancer. Ballet dancers are particularly susceptible to arthritis in their feet from years of standing on their toes. The real lesson for you: Activities that place constant strain on the same joints will likely harm them.

Likewise, don't play in the NFL. Many football players suffer from arthritis and other joint problems brought on by constant pounding. If you must play contact sports, at least wear protective pads to reduce the stress on your joints.

Don't be a weekend warrior. If you haven't played full-court basketball in five years, forget the "Just do it" slogan and don't. Intense exertion without preparation can hurt you bad. Get in shape before you play, start gradually and don't push yourself too hard. "Be reasonable when you get older," says Dr. Habusta. "People have to keep in mind that as they get older, natural wear and tear occurs in their bodies. You have to realize that's a natural part of aging."

Read your body's cues. If you experience problems with one type of exercise, such as running, switch to something that puts less strain on your joints. While you might be able to develop the muscles for the sport, your joints are far less likely to adapt to hostile challenges.

The Troubles of Joints

Movable joints are complicated structures made of varying types and amounts of cartilage, ligament and muscle, with specialized membranes and fluids to lubricate each joint and provide a cushion against stress. Given this complexity, it's hardly surprising that many different things can go wrong.

Sprains

You go for a run one evening along a tree-lined path. You can't see well in the shadows cast by the setting sun and step awkwardly on a tree root. You stumble and twist your ankle. It hurts. As you're limping home, it begins to swell.

Most likely, you've suffered a sprained ankle, a common joint injury. This means that you've stretched or torn a ligament, which holds adjoining bones together. Although it's possible to sprain any ligament in the body, those in the ankles, knees and fingers are most often injured because we tend to apply relatively greater force to them than to our other joints.

If you sprain a joint, apply ice in a 20-minutes-on, 20-minutes-off cycle during the first two hours following the injury. Continue the applications for about 8 to 10 minutes of every hour for the next day or so. Place a towel

Can Diet Fix Your Joints?

Some people claim to have developed miracle diets that cure arthritis. Well, hold your appetite: None of these diets has been proven to either cure or eliminate the symptoms. The evidence is too contradictory.

But some studies do suggest a correlation between diet and the severity of arthritis symptoms, and some people may find that their conditions improve when they change their diets.

The most essential advice is basic: Eat a well-balanced diet, making sure that you get the recommended amounts of nutrients, as detailed in the chapter on nutrition (page 2). Some diet strategies to consider:

Eat for relief. A study in Finland suggests that rheumatoid arthritis sufferers may get some relief by eating foods rich in vitamin E, zinc and beta-carotene. Vitamin E is plentiful in almonds and wheat germ; zinc, in lean meats and whole grains; and beta-carotene, in yellow, orange and dark green, leafy vegetables.

Learn your triggers. Several studies suggest that for some people, symptoms worsen when they eat certain foods. In a nationwide survey of more than 1,000 people with

between your skin and the ice to avoid burning your skin. Rest the joint and keep it elevated as much as possible to help reduce swelling. Use an elastic bandage for support. Begin exercising soon, but without putting weight on the injured joint, says Dr. Habusta.

If the pain is severe or lasts for more than a couple of days, see your doctor. It's often difficult to tell the difference between a sprain, which will usually heal by itself, and a bone fracture, which must be set in order to heal correctly. Another warning sign: Lots of bruising (bleeding beneath the skin) might signal a major ligament tear or fracture. In rare cases, a doctor may have to operate.

Tendinitis

Tendons, as explained earlier, attach muscle to bone. When you damage or tear a tendon, usually from injury or overuse, the adjoining area swells and hurts. If you continue to use the muscle and tendons, they will continue

arthritis, 10 percent said they were sensitive to or intolerant of specific foods. Of these foods, red meats were most often associated with flare-ups of arthritis pain. Some others: sweets, fatty and fried foods, salt, caffeine, dairy products, alcohol, processed meats and foods with additives and preservatives. Depending on your medical condition, some diets could be dangerous for you or could interact adversely with your medication.

In many of these studies, subjects first fasted, then gradually reintroduced foods in an attempt to identify those that bothered their arthritis. You might try something similar, charting your reactions to foods in a diary. But be careful and work with your doctor; fasting can be dangerous.

Eat more fish. Studies show that large amounts of fish oil, which contains omega-3 fatty acids, can help reduce the number of painful joints and increase energy levels in some people with rheumatoid arthritis. The best way to do this is to increase your consumption of cold-water ocean fish such as tuna, salmon, mackerel and sardines, says Fred G. Kantrowitz, M.D., author of the book *Taking Control of Arthritis.*

to be injured and will take longer to heal, says Dr. Habusta. In older people especially, tendinitis pain sometimes lasts for weeks or months.

Though you can injure any tendon, tendinitis develops most frequently in the shoulders, ankles and elbows. Tennis elbow, for example, is a form of tendinitis in which you strain the tendon on the outside of the elbow.

For tendinitis, apply ice to reduce swelling and rest the affected joint for several days. Take aspirin or ibuprofen to relieve pain and reduce swelling, says Dr. Habusta. Begin exercising the joint soon, so it doesn't become stiff, but avoid activities that put undue strain on the tendon. In other words, if you hurt your elbow playing tennis, don't play tennis for a while, meaning a week or two.

Bursitis

The layman's terms for several of the more common forms of bursitis—housemaid's knee, clergyman's knee and student's elbow, for example—hint at the nature and origin of this condition. Put pressure on a joint for too long, and it will often swell.

Bursae are tiny sacs filled with fluid that absorb pressure and reduce friction, usually within joints. When you apply too much pressure to a bursa, it sometimes becomes inflamed or fills with fluid. Bursitis occurs most often in the knees, elbows, hips and shoulders, where, at its most extreme, it results in a condition called frozen shoulder.

If you continually irritate the same bursae, they will sometimes scar, and bursitis can become a chronic problem. That's why men who constantly put pressure on the same joints—roofers, for example, who spend lots of time on their knees—should wear protective padding.

Bursitis is sometimes painful, but it isn't usually serious. With rest, the problem usually clears up on its own. If necessary, apply ice to relieve pain as you would with a sprain, says Dr. Habusta.

Damaged and Torn Cartilage

Cartilage covers the surfaces of bones that would otherwise touch within a joint. If you constantly put excessive pressure on a joint—the knees of football players are a prime example—the cartilage, which is ordinarily smooth and marblelike, will sometimes flake off, leading to grinding and pain. Often this sort of damage is a precursor to arthritis.

Each knee has an additional piece of cartilage that can be torn, especially when suddenly twisted. This injury is often felt as a sharp, intense pain. In contrast to a strained ligament, damaged cartilage won't heal itself, so it's important that you see your doctor. Some common warning signs: Fluid builds up in your knee, your knee locks or makes a clicking sound, and pain persists for more than a couple of weeks or becomes chronic.

Arthritis: The Big One

Of all of the problems that can afflict human joints, arthritis is surely the most common and the most frequently disabling. Literally, the word means inflammation of a joint. In practice, "arthritis" refers not to a single disease but to a collection of more than 100 different conditions, including gout, lupus, ankylosing spondylitis, rheumatoid arthritis and, most common of all, osteoarthritis. Their common denominator: All cause swelling, pain and/or loss of motion in joints.

Arthritis is by no means solely a modern, or even a human, ailment. Paleontologists have found evidence of osteoarthritis in the skeletons of dinosaurs. (Lesson number one in staving off the ravages of osteoarthritis, also known as degenerative bone disease: Don't get too big.) Researchers have identified chronic arthritis of the spine in human ancestors who lived two million years ago.

To some extent, arthritis is an inevitable part of the aging process. You lose hair. Your skin wrinkles. Your joints deteriorate. It's only logical: Over time, the moving parts of a machine break down. Your body is no different.

The Arthritis Foundation estimates that some 14 million American men—that's nearly one in six of us—have some form of arthritis. Although most of these suffer only variable levels of stiffness and pain, more than 2 million men must somehow restrict their everyday lives because of their arthritis. As the population grows older, the prevalence of

---

Is It Rheumatoid Arthritis?

You wake up stiff. As you walk downstairs, your knees hurt; you clutch the railing for support. At breakfast, your fingers ache. Is it rheumatoid arthritis? Here are some things to look for.

How old are you? Rheumatoid arthritis (RA), an immune system disorder in which white blood cells collect in joints, usually strikes men when they're 20 to 40 years old.

How long does your stiffness last? With RA, it usually persists for 30 minutes or more per day over a period of several weeks.

Where does it hurt? RA can strike both large and small joints, but most people first notice it in their fingers.

Are your stiffness and pain symmetrical? The knuckles of both hands hurt, for example. Or you have pain in both knees, rather than in the one you might have bumped on the dresser last week.

Other signs are more subtle: You feel listless, you feel vague muscle pain, you have a low-grade fever, you don't have an appetite, or you lose weight.

---

arthritis will likely increase.

When doctors speak of treating the most common forms of arthritis, they speak of control in most cases and of cure in only some, says Doyt Conn, M.D., senior vice-president for medical affairs of the Arthritis Foundation. The earlier you catch the trouble, the more you can limit its damaging effects. Typically, doctors treat arthritis with some combination of anti-inflammatory drugs, physical therapy and recommendations for lifestyle changes.

Because of both the nature of the disease and the limitations of existing remedies, many people with arthritis are disappointed with the results of traditional treatment methods. This may explain the vast array of ostensible "cures"—everything from cow manure and the light of a full moon to copper bracelets and bee venom—that quacks and hucksters have promoted over the years. In fact, such "cures" are so numerous that the Arthritis Foundation is in the process of evaluating these alternative treatments. (Actually, there is evidence that bee venom may help. One study of beekeepers, who are stung an average of 2,000 times a year, found that the prevalence of arthritis among beekeepers is less than half of what it is among the general population.)

Many health professionals believe that a combination of natural methods and more traditional Western techniques can be the best strategy. Alternative treatments that have at least some medical support range from aromatherapy and acupressure to juice therapy and reflexology. Get your hands on an alternative healing guidebook for an introduction to these therapies. Most books offer a list of resources that you can contact for more information. Just let your doctor know what you are doing.

Here are the major types of arthritis and what you need to know about them.

Osteoarthritis. If you're over age 40, chances are that your joints show signs of osteoarthritis, which results from the breakdown of cartilage between bones. That's a condition shown by x-rays, though not everyone experiences the swelling, stiffness and pain that characterize this disease. What the x-rays show is part of the aging process: As you grow older, cartilage hardens, becomes brittle and breaks down.

This is the form of arthritis most closely linked to age. Ironically, it is also the form that you may be able to affect most dramatically. "If you learn good body mechanics, have good muscle strength, are near ideal weight and continue to exercise, there's good evidence that you can stave off osteoarthritis or at least lessen its severity," says David Pisetsky, M.D., Ph.D., professor of medicine at the Duke University Medical Center and co-director of the Duke University Arthritis Center, both in Durham, North Carolina. Indeed, exercise is the closest thing that you have to the Tin Man's oil: It keeps your joints strong and flexible, strengthens your muscles and bones and keeps your weight down.

If you already have osteoarthritis, however, there's a lot you can do besides exercise.

• Aspirin, ibuprofen and other drugs can relieve pain while reducing the swelling and inflammation that often accompany osteoarthritis. Just be sure to limit your dosage to what is recommended on the bottle or by your doctor, says Dr. Pisetsky. Gobbling aspirin every time you feel arthritis pain can do a real number on your stomach. In extreme cases, a doctor may inject corticosteroids directly into a joint. Corrective surgery can also be used to restore function as well as relieve pain, says Dr. Pisetsky.

• Exercise without jarring diseased joints. Swimming, walking and riding a stationary bicycle are some of the best exercises for people with osteoarthritis to build endurance, arthritis experts say.

• A hot shower in the morning can help you loosen up. Towel-wrapped ice or a cold compress can help relieve pain in a particularly troublesome joint. So can a topical pain reliever, which dulls nerve endings in your skin, says Dr. Pisetsky. Ask your doctor for a recommendation. Examples of these, available in your drugstore, are capsaicin (Zostrix) and liniments such as Ben-Gay.

• Use your joints properly. Sitting up straight, for example, and walking upright can reduce pressure on your back, a common arthritis site, say arthritis experts.

Rheumatoid arthritis. Also known as RA, this is potentially the most severe and debilitating form of systemic arthritis. Its cause is not known. RA is an immune system disorder in which white blood cells collect in joints. In about one in ten people, RA seems to come and go; in others, the disease persists for years, eventually damaging cartilage and bone. Some joints wind up deformed and disabled. RA can be inherited, and genes seem to play a role in determining its severity. Unlike osteoarthritis, RA tends to affect people when they are younger—in men, usually between the ages of 20 and 40.

Given RA's potential severity, it's not surprising that RA has become the subject of intensive research. There are many excellent pharmaceutical treatments that can slow or even stop the progress of the disease, says Dr.

Pisetsky. Scientists are also investigating the healing effects of other natural substances, from borage seed oil and chicken collagen to capsaicin, the chemical that puts the heat in hot peppers. Some have shown some promise, but that doesn't mean it's time to begin swallowing peppers whole, says Dr. Pisetsky. The point is simpler: By the time you read this, doctors may well know more about RA. So if you have RA, see a specialist.

Gout. This is one of the few forms of arthritis that afflict men more than women. It is also one of the best understood and most treatable.

Gout is a metabolic disorder in which uric acid crystallizes in a joint, often the big toe. Doctors typically treat gout with a nonsteroidal anti-inflammatory drug such as ibuprofen or indomethacin or another medicine. Don't take aspirin, says Dr. Pisetsky; it will affect your body's process of ridding itself of uric acid. Also, eating less meat will slow the accumulation of uric acid in your joints, says Dr. Habusta.

Though diet alone doesn't cause gout, the wrong diet can trigger an attack. Especially if you've ever had gout, avoid foods high in purines (chemicals that turn into uric acid in the blood). Skip the alcohol, anchovies, fish roe and mussels and just about any kind of organ meat. All have extremely high levels of purines.

Even though gout is more common with age, you don't have to be old to be shot down in its flames of pain. Most men experience their first attacks in their forties, but bouts can occur much earlier. And forget the old notion that gout is a disease of the rich and royal; gout crosses all class and social lines. The primary target is a sedentary middle-aged man who eats and drinks in abundance and whose weight and blood pressure are on the rise.

⚒ Kidneys

- **Water, water, water.**
- **Check blood pressure regularly.**

Dirty blood going in. Clean blood going out. Waste in. Waste out. This, in a nutshell, is your kidneys. Treat them right, and they'll work fine.

Masters at recycling before it was hip, the kidneys filter every drop of bodily fluid, recycle what's worth it and dispose of the rest. For a guy who weighs about 155 pounds, blood flows through the kidneys at the rate of about 40 ounces per minute.

"They're two of the most durable organs we have," says Tom Peters, M.D., director of the Jacksonville Transplant Center at Methodist Medical Center in Jacksonville, Florida, and clinical professor of surgery at the University of Florida in Gainesville. "They're not affected by tobacco—directly. They're not affected by alcohol—directly. Not affected by exercise—directly. There's not a whole lot you need to do—directly—to maintain your kidneys' health."

This is stuff men love to hear: a low-maintenance piece of machinery. But (of course there's a but) . . . indirectly, high blood pressure, which is related to tobacco and alcohol use, and a high blood sugar level can wreak havoc on the kidneys. So if you have high blood pressure or diabetes, listen up: You should have your condition regularly monitored by your physician, and you gotta get rid of your vices—cigarettes, booze, fatty foods, salty foods, couch camping—or else you might damage your kidneys bad. And guess what? Even if your blood pressure or blood sugar level isn't high, all of this advice is still good.

Tale of Two Kidneys

Let's get the unanswerable question out of the way first: So why do we have two kidneys?

Donald Wesson, M.D., chief of the nephrology section at Texas Tech University Health Sciences Center in Lubbock, passes the buck on that question.

"That's a question for God," he says. "Fortunately, He has given us much more kidney function than we need. We can live on one kidney. In fact, patients who donate kidneys and those who receive kidney transplants do it all of the time. We have to lose the majority of our kidney function before we get into problems."

It's not as though there isn't enough work for two. The fist-size, bean-shaped kidneys contain millions of tiny filtering units called nephrons (that's why kidney doctors are called nephrologists). A nephron consists of a tuft of small blood vessels with convoluted tubing that would make the construction of a French horn look simple. "They're like the filters in fish aquariums," explains Dr. Wesson. "If the filter stops working or gets clogged, the water looks yucky."

In every 24-hour period, the kidneys process roughly 42 gallons of fluid. All but one to two quarts are returned to the bloodstream. The rest is waste, better known as urine. It leaves the kidneys through tubes called ureters. They lead to the bladder, where the pee waits most patiently for its opportunity to exit the system.

Among the kidneys' other chores: regulating the body's salt, potassium and acid content, making hormones that stimulate red blood cell production, regulating blood pressure and controlling calcium metabolism.

Preventing Kidney Disease

The trouble with kidney disease is that you typically don't get any symptoms until severe damage has been done. So we'll use this analogy: You willingly pay for auto insurance in the hope that you'll never need to use

it. Consider kidney care in the same way, with one big difference. Taking care of your kidneys, as outlined below, has many tangible benefits throughout your body that go far beyond not getting diseased. So be smart and do the following.

Keep your blood sugar level in check. The chapter on the pancreas explains why and how to contain the amount of blood sugar you allow in your body. Why is that relevant here? Diabetes is the leading cause of kidney failure in the United States.

If you don't want to flip there now, keep in mind that carbohydrates as well as sugary foods, candies and desserts can create a glut of blood sugar, taxing your pancreas beyond its normal functioning. (The pancreas makes the

Locating Your Kidneys

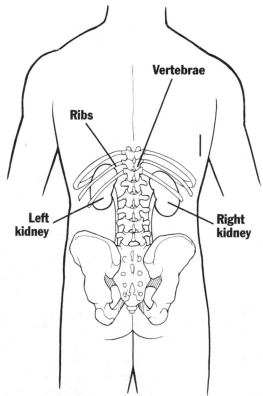

Can you feel the bottom ribs on your back? Your kidneys are tucked under them, a few inches above where your tailbone starts.

chemicals that help your body process blood sugar.) This, in turn, ricochets onto your kidneys. Specifically, a persistently elevated blood sugar level appears to be toxic to those kidney cells that filter dietary protein. When your kidneys' filtering system fails, the protein escapes into your urine without giving your body a chance to use it. That's why doctors start worrying about kidney disease when they find large amounts of protein in urine samples.

Don't fear protein. It has often been thought that too much protein in your diet might be harmful to your kidneys. "For years, people have been put on low-protein diets because traces of protein have been found in their urine. But protein is not necessarily the evil one," says Michael E. Eades, M.D., a family physician in Little Rock, Arkansas, and co-author of *Protein Power: The Metabolic Breakthrough*. If your kidneys are normal, protein shouldn't harm them. The evil is food that increases your blood sugar level excessively, Dr. Eades says.

Don't jump to kidney conclusions. "In some 20-odd years of practice, I have found that when people come in with back pain that they believe to be a kidney problem, 95 to 98 percent of the time it turns out to be a back problem," says William McGuffin, M.D., a nephrologist at Baptist Medical Center in Montgomery, Alabama. The confusion is understandable. Your kidneys are located toward the back of your midsection between your pelvis and your ribs, just about where you put your hand when your lower back starts to ache. Before you get too nervous, Dr. McGuffin

---

Heed Those Warning Labels

In 1985, when ibuprofen went over-the-counter, kidney specialists recommended that the drug carry an explicit warning that using it could have an adverse effect on the normal function of kidneys. The Food and Drug Administration has yet to act on that recommendation. It should have, says William Henrich, M.D., chairman of the Department of Internal Medicine at the Medical College of Ohio at Toledo and a member of the scientific advisory board of the National Kidney Foundation.

If you habitually load up on a drug such as ibuprofen, indomethacin (Indocin) or ketoprofen (Orudis)—all members of the family called nonsteroidal anti-inflammatory drugs—for run-of-the-mill pains such as tennis elbow, runner's knee, tendinitis and other joint aches, you may significantly increase your chances of developing kidney failure, Dr. Henrich says. These drugs, he explains, diminish the filtering capacity of your kidneys by decreasing kidney blood flow.

"After years of taking these drugs, you can develop chronic problems and scarring of your kidneys," he says. "Many people believe that because these drugs are available over the counter and on supermarket shelves, they are inherently safe and can be taken without paying much attention to side effects." His message is simple: "Don't believe it. Read the labels. Heed the warnings. It's primarily your responsibility, and you should consult your doctor if you have any questions about whether to take the medicine."

---

suggests that you have your back checked. If you do have a kidney problem, warning signs include difficulty urinating, pain or burning when urinating and blood in the urine.

Check it out. Have your blood pressure and urine checked once a year, recommends Saulo Klahr, M.D., chief of medicine at the Jewish Hospital in St. Louis and editor of the *American Journal of Kidney Diseases*. "Kidneys are both the villain and the victim when it comes to high blood pressure," he explains. "They can be the source of an increase in blood pressure, and high blood pressure can cause damage to the kidneys." Elevated blood pressure "upsets the delicate balancing act of

Leave This Stone Unturned

You don't want to get them. They hurt. Check that: They really hurt. To amplify: They really hurt very much. A half-million Americans a year—four in five of them men—can attest to that. Eventually, up to 10 percent of American men will develop kidney stones.

Though there are several types of stones, the most common are formed when there's a chemical imbalance between calcium and oxalate waste products. Too much of one or the other, and they crystallize in the kidneys into hard, insoluble little pebbles. "Like salt water that's allowed to evaporate, the crystals form rocks," explains Donald Wesson, M.D., chief of the nephrology section at Texas Tech University Health Sciences Center in Lubbock. If one of those rocks plugs a ureter, which leads from the kidney to the bladder, it will cause a pain in the area of your flank, pubic region or genitalia. Here are some strategies for encouraging kidney stones to roll in another direction.

Keep the calcium coming. Calcium used to be considered the culprit. Now that theory has been put to pasture. Calcium was blamed because it's a major component of most stones, and further, up to half of the people who develop stones have high levels of calcium in their urine. But not long ago, Gary Curhan, M.D., chief of clinical nephrology at the Veterans Affairs Medical Center in West Roxbury, Massachusetts, and his colleagues from the Health Professional Follow-Up Study at Harvard School of Public Health made a surprising discovery. In a giant study, they found that those who consumed the most dietary calcium were actually the least likely to form stones. Dr. Curhan's theory: Calcium may reduce the body's supply of urinary oxalate, and that oxalate may be more important to stone formation than calcium. Dr. Curhan recommends getting 800 milligrams of dietary calcium daily.

Drink to shrink your stones. "Be well-hydrated," advises Saulo Klahr, M.D., chief of medicine at the Jewish Hospital in St. Louis and editor of the *American Journal of Kidney Diseases*. "Drinking a lot of fluids will help dilute the concentration of calcium and magnesium salts in your urine." Dr. Curhan adds, "Picture urine as a beaker of water. Now add two teaspoons of sugar. If the sugar doesn't dissolve, add more water, and it probably will." More water in your kidneys will keep calcium dissolved.

several kidney hormones that regulate blood flow and pressure. When one goes out of whack, so do the others, causing serious kidney damage." Similarly, when your kidneys are diseased, the whole act goes haywire, sending your blood pressure through the ceiling.

As for the urine sample, doctors are looking for protein, which, as noted above, indicates that the kidneys are filtering it. "It's normal to find some small traces of protein in your urine," Dr. Klahr explains. "But large amounts of protein over time are a sign that there's some degree of kidney damage, and it could suggest any number of renal diseases."

Check it all out. An enlarged prostate can lead to kidney disease by obstructing urine flow. The increased pressure can eventually damage your kidneys. But removing the obstruction and restoring urine flow can potentially return kidney function to normal. Yet another reason to get the walnut-size vice that's wrapped around your urethra checked out on a regular basis. (For more information on this important gland, see page 265.)

Don't hit 'em where it hurts. Here's why people have been telling you, ever since you were a kid, that you shouldn't hit even your worst enemy in the kidneys: It's as painful as pain can be. "There's not a lot of fat protecting that area of the body, exposing some very sensitive nerve endings," says Ted Steinman, M.D., professor of medicine at Harvard Medical

School and director of the dialysis unit at Beth Israel Hospital in Boston. "A hard blow with a club or baseball bat, for example, would be very painful and could seriously traumatize your kidneys." If you must vent, hurl epithets, not hard objects, in the direction of your foe's kidneys.

Order a (virgin) Cape Codder. That's vodka and cranberry juice with a twist of lemon, but hold the vodka. This old wives' remedy for bladder infections may work after all. And for men, too. But it's not the high acid content or the vitamin C that makes cranberry juice work, as many have believed, according to Anthony Sobota, Ph.D., chairman of the biology department at Youngstown State University in Ohio, who since 1982 has been studying the effects of the red fruit juice on bladder infections. "It's still somewhat of a mystery, but we find that cranberry juice prevents bacteria from attaching to the lining of the bladder." Since bladder infections can move backward up to the kidneys, it is also helpful to drink cranberry juice for bacteria-free kidneys. Dr. Sobota suggests drinking about four ounces a day.

Don't add salt to the wound. Because sodium is related to high blood pressure (and you already know the relationship between high blood pressure and kidney disease), "it makes a lot of sense to reduce your salt intake," suggests Dr. Klahr. "Especially, but not only, if you have a tendency toward high blood pressure." Dr. Peters adds, "What we're saying is to use salt in moderation, whether it's table salt or salt contained in processed foods. Country ham seasoned with salt and pepper would not be a good idea." And by the way, canned vegetables usually have more sodium than fresh or frozen.

Understanding Kidney Disease

The disorders are many: infections, inflammations, obstructions and tumors, among others. "There are dozens of them," says Dr. McGuffin. We'll spare you an oration on the offenders. What you need to know is that kidney disorders beget kidney disease. And kidney disease begets kidney failure. And as folk prophet Bob Dylan sagely stated, failure is no success at all. In this case, failure is called end-stage renal disease. That's when you've lost 90 percent of your total kidney function.

Age works against your kidneys. As your thirties become a fond memory, you suddenly begin losing about 1 percent of your kidney function a year, says William Henrich, M.D., chairman of the Department of Internal Medicine at the Medical College of Ohio at Toledo and a member of the scientific advisory board of the National Kidney Foundation.

There are seven basic warning signs that your kidneys are not happy campers.
- A burning sensation while you are urinating
- More frequent urination, especially at night
- Blood in the bowl after you urinate (and it's not your nose that's bleeding)
- Puffiness around your eyes for no apparent reason
- Pain that feels like someone just hit home with a couple of swift jabs to the small of your back, below your ribs, and that is independent of movement
- Swollen hands or feet
- High blood pressure

Knowing these signs is a good thing. There's just one problem: By the time you start showing any of them, "it may be too late," according to Dr. Peters. "Kidney disease is often asymptomatic." Translation: There are no highway flares that go up in its early stages. In fact, "warning sign" may be a misnomer. By the time you get a warning . . . bingo! You may already have kidney disease.

If your kidneys do fail, you have two choices. One is dialysis. That's when you're hooked up to a machine that artificially does the cleanup duties that your kidneys have bailed out on. The other is kidney transplant surgery.

⋀Knees

- **Strengthen the surrounding muscles.**
- **Close your desk drawers.**
- **Flex often and keep them moving.**

Whether we're weekend runners or NBA forwards, file clerks or chief executives, most of us work and play at the expense of our knees. Even the fittest among us have knees that are tracked with surgery scars, wrapped in elastic supports, soaked each night in warm water, then packed in ice like fragile produce. Regular exercise makes the rest of our bodies stronger and tougher, but our knees, it seems, just won't get with the program.

And the deskbound among us are even worse off: Research shows that extended sitting can also lead to serious knee problems or exacerbate pre-existing symptoms. Knees have surpassed the back and all other parts of the body in terms of work-related injuries. "They are by far the weak link in the human anatomy," says James M. Fox, M.D., senior partner at the Southern California Orthopedic Institute and Medical Group in Van Nuys.

That's one way of looking at the knee dilemma. But then there's the shiny, happy way to view the issue: With a little thought and care, your knees need never hurt. There are plenty of proven ways to prevent knee injury and several ways that you can treat minor knee problems yourself. It requires commitment and self-discipline, but as the saying goes, you're only as strong as . . .

We, the Tin Men

Blame aching knees on evolution. The largest and most complex joint in your body is also the most poorly constructed. The hip and shoulder joints sport nifty ball-and-socket designs, but the knee joint is a snarl of bone, sinew and cartilage.

In the knee, the two knobby ends of the thighbone, or femur, meet the nearly flat surfaces of the shinbone, or tibia. All that comes between them are semi-attached disks of cartilage called menisci, which form a shallow socket for the femur to plug into. This mechanism is lashed together with a cross-hatching of ligaments and tendons, then covered up by the kneecap, or patella. "The

---

Ranking the Sports

Go ahead and play hard. Get it out of your system. Just be aware that certain sports provide more opportunity for knee injury than others. James G. Garrick, M.D., an orthopedic surgeon and director of the Center for Sports Medicine at St. Francis Memorial Hospital in San Francisco, has ranked the sports in tiers, matching the activity with its likelihood of injury.

- Tier one: On the top of the heap are basketball, football and wrestling, which earn orthopedic surgeons a good living repairing torn ligaments and damaged cartilage. Indeed, reports to the Consumer Product Safety Commission by the National Electronic Injury Surveillance System ranked basketball first on a list of injury-causing sports.
- Tier two: Soccer, volleyball, skiing and lacrosse are good sources of knee sprains. Injuries caused by these sports are less difficult to repair than those caused by the sports in tier one.
- Tier three: Track and field, aerobics, step aerobics, stair climbing and running all account for injuries from overuse, such as runner's knee and jumper's knee.
- Tier four: Tennis, racquetball and handball come last. They can lead to runner's knee and sprains, but not nearly as frequently as the other sports.

whole knee joint is basically just a ball on a flat surface," says Dr. Fox. "I don't think God figured on American football."

Maybe not. But the contraption does have its strong points. Stand in front of some stairs, stiffen your knees and try going up. Your knee allows your leg to bend and straighten. It allows you to sit and, even more important, to spoon.

Now climb those stairs, turn around and jump. Your knees can absorb a vertical impact equal to seven times your body weight. (Jump, but don't fall. Your kneecap doesn't really protect your knee. Primarily, it provides leverage for your quadriceps muscle, whose tendons are attached to it.)

Bum Knees and Other Facts of Life

Old timers called them bum knees and stoically limped away on them. But nowadays, doctors can usually trace a knee ache to one of a handful of common problems, and they offer some fairly remarkable remedies. Here's a list of five common causes of "bum knee–itis."

Bruises. Just what it sounds like. You fall, you bang a door, you run into a car bumper. For a quick diagnosis, listen for a loud expletive escaping from your lips, then check for a black-and-blue mark, immediate pain and swelling. Rest your leg and apply an ice pack to your knee for 15 minutes, remove it for a few minutes, then reapply, says Dr. Fox. Be sure to place a towel between the pack and your skin to avoid having to consult a book on skin grafts, he adds.

Squatter's knee. This means that your

Knee Stretches

Yes, you can improve upon nature. Knees that aren't stretched and strengthened tend to rust, says James M. Fox, M.D., senior partner at the Southern California Orthopedic Institute and Medical Group in Van Nuys. So keep them moving. Part 3 of this book offers several stretches and exercises for the thighs and calves that are also good for the knees. Here are three more exercises that Dr. Fox recommends for this most vulnerable of joints.

Hamstring stretch. Keeping your back straight, place your leg on a low table or stool. Bend forward from your

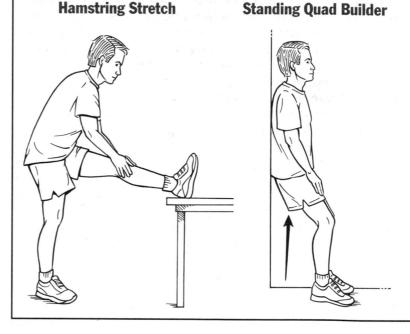

Hamstring Stretch   **Standing Quad Builder**

kneecap doesn't track well on your thighbone. The causes are genetic, but it's exacerbated by stair climbing, squatting, prolonged sitting and, frequently, running. You'll feel a dull ache behind your kneecap that usually subsides when you straighten your leg. Simple strength exercises such as leg lifts, stretches for the hamstrings and quadriceps and applying ice before and after workouts will help relieve the pain, Dr. Fox says. If it persists, your doctor may put you on a short program of anti-inflammatory drugs.

hips until you feel tightness, not pain, in your hamstrings. Hold for 10 to 20 seconds without bouncing. Do five repetitions with each leg.

Quad builders. Perhaps the most important of the bunch because it strengthens the quadriceps. Stand 1½ feet from a wall and lean back against it. Bend your knees and lower yourself four to six inches. (If you feel pain, you're too low.) Hold for five to ten seconds, then slowly rise. Start with 10 repetitions and increase to 35.

More quad builders. Lie on your back and bend one knee so that your foot is flat on the floor. Stretch out the other leg, and keeping it straight, lift it a few inches off the ground. Hold for five seconds, then slowly lower and relax. Start with 10 repetitions per leg and increase to 35. Add a two-pound ankle weight when the exercise is easy and keep adding weight as it gets easier. You can also do this exercise sitting against a wall if you suffer from lower back pain.

Lying Quad Builder

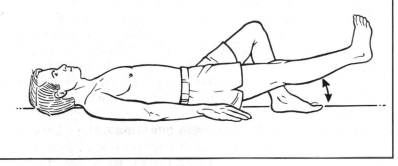

Sprains. Your knee moves fine from front to back, but it's not so hot at going from side to side. That's why clipping is penalized in football. A torn or overstretched ligament, otherwise known as a sprain, results from a sideways blow to the knee. The same blow can cause your menisci (the cartilage disks in your knee) to tear. In either case, you'll feel knee pain immediately and see swelling by the day's end. A less serious sprain can be treated by immobilizing your leg, applying ice packs and, with your doctor's approval, doing simple

rehabilitation exercises such as isometric leg raises, where you tense and then lift your leg while lying on a table or the floor, says Dr. Fox. For a more serious injury, you'll need arthroscopic surgery to remove torn cartilage and to repair or replace damaged ligaments, he adds.

Housemaid's knee. Also called water on the knee, this happens when you fall too hard or kneel too long. Small sacs surrounding your knee joint become inflamed. Check for redness, swelling and pain atop the kneecap. Ice packs and rest are the primary treatments, says Dr. Fox. But if you're not better in a day or so, see your doctor. You might also need a doctor to extract fluid buildup or to prescribe drugs to reduce swelling.

Jumper's knee. This is regularly visited upon basketball players, volleyball players and anyone who overuses the tendon connecting the kneecap to the front calf bone. You'll feel pain just below your kneecap, and you'll wince when you kneel. Again, ice packs and rest help, as may taking aspirin or another anti-inflammatory drug and wearing a knee brace, says Dr. Fox.

Your knees are also susceptible to all of the usual joint maladies, such as tendinitis, bursitis and arthritis. (For a full discussion of these conditions, see page 210.)

Building Better Knees

Delicate critters that they are, knees need your TLC. No one ever got himself on a beefcake calendar for having buff knees, but attending to your joints will help keep the rest of you fit and active. Follow a few simple instructions, and you'll go a long way toward preventing the most common knee injuries.

Exercise! A simple exercise program will help prevent repetitive-motion afflictions such as squatter's knee and runner's knee (also called tennis knee, this is a softening or breakdown of the cartilage below the kneecap). Strengthening the quadriceps muscle, which runs the length of your thigh, will help stabilize your knee against jarring blows. Even after you've been "cured" by surgery, exercise is crucial to recovery. "Knees don't heal themselves," says Dr. Fox. "You have to make it happen with exercise. People have to make a tremendous commitment to getting better."

Lighten your load. A lot of knee problems begin at the dinner table. You can do your knees a big favor by dropping excess weight. A few extra pounds up top won't immediately kill your knees, but one prestigious study has shown that serious obesity can lead to osteoarthritis, a painful degenerative joint disease.

Close the drawer. No kidding: A great number of patients who visit Dr. Fox's practice go there because they've banged their knees into their desk drawers. The resulting bruise can be painful and can indicate water on the knee, Dr. Fox says. The majority of knee injuries occur on the job or in non-sports-related accidents (car wrecks and falls, for example). The lesson: Be careful and close your desk drawers.

Warm up. Start exercising slowly to give your leg muscles a chance to stretch. If you're a weekend athlete, take extra time to get loose and warmed up, advises Dr. Fox.

Go against the tide. If your winter workout routine has you running around a short, circular indoor track, reverse direction after every lap to avoid a repetitive-motion injury. "You can always tell which runners are my patients," says Dr. Fox. "They're always going the wrong way on the track."

Try seeking support. The various knee supports available in pharmacies and sporting goods stores might give some benefit and help you feel more comfortable, says Dr. Fox, but

they should not be relied on as your sole protection. Do they really work? One three-year study followed hundreds of braced and unbraced college football players to determine whether braces decreased injuries. The results suggest that wearing a brace may be a good idea only in certain situations. (Customized braces, like those used in this study, should be used only after consulting a doctor, advises Dr. Fox.) But doctors report that some patients find various knee supports helpful.

Heal thyself first. About 25 percent of all knee injuries are simply repeats of unresolved problems. "Making sure that your previous injury is healed is the best way to avoid future injuries," says James G. Garrick, M.D., an orthopedic surgeon and director of the Center for Sports Medicine at St. Francis Memorial Hospital in San Francisco.

For lesser conditions, stop all painful activities for at least two to four weeks when your knee starts to ache, says Dr. Garrick. Post-surgical healing can take from one to six months, he notes. Arthroscopy, which involves operating on the knee via a small set of fiber-optic tubes, may be classified as minor surgery, but it requires major effort to strengthen your knee in the months following the procedure. Be sure to follow a physician-prescribed exercise regimen after arthroscopy or knee surgery, Dr. Garrick says.

Ask the right questions. Many knee problems are easy to diagnose, such as when you take a header down the stairs. But in other cases, the underlying problem isn't so obvious and may eventually require an expert's care. Don't waste your doctor's time or your money by hobbling into his office unprepared. According to Dr. Fox, here are a few questions that you'll want to ask yourself—and that your doctor will want answers to.

1. Why does it hurt? Think back 24 hours. Did you fall or get hit?
2. What does it look like? Is it black and blue? Is it swollen and red? Is it misshapen?
3. Where does it hurt? Gently press around the kneecap, the sides and the back to locate the source of the pain.

Lips

- **Keep your tongue inside your mouth.**
- **Keep your lips out of the sun.**
- **Use balm for moisture.**

Lips were not created to flap at abusive phone solicitors or to blow raspberries on a baby's belly. Nor did evolution intend them to murmur sweet nothings and otherwise delight your sweetheart.

Truth is, your lips are nothing more than gatekeepers for your mouth. They exist primarily for chewing and to help you rate the taste, touch and temperature of whatever comes into your mouth, be it food, flesh or fingernail, says Neil Sadick, M.D., clinical assistant professor of dermatology at Cornell University Medical College in New York City.

Your lips are made of a thin membrane, meaning that they lack the tough outer layer that protects the rest of your skin. They're red because blood vessels are so close to the surface.

The main problem with lips is that they dry out. Blame that on the weather. Just as the sun burns your skin, it also burns your lips.

Lips don't face too many other serious problems. The worst are cold sores and skin cancer. The former are pretty easy to care for if you are prone to getting them, and the latter is easily prevented (essentially, limit their exposure to the sun).

Don't Lick Your Troubles Away

It's easy to take care of your lips. Keep 'em moist, keep 'em protected from the sun, and they'll most likely grant you the kiss of health. Here's how to maintain those ruby reds.

Put on the balm. When you go outside, apply a lip balm containing a sunscreen with a sun protection factor (SPF) of 15 or higher, such as Blistex, or a moisturizer such as Chap Stick or petroleum jelly. This should go a long way toward protecting your lips from the sun and heat, according to Dr. Sadick.

Hold your tongue. In other words, don't lick your lips. It's a vicious circle, says Rodney Basler, M.D., assistant professor of internal medicine and a dermatologist at the University of Nebraska Medical Center in Omaha. "You lick your lips to make them feel better, but the moisture evaporates, so you lick more," he says.

But don't go to the other extreme by getting hooked on lip balms. "I've run into situations where people are essentially Chap Stick junkies," Dr. Basler says.

Instead, other moisturizing habits can help keep your lips kissably soft and unscaly.

Drink water frequently. What's good for your innards is also good for your lips: Drink lots of water throughout the day. No specific amount is required, but particularly in hot, dry weather, keep the fluids flowing, says Dr. Basler.

Wash with a gentle soap. You don't want washing to dry out your lips. So use a gentle soap that doesn't dry out your skin, such as Basis or Purpose, suggests Dr. Sadick.

Let it cool. Don't gobble down that chicken while it's sizzling or gurgle down the java while it's still steaming. Let it cool down, so you can enjoy what you ingest instead of burning your lips.

When to Get Help

Some lip ills are not so easily prevented or dampened. But take heart: Lip tissue heals more rapidly than skin. Unless you have cancer, most lip ailments heal in four days or fewer, even without treatment.

Here's what to look for.

Cold sores, also known as fever blisters, are caused by the herpes simplex virus (it's related to, but not quite the same as, the virus that causes genital herpes). Cold sores can be triggered by a number of things, including sun, stress and dental work, says Diana Bihova, M.D., a dermatologist in New York City. The good news: They can be treated with a prescription drug called acyclovir (Zovirax).

If it's your first sore, go to your doctor right away for a diagnosis, says Dr. Sadick. If you've already been prescribed acyclovir, resuming the medicine when an outbreak occurs should stop the sore in its tracks. Dosage differs by body weight, but an average-size guy might get a prescription for one 200-milligram tablet five times a day for ten days.

Infections can occur when lips become unusually dry and cracked. Doctors recommend using an over-the-counter antibiotic ointment such as Polysporin or Bacitracin. Apply a thin layer as needed (that can be several times a day) until your lips heal. If the infection doesn't go away in a week, see your doctor.

Allergies can make lips swell. Toothpaste is sometimes the culprit. Some toothpastes contain a compound called cinnamic aldehyde, which can cause your lips to get hot, swollen and tender. If that happens, pick up an over-the-counter hydrocortisone cream such as Cortaid from your drugstore, advises Dr. Sadick. To ease the ache, apply a thin layer of the cream as often as you need to, he says. And stop using whatever made your lips react. If you can't figure it out what that was, or if the swelling doesn't go away in a week or your lips get infected, visit your doctor.

Broken blood vessels are not uncommon, especially when you have the nervous habit of biting your lip. The best solution: Don't bite your lip. If you can't beat the habit, don't fret. Your lip will probably heal on its own without leaving a scar, says Dr. Sadick. But if the big red spot gets bigger or starts bleeding, or if you have a hot date and you'd rather not sport a red lip bump, your doctor can whisk it away with a laser.

Cancer, most often caused by extreme exposure to the sun, remains the worst-case scenario. "Your lower lip is like a shelf. It gets more direct rays of sun than the rest of your face," Dr. Basler says. This is particularly true for smokers because of the way heat combines with tobacco's residual chemicals.

How can you tell if you have lip cancer? A thin white film on your lower lip is a dead giveaway, Dr. Basler says. So is a brownish bleeding lump or a freckle or mole that is changing over time. If you have a suspicion that your lip is cancerous, see your doctor immediately.

Liver

- Be reasonable with alcohol.
- Don't mix your toxins.
- Avoid strange needles.

The Mick. That's all you need to hear. And instantly, even if you aren't old enough to have seen him play, you conjure up the immortal image: number 7 in a pinstripe uniform. The bull-strong body clobbering another ball out of the park, beating out another infield grounder, chasing down yet another long fly into deep center field. The blond crew cut, that boyish Oklahoma-sunshine smile, the humility with which this son of a zinc miner bore his heroism. This is why he became the American icon: Mickey Mantle.

And then all of the records, including the 18 World Series homers, were suddenly eclipsed by a new image. We learned in 1995 that the Mick was not immortal, that 40 years of heavy drinking had left him with cirrhosis, which led to liver cancer. And the image of the consummate athlete gave way to the image of a consumed liver. Not even a liver transplant could save him from reported indulgences such as his version of the Breakfast of Champions: two shots of brandy and a shot of Kahlua and cream.

But even in death he set a record of sorts, though not the kind anyone would want to beat. "It ranks up there as one of the worst cases of recurrent liver cancer that anyone on the medical team has ever seen," says Robert Goldstein, M.D., a transplant surgeon at Baylor University Medical Center in Dallas, who was part of that team.

After first examining Mantle, Dr. Goldstein told the press, "There is no doubt that his lifestyle has played a part in his condition today. Maybe people should reconsider their drinking habits, as Mickey has pointed out." It was an understatement. Perhaps Mantle himself put it best: "If I'd have known I was going to make it to 50, I'd have taken better care of myself."

Okay, so you're not Mickey Mantle. Okay, maybe you haven't been on a 40-year binge. But the take-home lesson still hits home: Be good to your liver, or you could be benched long before you're ready to quit the game on your terms. "Drinking in moderation will not necessarily lead to liver disease," says Dr. Goldstein. "But if you overindulge like Mickey Mantle, you'll end up like Mickey Mantle."

It Works Hard, It Plays Hard

Talk about overcommitted. More than 500 functions of this three-pound gland, located in the upper right side of the abdomen and shaped roughly like an NFL football, have been identified.

"The liver is a powerhouse," says Dr. Goldstein. "It is the engine that drives your body. It generates so much energy that body temperature surges up when we put in a new liver."

All blood that leaves the stomach and intestines passes through the liver before moving to the rest of the body. In the liver, nutrients in the blood are further broken down into glycogen, the fuel that cells use to create energy. What else does the liver do? Glad you asked. The liver:

- Processes drugs absorbed from the digestive tract into forms that are easier for the body to use
- Detoxifies blood and excretes substances that would otherwise be poisonous
- Produces bile to aid in the breakdown of fat
- Stores certain vitamins, minerals and sugars
- Helps make sure that blood clots
- Metabolizes alcohol

Besides all of that, the liver is the only vital organ in the body that is able to fix itself—that is, unless you drink too much alcohol. Alcohol damages not only the liver but also the liver's natural ability to repair itself.

It's a good bet that the Greek Titan Prometheus wasn't a drinker; otherwise, he would have long been dead, and happily so. In case you slept through Greek mythology class, it is Prometheus whom the god Zeus punished for stealing fire from heaven and giving it to mankind. The punishment: He was chained to a rock, where a bird of prey ate his liver. Again and again. Thanks to the regenerative powers of the organ, poor Prometheus was doomed to eternal torture rather than death.

As further demonstration of the liver's incredible complexity, it cannot be replicated. There are kidney, heart and lung machines. There are artificial legs and arms. But there is no mechanical liver as yet that can sustain human life.

That's one more reason why you should lavish your liver with love and attention. Some doctors have circulated a number of theories about how to do exactly that. Suggestions range from curtailing caffeine to being wary of excess beta-carotene to freeing yourself from fatty foods. But alas, there is little consensus short of maintaining a balanced diet and avoiding heavy drinking. With these obvious tips in mind, here are some others you may not have considered.

Don't take pain relievers when you're feeling no pain. In other words, while it's never a good idea to mix drinking and drugs, it's particularly unfair to your liver. We're talking about legal drugs such as acetaminophen and aspirin. In fact, avoid any analgesics, even prescribed ones, when drinking alcohol. You're asking your liver to pull a double shift and filter two toxins at once. "You throw your liver into turmoil," warns Frederick Whitcomb, M.D., a gastroenterologist and hepatologist who is a consultant to the Lahey Hitchcock Clinic in Burlington, Massachusetts. "Be cautious with any kind of sedative. It can send you into a hepatic coma." Hepatic coma, which occurs when the liver fails to detoxify ammonia, can lead to disorientation, slurred speech, tremors and flapping hands.

Steer clear of steroids. Anabolic steroids may beef you up, if you're after the Schwarzenegger look. But you'll pay a Hollywood-high price. "In large doses, they may be highly toxic to a variety of cells," says

Dr. Whitcomb. "They can cause liver disease. They're not worth the gamble."

Flush it down. If you're looking for an alternative, all-natural approach to keeping your liver machine-clean, try what's known as the liver flush. Combine the juice of one fresh lemon, a tablespoon of olive oil (preferably cold-pressed) and one clove of garlic, minced. Sweeten with honey, so you can get it down. While most doctors trained in Western medicine will at best look skeptically at this concoction, those experienced in holistic and Oriental medicine—among them Willard Dean, M.D., a holistic physician in Santa Fe, New Mexico— highly recommend it. The mixture can be used once a month or every six weeks.

"The lemon juice is high in acid, which helps break down crystallized substances," explains Dr. Dean. "The fatty olive oil forces the gallbladder to squeeze down, eliminating toxic bile secreted by the liver. Garlic stimulates the immune system by activating white blood cells to surround foreign matter (such as drugs and alcohol). Like voracious little Pac-Men, the white blood cells gobble up those toxins."

Don't drink on an empty stomach. "Drink spirits with food if you want to protect your liver and the rest of your physiology," says David Whitten, M.D., author of *To Your Health: Two Physicians Explore the Health Benefits of Wine*, assistant professor of physiology at the University of California, San Francisco, and chief of emergency services at Kaiser Foundation Hospital in Santa Rosa, California. You'll slow the rate at which the alcohol is absorbed into the bloodstream. Even so, he says, hard liquor is absorbed faster than beer or wine. So that scotch before dinner will do more harm than the wine or beer with dinner.

The Price of a Round or Two

Here's the question asked by any man who enjoys a couple of rounds after work: How much drinking is considered "heavy"? If you're into complete self-destruction, 80 grams of alcohol a day for 15 years should do the trick, says Dr. Whitten. That translates into bellying up to the bar every day and putting away any

of the following: about a liter of wine (that's a little more than a regular-size bottle), a half-pint of whiskey or eight 12-ounce bottles of beer.

No one you know? Perhaps the better question to ask is: How much can you drink and still safely make it around all of life's bases? On this one, you'll hear some differences of opinion.

"When you start talking about what alcohol does to the liver, you'll hear all sorts of misconceptions," says Dr. Goldstein. Like "Oh, I drink only the good stuff, and that's better for you than the bad stuff." Or "Beer is better for you than wine." Or "White wine is better than red wine."

Dr. Goldstein clarifies the situation: "All of it is old wives' tales. All that matters is the volume of alcohol intake." With that as the criterion, he recommends no more than the equivalent of two drinks a day. (A drink is a 12-ounce beer, a 5-ounce glass of wine or 1½ ounces of hard liquor.) At that level, he suggests, the chances of doing serious, permanent damage to your liver are slim.

For those who are always trying to beat the system, that doesn't mean filling your weekly quota all on Saturday night. "Binge drinking results in toxic blood levels of alcohol and could be seriously harmful," warns Dr. Whitten. "But the capacity of the human liver to detoxify is enormous."

It does, however, have its limits. When the liver becomes injured or scarred, the resulting condition is called cirrhosis. The loss of normal liver tissue slows down and backs up the assembly line, affecting everything from blood flow to the processing of nutrients, hormones, drugs and toxins to the production of proteins and other substances. Cirrhosis is the seventh leading cause of death by disease in the United States; 25,000 people die of it each year.

Most cases of cirrhosis are caused by heavy drinking. The rest are caused by hepatitis, genetic diseases such as cystic fibrosis and other relatively rare problems. Cirrhosis has few symptoms at first. Later, you'll experience fatigue, weakness, exhaustion, loss of appetite, nausea and weight loss. Bile products deposited in the skin may cause intense itching. And while we're on the subject of skin, cirrhosis could also cause a yellowing effect called jaundice. Jaundice occurs when bile—which, when not digesting fat, moonlights at bringing that rosy pink tone to your skin—gets backed up and passed to the intestines by a lousy liver.

Hepatitis Happens

Hepatitis is an inflammation of the liver that is most often caused by a virus. Now there's also a nonviral hepatitis that is caused by ingestion of or exposure to toxic substances such as poisonous mushrooms and many types of drugs, including alcohol and cholesterol-lowering medications.

But generally, it's the viral variety that you have to worry about. This type of hepatitis comes in a number of lettered disguises. A, B and C are the most common, but new research has uncovered D and E strains, with more to come. A is spread through contaminated water and food. B is acquired through exposure to blood and other bodily fluids and is spread by simple acts such as kissing, ear piercing, tattooing and sexual contact. C is spread through infected blood.

While there is no clear accounting for the number of hepatitis cases in the United States, the American Liver Foundation estimates that there are more than a million carriers of hepatitis. These are people who are not ill but who may pass the disease on to others.

Acute viral hepatitis destroys liver cells. It can take months for the liver to repair itself. Meanwhile, you're left with flulike symptoms: loss of appetite, nausea, vomiting, jaundice, dark urine, abdominal pain and clay-colored stool. Most people recover without treatment.

Chronic hepatitis does not occur with hepatitis A and occurs in only about 5 to 8 percent of cases of hepatitis B. In contrast, 80 to 90 percent of those with hepatitis C will develop chronic hepatitis, and a bit more than one-third of them will develop cirrhosis.

While several effective antiviral medications are available, the best option is avoiding the problem altogether by following these preventive suggestions.

BYO blood. Prior to 1990, anyone who had a blood transfusion ran a 7 percent chance of contracting hepatitis C, because a test hadn't been developed and blood couldn't be screened for it effectively until then. "This was an unfortunate situation for those people," explains Bruce R. Bacon, M.D., professor of internal medicine and director of the Division of Gastroenterology and Hepatology at St. Louis University School of Medicine. Mickey Mantle was among the unlucky; hepatitis C caught during an early knee surgery added to the liver complications that took his life. Today, blood transfusions account for only a very small proportion of cases of hepatitis C. But if you are concerned in the event that you need blood for surgery, consider storing your own.

Keep away from nasty needles. Both hepatitis B and hepatitis C are frequently spread by intravenous drug users who share dirty needles. Keep them and their paraphernalia out of your life, says Dr. Bacon.

Avoid sexy strangers. Almost one-third of the reported cases of hepatitis B are thought to be sexually transmitted. Even if you use a condom, "avoid high-risk promiscuous sex with people whose history is unfamiliar to you," recommends Dr. Bacon.

Don't procrastinate—vaccinate. There is a "very effective and safe" vaccination called Havrix that international travelers should get as a safeguard against hepatitis A, according to Raymond Koff, M.D., chairman of the Department of Medicine and chief of the hepatology section at MetroWest Medical Center in Framingham, Massachusetts, and professor of medicine at the University of Massachusetts Medical School, also in Framingham. "Two doses will protect you for 10 to 25 years," he says. "Gamma globulin continues to be used for postexposure protection against hepatitis A." He also suggests getting vaccinated against hepatitis B if you have multiple sexual partners, share needles or are likely to need blood products. So far, there's no vaccine for hepatitis C.

Lungs

- **Breathe deeper and less often.**
- **Avoid irritants such as smoke, pollution and pollen.**
- **Keep good posture.**

Gawkers in 1912 must have thought Harry Houdini's lungs reached to his toes. The escape artist's most popular feat involved being locked upside down in a "water torture cell." It usually took him about 20 minutes to escape.

How did Houdini do it? He cheated. His body usually displaced enough water to create an air pocket at the top of the tank. He pulled himself into a fetal position, so his mouth could reach the air. Then he undid the shackles.

Had he wanted to, however, Houdini could have trained himself to hold his breath for 5, 10 or even 15 minutes. But then he may not have been able to free himself from the tank.

How Breathing Works

The lungs take in roughly a pint of air each time you breathe, which averages once every five seconds. That multiplies out to more than 17,000 breaths a day. Your breathing rate jumps to about once every three-quarters of a second during exercise, with those heavy heaves sucking in from two to four quarts of air.

That seems like an incredible amount of work for a pair of spongy balloons encased in the chest. But the lungs actually get too much credit. Without various other muscles, the lungs would be failures.

The lungs are encased by ribs and muscles and sit on top of the muscular diaphragm. They're covered with a thin liquid lining that acts like glue, so when the surrounding ribs and muscles move, the lungs get pulled along with them.

When we breathe in, the diaphragm contracts from a dome to a saucer shape, stretching the lower lung lining downward to about the tenth of the 12 ribs. Meanwhile, other muscles make the rib cage swing up and out, pulling the sides of the lungs with it. As the lungs expand, they form a vacuum. That causes air to rush in.

When we breathe out, the diaphragm relaxes, expanding upward to just below the nipples. The ribs contract, squeezing air out.

Inspiration

Ribs elevate.
Breastbone flares.
Rib muscles
contract.

Diaphragm
moves
downward.

Expiration

Ribs and breastbone
depress to normal
position. Rib
muscles relax.

Diaphragm
moves upward.

Into the Tunnel

Air enters the body through the nose or mouth, obviously. Then it travels down the back of the throat and into the ten-inch-long windpipe. At the end of the windpipe, air takes one of two tunnels that lead into passageways called bronchi. The bronchi lead into the lungs.

Inside the lungs, the air travels into smaller and smaller passageways. The bronchi branch into smaller bronchi, then into more than 250,000 smaller bronchioles. Those bronchioles divide into alveolar ducts, which lead to cell-size air sacs called alveoli.

Your 300 million alveoli represent oxygen's last stop in the lungs. Capillaries, the smallest of the blood vessels, form a web around the alveoli. As the dark, oxygen-thirsty blood passes through those capillaries, it drops off carbon dioxide and picks up oxygen from the alveoli. The bright red, oxygenated blood then heads to the heart so that it can be pumped to the rest of the body and used to make energy.

How to Breathe Correctly

When you were a cute, chubby-cheeked baby, you were the epitome of perfect breathing. You let your diaphragm, the largest breathing muscle, do most of the hard labor.

But as you grew, life's daily stresses—from accidentally knocking over glasses of milk to confronting bullies who stole your lunch money—took their toll on your respiratory system. As you grew more tense, your breathing became more shallow. If you're like most people, you barely use your diaphragm these days. You breathe just enough to get by, says Jeffrey A. Migdow, M.D., a holistic physician and director of the Kripalu yoga teacher training program at the Kripalu Center for Yoga and Health in Lenox, Massachusetts.

By breathing inefficiently, you're putting your lungs through unnecessary toil. You're probably breathing between 12 and 16 shallow breaths a minute when it's possible to take as few as 8 to 10 deeper, more satisfying, healthier breaths in the same amount of time. It only makes

sense: The less you breathe, the longer your lungs will last.

Fast, shallow breathing has been linked to a number of health problems. One is stress. One study, at San Francisco State University, asked some anxiety sufferers to breathe shallowly. The participants became more anxious. And stress has been linked to various sicknesses, from cancer to ulcers to heart disease.

Our breathing can even dictate how well we learn. One study, from Wheeling Jesuit College in West Virginia, found that students who breathe less have higher grade point averages. Another study from the same school showed that those who breathe less can better remember a series of words.

And stronger lungs increase your endurance, whether you need it to help you run a marathon, bike up a hill or have sex all night long.

The Lung Expander

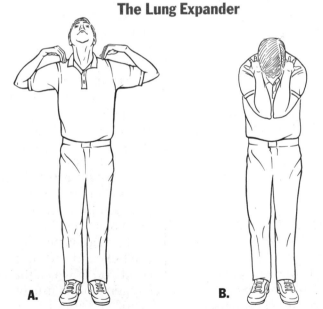

A. **B.**

Use this exercise to increase the flexibility of the muscles that help you breathe.

A. With triceps parallel to the ground and fingers on shoulders, breathe slowly and deeply through your nose, tilting your chin to the ceiling and pulling your elbow back.

B. Then inhale through your mouth, bringing your elbows together and your chin to your chest. Repeat five to ten times.

That's Incredible Expansion

Houdini may have been a cheater. But for some people, holding their breath for a half-hour is child's play. When not showing off their breath-holding skills, they breathe only four to six times a minute.

"Our breath is simply constricted by tight physiology," Dr. Migdow says. "People in India who have been practicing breathing exercises since they were children can expand their lungs to up to ten times normal capacity because they have so much flexibility in the diaphragm and the chest muscles. They can just inhale and inhale and inhale."

You may not be able to train yourself to survive for a half-hour on one inhalation. But you can increase your lung capacity once you learn to breathe correctly.

In their book *Take a Deep Breath*, Dr. Migdow and James E. Loehr, Ed.D., suggest lying on your back and putting your hand on your tummy. Then push your tummy against your hand when you breathe in. When you breathe out, let your tummy relax toward the ground naturally. That's called abdominal breathing. It forces you to use your diaphragm and gets you away from relying on smaller, weaker chest muscles. And it makes you fill your lungs to capacity, exhaling all of the stale air and inhaling more oxygen.

Once you understand how

Deadly Lung Diseases

If the government, your doctor, your boss, your wife and the guy next to you on the bus could agree on just one thing, it would be this: You should stop smoking. Here's why you should agree.

Lung cancer is the most common fatal malignancy in the United States. It makes up 16 percent of male cancer cases and 3 percent of male cancer deaths. Lung cancer is a killer mainly because early detection is difficult. Often the only symptom is a persistent cough, and by then the cancer could have spread, says Peter Greenwald, M.D., director of the Division of Cancer Prevention and Control at the National Cancer Institute in Bethesda, Maryland. Approximately 80 to 90 percent of cases are caused by outside contaminants or carcinogens that generally are easy to sidestep.

Cigarette smoke is responsible for 90 percent of lung cancer cases among men. Radon exposure may play a role, especially in smokers. Family history of the disease also puts you at slightly higher risk.

The basic treatment plan is to surgically remove the tumor, which generally means taking out either a lobe of one lung or the whole lung. Essentially, you could be left with only half of your lung power, and if you've been a smoker, the half that you have left might also be diseased or damaged.

If surgery is not an appropriate option (because, for example, there's another respiratory problem such as pneumonia or the cancer has spread to other parts of the body), doctors may instead prescribe radiation or chemotherapy.

Emphysema affects about 10 of every 1,000 men and kills 16,000 men a year. Sure, it can be caused by air pollution. But the likely culprit, again, is smoking. It develops from the assault on the lung tissue. The lung's walls break down, become too large, lose elasticity and can't expand and contract correctly. It's an irreversible condition in which the victim becomes dependent on an oxygen tank. It usually results in death from a damaged heart.

There's very little you can do once you get it. You can exercise your chest muscles to help you get a little more air. Other than that, the only option is a lung transplant.

to breathe with your diaphragm, practice it for a couple of minutes each hour. Do a longer session in the morning and at night, Dr. Migdow says.

"If you can do that consistently for six to eight weeks, what will happen is that more and more during the day you'll start breathing that way automatically. Then when you get into stress, it'll automatically kick you into deep breathing because you've practiced," Dr. Migdow says.

Once that becomes automatic, you're ready for the lung expander. This exercise boosts your lung capacity by increasing the flexibility of various breathing muscles. If the muscles expand more, they'll pull the lung tissue farther apart, allowing more air to flow in.

Here's how to do it, according to Dr. Migdow.

1. Stand and relax by spending a few minutes breathing abdominally.
2. With your arms bent and your triceps parallel to the floor, put your fingers on your shoulders.
3. Inhale through your nose as you tilt your chin toward the ceiling, spreading your elbows apart from each other. As you inhale, pull your elbows back. Spreading your arms apart helps you expand your chest cavity.
4. Then exhale through your mouth, pulling your elbows together by your

Ditching the Butts for Good

Probably no other modern health concern has been attacked as thoroughly, viciously and consistently as smoking. And yet 28 percent of men still smoke, according to one counting.

Why? Rather than being hardheaded or ignorant of health facts, most smokers are addicted, both physically and psychologically.

In fact, one report from the U.S. Surgeon General compared the mechanics of nicotine addiction with those of heroin or cocaine addiction. The conclusion: "It's often more difficult to withdraw from nicotine than any of the others," says Thomas Glynn, Ph.D., chief of the Cancer Prevention and Control Research Branch at the National Cancer Institute in Bethesda, Maryland.

In fact, of the 15 million Americans who try to quit smoking each year, only 3 percent stay off cigarettes. Dr. Glynn says you should realize that you are likely to relapse while trying to quit, since most people have to make three or four attempts. Don't give up, he urges. Each attempt is actually a learning experience.

Here are a few of Dr. Glynn's top tips.

Go cold turkey. Cutting down doesn't seem to work. When most people get down to about eight to ten cigarettes a day, they resume again.

Prepare yourself mentally. You should be adamant about wanting to quit and know exactly why. Some people like to write down their reasons for stopping and ask friends and family to help them. It's also good to pick a specific date, particularly a birthday or anniversary, as Quit Day.

Ditch smoking souvenirs. Get rid of all cigarettes, matches, lighters and ashtrays in your home and office. Also, have smoky clothes cleaned professionally, or have your tobacco-assaulted teeth polished by the dentist.

Wean yourself with the patch. A doctor can give you a prescription for a nicotine patch, which is worn like a bandage and releases some nicotine for your skin to absorb. The patch goes on your upper arm, upper torso or shoulder and has to be replaced every 16 or 24 hours. These devices, which you wear for 12 to 16 weeks, help release you from nicotine addiction. Nicotine gum works the same way, but unlike the patch, it has a couple of drawbacks: You have to chew about 12 pieces a day, and some people gripe about the taste.

chest and bringing your chin to your chest.

5. Repeat five to ten times.

This exercise allows you to take in as much air as possible by expanding your chest. Then when you pull your elbows together, you contract your chest, pushing the air out. This relaxes the muscles between the ribs that, together with the diaphragm, help you breathe.

How to Get Stronger

In addition to strengthening your breathing muscles, you can ensure longer use of your lungs by keeping them free of disease. With each breath you take, a bunch of bad invaders gets in, including pollen, dust, viruses and other particles.

For the most part, your body has an arsenal of germ-fighting weapons that continually cleanse air as it travels to your lungs. Hairs called cilia inside the nose, windpipe and bronchial tubes push the bad guys north, where they are sneezed out, coughed up or swallowed into the stomach. Mucus that lines the passageways also catches bacteria, dust and other debris. And if a germ gets as far as the alveoli, scavenger white blood cells attack it.

But as you age, your lungs do a poorer job of cleaning themselves. In people over age 35, the cilia don't respond as well. Breathing is also hampered by less flexible ribs.

But you can prevent sickness and loss of lung function by eating right, exercising and relaxing. Here are some ways to do that.

Don't smoke. Okay, you've heard this a gazillion times. Go ahead and groan. Then skim through this very short lecture. You might find something you haven't heard before.

Everyday Diseases

Lungs suck in a lot of nasty funk. That means they are susceptible to a host of medical problems. Here are the most common ones.

Acute bronchitis affects about four to five million American men annually. In most cases, it is caused by the same viruses that cause colds and flus, except that they travel farther south in the body than the usual landing sites (the sinuses and the throat). The virus causes the airways connecting the windpipe to the lungs to inflame. To protect itself, the body produces secretions along the airways. As the secretions build up, breathing gets harder, and you start to cough up the secretions, usually in the form of green or yellow phlegm. In most cases, bronchitis clears up within a week as the germ colony dies off.

If your bronchitis is caused by a virus, rest, drink lots of hot fluids such as soup and tea and keep clearing out the phlegm, says Diana Decosimo, M.D., director of the Division of General Medicine and Geriatrics in the Department of Medicine of the University of Medicine and Dentistry of New Jersey–New Jersey Medical School in Newark. See a doctor if you have a temperature above 101°F, if you are short of breath or if your sputum contains blood.

Sometimes bronchitis can be caused by bacteria; in these cases, a doctor might prescribe an antibiotic to kill the germs.

Another six million men have chronic bronchitis, also known as smoker's cough (for the obvious reason that it is almost always caused by smoking). This type of bronchitis can last for months or even years. The remedy, of course, is to stop smoking. If you don't, chronic bronchitis can lead to emphysema and even heart failure.

Asthma affects about five million American men. It is caused by hyperactive bronchial tubes. The tubes go into spasm when the person breathes particles such as smoke,

When you inhale smoke, you're doing a number of things to hurt your lungs. Smoking dries out the linings of your air passageways, making them sore. The nicotine cuts down on oxygen flow by narrowing your blood vessels and, along with other gases, paralyzes the hairs in your passageways that catch germs.

Without the germ-fighters, more smoke gets in your lungs, creating more mucus and clogging airways. The carbon monoxide in smoke sucks oxygen from your blood. Also, irritation from smoke can destroy your alveoli. They can't be repaired.

Smoking has been linked to cancer, heart disease, allergies, gum disease and impotence, among other things. Lung cancer is the number one killer of men among all cancers; about 94,000 men die of it a year.

Stay away from butt heads. When people smoke, they release poisons such as carbon monoxide, benzene and formaldehyde into the air. Then you inhale them. And you're actually inhaling worse cancer-causing substances than the smoker because second-hand smoke goes through a different chemical process than inhaled smoke, says David Mannino, M.D., medical epidemiologist for the Centers for Disease Control and Prevention in Atlanta. Studies have shown that about 1 in 1,000 people who are exposed to secondhand smoke develops lung cancer. That rate is about 1,000 times worse than for any other air pollutant associated with lung cancer, Dr. Mannino says. To avoid secondhand smoke, you need to avoid smokers.

Get your vitamins. There's some evidence that antioxidants—vitamins C and E, beta-carotene and selenium—can protect the lungs against cancer, says Dr. Migdow. Though taking supplements

mold and pollen. Exercise and even stress can trigger the wheezing attacks. Asthma sufferers gasp for breath as their airways constrict.

If you have one parent with asthma or allergies, you have a 30 percent chance of having the same. If both parents have asthma, your risk jumps to 60 percent.

The best way to control this chronic condition is with inhaled medication such as bronchodilators and with corticosteriods, which reduce inflammation. Both need a doctor's prescription.

Pneumonia affects about 1.8 million American men annually, particularly those with weak immune systems, such as the elderly, the very young and alcoholics. Pneumonia is usually the result of a cold or flu complication. With pneumonia, the air sacs in the lungs fill with pus, hampering oxygen from reaching the blood. Those who suffer from pneumonia may produce large amounts of thick gray-green or bloody mucus when they cough or sneeze.

There's no medicine that kills the viruses that cause pneumonia. Bacterial pneumonia can be treated with antibiotics. In either case, it may take several weeks to fully recover, so you'll need to be patient. Drink lots of fluids, avoid vigorous exertion, get rest, take two standard-strength aspirin or acetaminophen every four hours to lower a fever and reduce discomfort and consider using a heating pad on your chest—that relaxes sore muscles, says Gary Gross, M.D., clinical professor of internal medicine at the University of Texas Southwestern Medical Center at Dallas Southwestern Medical School.

We know you probably hate doctors, but pneumonia is serious enough to make the trip. You want to get rid of the disease as soon as you can, and professional help makes a difference.

could be helpful, research has proved only that foods containing these nutrients may protect your lungs against cancer. The Daily Value for vitamin C is 60 milligrams; for vitamin E, 30 international units. "It's not a good idea to take supplements of selenium," advises Dr. Migdow. "Instead, make sure to include the Daily Value of 70 micrograms in your daily diet." You can get beta-carotene and vitamin C from fruits and vegetables, vitamin E from nuts and wheat germ and selenium from seafood, says Dr. Migdow.

Don't let your job kill you. Many guys have dirty jobs. Drilling, sawing and even farming can wreak havoc on your lungs. In any occupation where particles or fumes fly through the air, you should wear either a protective mask or a breathing apparatus.

Often workers don't like to wear respiratory devices because they are hot and clunky. "It's possible to make the workplace more friendly to your lungs by installing improved ventilation and hoods," Dr. Mannino says. "Also, changes in engineering can decrease the dust. That way, the person doesn't have to mess with a respirator face mask."

Watch for horrible hobbies. Though most people think of the great outdoors when they think of air pollution, they have more to worry about from the great indoors. Many people slowly poison their lungs from things they do inside the house. Any hobby or activity that involves using chemicals should be done in a well-ventilated room. That means opening

---

Is It Asthma or Allergies?

You're huffin' and wheezin', and you're not sure why. Well, don't try to figure it out on your own. Instead, head to your doctor, who'll run a series of tests to unravel whether you have asthma, allergies or both.

The best way to determine if someone has allergies is with skin-prick tests, says Garrison Ayars, M.D., an allergist and clinical associate professor of medicine at the University of Washington in Seattle. With these tests, various allergens are pricked into the skin. If a hive develops, you're allergic to that substance. (People who have intrinsic asthma won't get any reaction.)

Allergists also check to see whether you have symptoms in addition to wheeziness or shortness of breath. Allergies that involve the nose and eyes, such as hay fever, can also cause asthma.

The doctor may also test your lung function with a machine called a spirometer, which measures the amount of air you breathe in and how fast you can breathe it out.

One important key to finding answers is discussion with your doctor, says Gary Gross, M.D., clinical professor of internal medicine at the University of Texas Southwestern Medical Center at Dallas Southwestern Medical School.

"You talk about when your first attack took place and what it was like, what your job is like and what allergens you're exposed to at work and home," he notes. After you've found out whether you have asthma—and, if so, what kind—you can work with your doctor to find the best treatment.

---

the windows when you paint furniture or polish your shoes, Dr. Mannino says.

Avoid air pollution. If you live in an area where air pollution is a problem, don't exercise in the late afternoon, says Dr. Mannino. That's when air pollution levels are highest. Go out early in the morning or in the evening after the sun goes down. That's when ground-level ozone, an irritating form of oxygen formed when sunlight hits car exhaust and other pollutants, is lowest.

You can find out your area's smog level

by checking the weather page of your local newspaper; it's reported as a pollution standard index on a scale of 50 to 500. Any time it reaches 100, there's a potential for problems. "Clearly, one has to weigh the benefits of exercise versus the potential health consequences of that exercise," says Ira Richards, Ph.D., associate professor of toxicology at the University of South Florida College of Public Health in Tampa. "Stay indoors if there's a smog alert. If the level is high, it would be much more advantageous either to not exercise or to do something indoors."

Steer clear of cars. You'll inhale the same amount of carbon monoxide by running near an urban highway as you would by smoking a pack of cigarettes in one day.

Relax. Bring your hand to your shoulder as if trying to do a curl. Then try to flex your biceps. It's hard because your biceps is already tense. That's why breathing is hard when you're tense: Your muscles are stiff. Here's one relaxation exercise. "Sit in a chair, and as you inhale, clench your fists, shrug your shoulders and tighten your arms," suggests Dr. Migdow. "Then as you exhale, let your shoulders fall down, open your hands and let your arms hang straight down. Tighten your legs and feet, then relax them the same way."

Sit up. Your lungs need room to expand. If you sit hunched over, with your shoulders pulled forward and up, you're constricting your breathing muscles. To teach yourself proper posture, try this Chow Chinese qigong exercise from *Miracle Healing from China . . . Qigong*, by Charles T. McGee, M.D., and Effie

---

Wheezing on the Run

Some men have difficulty breathing only when they're active. It doesn't necessarily mean they are out of shape; the problem could be exercise-induced asthma (EIA), a very real medical condition independent of fitness level. Here's what doctors recommend if you regularly have trouble breathing shortly after getting active.

Ease into it. Warm-ups are very important, according to Phillip Corsello, M.D., staff physician at the National Jewish Center of Immunology and Respiratory Medicine in Denver. "About ten minutes of walking at a gradual pace or other gentle aerobic exercise may help prevent or reduce the severity of EIA," he says. "Also, don't exercise in cold or polluted air. These conditions can irritate airways."

Spray before you play. If you use an inhaler before you exercise, it might help prevent an attack. "It's good to use your inhaler about five to ten minutes before you start," says Garrison Ayars, M.D., allergist and clinical associate professor at the University of Washington in Seattle. "With exercise-induced asthma, if you premedicate, you'll do fine."

Shape up. With regular aerobic exercise, you may find that you have asthma less often. "If you get into better aerobic condition, you'll eventually have less of a problem with exercise-induced asthma," says Dr. Ayars.

Poy Yew Chow, Ph.D. While you're standing or sitting, visualize a thread extending from the ground through your tailbone and up your spine to the top of your head. Imagine the thread is pulling you up. Allow it to stretch your spine. Roll your shoulders back and down away from your neck, so your shoulder blades drop down.

It may feel awkward at first. But eventually, you'll get used to it. "If you're used to having your shoulders caving in, of course it's going to feel uncomfortable. Your muscles have all contracted. So you must begin working at loosening up those muscles," says Dr. Chow, who is also president of the East West Academy of Healing Arts/Qigong Institute in San Francisco.

Lymphatic System

- **Percent of lymph that is water: 95**
- **Amount of fluid that leaks from the bloodstream and must be picked up by the lymphatic system each day: 3 liters**
- **Length of a lymph node: 1 inch**
- **Amount of body weight accounted for by lymphocytes: 2 pounds**

The ABCs of Drainage

Even if the closest you've ever come to an anatomy class is putting on a skeleton costume for Halloween, you know that fluids course through your body via two types of pipes: veins and arteries.

What you may not know is that there's a third system for transporting fluids. It's called the lymphatic system. Essentially, it runs parallel to, but separate from, the bloodstream.

The lymphatic system has two main tasks. It collects fluids that have spilled from the bloodstream and returns them to circulation. (Once the fluids are picked up, they're known as lymph.) At the same time, it stores and produces a variety of lymphocytes, which are infection-fighting white blood cells that help protect your body from bacteria, viruses and even cancer cells.

The lymphatic system is a remarkable piece of plumbing. Unlike the circulatory system, which is a high-pressure engine powered by the heart, the lymphatic system acts more like the roots of a plant. All day long its various tributaries sip fluids—up to three liters in a 24-hour period—that have been lost in the body's tissues, and all day long it slowly pushes those fluids upstream in the direction of the heart.

The system is so gradual, in fact, that it doesn't even need its own pump. It depends on the movement of muscles and the pulsations of nearby blood vessels to drive its cargo uphill.

There's more to the lymphatic system than just a series of pipes. As lymph moves upstream, it passes through hundreds of organs called lymph nodes. Each node is like a small storage sack, stuffed to the brim with voracious cells called macrophages.

The word *macrophage* means big eater, and that's exactly what these cells are. Whatever passes through the lymph nodes—bacteria, fungi, cancer cells and anything else—is engulfed and destroyed by macrophages. This is how the lymphatic system filters fluids before passing them back into the bloodstream.

Other lymphatic organs include:

Tonsils. If you haven't had yours removed, your tonsils form a ring around your throat. It is their responsibility to destroy inhaled or swallowed microbes before they get into your system.

Spleen. The largest organ in the lymphatic system, the spleen produces and stores infection-fighting lymphocytes (a type of white blood cell) and also cleanses the blood of bacteria, viruses, toxins and old and discarded blood cells.

Thymus gland. Most active in children, this gland releases hormones that activate immature immune cells (the T cells). Essentially, it arms the young cells and instructs them to respond only to specific targets. As we age, the thymus gland gradually loses function; by the time we reach old age, it's withered and difficult to even find. ∎

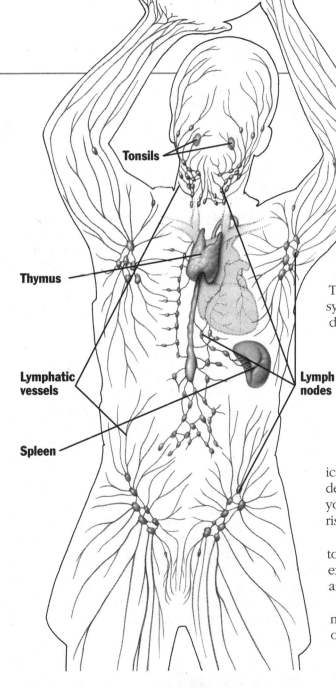

Tonsils

Thymus

Lymphatic vessels

Spleen

Lymph nodes

Elsewhere . . .

- **Blood**   **Page 104**
- **Immune System**   **Page 200**
- **Spleen**   **Page 309**
- **Tonsils**   **Page 334**

How to Help the Fight against Disease

The immune system, which protects your body from foreign substances such as viruses and bacteria, is a complicated system unto itself. But in many ways, you can't separate it from the lymphatic system, since the lymph organs are the seedbeds and programming sites for the immune cells and provide crucial vantage points for monitoring foreign substances in the body. The following tips will help your lymphatic system better contribute to the fight against disease.

Quit. Here's yet another reason to stop smoking. Smoke suppresses the lymphatic system, increasing your risk of infection.

Exercise. Studies show that exercise improves immune function. Three times a week for 30 minutes at a stretch is enough to boost your lymphatic system as well.

Learn to cope better. Severe, chronic physical or psychological stress is probably detrimental to your lymphatic system. When you're stressed out, levels of certain hormones rise, suppressing immune function.

Watch the beer. Alcohol may be devastating to your lymphatic system. Even single bouts of excessive drinking tax both your immune system and your lymphatic system.

Skip steroids. Anabolic steroids stimulate muscle growth by changing the metabolic state of muscles, a process that kills lymphocytes.■

▣Moles

- **Avoid sun.**
- **Monitor closely for changes.**
- **Leave 'em alone.**

A few years ago, a couple of pool-playing guys in a television commercial revived an ancient argument that has plagued man ever since *Gilligan's Island* began its endless cruise of reruns. Whom, they asked, would you rather be stranded with: Mary Ann or Ginger?

For years, the consensus was Mary Ann. Sure, Ginger had those glamorous curves, but she also had that peculiar mole on her left cheek. Then came the rise of Cindy Crawford. Probably the most lusted-after model in America, she also has a mole, above her lip. Ginger's stock, we imagine, must be skyrocketing.

Of course, such pickiness is a bit absurd. Almost all of us have a few moles somewhere on our bodies. What's the big deal?

Moles are little hitchhikers that ride along on your arms, back, legs, scalp and face for years or even decades and then may mysteriously disappear. Usually harmless, these brownish black growths—doctors call them pigmented nevi—begin forming in early childhood. Most appear by age 40. At first, they look flat, like freckles. As they mature, they can enlarge, become elevated and develop hairs. The average man has between 25 and 40 moles during his lifetime.

Although doctors aren't sure why moles appear, they do know that excessive sun exposure increases the risk that a mole will become cancerous. Moles can develop into both a benign cancer or the more serious form, known as malignant melanoma. If one of your parents had a mole that developed into a melanoma, your risk of having the same thing happen on your body is almost 100 percent. Early detection that a mole is changing reduces your risk of skin cancer spreading to other parts of your body. When a melanoma gets larger than a dime, it has more than a 50 percent chance of spreading.

Here's what Michael Kaminer, M.D., director of cosmetic dermatologic surgery at New England Medical Center in Boston and assistant professor of dermatology at Tufts University in Medford, Massachusetts, suggests you do to protect yourself.

Stay in shadows. Avoid the sun between 10:00 A.M. and 3:00 P.M., when the sun's rays are most intense, and minimize your exposure at other times of the day. When you are in the sun, wear a hat, long pants and shirt and cover yourself with a sunscreen with a sun protection factor (SPF) of at least 15.

Do a once-over once a month. Inspect your skin from head to toe every four weeks. After a shower is the perfect time, since you're naked anyway. Use a full-length or handheld mirror to examine hard to see spots such as the top of your head and your buttocks. Look for new growths as well as changes in any existing moles.

Remember your ABCDs. When you do your skin inspection, keep these rules in mind.
- *A* is for asymmetry. Both halves of the mole should look the same.
- *B* is for border. Be on alert for moles that have ragged, irregular edges.
- *C* is for color. Look for pigmentation changes such as a dark spot arising in a mole.
- *D* is for diameter. The mole is growing or is bigger than a pencil eraser.

Any of these changes should be brought to your doctor's attention.

Get it off. If a mole is bigger than a pencil eraser, if you nick it frequently while shaving or if it is in a hidden location where it can't easily be monitored for changes (such as on your scalp), ask your doctor about removing it.

⌘ Mouth

- **There's more to it than teeth and gums, so keep it all clean.**
- **Fight bad breath with flossing, rinsing and smart eating.**

The mouth is a huge source of wonder for children. It's the one place where they can easily see what their insides look like, full of pink, wet flesh and veiny, quivering membranes. Then there's the mystery of food and drink going in and disappearing and of weird sounds emerging from the back.

Adults are different. We romanticize the mouth as the expressway of emotions, the gateway for kisses and sensual pleasures. But kids may have a more accurate take: The mouth is a pretty complex machine. It is home to your teeth, gums, tongue and salivary glands, all of which participate in an intricate dance whenever you eat or speak. Each of these parts is discussed in its own chapter. What else is there?

The roof of your mouth is called the palate. The front part, or hard palate, keeps you from sticking your tongue through to your nose. The fleshy back part, or soft palate, separates your nose from the top of your throat. When you swallow, the back of the soft palate swings up and makes sure the food goes down, not up. The uvula, the fleshy lobe in the middle of your mouth, keeps your tongue tied in there. And farther back lies the epiglottis, doorway to digestion and speech.

Got that down?

If you keep your mouth healthy, you'll never get tested.

The Clean Routine

Moms who threatened to "wash your mouth out with soap" might have been onto something—though bad hygiene, not language,

is what generally needs correction in the adult male.

The mouth is surprisingly dirty. "A human bite often is more dangerous than an animal bite," says Richard Price, D.M.D., clinical instructor of dentistry at Boston University's Henry Goldman School of Dentistry and consumer adviser for the American Dental Association.

More than 300 types of bacteria live in our mouths. Some are good, keeping down the population of nasty fungi such as *Candida albicans*, a common fungus that can produce a yellow mouth coating called oral thrush. On the other hand, many of the bacteria are bad and can lead to infection. So if you bite someone, you have a high chance of infecting that person.

Essentially, what is good for your teeth and gums is good for the rest of your mouth. So brush and floss. Floss and brush. Get regular dental checkups and cleanings. These are the main ways to keep your mouth clean and healthy. (For detailed discussions of brushing and flossing techniques, see "How to Brush Your Teeth" and "How to Floss Your Teeth" on page 320.)

Banishing Bad Breath

Then there's bad breath. It can be caused by a noxious food such as garlic or pepperoni, poor oral hygiene or a medical problem such as a sinus infection. In the first two cases, you can usually vanquish bad breath yourself. Here's how.

Attack plaque. Your mouth can be a haven for plaque, a soft, clear film that those hundreds of living and dead bacteria love to glom on to. Brushing three to five times a day, or at least after breakfast and before bedtime, and flossing at least once a day can help keep your gums in the pink and your breath in the comfort zone.

Brush your tongue. After you've brushed your pearly whites, run a toothbrush

(continued on page 242)

◥Muscular System

- **Percent by which the average untrained man can increase his strength: 300**
- **Number of movements the eye muscles make in a day: 100,000**
- **Percent by which muscle strength decreases each day during complete immobilization: 5**

How Muscle Growth Works

Sure, muscles give you strength. But how? The next time someone asks, say this.

A muscle is a bundle of long, slender cells (also known as fibers) that contract upon demand. Muscles can be attached to other muscles, to bones or to skin (muscles pulling on skin is what makes you smile). What tells the muscles to contract? Nerves, of course. Each muscle fiber gets independent nerve impulses telling it when it needs to move. Some muscles move voluntarily, such as when you decide to kick over a chair, while others move involuntarily, such as when your stomach muscles act automatically to churn food.

When a muscle gets the message to move, the fibers take glycogen (a form of stored energy) and oxygen and, in a chemical reaction, convert them to mechanical energy. Voilà—motion! Glycogen and oxygen are delivered to the muscles in blood, which also carries away the by-products of the energy chemical reaction, such as carbon dioxide.

So how does exercise work? Muscles have this amazing capacity to rebuild themselves after injury. To become stronger, we deliberately cause muscles to strain at a microscopic level. In the hours and days after straining, they rebuild themselves, but with slightly greater size and capacity. Repeat this process, and the pulling power of your muscle fibers grows.

The amount you can advance is limited, however. The length of your muscles, measured from tendon to tendon, is the single most important factor in determining potential muscle size. Only one in a million men is born with either super-long muscles (Arnold Schwarzenegger) or super-short ones (Woody Allen). As for the rest of us, we can likely realize modest body-shaping dreams through a well-balanced program of weight lifting, aerobic exercise and nutrition.■

Name That Pain

Complain, complain—that's all we do. Here is what all of those achy muscle terms mean.

Charley horse. Slang term for a painful involuntary spasm in one of the calf muscles.

Cramp. A spasmodic muscle contraction.

Delayed-onset muscle soreness. Ordinary all-day stiffness in a muscle that peaks a day or two after the muscle has been exercised.

Heat cramp. Cramp caused by overexertion in hot weather. It could result from lack of water, an overheated body or electrolyte imbalance.

Muscle tension. The measure of actual force in a muscle at a given time. In popular lingo, it describes pain from maintaining extremely taut muscles, often involuntarily, often due to stress.

Muscle fatigue. A state in which muscles are increasingly uncomfortable and less efficient as a result of extended exertion.

Plateauing. Weight lifters' term for when you cease making gains in muscle strength.

Sore muscle. General term referring to a muscle pain that could come from anything—a bruise, overuse or strain, for example.

Sprain. Wrenching or twisting of a joint that could include tearing of a ligament.

Strain. Overstretching or overexertion of a muscle that could include tearing of a muscle or tendon (tendons connect muscles to bones).■

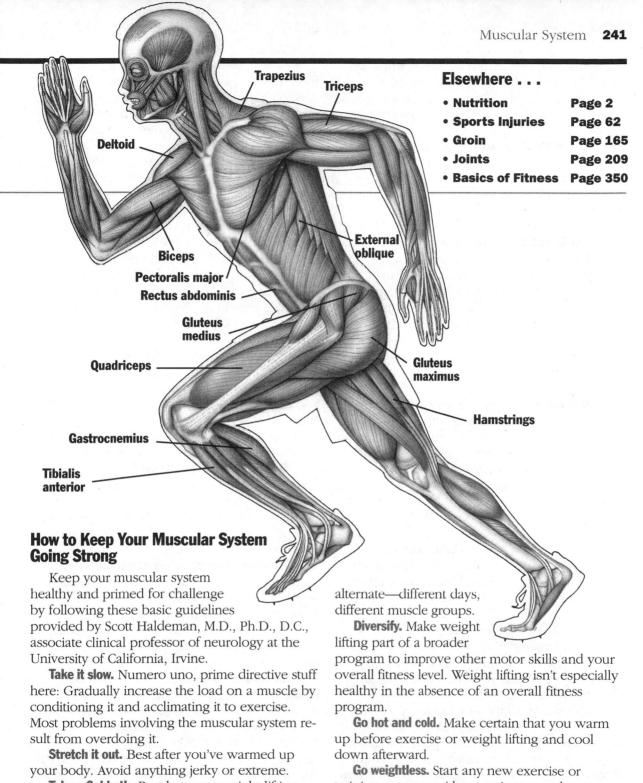

Trapezius

Triceps

Deltoid

Biceps

Pectoralis major

Rectus abdominis

Gluteus medius

Quadriceps

Gastrocnemius

Tibialis anterior

External oblique

Gluteus maximus

Hamstrings

How to Keep Your Muscular System Going Strong

Keep your muscular system healthy and primed for challenge by following these basic guidelines provided by Scott Haldeman, M.D., Ph.D., D.C., associate clinical professor of neurology at the University of California, Irvine.

Take it slow. Numero uno, prime directive stuff here: Gradually increase the load on a muscle by conditioning it and acclimating it to exercise. Most problems involving the muscular system result from overdoing it.

Stretch it out. Best after you've warmed up your body. Avoid anything jerky or extreme.

Take a Sabbath. Rest between weight-lifting sessions to give those muscles a chance to repair. It's okay to lift up to seven days a week. Just alternate—different days, different muscle groups.

Diversify. Make weight lifting part of a broader program to improve other motor skills and your overall fitness level. Weight lifting isn't especially healthy in the absence of an overall fitness program.

Go hot and cold. Make certain that you warm up before exercise or weight lifting and cool down afterward.

Go weightless. Start any new exercise or training program without resistance to learn proper technique. Gradually add weights only after you've mastered the technique.■

over your tongue to wipe out the hard-to-get food particles and plaque harbored there, suggests Dr. Price. If that feels too much like chalk on a blackboard, use a spoon on your tongue (bowl side up).

Rinse your mouth. You may not have a toothbrush, but you can probably find some spare water. Bad breath often results from dry mouth, and odors from food and drink ferment in a dry environment. Swishing helps flush them away, says Dr. Price.

Chop out the onions. Stay away from onions and garlic, says Dr. Price. They may taste great, but they'll recirculate in your body for 24 hours afterward. Instead, eat an apple. It'll give your breath the come-hither appeal that more pungent foods can't.

Other Issues

Here are some other ailments that may lie in the dark hole.

Dry mouth. Most everyone has experienced this sticky, desertlike sensation at one time or another. This feeling is common when you're acutely anxious—for example, "when you've just missed being run over by a bus," suggests Vernon Brightman, D.M.D., Ph.D., professor of oral medicine at the University of Pennsylvania School of Dental Medicine in Philadelphia.

But while situational dry mouth can be eased with a drink of water and a little time to chill out, the chronic kind has different causes and solutions. It can result from diseases as disparate as diabetes and depression, but it most often is a side effect of medication. If dry mouth isn't treated, you can end up with extensive dental decay or thrush. Also, when your saliva stops flowing, you often lose some of your ability to taste.

In some patients, persistent dry mouth can be eased with pilocarpine (Salagen), a prescription drug. Frequent sips of a sugar-free liquid, particularly hot lemon tea, might do the trick. For some, artificial saliva solution purchased from a pharmacy also helps relieve the discomfort and dry feeling.

Note: Stay away from candy and other foods that cause dental decay. "Many people suck on hard lemon candy to relieve dry mouth but end up with rampant tooth decay, an event referred to in the medical literature as sour-ball syndrome," says Dr. Brightman.

Canker sores. No one knows what causes these ulcers that affect the lining of the mouth, although they probably result from an inherited abnormality in the patient's immune system, says Dr. Brightman. Stress and lowered resistance to infection, sometimes because of illness, are two other possibilities, says Dr. Price.

"Size-wise, these ulcers are the most painful lesions in the human body," Dr. Price says. And they often last as long as two weeks, especially if they are larger than usual. In these cases, medical treatment might include a prescription for a steroid cream. Be sure to see your dentist or physician if the frequency or severity of your canker sores increases, says Dr. Brightman.

There are other ways to cut short these nasty sores or to avoid them altogether.

Baste it with Orabase-B. This over-the-counter remedy gets a thumbs-up from Dr. Price as the best relief money can buy in your neighborhood drugstore. You put it directly on the sore to stop the pain. Zilactin, a medicated gel, is also recommended.

Avoid sharp or spicy foods. That means holding not just the salsa, which can make a sore burn, but the chips, too, says Dr. Price. Their sharp edges can puncture the skin and cause sores. Acidic foods such as pineapple can also make you yowl with pain, so avoid them as well.

Cancer. Mouth cancer has a higher incidence among people who smoke, chew tobacco or drink heavily over the long term, says Dr. Price. Two lessons: First, here's one more reason to stay away from these vices; and second, if you must smoke or imbibe, be smart and see your doctor immediately if an unusual sore comes along in your mouth. He can check it to see if it's cancerous.

⟩ ⟨ Neck

- **Keep it stretched.**
- **Maintain good posture.**
- **Stop gazing at stars and ants.**
- **Massage often.**

Women have bad necks; men have bad backs. No one knows exactly why. But one physical therapist just may have stumbled onto something: Women have breasts. And men have chests.

Physical therapist Wayne Rath, co-director of Summit Physical Therapy in Syracuse, New York, speculates that the sheer weight of women's breasts pulls their heads and shoulders forward. And that strains their necks. Men's bad backs, however, might be caused by their less curvy lumbar curves and heavier bellies.

There's also the tension-of-the-sexes explanation. Men are often a pain in the neck for women, and women can be a pain in the behind for men, jokes Rath.

It's All in Your Head

Stereotypes aside, plenty of men suffer from neck pain, too, mostly because of their big heads. The typical head weighs between 10 and 12 pounds. Some weigh as much as 25 pounds, which is three times the weight of a newborn baby. And it's the job of the neck's seven vertebrae, 32 muscles and assorted ligaments and nerves to balance and rotate that weight.

Big heads have big necks. No-necks. Pencil-necks. That's all a matter of heredity. Though everyone's neck has exactly seven bones, some people's bones are bigger than others', says William Stauber, Ph.D., muscle physiologist at West Virginia University in Morgantown. And people with big neck bones tend to have big bodies.

The neck is happiest when it's aligned with the rest of the body. When your ears are above your ankles, your entire body helps hold up your head. But when you slouch, you make your neck muscles work harder to hold your brain aloft.

Imagine, for example, holding your arm up and balancing a bowling ball in your hand. If the ball tipped forward just a tad, your arm muscles would tighten to keep the ball from falling off. The farther forward or backward the ball moved, the tougher it would be to hold it up straight. Similarly, if you tip your 12-pound noggin, you have neck muscles straining to keep it from kerplopping onto the cement.

You would think that after 14 million years of uprightness, we would have the hang of this standing and sitting thing. But evolution apparently takes a long time to reach perfection. We're a bunch of slouchers. And gravity is only too happy to pull us down.

"Oftentimes Mother Nature sort of collides with all of the wrong ways we do things," says Annie Pivarski, an orthopedic physician's assistant and ergonomics and prevention supervisor at St. Francis Memorial Hospital in San Francisco.

Don't Follow Your Nose

According to one Norwegian study, about 15 percent of the male population suffers from neck pain. And the main culprit is poor posture. So listen to your mother and stop slouching. Line yourself up against a wall. Feel your head over your shoulders. Then keep yourself that way. Once you start paying attention to where your neck is, you'll realize only too painfully that your head is tipped forward far too often.

One of the primary slouching havens is the workplace. "People today tend to do work that's fairly static. They stay in one place all day long," says Pivarski. But you can arrange your office to fit your neck's needs.

• Your body should not turn into a statue. Don't sit still for longer than an hour. Change positions, especially when you feel tense. Walk around. Get the kinks out. "Do the opposite of what you're doing all day long. So if your head is leaning forward, you want to tuck it back," says Pivarski.

• Your chin should be in line with the center of your computer screen. The distance from the screen to your eyes should be 20 to 28 inches. You should not have to lean forward to work. Your arms should be in straight lines with your wrists. Your elbows should be bent at 90-degree angles, Pivarski says.

• Your chair should support your lower back. Your hips should be level with your knees, says Pivarski. If you feel pressure on your tailbone, the chair is too close to the floor. If you feel pressure in your thighs, the chair is too high.

• Your reading material should be at the same height as your computer screen to avoid craning your neck, Pivarski says. An adjustable copyholder can help you do that.

General Maintenance

Here are some other things you can do to keep your neck from fighting back.

Get off the foam. A foam pillow makes you bounce when you roll over at night. Your pillow should fit the contour of your neck, Pivarski says. For instance, if you're lying on your side, your neck should be in alignment with your body.

Sleep on your back. You wouldn't walk around all day with your head turned to the side. But that's what you do to your head when you sleep on your stomach. Your neck will like you much more if you roll over on your back, says Rath.

Be true to your height. If

Giving Yourself a Massage

Once you get a neckache or a headache that won't quit, you can beat the tension out of the area with massage. Massage improves circulation, which carries oxygen in and waste out. And that releases tension. But you don't have to part with a chunk of your paycheck to get a massage. Here are some simple things you can do to massage your own neck.

1. Put one hand on the opposite shoulder. Use your thumb and index finger to grip the thick muscle that runs from your neck to your shoulder. Then press and roll down the muscle. "Very often what people find is that they hit several tender spots. But they probably hit some that fire into their heads, creating a headache effect. These are 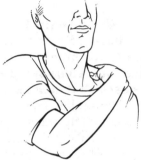 trigger points," says Betsy Bickel, a certified massage therapist at the Duke University Diet and Fitness Center in Durham, North Carolina. Trigger points radiate sensation to other parts of the body. When you find one, hold pressure for 10 to 12 seconds. Usually, the muscle will soften, and the headache sensation will melt away.

2. Put your hands behind your head and use your thumbs to circle across the base of your skull. Then cross your hands and use your thumbs and fingertips to grip and knead the thick muscle that runs up each side of your neck.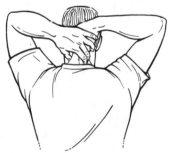

3. For those hard-to-reach places, a tennis ball comes in handy. Lie on top of the ball and position it around your shoulder area, making sure it is not directly on your spine. You can change pressure by moving your arms over your head and down by your sides.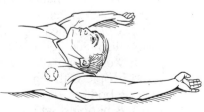

Head-Bangers' Ball a Bad Call

Ozzy's onstage biting the head off a bat. The music pounds. And you're hip. You think you're Iron Man. Your chin flips toward your chest, then whips backward. Then forward. Then backward.

Hours later, you awake groggy. You lift your head ever so gingerly off the pillow. *Yeeow!* You have head-banger's whiplash.

The phenomenon was discovered in 1993, when one day a severely neck-pained girl knocked on the front door of Boston neurologist Marilyn Kassirer, M.D. The girl had been head-banging during a seven hour benefit dance the night before. And Dr. Kassirer, who is assistant clinical professor of neurology at Boston University School of Medicine, soon learned that most of the other young head-bangers had similar symptoms: killing, aching, twinging pain in the back of the neck.

The pain was a result of hyperextension of the neck. This often occurs in car accidents, when a rear-end collision makes the driver's head snap backward and then forward. The only difference between an accident and the dance is that the dancers whip their heads voluntarily.

"Actually, the head-banging took place during only three songs within the whole seven-hour time. It doesn't take a lot of time to get this activated," says Dr. Kassirer.

It seems the longer the hair, the worse the damage. More girls got whiplash than boys. "If you think about how they extend and flex their heads with that extra whipping action that they do in this head-banging dance, the girls' hair propels a little bit farther forward and a little bit farther backward than the boys' hair," she speculates.

Children's necks are more flexible than adults. So for any child to suffer from whiplash is very unusual, Dr. Kassirer says. An adult who head-bangs would probably suffer a worse fate. "I wouldn't want to see what would happen to many grown-ups if they were to do head-banging," she says.

The best way to avoid head-banger's whiplash is to not do the dance, Dr. Kassirer say. But if you can't stop yourself, try building up the muscles around your neck—the trapezius and assorted back muscles—to give your spine more support. And keep your neck as flexible as possible by stretching the muscles. (For a how-to on neck exercises, see page 360.)

you're short, don't stand around all day admiring the world above you. And if you're tall, don't spend all of your time watching ants. Tipping your chin upward or slumping your shoulders down strains your neck.

Get up. Don't read in bed or slouch in a low chair with most of your weight on your neck. You also shouldn't read while lying on your stomach with your head extended backward. All of these positions stress your neck.

Avoid the front. When you're at the movies, sit in the middle or the back of the theater. The first few rows of seats may cause you to sit for two hours with your chin toward the ceiling. You want the screen to be at or below eye level.

Make headgear fit. If your bicycle helmet is wobbly, you'll strain your neck trying to keep it on your head.

No crash tests, dummy. About 85 percent of all neck injuries are caused in rear-end collisions. When someone slams into the rear bumper of your car, your head whips backward and then forward. Your neck hyperextends, straining neck muscles and spraining ligaments. A head restraint can prevent this injury if you adjust it correctly, says Dr. Stauber. The top of the headrest should reach the middle of the back of your head. Taller drivers (about six feet) should pull it all the way up. Shorter drivers (about five feet two inches) should push it all the way down.

Nervous System

- **Maximum speed of nerve impulses: 223 miles per hour**
- **Percent of stimuli ignored by the brain to prevent overload: 99**
- **Number of cold receptors per square centimeter of the lips: 15 to 25**
- **Longest nerve in the body: the sciatic nerve, at 2 to 3 feet**

Your Body Online

A walk down a crowded city street on a warm spring day can bombard even the most organized guy's brain with information overload.

Just how does your brain process all of that information and filter out the beautiful from the banal? It's not easy. Your body is wired with sensors, processors and high-speed, high-capacity cables. It's called the nervous system, and for sheer complexity, it puts Ma Bell to shame.

Your nervous system consists of the brain, the spinal cord and a gazillion individual nerve cells called neurons. The three work in tandem to achieve three different but interrelated tasks: to monitor signals arriving from inside or outside your body; to interpret the information so that you know what it means; and to activate the appropriate muscles or glands to respond to it.

The nervous system has two main parts. The brain and the spinal cord make up the central nervous system. This is the command center that interprets incoming signals and marshals the appropriate response. The peripheral nervous system consists mainly of the nerves that extend from the brain and spinal cord to virtually every corner of the body. It tells the brain what's going on.■

Make the Connection

To keep your nervous system working well, here's what experts advise.

Mind your minerals. Neurons can't function without calcium, magnesium, sodium and potassium. Fortunately, these minerals are readily available in foods and even in water. Experts advise getting 1,000 milligrams of calcium, 400 milligrams of magnesium and 3,500 milligrams of potassium a day. For sodium, keep your intake to around 2,400 milligrams a day.

Get the lead out. In small amounts, it's invisible and tasteless. Yet it's a terrible toxin that can severely damage the nervous system, even in minuscule amounts. Lead water pipes should be stripped out and replaced. And be cautious about using lead-glazed dishes and cups from Mexico, China and other developing countries, since in many cases the pottery isn't fired at sufficiently high temperatures to lock in lead and prevent it from leaching into foods.

Protect your brain box. Some of the most severe nervous system problems are caused by accidents. Wear your bicycle helmet. Buckle your seat belt. Take every reasonable precaution to protect your brain and spine from trauma.

Don't neglect these nutrients. Other nutrients that can help keep your nervous system strong include the B vitamins and copper. Try to get the Daily Values of two milligrams of vitamin B_6 and six micrograms of vitamin B_{12}. Foods rich in vitamin B_6 include potatoes, bananas and chicken breast. You'll find significant amounts of vitamin B_{12} in meats, seafood and dairy products. While you're at it, try to get the Daily Value of two milligrams of copper, since a shortage can bring on nervous system disorders. You get copper from nuts, fruits, peas and beans and oysters and other shellfish.■

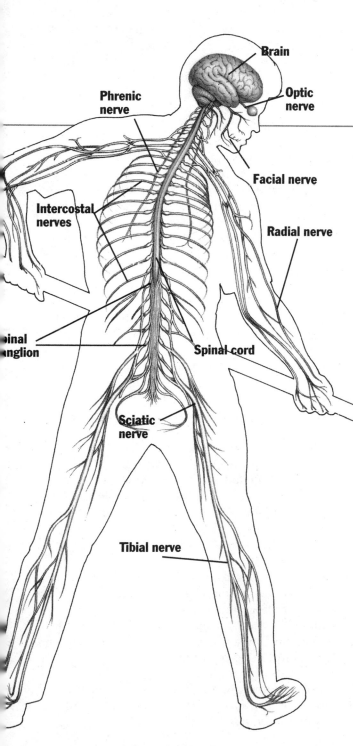

Brain
Optic nerve
Phrenic nerve
Facial nerve
Intercostal nerves
Radial nerve
inal nglion
Spinal cord
Sciatic nerve
Tibial nerve

Elsewhere . . .
- **Brain**   **Page 110**
- **Touch**   **Page 180**
- **Lips**   **Page 223**
- **Spinal Cord** **Page 307**

Weird Wiring

A simple question, and your mind goes blank. What's going on? Does anyone study these things?

Enter Alan P. Xenakis, M.D., author of *Why Doesn't My Funny Bone Make Me Laugh? Sneezes, Hiccups, Butterflies and Other Funny Feelings Explained*. He takes a close look at some of life's curious and not always pleasant sensations and tries to understand why they make us feel the way they do. For example:

Your mind goes blank. Neural pathways at the base of the brain are responsible for controlling strong emotions. When you're nervous, this area can get overloaded, making the system unable to respond. Recovery usually occurs within a few seconds. You'll answer the question and keep your job.

Your arm goes numb. Placing your arm around your girlfriend's shoulders (or in a similar position) for two or more minutes may result in a compressed nerve and blocked blood supply. Once you move your arm, it can take up to ten minutes to restore normal blood flow and nerve impulses.

Your feet fall asleep. This is another example of reduced nerve function. Keeping your feet in one position can reduce the normal and essential exchange of potassium, sodium and chloride among the nerves. When you stand up, there's a sudden surge of ions, which results in painful tingling. ■

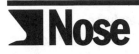

Nose

- **Keep it moist.**
- **Keep your fingers out.**
- **Keep out of harm's way.**

Through the ages, a man's nose has been linked to another protruding, though far more private, part of his anatomy. The Roman historian Lampridius described big-nosed men as being especially well endowed underneath their togas. Then there was Rostand's Cyrano de Bergerac, whose protracted proboscis was exceeded only by his . . . uh, sword. And the myth survives even today. Actress Linda Fiorentino, in an interview with *Esquire* magazine, said she uses a man's extremities—his nose, hands and feet—to gauge his penis size. "You take an average-size man—six-foot-one, long aquiline nose— and you're talking about an 85 percent accuracy rate," she enthused.

Before you panic, wondering how you wound up in the 15 percent minority, rest assured that there is no scientific correlation between nose size and penis length. The phallic fascination is merely an indication of the misplaced emphasis we lavish on how a nose looks. After all, rhinoplasty, more commonly known as a nose job, is the most popular form of plastic surgery among men. But what really matters—and this is one trait the nose truly does share with the penis—is the way it works.

A Well-Oiled Machine

Your nose does a lot more than merely give women something to look forward to. This intake chamber has to warm the air that comes in, filter it and pump up the humidity before passing it along to your lungs.

Blood vessels in the nasal cavity are the space heaters that warm the air to about 95°F.

For the cleaning work, you have mucous membranes that secrete about a quart of gooey mucus every day. You also have millions of minute hairs called cilia. The cilia are relentless mucus movers, thrashing away at all of that goop at the rate of 12 to 15 beats per second as they move it along toward your throat. Like a miniature wet-dry vacuum, the moving mucus flushes dust and debris away from your lungs.

In addition to heating, moistening and vacuuming, your nose functions as your olfactory operations center, able to detect the scent of a woman wearing Bijan perfume, a sizzling steak on the grill or, almost as pleasant, the aroma of a brand-new car. And these are just a few of the 4,000 or so distinctive odors that your alert schnozz can detect.

The nasal hound dogs that track down fragrance are two smell receptor sites, each about the size of a nickel, stuck way up near the top of your nasal cavity. The scent perception is done by millions of nerve fibers, which pick up distinctive smells as odor-filled air swirls around them. Signals shout to the sprightly limbic system and hypothalamus in your brain, which quickly sort things out to make sure you don't try to take the steak out for a test drive or fry up the car for breakfast.

The Trouble It Sees

The poor nose. It's blown, rubbed, picked, scratched and subjected to smoke, air pollution and dry air almost on a daily basis.

Problems with your proboscis are often with the mucous membrane that lines its interior. This lining is very thin, which means that when air gets dry, the lining can become irritated and cracked, says Anthony Yonkers, M.D., professor and chairman of the Department of Otolaryngology–Head and Neck Surgery at the University of Nebraska Medical Center in Omaha. The result is troubles ranging from crusting to recurrent bleeding.

Although most nosebleeds tend to be spotters rather than frightening gushers, they can still be annoying. Here are a few tips for stopping them before they start.

Humidify. Using a hot-air humidifier in your bedroom helps keep your nasal tissues moist, notes Alexander C. Chester, M.D., clinical professor of medicine at Georgetown University Medical Center in Washington, D.C. "Many of the new office buildings have no humidifiers at all, so you could take a humidifier to work as well," he notes.

Pass the jelly. Wiping a thin layer of petroleum jelly just inside your nose is another good membrane moistener, notes Dr. Chester.

Measure your pressure. If you get chronic nosebleeds, it is important to have your blood pressure checked, advises Dr. Yonkers. "Nosebleeds may be an indicator of high blood pressure," he notes.

Pinch an inch. If the blood flows despite your best preventive efforts, Dr. Yonkers recommends holding your head level while pinching your nose closed, with a towel or handkerchief under your nostrils to stop the dripping. "If it keeps pouring out after 10 to 15 minutes, seek a doctor's help," he says.

Trimming the Undergrowth

Another troublemaker is the nasal polyp, a benign growth in the mucous membrane of the nose that can lead to sinusitis and nasal obstruction, notes David Zwillenberg, M.D., an otolaryngologist at Thomas Jefferson University Hospital in Philadelphia.

(continued on page 252)

Setting a Pick

Jerry Seinfeld's girlfriend breaks up with him because she thinks she saw him pick his nose while he was driving.

It's a case of sitcom imitating life. According to the first population survey of nose picking, men are more likely to consider public nose picking to be normal. The automobile and office are the most common places to pick, as cited by the 254 Dane County, Wisconsin, residents involved in the survey. And more than half of the men admitted picking their noses daily.

Among both sexes, private nose picking is so pervasive—more than 90 percent of those interviewed admitted to being active nose pickers—that the study concluded that nose picking is an almost universal, benign practice in most adults.

But exactly what constitutes a pick? Throughout the *Seinfeld* episode, Jerry passionately defends his actions, insisting that his finger was "on the outside." The co-authors of the nose-picking survey, James W. Jefferson, M.D., and Trent D. Thompson, M.D., would have to side with the famous comedian. Their questionnaire defined nose picking as "insertion of a finger (or other object) into the nose with the intention of removing dried nasal secretion."

You won't find a discussion of nose picking in standard etiquette books. But when something inside your nose begs for removal, Thomas Pasic, M.D., assistant professor of otolaryngology at the University of Wisconsin-Madison, suggests the following:

• Try to blow it out into a tissue rather than manually removing it.

• If that fails, try using a handkerchief and your little finger. It's still nose picking, but in a more dignified, covert way.

• Don't keep rubbing the outside of your nostril. Sure, you might be able to break up the clog and move the debris closer to the edge, but nose rubbing is pretty ugly to watch, too. More important, nose picking and rubbing can lead to a nosebleed.

• Use spray. A shot or two of saline spray into the nostril can help loosen crusting or debris, so it can be blown out easily.

• Forget about it. Your nose will automatically process the material without your help.

Smell

- **Percent of taste that is actually smell: 80**
- **Number of chemicals that the sense of smell can pick up: 10,000**
- **Number of receptors in the nose for the sense of smell: up to 100 million**

How Smell Works

Your sense of smell is your chemical readout on your environment. It is astonishingly sensitive; you can detect as few as three to five molecules of a certain airborne substance. Smell nerves are thousands of times more sensitive than taste buds, which is why smell is such a big part of taste.

Here's how smelling works: A molecule enters your nose and ascends through a narrow passageway to a region of smell nerves high up in your nose. This is the only place where nerve cells are on the external surface of your body (the inside of the nose is considered the outside of the body).

The molecule comes into contact with the nerve cells and, if it provides enough stimulation, triggers an electrical signal to be sent to your brain. There, the signal gets passed farther on to where the actual perception of smell occurs.

This is not a static process. Various controls regulate your smell nerves based on your body's needs and environment. Food smells are more intense when you're hungry, because the hunger center of your brain sends messages to the smell region to heighten its sensitivity. But if you were rescuing someone from fire, you probably wouldn't notice the waft of cinnamon buns cooking next door, not even on an empty stomach.

Your reaction to some smells, such as skunk, are preprogrammed in your brain. But the loveliness or putridity of most other odors is strictly personal. Why? Memory and emotions evolved from the same part of the primitive brain that governs smell. That's why memories and emotional responses are intrinsically linked to your sense of smell.■

How to Be a Power Smeller

It's inevitable that your sense of smell will deteriorate with age. But you can help prevent premature deterioration and enhance your smelling prowess.

Be a bloodhound. To smell more accurately, take several small sniffs rather than one big one, says Harry Fremont, a perfumer for Firmenich in New York City. If you smell something very fully, your brain has a built-in capacity to tune out a powerful scent (that's why dinner smells so great when you first walk in the door but you don't smell it as strongly after a few minutes). "If you sniff, you take in only a little bit of the scent, so you won't tune it out," says Fremont.

Taste that smell. Smell and taste are the kissing cousins of the sensory set; one improves your appreciation of the other. So when you smell something, Fremont recommends sniffing with your mouth open. Drawing the odor in through your mouth as well as your nose adds dimension to it.

Practice, practice, practice. When was the last time you went outdoors, shut your eyes and smelled deeply? There's a world of odors all around us, and yet we rarely bother to sort them out. Want to be a great smeller? You'll have to work at it. Perfumer Fremont's pastimes revolve around activities that will get him smelling more. "I garden and I walk. When I do these things, I am in contact with a variety of scents. When I am

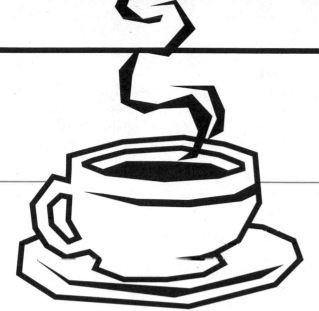

at the store, I smell the different foods," he says.

Use it or lose it. Experts say that the more you smell, the more you can smell. "Experiments have shown that if you're in a room devoid of odors, the receptors that govern smell shut down over time, and you can lose your ability to smell," says Alan Hirsch, M.D., a neurologist, a psychiatrist and director of the Smell and Taste Treatment and Research Center in Chicago. "But the more scents you're exposed to, the healthier those nerve endings are."

Stay fit. The healthier you are, the less often you'll get colds and flus. A full one-third of the

cases of smell loss result from colds and viral infections, making them the most common causes of smell loss, says Dr. Hirsch.

Avoid allergens. Chronic sinus infections and allergies account for one-quarter of the cases of smell loss. If you suffer from allergies but aren't sure what you're allergic to, get tested.

Go easy on the antihistamines. Although a clogged nose is going to have a tough time smelling, the steps you take to unstuff that nose may be just as bad for your sense of scents. "I find that antihistamines and decongestants dry out the nose too much," says Fremont. The best nose for smelling is a moist nose, he says. If congested, he uses a nasal spray, which unstuffs the nose and keeps it moist.

Don't smoke. Smoking has been shown to diminish the sense of smell across the board.

See red and yellow. Fruits and vegetables in these colors are high in vitamin A, which is vital for maintaining a healthy nasal lining. ■

Healing through Smell

In recent years, medical research has concluded that the odors we smell have a significant impact on the way we feel. Some doctors are beginning to believe that smell acts directly on the brain, like a drug, says Alan Hirsch, M.D., a neurologist, a psychiatrist and director of the Smell and Taste Treatment and Research Center in Chicago.

Thank you, modern medicine, for confirming a practice that is merely several thousands years old: using soothing odors from aromatic plants to help the body heal. Ancient Egyptians were among the first to use fragrant oils for healing. But it wasn't until the eleventh century A.D. that European healers began working with plant ex-

tracts to create highly concentrated, volatile "essential oils" for medicinal purposes.

Fast-forward to today. The concept of aromatherapy has been quickly growing in popularity in the United States, helped in part by some validation through modern research techniques, says Dr. Hirsch. Now it's not exactly in character for an old-fashioned guy to smell lavender oil to relieve stress, but even old-fashioned doctors are becoming more open to using such oils to relieve pain, care for the skin, alleviate tension and even treat illnesses, says Dr. Hirsch. There are lots of new books out on the topic, and stores such as the Body Shop are beginning to carry essential oils. ■

"It's an inflammatory reaction," he says. "The lining of the nose gets so swollen from irritation that it herniates downward."

About half of all polyps develop as the result of allergies, so managing sniffles and congestion is a key to treatment, Dr. Zwillenberg says. Another polyp aggravator is aspirin, Dr. Chester says.

Often polyps can be treated with nasal steroids. They can also be removed surgically, but about half of the time they'll grow back.

A Bad Curve?

Another nose plugger is a deviated septum. The septum is the partition separating the two nasal cavities from each other. When the partition is bent or twisted, it's called a deviated septum.

Any of life's blows, from your trip down the birth canal to a right hook you never saw coming, can cause the septum to deviate. The most common problem resulting from a deviated septum is an inability to breathe well through the nose, which can cause problems with snoring and dry mouth, says Randy Oppenheimer, M.D., part-time clinical instructor of otolaryngology at the University of California, San Diego.

How easy is a diagnosis? "We just look up with a nasal speculum and can tell in one second," Dr. Oppenheimer says. "It's a very common problem. A lot of people have deviated septums and don't even know it."

To straighten a deviated septum, doctors remove or restructure the pieces of cartilage and bone causing blockage.

Opening the Airways

The first time you saw a pro football player wearing one, you probably figured that he had suffered a bad cut on his nose. Turned out that the strip across the bridge of his nose, now popping up on athletes everywhere, was a nasal dilator. Players swear that this device aids breathing on the field. But the question is whether it works for its original purpose: to improve nasal airflow to prevent or diminish snoring.

Apparently not. Two studies have found no direct relationship between increased nasal airflow and decreased snoring.

Researchers at St. Michael's Hospital in Toronto monitored eight normal male snorers during sleep. The men did not experience significant decreases in nasal airflow during any phase of sleep. Also, there was no relationship between how much or how loudly they snored and the minor fluctuations in nasal airflow that did occur while they slept.

The researchers concluded that the amount of nasal obstruction isn't related to either the frequency or the intensity of snoring when men are breathing exclusively through their noses. This suggests that increasing nasal airflow with a nasal dilator will not cut snoring.

A University of Toronto study reached a similar conclusion, finding that a nasal dilator had no impact on snoring for any of the 15 study participants.

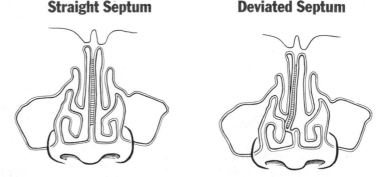

Straight Septum   **Deviated Septum**

Behind each nostril is a single cavity that leads to the sinus cavities. The main partition between the two nasal cavities is the septum, a thin wall of cartilage and bone down the center of the nose. A crooked, bent or off-center septum is said to be deviated. The impact: difficulty breathing out of one nostril.

It's a simple hour-long procedure done on an outpatient basis, Dr. Oppenheimer says.

🖰 Pancreas

- **Eat a balanced diet.**
- **Exercise regularly.**
- **Get checked for diabetes.**

The islets of Langerhans sound like a great vacation hideaway off the coast of Germany. But don't call your travel agent. You're already there. Or more accurately, they're already here.

The islets of Langerhans are 100,000 tiny bits of tissue located at the tail end of the pancreas, the small cone-shaped gland that hides below and behind the stomach. On each islet are clusters of hard-working cells—they're definitely not on vacation—secreting hormones and enzymes that make sure we digest food and convert it into energy.

Even if you could visit the islets, you wouldn't want to; they and their surrounding areas are strictly industrial. "The pancreas is a chemical factory," says Howard Reber, M.D., vice-chair of the Department of Surgery at the University of California, Los Angeles, UCLA School of Medicine, chief of surgery at Sepulveda Veterans Administration Medical Center, also in Los Angeles, and past president of the American Pancreatic Association. "Every time you eat a meal, the pancreas is stimulated to release enzymes vital to digestion into the intestines."

Making Chemicals

The pancreas works two jobs. One, part of what is called the exocrine system, is to make the digestive enzymes: lipase to digest fat, amylace for carbohydrates and trypsin for protein. These pancreatic juices are secreted into the small intestine through a duct called, not surprisingly, the pancreatic duct.

The pancreas's other job is to manufacture chemicals for the endocrine system. That's the system that produces and distributes essential hormones and other chemicals throughout

your body via the bloodstream. Of the three such chemicals that the pancreas makes, the hormone insulin is probably the most important, followed by the hormone glucagon.

You hear of insulin all of the time, but can you explain what it does? Trust us, it is very important. Here's the simple answer.

During the digestive process, carbohydrates such as breads, pastas, fruits and vegetables break down into a simple sugar called glucose. The glucose (or blood sugar) passes through the walls of your intestines into your bloodstream, to be carried to fuel-hungry cells throughout your body. But cells don't have mouths; each is protected by a thin wall, or membrane. In order to let the glucose pass through that wall, the cell needs a key. That key is insulin, which responds to the presence of glucose by commanding the cell: "Open sesame!" Once inside, the glucose is burned by the cell—*metabolized* is the expensive word for it—firing up your energy pistons.

While insulin lowers glucose, glucagon raises it. Together these hormones perform a balancing act, keeping your blood sugar level normal (for you chemistry nuts, that's about 60 to 110 milligrams of sugar per deciliter of blood).

Diabetes, without the Sugar Coating

When certain cells in the pancreas go on the blink, one of two things can happen. They can produce too little insulin, which is called Type I diabetes. Or the insulin they produce does not help glucose get into your cells; that's Type II diabetes. Robert McEvoy, M.D., director of the Division of Pediatric Endocrinology at Mount Sinai Medical Center in New York City, describes those with Type I diabetes as "skinny young people" and those with Type II diabetes as "fat old people."

People with Type I diabetes are usually children and young adults. They are insulin-dependent, meaning that they must get daily doses of the hormone by injection. They account for between 5 and 10 percent of all people with diabetes.

Type II diabetes, also called non-insulin-dependent diabetes, is more common and occurs in people 40 years of age and older. Here the pancreas produces insulin, but for unknown reasons, the body resists its effects, almost as though someone changed the locks when you weren't looking.

There are 14 million people walking around with diabetes, but only half of them know it, "because they are ignoring the symptoms or are unaware of them," says Wahida Karmally, R.D., a registered dietitian, a certified diabetes educator and director of nutrition at Columbia University's Irving Center for Clinical Research in New York City. Without proper treatment, the symptoms of diabetes, whether Type I or Type II, are about the same: lack of energy, constant hunger, weight loss, frequent urination, excessive thirst and blurred vision. Up to half of men with diabetes may develop impotence, because high blood sugar damages the nerves controlling the flow of blood into the penis.

Who gets diabetes? One answer can be found at the Great Genetic Roulette Wheel. With Type I diabetes, if both of your parents have it, there's a 20 percent chance that you'll get it, Dr. McEvoy estimates. If your brother or sister has Type I diabetes, your risk is 4 to 5 percent, he adds.

With Type II diabetes, the numbers game becomes a little more complicated. But simply, if a first-degree relative (your mother, father or sibling) has it,

Wild about Sugar

It's almost noon at the office, and people are bouncing off the walls. Or so it seems. Isn't there always someone who claims that the lack of sugar in his blood is turning him from a friendly Dr. Jekyll into a hell-realm Mr. Hyde? He says he needs a snack, not a shrink. He says he's hypoglycemic. Or is it hy*per*glycemic? Let's get this straight.

Hypoglycemia

Hypoglycemia is a condition marked by a low level of sugar in the blood. If you skip a meal or are late to the feeding trough, your body may suffer from insulin overload. There's too much of the hormone in relation to the amount of sugar in your body. Early signs of hypoglycemia are shakiness, nervousness, sweating, dizziness, weakness, irritability, hunger and a pounding heart. If it gets worse, you may stagger around, cry or get angry, drowsy or confused. Your vision can blur, and it's possible that you'll get a headache. You will definitely not feel like working.

Other causes: eating too much of a high-sugar or high-carbohydrate food such as caramel corn, marshmallows, hard candy or pancakes with maple syrup. Or a too-fast blood sugar drop in too short a time after an intense workout.

"Frequently, the symptoms of hypoglycemia are confused with the symptoms of panic or anxiety disorder: a pounding heart, profuse sweating and impaired vision," says Susan Thom, R.D., a Cleveland-based registered dietitian and certified diabetes educator who is a spokesperson for the American Dietetic Association. If it is hypoglycemia, try these quick remedies.

Fuel up. To help break the funky feeling, eat or drink one of the following: four ounces of fruit juice, five to six ounces of ginger ale or cola, three teaspoons of sugar dissolved in water, a tablespoon of honey or maple syrup, two tablespoons of raisins, a portion of fresh fruit or a bunch of hard candies. Don't chew a chunk of chocolate or a handful of nuts; they're full of fats that interfere with the absorption of sugar.

Be prepared. Keep pieces of fruit in your desk drawer, glove compartment and gym bag. A snack will go a long way

your chances of getting it are three to four times greater than the chances of someone without the family connection, according to Pat

toward making you feel like rejoining the human race.

Lay low. Admit it: When you have the low-sugar blues, you're no day at the beach. So distance yourself from those you work or live with, says Thom. While you're waiting for your blood sugar level to rise, excuse yourself. Take a short nap. Disappear behind a newspaper. Don a headset and chill out. Just eat something first, adds Thom.

Hyperglycemia

Hyperglycemia is high blood sugar. Proof that too much of a good thing is not necessarily a good thing, it usually kicks in after you've binged on too much food. It can also be triggered by some big-time mental or physical stress such as a major deadline, an acute illness, a car accident or surgery. "What happens in these cases is the release of the same hormones that respond to high-stress situations. They are all antagonistic to insulin," explains Thom. "So the body is less able to tolerate the same amount of carbohydrates." The result: less insulin, more blood sugar.

Symptoms of hyperglycemia include a flulike, achy feeling, blurred vision, thirst, lots of pit stops and tiredness. Here are some ways to give hyperglycemia the heave-ho.

Don't eat sugar solo. If you do eat high-sugar foods, eat them in the context of a meal—hopefully, a well-balanced meal that include fats and proteins, says Howard Reber, M.D., vice-chair of the Department of Surgery at the University of California, Los Angeles, UCLA School of Medicine, chief of surgery at Sepulveda Veterans Administration Medical Center, also in Los Angeles, and past president of the American Pancreatic Association. They'll blunt the absorption of sugar into your system. In other words, eat dessert when you're supposed to—after a meal, not by itself.

Don't push your pancreas. If you skip breakfast and lunch and then gorge yourself for dinner, you're asking your pancreas, which has been on a mini-vacation, to suddenly go back to work. "Now your poor pancreas has to work overtime, and it actually works too hard, producing too much insulin," explains Thom. Instead, spread your carbohydrate intake throughout the day by eating at normal intervals.

Who else gets it? Men get it: 49 percent of those with diabetes are men, says Susan Thom, R.D., a Cleveland-based registered dietitian and certified diabetes educator who is a spokesperson for the American Dietetic Association. "For a long time, we were told that diabetes is a disease of women. But men are catching up real fast," she notes. African-Americans, Native Americans and Hispanics are at greater risk than Caucasians for getting Type II diabetes. Obese people have a greater risk of getting it as well.

Pampering the Pancreas

There's no cure for diabetes once you have it; there is only managing it. But it is manageable. Whether you have diabetes, are at risk for getting it or just want to remain a normal, red-blooded specimen, take the following tips to heart, and your pancreas will benefit.

Pump that heart. "Daily aerobic exercise can stave off the development of Type II diabetes, even if someone in your family has it, even if you are overweight, suffer from high blood pressure and have a lousy diet," says Thom. We're not talking about a Jane Fonda workout here. Simply walking the dog, working in the garden or a short bike ride "might add ten healthy years to your life,"

Concannon, Ph.D., a researcher at the Virginia Mason Research Center of Virginia Mason Medical Center in Seattle.

she points out.

"It's fairly clear that exercise decreases cardiovascular risk, a problem for those with diabetes," adds William W. Fore, M.D., director of the Joslin Clinic of Diabetes at Wills and Jefferson in Philadelphia. Also, he says, exercise improves the way insulin works and can delay the onset of diabetes. "The key is finding something you enjoy doing and doing it."

Balance your eating act. First, forget the myths. "Eating carbohydrates is not going to give you diabetes," says Karmally. "Eating sugar won't give it to you." Rather, she suggests, don't pile up on foods without many nutrients, even if they're fat-free. Eat a variety of foods, including complex carbohydrates, fiber-containing grains, legumes and vegetables. And cut down on fat. If you eat chicken, remove the skin; trim the fat off meats; and stay away from those marbled steaks. She adds, "Eat more of the best and less of the rest."

"Diet is a negotiation," says Thom. "What would you be willing to give up, such as rolls and butter, in order to eat something else, such as red meat?"

Drop a few pounds. If you don't have diabetes now, "your chances of getting it in the future can be decreased by not gaining weight," according to Frank Vinicor, M.D., president of the American Diabetes Association and director of the Division of Diabetes Translation at the Centers for Disease Control and Prevention in Atlanta.

Make small strides. Start somewhere in building up your exercise regimen, and cut down on fats and other foods that aren't good for you. Remember that some exercise is better than none. Start with a walk halfway down the block, Thom suggests; then increase your goal. If you can burn 600 to 800 calories a week, you're making headway. "Guys who eat 1 to 1½ pounds of meat a day should try to cut back to 8 ounces—for starters," Thom recommends.

Be a man about it: Get checked out. "The real issue is not being afraid to find out once and for all if you have diabetes," says Richard Beaser, M.D., assistant clinical professor of medicine at Harvard Medical School, chairman of the patient education com-

mittee at Joslin Diabetes Center in Boston and co-author of *The Joslin Guide to Diabetes.* "There's this macho thing men have about not liking to show their weaknesses. In this case, that type of behavior can be deadly."

Study your family tree. Diabetes can be hereditary. Knowing if someone in your family has it or had it "is critical," according to Dr. Beaser. "The best advice for people with family histories of diabetes is: Don't let yourself get overweight, as obesity worsens insulin resistance."

Other Pancreas Issues

Like many of the other digestive organs, the pancreas is pretty much on autopilot. It does not require special feeding and handling. Rather—and this holds true for virtually every body part—lead a healthy lifestyle, and the pancreas is happiest.

"What you can do to keep your pancreas healthy is eat a well-balanced diet, drink moderately if you drink at all and exercise regularly," suggests Thom.

There are few things that can go wrong on the pancreas's digestive shift. One of them is pancreatitis. This inflammation occurs when the pancreas fails to produce the enzymes it needs to protect itself from its own powerful juices. Basically, the thing starts to eat itself and everything around it. About 80,000 cases of acute pancreatitis are reported in the United States each year, many the result of a gallstone getting stuck in the bile duct. (For more on that unpleasantry, see page 163.) But we mention pancreatitis to make a point: In more than 90 percent of adult patients suffering from chronic pancreatitis, the cause is long-term overdrinking. And the disease is more common among men—especially men between the ages of 30 and 40—than among women.

"The point is clear," warns James George, M.D., a physician in the Division of Gastroenterology at Mount Sinai Medical Center. "Drinking in excess causes irreversible damage to the pancreas and leads to chronic pancreatitis."

Penis 257

Λ\Penis

- Pamper it.
- Use it often.
- Be satisfied with what you have.

In 1879, in one of serious medical literature's earliest studies of penis size, a doctor named W. Krause reported that "in most cases," an erect penis is just under 8¼ inches long.

He was over the mark by only about 2½ inches.

More than a century after Dr. Krause's lengthy pronouncement, we still traffic in myths and misinformation about this most-prized organ. We men don't talk to one another openly, honestly, matter-of-factly about our penises. We follow the lead not of Masters and Johnson, the famed sex researchers, but rather of Lyndon Johnson, the U.S. president. We talk about Jumbo, as LBJ called his male member, in locker-room lingo. We brag. We joke. We gather and pass on lines, legends and lies, sometimes mixed in with facts.

That's counter to good health. The real key to building and maintaining penis vitality, health and fitness is maintaining an informed, respectful attitude about this most private and pleasurable appendage.

So here's some straight talk, right up front.

Most of us didn't get the foot-long model. One study of 200 Caucasians tagged the median-size penis at a little more than 5⅝ inches long when erect, reports Brazilian researcher Claudio Teloken, M.D. Seventy-six percent of the 200 penises measured ranged from about 4⅜ to 6¼ inches long when erect. Anywhere in that 1½-inch range is normal.

Twelve percent were shorter; 12 percent were longer.

Compare apples to apples. Don't use X-rated films as a gauge, warns Abraham Morgentaler, M.D., director of the male infertility and impotency program at Beth Israel Hospital in Boston and author of *The Male Body: A Physician's Guide to What Every Man Should Know about His Sexual Health*. Porn stars and nude male models are selected for their bigger-than-life equipment, just as girlie-mag models are selected for overly ripe lips and breasts. How many Pamela Lees do you know?

It all comes out in the wash. Give or take an inch, most penises inflate to about the same length when erect, regardless of flaccid length, says Dudley Seth Danoff, M.D., senior attending urologic surgeon at Cedars-Sinai Medical Center in Los Angeles and author of *Superpotency*.

Women, for the most part, couldn't care less about penis size. Average is fine with them, says Irwin Goldstein, M.D., professor of urology at Boston University School of Medicine. It's men who make the trek from the locker to the shower a game of inches.

The penis is a barometer. Sometimes it's up; sometimes it's down. It reflects your emotional state, comfort level and stress level, writes Dr. Danoff. When you're up, your penis is perky. When you're in the dumps—depressed, frazzled or uneasy—your penis

---

How to Measure

Not all doctors agree on where to hold the yardstick. Some place it above the penis, some below. You'll get the most satisfying measurement if you do it like this.

Start with an erection, then slide a ruler under your penis. Press the ruler firmly against your body just beneath where the penis shaft protrudes from the groin. Gently lay the erect penis atop the ruler and record the measurement.

This method offers the benefit of the doubt, says syndicated sex columnist Isadora Alman, because measuring from the top side of the base of the penis will yield a number that's approximately an inch less.

slumps. Accept it. All men limp along at times. Learn to talk about it instead of worrying.

We mellow with age, but we don't wither and die. A large study showed that half of all men over age 40 find it isn't always easy to be hard, says Dr. Goldstein. As we mature, our penises are less easily impressed. They want more stimulation before they stand up and dance. The solution: Devote more time and effort to sex. What's wrong with that?

We're not alone when we're alone. Pioneering sexologist Alfred Kinsey, D.Sc., found that 92 percent of us masturbate regularly. Married men are included in the count.

Obviously, there is much to learn about this intimate, precious organ. In a minute, we'll talk about care and maintenance tips for peak functioning. But first let's look at the miracle of hydraulics, just what this thing is and how and why it works the way it does.

Mechanical Wonder

We may think of the penis as an expandable, flexible rod, but it's really wishbone-shaped. We see only about half of it: the shaft portion that hangs outside the body. The remainder is inside the abdomen. It splits into a Y and attaches to the underside of the pubic bone. That anchors the penis, so it doesn't flop around excessively when erect and can be steered gently with . . . look, Ma, no hands!

The penis has three primary jobs, says Dr. Morgentaler.
1. To squirt urine where you point it
2. To fill with blood and become firm enough to enter a vagina
3. To dump sperm where it counts for making babies

Three chambers, running the length of the shaft, allow the penis to accomplish these tasks. Two are side-by-side erectile chambers. These are full of spongy tissue, which soaks up blood and expands when the brain signals certain arteries to begin pumping. The other, much smaller chamber runs along the bottom of the penis and houses the urethra, a tube that acts as the bladder's drainpipe and also as a

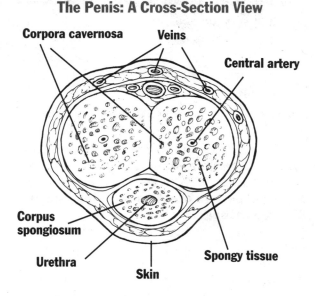

The Penis: A Cross-Section View

Corpora cavernosa — Veins — Central artery — Corpus spongiosum — Urethra — Skin — Spongy tissue

Blood floods the spongy chambers of the penis to create an erection. A leading cause of impotence is fatty deposits in the penile arteries, which diminish the flow of blood.

conduit for sperm, seminal and prostate fluids.

The erectile chambers are called corpora cavernosa and account for most of the penis's bulk, from its tippy-tip-tip to its anchors at the pubic bone. Each erectile chamber has a major artery that floods it with blood during arousal. As the blood pours in, the spongy tissue inside the chamber expands, slamming little veins that act as drains firmly against the chamber wall. That effectively clamps off the drains. So more blood in, less blood out, and soon you end up with a serious case of big stick.

It's up to the mind whether to start pumping blood into the erectile chambers and whether to keep it up. If the mind likes what it's seeing, thinking, feeling and dreaming, the penis stands up and stays up. The process is updated second by second. If the mind is distracted, irritated or discouraged at any point, the launch is aborted, and the penis deflates. Just like that.

When you climax, an enjoyable spurt of adrenaline races through your bloodstream. Adrenaline shuts down the erection quickly. It contracts the big arteries and the spongy tissue inside the erectile chambers. That loosens the clamp on the drain veins and lets them dump blood into a main drain called the deep dorsal vein. Then it's good-bye erection until the adrenaline dissipates or until your brain experiences enough sexual stimulation to overcome it.

The downtime is called the refractory period. It can be a momentary lapse for a teenager or a 24-hour waiting period for an older fella.

Downtime or not, all healthy men experience four or five erections while they're sleeping—up to about 180 minutes' worth per night for those in their teens and twenties. These erections seem to take place during dream periods but are not related to sexy dream content. Dr. Goldstein believes that this is your body's way of ensuring that your penis gets an adequate inflow of oxygen-rich blood, which is necessary for the production of prostaglandin E_1, a substance that keeps penile arteries clear. Nocturnal erections taper off some as a man ages. So for optimum penis health, a man needs to see that his penis experiences and sustains regular erections—at least three a week, says Dr. Goldstein. You don't have to tell us how you accomplish that.

That's how the machine works. There's a lot you can do to keep it working well.

Penis Power

A healthy flow of blood is essential to good penis function. Equally important is healthy self-esteem and the ability to diffuse stress, says Dr. Danoff.

Here are nine easy ways to improve penis vitality and assure optimum penis power for life.

Clean your pipes. Cut out fatty foods that clog the arteries of the penis as well as the heart and prevent healthy blood flow where it matters. Clogged arteries are linked to erectile weakness in older men. Experts say that by the time most men reach age 30, their penile arteries are clogged enough that erections are no longer as firm as they once were.

You can undo the damage and strengthen your erections with a low-fat, high-fiber diet, says Dr. Danoff. Limit your total daily fat intake to 30 percent or less of your calorie intake. And watch your cholesterol levels. Higher levels of HDL, the good cholesterol, have been linked to strong erections. Up your HDL by trading fats. Swap the saturated fat found in butter, meats and fried and processed foods for the monounsaturated fat found in canola oil, olive oil, nuts and avocados.

Get aerobic, get erotic. Run, row, bike. At least 30 minutes of heart-pumping exercise three times a week keeps the blood and oxygen flowing to your penis and throughout your body. Plus aerobic exercise builds stamina. You won't huff and puff and have to stop for breathers during prolonged sexual encounters.

Make like Elvis. Do the hula. Dr. Danoff claims a limber pelvis gives you more control over your penis during intercourse. And pelvic exercise increases circulation in the whole region. A few minutes a day working out with a hula hoop is ideal. Absent the toy, just try thrusting and gyrating like a hula dancer. A little music makes it more fun. You might want to draw the shades.

Ejaculate often. It is a wonderful stress reliever and is said to keep sperm from stagnating. And while not all doctors agree, some believe it can relieve or prevent prostatic congestion.

Stop smoking. Nicotine constricts blood vessels. That means each puff makes it harder for blood to get to the penis. And smoking leads to plaque buildup in the arteries, including those that serve the penis. Certainly, if you must smoke, it's better to wait until after sex, like in the movies.

Feel good about your body. You gain pride by taking care of yourself: exercising, stretching, grooming, feeding yourself healthfully. You don't have to look like a Hollywood hunk to feel like a million dollars, says Dr. Danoff. When you feel good about yourself, your penis knows and repays you in kind.

Relax and let go. Letting troubles get the best of you withers your penis's confidence, says Dr. Danoff. It's hard to convince a penis to stand up straight and look the world in the eye when its owner is slumping like Atlas. If you're particularly tense, you can relax your way into lovemaking with a hot bath, either by yourself or with your partner. Besides soothing you all over, the hot water increases blood flow into your penis.

Physical exercise is another wonderful stress buster. Working out works it off.

Here are two one-minute stress-diffusing relaxation exercises that you can use throughout the day.

1. Close your eyes and take five slow, deep breaths. Hold each breath for a few seconds, then release it fully, slowly. Pause and repeat. Picture, as vividly as possible, a peaceful, pleasing scene.

2. Either lying on your back on the floor or standing, stretch your arms above your head and spread your toes and fingers as far as you comfortably can. Stretch, first tensing every muscle in your body for five seconds, then going limp for five seconds. Repeat six times.

Don't abuse it. Be gentle to your penis. It's made to last a lifetime when treated right. Don't force it to make U-turns when erect, don't coat it with caustic substances and avoid excessive friction, advises Paul Gleich, M.D., chief of urology at St. Paul–Ramsey Medical Center in St. Paul, Minnesota.

Consume chromium. This trace element stabilizes blood sugar and may prevent penis-crippling diabetes in adults. Get it from broccoli, wheat germ and bran cereals. You might want to take a supplement to ensure that you get the recommended 50 to 200 micrograms daily, says Dr. Gleich.

Get Physical

In an old joke, Sensitive Guy wants to work out a simple signal so that his bride can let him know when she does and doesn't want his amorous advances. "If you're in the mood," he tells her, "just grasp my penis and tug on it three times."

"And what should I do if I'm not in the mood?" she asks.

"Oh, same thing," says Sensitive Guy. "Just grasp my penis and pull on it a hundred times."

Here's our humorless response: Repeated tugging, rubbing and stroking, enlightening and satisfying as it may be, can rub a penis raw if lubrication is not adequate. "You'd be amazed at how many men come into my office with sore skin," says Dr. Gleich. "They're just having a lot of intercourse or masturbating frequently. Men can get scratched up and sore from vigorous sexual activity."

The sexually sophisticated man keeps a lubricant within reach of his lair and employs it when needed. Oils are fun to experiment with but may stain bedding and clothing, contribute to vaginal infections and cause latex condoms to disintegrate, says marriage and family therapist Patricia Love, Ph.D., co-author of *Hot Monogamy: Essential Steps to More Passionate, Intimate Lovemaking*. Commercial water-soluble lubricants are less messy and are compatible with latex. Dr. Love recommends Astroglide as "the premier lubricant."

Besides rubbing your penis the right way, here are some other tips for keeping it in tip-top physical shape.

Keep it on a leash. Be careful where you put that thing. Genital warts, genital herpes, AIDS—need we say more?

"Monogamy is probably the healthiest behavior a penis can practice," says Dr. Gleich. But for some reason, it's not a choice everyone makes, so beyond monogamy, be sure to wear a latex condom. (For much more on this, see page 31.)

Steer carefully. Overall, the penis is quite durable. Still, an erect penis should not be bent severely, or slammed headlong into an unforgiving surface, or smashed with a hammer. You can wind up with what's called a penis fracture. This isn't really a fracture, because the penis has no bones. Instead, tissue in the wall of an erectile chamber rips.

"When it rips, you may hear a crack, pop or tearing sound," says Dr. Gleich. "You suddenly lose your erection, and your penis becomes swollen and discolored from the blood escaping the chamber. It does get your attention, but it's usually not painful." Most fractures heal on their own, but "current thinking is that we should fix them surgically by sewing the tears shut to make sure they don't heal crooked," says Dr. Gleich.

Fractures are a suspected cause of Peyronie's disease, a rare condition in which the penis severely lists to the left, to the right, upward or downward when erect. The fractures may occur when men roll over on erections while sleeping, doctors speculate. Scar tissue at the injury site eventually deforms the erectile chamber. Some curvature is common. But an extreme bend that prevents intercourse requires surgical correction and possibly the insertion of a prosthesis.

Jilt jungle rot. Heat and moisture can have caustic effects on the innocent penis, bringing on a case of heat rash, fungus or another skin infection. The remedy for each is similar, though, says Dr. Gleich. Keep the region clean and dry, avoid chafing, use talc when you know you'll be working up a sweat and zap jock itch quickly with an over-the-counter antifungal remedy.

Face the hard facts. A solid hard-on that just won't go away might seem like a great conversation piece. Fact is, it's dangerous. After a couple of hours, the oxygen-starved blood in the erectile chambers starts to thicken, penis tissue that's hungry for nutrients suffers, and serious damage takes place. Not to mention pain: The big guy aches.

This condition, called priapism, once was quite rare. But with the advent in the 1980s of papaverine and prostaglandin E_1 injections to induce erections, priapism is back in a big way, so to speak.

Men with erection difficulties are trained to inject the drug no more than once a day. A designated small dose produces an erection for about a half-hour. Those tempted to abuse the drug end up with big, aching, stagnant hard-ons to explain to the emergency room doctor.

Treatment is simple: a penile injection of adrenaline or the blood vessel–constricting antihistamine phenylephrine hydrochloride, says Dr. Gleich.

You don't have to shoot up to get priapism. It's a possible side effect of a long list of oral medications. And using a so-called cock ring that is too small can do it, too. If you can't coax the friendly fella down within two hours, call your doctor or get to an emergency room. What goes up must come down, or gangrene will set in.

A perpetual hard-on is a problem that most of us will never face. But sooner or later, all of us deal with a glum Mr. Happy, as comedian Robin Williams calls it. Penises don't automatically rise to the occasion on every occasion. And there are many reasons.

Standing Tall

While President Calvin Coolidge and his wife were visiting an egg farm, the story goes, Mrs. Coolidge noted how many sitting hens there were and how few roosters. The roosters, she commented, must really get around.

Oh yes, said the farmer, they perform their duty dozens of times a day.

"You might point that out to Mr. Coolidge," the First Lady said.

The president was intrigued.

And does the rooster mate with the same hen every time? the president asked.

Oh no, said the farmer, the roosters are free to mount any hen they feel like.

"You might point that out to Mrs. Coolidge," the president said.

That, they say, is how the Coolidge Effect worked its way into medical nomenclature. The term describes a situation many men encounter sooner or later: At some point, the old penis tires of the same old sex with the same old lady. It has trouble getting worked up. But it perks right up when some new babe walks by.

The Coolidge Effect is perhaps the greatest reason that men in long-term relationships experience erection failure, Dr. Danoff says. And anxiety, he says, is the leading cause of erection difficulty with a new partner. Most erection problems, says Dr. Danoff, are the result of boredom or of psychosomatic factors such as stress and anxiety, which increase the flow of adrenaline in the body. We've already seen what a downer adrenaline is to erections.

Dr. Morgentaler is less convinced that most erection problems are psychologically based, though he agrees that many are. He says that if erection difficulty gets progressively worse over a long period of time, the problem is most likely physical. If it occurs suddenly, he suspects stress or other psychophysical factors—or the onset of an illness.

We will deal with the physical causes of erectile dysfunction in a moment. But first, here are some ways to perk up a penis that is suffering from anxiety, or low self-esteem, or boredom.

Shake things up. Break the routine. Change anything. Change everything. Sameness breeds boredom and disinterest and diminished desire. Try different locations, times, clothes, scents, positions, oils, toys, lighting, music, foreplay, words, fantasies, erotica. Commit to keeping things fresh and restoring surprise and mystery.

Pamper your penis. No matter how exciting we find life, our erections soften some as we get older. This often begins by age 30. Testosterone levels are down, diminishing sexual desire. Plaque levels in the arteries feeding the penis are up. And Little Elvis doesn't twitch with quite the same conviction as when he was 18.

No need to send your penis out to pasture. Instead, Dr. Danoff says, enjoy the slower pace, increase stimulation, use lubricants to heighten sensation and, for great blood flow, follow the diet and exercise tips offered earlier.

And remember, you don't need to maintain a steel-hard erection for the full duration of a sexual interlude. Your erection can come and go while you and your partner explore other pleasing possibilities and oppor-

tunities. Good sex is more than just penetration and humping and pumping.

Deal with depression. If you are down or have the blues, your penis is likely to be down, too. And that's okay, says Dr. Danoff. If you're chronically depressed, seek professional help. You can get over it.

Check your meds—at the bedroom door. Read the fine print. An amazing number of prescription and over-the-counter medications interfere with sex drive and sexual functioning. Among the most common offenders are some popular antidepressants and blood pressure regulators. Often you can switch to a different drug if the one you're on turns your penis off.

Sleep now, play later. When you're physically or mentally exhausted, your penis may be, too. Sometimes you should just give it a rest.

Plug performance anxiety. Nobody bats 1,000. And if you start to think you're going to miss every time you swing, you start to dread hearing "Batter's up." In sex, it's the same. Worry about this time based on last time, and soon you're in trouble every time. The key is to face up to it immediately and talk about it, says Dr. Danoff. Admit you're stressed out, or unable to relax, or whatever. Suggest a massage or something else fun and relaxing besides intercourse. And then forget about it. Really.

Talk about it. If Snoopy has gotten droopy and never comes when called, talk to a psychotherapist or sex counselor, says Dr. Morgentaler. Just talking about the situation loosens you up, and a counselor can help you develop positive strategies and penis pep talks that work.

Avoid excessive drinking. A few sips may warm desire and drop inhibitions. More may numb the penis-brain connection and drown any possibility of an erection. And regular excessive drinking causes hormone and brain chemical changes that put the damper on both sexual desire and wherewithal.

Opt for the oral alternative. Encourage

your partner to suck on your penis. Besides feeling quite nice, actual sucking (not licking, which is sometimes referred to as sucking) creates a vacuum in the corpora cavernosa and literally draws blood into the chambers, says Dr. Danoff. Relax and enjoy it. This can stimulate an erection.

Stamp out ignorance. A healthy man has several erections each night during periods of deep sleep. Of course, short of waking with a hard-on, you have no way of knowing for sure whether this is happening. But if it is, you can probably rule out physical causes of any erectile dysfunction that you may be experiencing. To find out, take Dr. Danoff's do-it-yourself postage stamp test. Glue a strip of stamps around your penis before falling asleep. (Bend the perforations back and forth a couple of times first.) If the perforations are torn in the morning, you know your equipment is working. If not, a urologist can run more sophisticated tests and recommend ways to restore erectile function.

Mechanical Problems

A penis will not stand up if it does not have a strong inflow of blood or if it cannot shut down the drains and hold on to the blood that is pumped in. A penis won't respond to mental or physical stimuli if nerves carrying signals between it and the brain are damaged.

Injuries as well as diseases such as diabetes and multiple sclerosis can cause nerve damage. Diabetes also often causes hardening of the arteries, which interferes with blood flow.

Using ultrasound and other high-tech devices, doctors can watch for and identify problems with blood flow. And often they can correct them. Here are some alternatives.

See a surgeon. If blood flow is impaired by an injury, plaque buildup or hardening of the arteries, it can be improved by routing another artery to the penis. This is called a

---

Lengthening Your Penis

Porn star Long Dong Silver has posed for publicity photos with his 18-inch-long breadwinner tied in a knot. We don't advise you to try this at home.

Most of us wouldn't want to. We wouldn't want to do anything that would make our penises look shorter. In fact, there are those among us who would like to add an inch or two. If this is truly important to you, it can be done. Here are two ways.

See a surgeon. From 40 to 60 percent of your penis is concealed within your abdomen. The penis root, however, can be cut loose from the ligaments that anchor it to the underside of your pubic bone. When the penis is unhinged from the pelvis, more of it can protrude from the abdomen, usually an additional 1 to 1½ inches. A patch of skin from elsewhere on your body must be grafted onto the base of your penis to allow for a longer shaft. The longer penis that results may look a little odd and be a little wobbly. This procedure is recommended only for men with especially short penises, known medically as micropenises, according to Paul Gleich, M.D., chief of urology at St. Paul–Ramsey Medical Center in St. Paul, Minnesota. For them, it could mean a gratifying 100 percent increase in length.

Some doctors are injecting fat cells to increase penis girth, but the results are lumpy and temporary. The procedure is not advised, says Dr. Gleich.

Lose weight. Fat in the pubic region actually results in a shorter penis. This condition is reversible! Some very obese men suffer what is called disappearing penis. Most of the penis lies rooted within the abdominal fat, with only the tiniest stub protruding. Most overweight men will gain an inch in penis length for every 35 pounds they lose—up to a point.

bypass, says Dr. Morgentaler.

Drain veins that leak consistently can be tied off. The tie-off surgery has about a 50 percent success rate, says Dr. Morgentaler, and is often combined with a bypass for better results.

Inflate with an implant. Inflatable tubes are inserted in the penis, a pump and an on-off switch are hidden in the scrotum, and a fluid reservoir is implanted in the groin. Push the button in your scrotum, the tubes fill with gel, and you have an erection. Push the button again, and the fluid drains back to the reservoir. No more erection.

A simpler implant, consisting of a couple of flexible rods, can be placed in the penis. With this option, though, your penis may look a little odd in the locker room. The implant never deflates; it just bends conveniently to fit in your shorts when you don't need your penis in an upright position.

Induce erections with injections. Injecting a drug directly into the side of the penis through a tiny needle increases arterial blood flow and shuts down drain veins in many men, providing a serviceable 30-minute erection. Injections are good for at-home use, but the drugs must be refrigerated, so they're harder to handle on the road, notes Dr. Morgentaler.

Operate in a vacuum. In letters to *Penthouse*, men have at times extolled the virtues of placing their penises in a vacuum cleaner hose (a dangerous practice that sometimes ruptures blood vessels). Modern medicine offers a safe hydraulic suction device that works on the same principle. A long plastic cylinder is placed over the penis and pushed, airtight, against the groin. A hand-squeezed or battery-operated pump attached to the top creates suction inside. This draws blood into the penis. When the penis is engorged, a tight rubber ring is slipped down to the base of the shaft to prevent blood from escaping. A vacuum device, while difficult to explain on a first date, could be a blessing in an otherwise rock-solid relationship.

For many men, the problem is not how to get it up but how to keep it from firing too soon. We look at that next.

How to Last All Night

In the teen ritual game of circle jerk, boys compete in a darkened room to see who can get themselves off the fastest. In the real world of sexual finesse and sophistication, speed demons win no prizes. Men are expected to withhold their ejaculate until their partners achieve some satisfaction and enjoyment from the coupling.

As enjoyable as prolonging sex can be, it doesn't seem to be innate in the male nature. But a skillful cocksman develops brain-body tuning and toning to hold off the inevitable. If you have never practiced holding back ejaculation, don't expect to be able to do it immediately. But practice will pay off. Here's how it's done.

Build endurance. Pay attention to how it feels as you near the point of no return while masturbating and while making love. Practice building up to and backing down from that point again and again, advises Dr. Danoff. Some men stop thrusting when they feel they are close to the edge. Some breathe slowly and deeply until the tension passes, then resume sex slowly. Others withdraw entirely for a while. Others shift gears, changing speed, depth, position or motion.

Tense up. Apply the brakes as you approach the danger zone by tensing the pubococcygeus muscle tightly until the urge to ejaculate passes. The pubococcygeus muscle is the one you tighten when you need to stop urinating midstream. Daily tensing and releasing of that muscle strengthens it and your control over it. The process is known as a Kegel exercise. (For more information on this, see the full description in "The Ooh-la-la Factor" on page 266.)

Squeeze it. Masters and Johnson teach another technique, called the squeeze or the choke method, for postponing ejaculation. Grasp your penis around the shaft and squeeze firmly, from underside to top, for about four seconds, then release. When the urge to ejaculate subsides, resume sex—slowly at first. This may be repeated as needed.

⚠ Prostate

- **Exercise a lot.**
- **Stand up a lot.**
- **Urinate often.**
- **Get regular exams beginning at age 40.**

When legendary country songwriter Hank Williams crooned "I'll Never Get Out of This World Alive," chances are he wasn't singing about his prostate. But he could have been.

This walnut-size gland, which helps us squeeze every ounce of pleasure from sex, secretly breeds cancer. Prostate cancer is the chart-topping cancer among men over age 50. One in 8 of us will develop prostate cancer, and 1 in 20 of us will die from it. By age 100, we all have it. Overall, it's the second leading killer cancer in men.

Sometimes it's a virulent cancer that runs by night, without lights and in perfect silence, then launches surprise attacks that take out some of the best and brightest. But usually, it develops slowly. When caught early, it can be zapped. If discovered after spreading, it can be treated—for a while. The object of this game is to snag it early.

What the Prostate Does

The prostate's job is to manufacture globs of milky fluid for sperm to surf through. About 90 percent of ejaculate is prostate fluid. The prostate secretes and stores the fluid during sexual arousal. The juice is squeezed and pumped into the urethra as you climax. It mixes with sperm from the testicles, and the whole wad spurts out of your penis.

It's a small but important job. Prostate fluid insulates and protects sperm from the hostile environments they encounter once they exit the penis and begin searching for an egg to fertilize.

And, researchers say, it appears as though prostate fluid carries flowers and talks sweetly to a woman's cervix. It somehow coaxes the cervix to relax, open up and pay no mind to the flotilla of sperm rapidly approaching.

Healthy and Happy

For a small gland with a rather limited role, the prostate has some big secondary effects, good and bad. Good: The prostate is rich with nerve endings that make you feel oh-so-fine during sex. Bad: The prostate not only is highly susceptible to cancer but often presents older men with other debilitating troubles as well. We'll get to all of these in a bit. But first, what matters most: what you can do to keep your prostate healthy for life, in six easy steps.

Walk, run, ride your bike. Men in good shape have less prostate trouble, plain and simple. So get more exercise.

Pee often. Dad may have considered it a virtue if you could hold it from St. Louis to Akron, but as they say in the commercial, "This is not your father's Oldsmobile." An overly filled bladder can relatively easily back up pee into the prostate. When that happens, you'll know it. Your prostate will get . . . well, pissed. So relieve yourself often.

In particular, "always empty your bladder before doing any exercise or lifting," says E. David Crawford, M.D., chairman of the Division of Urology at the University of Colorado Health Sciences Center and director of the Colorado Prostate Center, both in Denver. It's easy to irritate your prostate with urine during exercise.

Wag your tail. Get up and move around. Don't sit for too long. You're sitting on your prostate, squishing it. It's under enough pressure already.

Savor sex regularly. Tough medicine, we know. Regular ejaculation keeps your prostate from getting stagnant and inflamed from congestion. If you don't have an eager partner handy, take things into your own hands: Masturbate. Doctor's orders.

Truck drivers, motorcycle cops, bicycle riders and others whose genitalia are subjected to constant vibration are particularly prone to congestion. The vibration apparently teases the prostate into secreting fluid. It becomes engorged when there is no release.

Trim the fat. A diet high in fatty foods seems to irritate the prostate and increase cancer risk. Saturated fat seems particularly troublesome.

The best meals for prostate health are low in fat and cholesterol and big on vegetables, whole grains, leafy greens and fiber. Foods high in vitamins A, C and E are particularly healthy for the prostate. Good sources of vitamin A include carrots, squash, pumpkin, sweet potatoes, apricots, cantaloupe and dark green, leafy veggies such as spinach, kale and broccoli. For vitamin C, load up on citrus fruits and juices, strawberries, peppers (both red and green), broccoli, tomatoes, melons, brussels sprouts and cauliflower. Get your vitamin E from wheat germ, peanut butter, almonds, sunflower seeds, shrimp, vegetable oils and green, leafy vegetables.

Zig toward zinc-rich foods. Your prostate thrives on them. The jury is out on whether zinc supplements help or hurt, but foods high in zinc content definitely soothe and support your prostate. Zinc-rich foods include oysters, soy, nuts, pumpkin seeds, wheat germ, bran, milk, eggs, chicken, lentils, peas and beef liver.

Preventing Cancer

Prostate cancer is mercilessly sneaky. It shows no symptoms until it's serious. Reg-

The Ooh-la-la Factor

The pleasant tingling sensation you feel deep inside your crotch during sexual excitement? That's your prostate humming a love song.

Most of us pay no attention to the prostate until it malfunctions or becomes diseased. But the prostate deserves our gratitude. After all, it is largely responsible for some of our more delicious sexual sensations, says psychologist and sexologist John D. Perry, Ph.D., co-author of *The G-Spot*.

The prostate is sometimes referred to as the male G-spot because it is so sensitive to sexual stimulation. The nerve-rich organ tingles as it secretes fluid during arousal and ejaculation. The prostate also responds warmly to direct massage and muscular contractions. The prostate especially appreciates firm pressure in the perineum (the vacant land between the scrotum and the rectum), says Dr. Perry. And we're grateful.

Here are two fun things to do with your prostate, if you are so inclined.

Massage it. Gay men know that stimulating the prostate increases sexual pleasure. The gland gets quite a workout in male anal sex.

Dr. Perry suggests that all men take advantage of the heightened pleasure gained from stimulating the prostate. You or your partner can firmly press (as in deep massage) on the perineum or slide a lubricated finger in the anus and stroke the prostate.

Some doctors are wary of this and warn that any form of anal sex has the potential to spread disease. Dr. Perry thinks that's just hang-ups talking. "They're just trying to cover their butts," he says colorfully. A good cleanup following sex should be adequate, he says.

Exercise it. If you're uncomfortable with the finger-in-the-rectum suggestion, practice Kegel exercises, says Dr. Perry. They strengthen and tone the muscles that stimulate the prostate. The exercise also helps with sustaining erections and withholding ejaculation.

Do a round of ten Kegels several times a day—while driving, or sitting at work, or eating. Just don't do the Meg Ryan fake-orgasm movie bit, and no one will be the wiser. Simply contract the same muscles that you tense to stop in the middle of peeing. Hold tight for a count of ten, then release. That's one. Now do nine more.

Locating the Prostate

All men age 50 or older should have a digital rectal exam and a prostate-specific antigen, or PSA, test every year to check for prostate cancer.

ular exams are the only way to nip it in the bud. Cancer caught early can be stopped cold 91 percent of the time. Here are some suggestions from Dr. Crawford on how to do that.

Checkmate cancer with checkups. All men should have a digital/rectal exam every two years beginning at age 40 as well as a prostate-specific antigen (PSA) test every two years beginning at age 50, switching to every year at age 60.

The digital/rectal exam is where the doctor slips on a glove, lubricates his finger and says "Bend over the table and spread 'em." The doctor feels as much of the prostate as possible through the rectum wall, probing for lumps, growths, hardening and more.

The PSA test is a blood test. It finds cancer that the finger misses.

Don't delay testing until you're age 50 if you urinate blood, have a hard time urinating or are in a high-risk group.

Rate your risk factors. African-Americans and men who have family members with prostate cancer are at highest risk. They should get a baseline PSA in their early thirties

and then begin routine annual exams at age 40. "I've operated on people in their thirties with prostate cancer," says Dr. Crawford.

Dealing with Cancer

Television actor Bill Bixby survived life with a naive Martian and the travails of raising Eddie, but when he wasn't looking, his prostate killed him. Musician Frank Zappa survived a brain-spraining, larynx-smashing, leg-breaking fall off a concert stage, but he also met his match with prostate cancer.

In both men, the cancer was found too late to be stopped. But when prostate cancer is caught early, the cure rate is high.

So your annual exam indicates cancer. What next?

The urologist does a needle biopsy, an in-office procedure, to extract some prostate cells. The biopsy reveals how active the cancer is. Once that is known, a course of treatment can be discussed. Treatments vary drastically.

With a slow-growing cancer, the treatment often is to simply keep an eye on it. More than 80 percent of prostate cancers are in men over age 65. For most, it's unlikely the cancer will get out of control in their lifetimes.

Cancer in younger men often is more virulent because younger men have a longer risk time for the cancer to grow and spread. These men often require aggressive treatment. For cancer that hasn't escaped the prostate, doctors can:

- Blast the prostate with x-ray beams.
- Seed the prostate with radioactive pellets. This causes impotence 50 percent of the time and can cause incontinence.
- Freeze the entire prostate.
- Slice out the entire prostate or portions of it and possibly excise surrounding lymph nodes. But this procedure and the

one above result in infertility and cause impotence in many men and incontinence in a few.

If the cancer has spread beyond the prostate, forget prostate surgery. Expect radiation treatments, chemotherapy, hormone-blocking shots or castration.

Why the latter? The spread of prostate cancer cells is fueled by male hormones, says Grant Mulholland, M.D., chairman of the Department of Urology at Thomas Jefferson University Hospital in Philadelphia. Blocking testosterone production with drugs or by castration prolongs life 80 percent of the time.

If your cancer has spread, these treatments won't buy you life, but they will buy you time. Make the most of it.

BPH: The Main Squeeze

It's time to drain the alligator. You know it. The gator knows it. But for some reason, it just doesn't want to start. Then it starts. Weakly. You can't pee with force. Your bladder begins emptying, but like Mick Jagger, you can't get no satisfaction. You don't feel any relief as you relieve yourself. Instead, the pee stream sputters; it starts and stops more than a rush-hour commuter on an LA freeway. Then your penis says "That's all, Bubba. We're done now." But it doesn't feel like that's all, like you're done. But apparently, you are. You shake the thing and ring it out and slip it back into your trousers. Then it squirts. Or dribbles. Leaving a new challenge: how to hide the wet spot on your trousers.

Any of these symptoms, or any combination of them, can indicate benign prostatic hyperplasia, or BPH for short. Other symptoms include an increasingly frequent urge to whiz; waking often at night to pee, even when you haven't guzzled a quick-stop 44-ounce cola before nodding off; unexplained lower back pain; and possibly pain in the perineum or a sensation that you are sitting on a golf ball.

BPH starts around the time you celebrate the Big 4-0. That's when your prostate decides to embark on a little personal growth.

The growth itself would be of no

consequence were it not for location, location, location. The prostate surrounds the urethra, the hose that carries urine and sperm out of the penis. Often as the prostate swells in size, it chokes off the hose. And you can no longer pee with power. Sometimes you can't pee at all, even when you hop from foot to foot.

While prostate cancer will challenge about 12 percent of us, prostate enlargement will cause problems for about 50 percent of us.

Treatment is needed only if the condition is bothersome or if you really can't pee. If you can't pee, get to a doctor quickly. You'll damage your kidneys if your plumbing backs up for too long.

The type of treatment required for BPH depends upon the severity of the problem. It can range from doing little or nothing to emergency surgery, with lots of options in between. Here are some.

Cut the hormones. Doctors believe that prostate growth is activated by natural changes in hormonal balance as your body ages. The key to treating it, in most cases, is to cool your body's production of a certain constituent of testosterone called dihydrotestosterone (DHT).

"In the late 1800s, they used to castrate men for prostate enlargement," says Dr. Crawford. "It worked. It resulted in shrinkage of the prostate. Needless to say, that wasn't an extremely popular treatment.

"Now we have the ability to alter the male hormone action, to lower it with drugs, particularly the drug Proscar (finasteride). What it does is block the development of the DHT hormone."

Relax chemically. The muscles in the prostate tend to relax in response to high blood pressure drugs known as alpha-blockers. As the muscles relax, they loosen their grip on the urethra. "In about 24 hours, you have an improvement in your urinary flow," Dr. Crawford says.

Medicate with herbs. For 20 years, physicians in Europe have been prescribing herbal medications that seem to relax and shrink the prostate, according to their studies. Two commonly used herbal medications are extracts of saw palmetto (*Serenoa repens*) and *Pygeum africanum.*

Some holistic health–oriented physicians in the United States dispense saw palmetto and pygeum herbal extracts and compounds containing them or refer patients to health food stores that sell them, says Willard Dean, M.D., a holistic physician in Santa Fe, New Mexico. The remedies seem to be effective in reducing symptoms in many cases of BPH, he says, and seem to have few, if any, side effects.

If all else fails, consider surgery. According to Dr. Crawford, surgical treatments are effective and may be required in serious or stubborn cases. Surgery comes with potential risks of impotence, reverse ejaculation (the ejaculate shoots backward into the bladder) and, in a tiny percentage of men, permanent incontinence.

Serious side effects are most common with the traditional prostate surgery, called open prostatectomy. Here, the surgeon slices through the abdomen or perineum to reach the prostate and then trims the area that is impinging upon the plumbing. Open surgery is the only option if the prostate has ballooned to extraordinary proportions.

Newer surgical procedures are exquisitely delicate. Using a scope or ultrasound guidance, a surgeon can direct tiny instruments through the urethra, find the obstruction and:

- Pop it open. A collapsed metal stent is guided up to the point where the prostate is squeezing the urethra. The tubelike, wire mesh stent is popped open and left in place.
- Microwave it. A microwave heating rod, slid up the urethra, cooks the swollen area for a few minutes. With repeated treatments, the swollen area relaxes its stranglehold on the urethra.
- Burn it with a tiny laser.
- Vaporize it with a miniature rolling pin that transmits high-frequency electrical current.
- Trim, slice or ream it. With tiny, tiny blades, the surgeon cuts away tissue impinging upon the urethra, slices the

inside of the prostate to open a little more room or reams out a circular core.

Infections: Doing a Slow Burn

Old Faithful down there suddenly starts to drip and burn when you pee or have an orgasm, just like in the scare films they showed in eighth grade. But you haven't been dirty dancing with strangers in years.

Before you rush off to the county clinic or hire a private detective to spy on your one and only, see a urologist. It could be that your old pal the prostate has gotten infected.

"Who knows why?" says Dr. Crawford. "If bacteria get into the prostate, they're difficult to eradicate. It can take three months of antibiotics."

Bacterial invaders such as chlamydia, *Escherichia coli* and staph lodge in and between crystalline stones in the prostate, then just lie back and wave at the antibiotics floating by. It takes a lot of antibiotics to swamp them.

But Dr. Crawford presents a worst-case scenario. In fact, most prostate infections and inflammations are nonbacterial. Some are viral. Others are chemical, such as from getting urine backed up into the prostate. High-risk activities include anal sex and wearing a catheter. But cooties can find you at the beach or in a pool, too. Or an infection can simply migrate from somewhere else in your body.

And then there are prostate infections caused by lifestyle. Men "use their prostates and bladders as end organs for stress," says Dr. Mulholland. The prostate has the same type of nerve fibers as the stomach, colon and other body parts that we tend to tense when we are stressed. In one large study, when men complaining of prostate pain were taught stress-management techniques, 89 percent experienced long-term relief of symptoms.

Prostate infections are most common between ages 30 and 50 but can hit any time after adulthood. Symptoms of a prostate infection can be identical to, or worse than, BPH symptoms. An acute infection can slam you with high fever and severe pain and land you in a hospital bed, sprouting intravenous tubes.

◤ Reproductive System

- **Temperature difference between the scrotum and the rest of the body: 4° to 7°F cooler**
- **Rank of testicular cancer among the most common cancers in young men: 1**
- **Number of frozen ejaculates for sale through fertility clinics in the United States: well over 100,000**
- **Number of sperm present per milliliter of semen: 50 million to 100 million**

The Real Reason for Sex

Sexual pleasure is a very good thing. But the male reproductive system has a more rational purpose: to produce and deliver sperm to the female reproductive tract, where they can fertilize a female egg, or ovum. The two concepts might not be unrelated, of course. Feeling good is a wonderful incentive to produce and deliver more sperm.

For sperm, the job calls for lots of travel. Produced within the testicles, sperm travel through some 20 feet of tightly coiled epididymis over the course of 20 days. During arousal, the sperm are expelled from the epididymis, heading north-bound through a 1.5-foot tube called the vas deferens, which wraps up and over the bladder. During ejaculation, sperm head back south through the roughly six-inch urethra before being blasted out of the body.

Accessory glands help the process along. The prostate's main job is to manufacture an opaque fluid whenever its owner gets sexually aroused. That fluid mixes with sperm in the urethra and makes up roughly 90 percent of semen. Other, smaller glands also secrete fluids into the urethra prior to ejaculation as part of the semen creation process. ∎

Sexual Averages

- Average number of times men have sex each month: 7
- Average volume of ejaculate: 2.75 milliliters
- Percent decline in average volume of ejaculate over the past 40 years: 20
- Average number of sperm a man produces daily: 400 million
- Percent decline in average sperm count over the past 40 years: 40
- Average amount a Caucasian sperm donor receives per donation: $45
- Average cost of one vial of sperm (enough for one artificial insemination): $100
- Average number of hours that sperm remain potent inside a woman's reproductive tract: 12 to 48 ∎

Keeping Your Reproductive System Healthy

Experts say these are ways to keep you (re)productive.

Take plenty of vitamin A. This vitamin is vital for keeping the adult reproductive system functioning properly. Deficiency causes glandular problems and sterility. Aim for the Daily Value of 5,000 international units.

Get your need of vitamin C. It is naturally found in high concentrations in sperm and is generally believed to protect genetic material from free radical damage. Get the Daily Value of 60 milligrams.

Eat enough zinc. At least one study has shown a direct correlation between adequate

Elsewhere . . .

- **Prostate**   Page 31
- **Sex**   Page 257
- **Penis**   Page 265
- **Sperm**   Page 304
- **Testicles**   Page 323

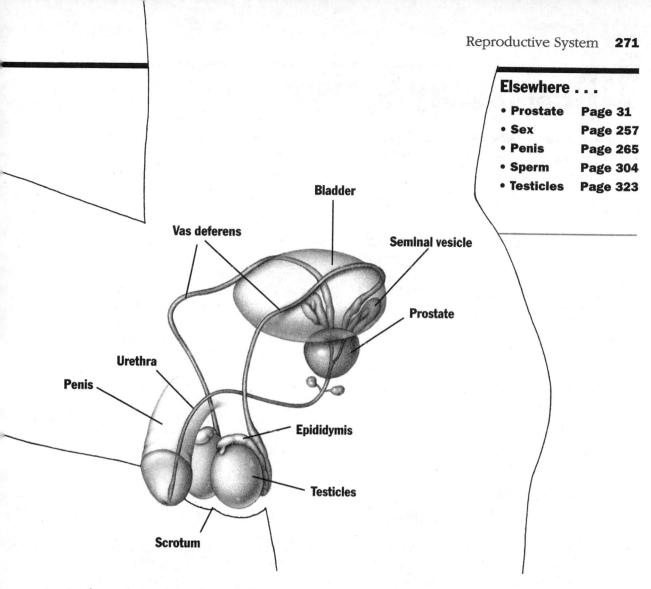

zinc intake and ejaculate quantity. Doctors recommend the Daily Value of 15 milligrams; get this amount from foods such as crab, oysters and lean beef or from supplements.

Nix nicotine. Nicotine helps destroy vitamin C and has been shown to diminish sperm concentration, motility and shape. Smokers need higher doses of vitamin C to offset these problems. In one study of 75 young smokers, those receiving 1,000 milligrams of vitamin C every day for a month experienced less sperm damage than those taking 200 milligrams a day.

Play it safe. Your sexual organs are easy targets for disease and infection. Put your penis in the wrong place, and you could die from it. So be smart about who you partner with and practice safe sex until you land in a monogamous relationship with a healthy partner.

Wear it. A latex condom creates a barrier that prevents the passage of microorganisms that cause sexually transmitted diseases. For added protection, use condoms coated with the spermicide nonoxynol-9 (such as Trojan-Enz), which has been shown to help kill HIV.

Don't drink to excess. Alcohol can affect the liver's metabolism of hormones, including testosterone. One large study suggests that higher consumption of alcohol is responsible for the poorer quality of semen among Europeans compared with middle-aged American men.■

🕮 Respiratory System

- **Percent of people who primarily breathe through only one nostril at a time: 80**
- **Number of breaths the average adult takes in an hour: 840**
- **Ratio of the number of alveoli in one lung to the number of residents of New York City: 41:1**

Gas and You

It's the grand recipe for human life: Provide your cells with glucose and oxygen, and voilà! Out comes energy plus some trash for the curb. Glucose you get from food. Oxygen you get from breathing.

So how does respiration work? Easy.

- Muscles pull your lungs down and out, creating a vacuum that sucks in air.
- Air is 20 percent oxygen and almost 80 percent nitrogen, plus some trace gases. The oxygen leaks through the lungs' membranes into extremely thin blood vessels called capillaries. There the oxygen binds with hemoglobin, a main ingredient of blood. Hemoglobin doesn't bind with nitrogen, so most of that gas gets exhaled.
- The oxygen-rich blood courses through the muscles and organs of the body. When it finds a cell that has built up a lot of carbon dioxide, a chief waste product of the energy chemical reaction, the oxygen enters the cell and switches places with the carbon dioxide, which, in turn, attaches to the hemoglobin.
- When the carbon dioxide–saturated blood returns to the lungs, the carbon dioxide switches places again, this time with newly inhaled oxygen. Then the carbon dioxide is ready to be exhaled.■

What Your Lungs Need

To keep your respiratory system healthy, be sure to eat a diet that includes the following.

Vitamin E. Studies have shown that this vitamin protects your lungs from the damage wreaked by the toxins found in almost all air pollution. The Daily Value for vitamin E is 30 international units.

Vitamin A. This crucial vitamin bolsters the cells in the lining of your respiratory tract, protecting you from respiratory infection. The Daily Value for vitamin A is 5,000 international units.

Iron. Every aspect of respiration involves iron. Without it, your body can't transport oxygen to produce energy. The Daily Value for iron is 18 milligrams.

Vitamin C. This nutrient is known to halt free radical damage in lung fluid. It is also associated with slightly higher lung function. The Daily Value for vitamin C is 60 milligrams.■

Powerful Lungs

Want to be able to blow out all of the candles in one breath at your 80th birthday party? Here are five tips for strong, enduring lungs from Harold S. Nelson, M.D., senior staff physician for the National Jewish Center for Immunology and Respiratory Medicine in Denver.

Don't smoke. Not smoking is the single most important thing you can do for healthy lungs.

Breathe deeper and longer. Deep, long breaths make your lungs last longer and help your body as well.

Breathe through your nose. Your nose warms

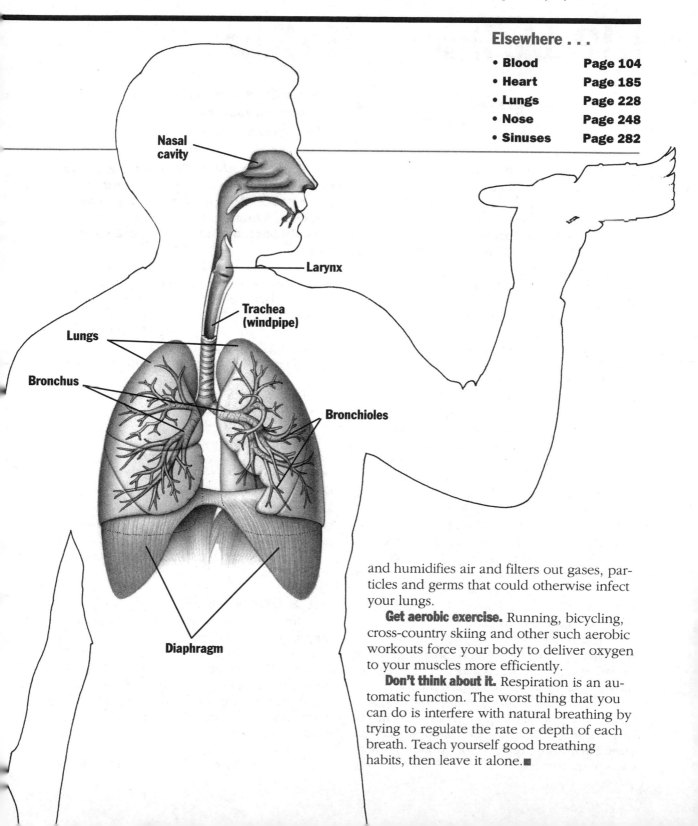

Nasal cavity

Larynx

Trachea (windpipe)

Lungs

Bronchus

Bronchioles

Diaphragm

and humidifies air and filters out gases, particles and germs that could otherwise infect your lungs.

Get aerobic exercise. Running, bicycling, cross-country skiing and other such aerobic workouts force your body to deliver oxygen to your muscles more efficiently.

Don't think about it. Respiration is an automatic function. The worst thing that you can do is interfere with natural breathing by trying to regulate the rate or depth of each breath. Teach yourself good breathing habits, then leave it alone.■

⋀ Pubic Hair

Why pubic hair? Certainly not so that we can style it, mousse it, spritz it.

In *The Bald Book: The Complete Book of Hair Loss and Regrowth*, science writer Walter Klenhard speculates that early in the species, when we were all naked and longhaired, it served as a means of immediate sexual identification from a distance.

The pubic hair patterns of men and women are distinctly different, Klenhard points out. Women's are triangular. Men's are rectangular. From across the jungle, you could identify the shape of a dark thatch and prepare to club someone, love someone or, if a bit psychotic, maybe both.

Klenhard also suggests that the hair was intended to sop up and sustain the unique musky scent exuded around the sex organs. This, he figures, encouraged men and women to copulate by causing them to think about sex whenever they caught a drift or got a whiff.

Pubic hair is coarse, curly, colored terminal hair, which means that the strands are genetically designated to grow only an inch or two long before falling out and being replaced by new growth. Pubic hair does not always match the color of the hair on your head, so don't make any assumptions about blondes.

Why is the region smelly? Apocrine sweat glands exist solely under the arms and between the legs. These glands create a unique, thick sweat that reacts with bacteria to cause a pungent, long-lasting body odor.

These days, most of us don't want to smell like cavepeople. Routine soap-and-water cleansing of the pubic area as part of a regular shower usually tames the primal odor.

If you want to shave your pubic hair, go with caution, warns Alex Comfort, M.D., in *The New Joy of Sex*. Don't use depilatories; they can burn. Finally, be prepared for the itch when it starts to grow back.

⋀ Ribs

- Do breathing exercises.
- Strengthen your abs.
- Quit smoking.

There's nothing like a smoky, sizzling rack of barbecued spareribs smothered in spicy sauce. Add some collard greens on the side, a hunk of warm cornbread, an ice-cold beer. Such moments are very good.

We conjure up this image for a purpose: When you think of your own ribs, you think mostly of bones. But it's the thin sheets of muscle between those bones that make the rib cage more than just a shield that protects your heart, lungs and digestive organs.

The muscles between the ribs regularly pull the lungs down and out, creating a vacuum to suck in air. When the muscles return to their resting positions, they force the lungs to exhale.

As for the bones, you have 12 pairs of them. They are curved to circle off your spinal column. Seven pairs curve around front and attach to your sternum, or breastbone. The 3 lower pairs, referred to by doctors as false ribs, curve around front and upward, attaching to the ribs above. The last 2 pairs of bones don't attach to anything in front, thus the name floating ribs.

It's a Snap

If you fracture one of these protective bones, you'll know right away. "It is extremely painful," says Bruce Janiak, M.D., director of the emergency center at the Toledo Hospital. A rib fracture usually results from a fall or a blow. If one area of your rib cage is extremely painful to the touch, a doctor will be able to confirm whether one or more ribs have been broken, sometimes without an x-ray.

If you've broken just one rib, there isn't

much your doctor can do to help you. Ice packs and anti-inflammatory medication will usually relieve the pain, says Dr. Janiak, and your doctor will advise you about rest and movement. But if your ribs have moved out of alignment, what's called a fragmented fracture, your doctor might have to perform surgery to wire your ribs in position.

What are "bruised ribs"? The term is actually a catchall for three different injuries. Unlike other bones, your ribs—especially the lowest pairs—can be bruised through direct impact. That's the first type of injury. The second is pulled or torn intercostal muscles, which are the muscles between two ribs. A third possible injury is a separated or strained joint between a rib and the sternum.

Keeping Your Ribs in Shape

Beyond the obvious advice to avoid the trauma that can cause broken, fractured or bruised ribs, the best thing you can do is condition your ribs' supporting muscles to minimize injury in the event of trauma. Here are some ways to accomplish that, according to Scott Haldeman, M.D., Ph.D., D.C., associate clinical professor of neurology at the University of California, Irvine, and adjunct professor in the research department at Los Angeles Chiropractic College.

Take a breath. A deep one. Deep-breathing exercises give your intercostal muscles a good workout. That's why breathing, coughing and even laughing are so painful when your ribs are injured.

Work those abs. Strengthen your abdominal muscles and the bracing muscles of your chest so that your ribs have as much support as they need. Your risk of injury from trauma is decreased if these major supporting muscles can provide strong padding. (See the exercises in the chest workout on page 362 and the abdomen workout on page 364.)

Once again, stop smoking. Smoking leads to chronic lung diseases that tax the intercostal muscles and cause your ribs to expand into a barrel shape.

Salivary Glands

- **Drink lots of water.**
- **Chew crunchy, fibrous foods.**
- **Watch your medications.**

In the dry, oppressive heat of Polynesia, swirling winds and pounding sun can parch an islander to death. So to whet their palates, Vanuatu tribesmen rely on a drink that you won't find at the corner store.

By chewing on a bitter root, Vanuatu women jump-start their salivary glands. They then spit the chewed root into a hollow gourd, dilute it with a little water and squeeze it through a coconut leaf. Over time, the plant material settles to the bottom of the gourd, forming a viscous black sludge, while the salivary slush, called *kava* by Polynesians, floats above.

During a ceremony called *yangonna*, Vanuatu men suck the kava up through wooden straws. One cup will send you howling at the moon; two cups can knock you out. "It's an acquired taste," admits Mac Marshall, Ph.D., professor of anthropology at the University of Iowa in Iowa City. "Kava doesn't really affect your head, but it packs a punch. The rest of your body just goes limp."

Saliva Made Simple

Saliva allows us to make kava, lick stamps and moisten envelope glue. An alkaline solution that is almost 99 percent water, saliva also softens food, lubricates the throat for speaking and swallowing and contains powerful enzymes that break down starch into glucose and other simple carbohydrates. These enzymes also enhance taste by converting flavorless starch into sugar, the reason saltines gradually become sweeter as you chew.

Saliva is your body's first line of defense against the more than 300 different types of bacteria that inhabit your mouth, making it critical in warding off mouth infections and tooth loss. "A decrease in saliva creates an ideal environment in the mouth for opportunistic bacteria. This can lead to ulcerations of the gums and infections," says Steven D. Vincent, D.D.S., professor at the University of Iowa College of Dentistry.

Also, by neutralizing the destructive acids in plaque, saliva helps prevent gingivitis, the first stage of gum disease.

Keeping the Well Full

Your body's three major sets of salivary glands—located on each side of the mouth, on the bottom of the mouth and under the jaw—crank out as much as a quart of saliva a day. Salivary glands stay in low gear at all times; you never know when you might be blurting out a comment or sucking in some fresh bacteria. But it's when they get the signal that food is coming that they really rev up for action.

Keeping your glands healthy means keeping them operating. Here's what you can do to help give your mouth the wet look.

Slurp it down. Because your body produces up to a quart of water-based saliva a day, you should drink at least eight cups of *agua* daily just to keep your saliva wells full, says Philip Fox, D.D.S., a senior investigator at the National Institute of Dental Research in Bethesda, Maryland. Copious amounts of water will not only keep your glands and mouth hydrated, he says, but also prevent bacteria from adhering to your gums and flush your mouth of food residue.

Graze veggies. Crunchy vegetables that require vigorous chewing, such as carrots and celery, also cause your mouth to be flooded with that protective salivary solution, says Dr. Fox.

Fuel your glands with fiber. Eat a balanced diet that's high in fiber to keep your salivary glands healthy. "The most active stimulus of your salivary glands is chewing and tasting food while eating. High-fiber foods are great stimulants of salivation," says Dr. Fox.

Chew gum. Sugarless chewing gum helps stimulate the release of saliva. Steer clear of gum and candy containing sugar, though. The sugar gives bacteria a medium in which to grow, advises Dr. Fox.

Vitalize with vitamins. A lack of key vitamins could also rob your mouth of precious moisture and leave it high and dry. Deficiency of vitamin A or vitamin C can cause your salivary glands to malfunction or turn off completely. Make sure that you get your Daily Values of 5,000 international units of vitamin A and 60 milligrams of vitamin C. "A daily vitamin supplement should keep your salivary glands on full charge," advises Dr. Fox.

When the Well Runs Dry

The only time you're likely to get concerned about your salivary glands is when the spit suddenly won't come. Cotton mouth, as a dry mouth is often called, is uncomfortable and unhealthy but relatively rare and usually short-term. If you experience chronic dry mouth, however, get checked out by a doctor. It may be an indication of a more serious health problem.

Xerostomia, the technical name for cotton mouth, results when the salivary glands don't produce adequate amounts of saliva. The resulting dry mouth not only impairs eating and talking but also makes the mouth vulnerable to bacterial invasion.

"Xerostomia is often a side effect of medication. Literally, more than 400 drugs, including antihistamines, decongestants and antidepressants, cause dry mouth as a side effect," Dr. Fox says.

Don't fret if your mouth seems to hit a dry spell for two to three days. It probably is just temporary. "Short-term dry mouth is not a problem. Long-term dry mouth, however, can cause serious dental problems," says Dr. Fox. So if after three days the monsoon season for saliva still hasn't arrived, see your physician or dentist.

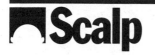

Scalp

- **Massage it.**
- **Cover it when cold.**
- **Wash it.**

Want to feel something wonderful? Try scalp massage. Let a professional massage therapist work your scalp for five minutes. You'll beg for more. Gently tease your own scalp with your fingertips, focusing on the sensations, and you'll get the idea. This is, without question, feel-good medicine. It increases blood flow and is invigorating. But does it do anything for your scalp? Does it promote healthy hair growth?

Many unproven and disproven baldness "cures" involve massage with various oils and creams. Special scalp vibrators have been marketed as miracle hair restorers. Here's the truth: Gentle fingertip massage does improve blood circulation to the scalp, encouraging new hair growth, says Sarah Brewer, M.D., in *The Complete Book of Men's Health.*

But don't take any leaps of logic here. "There's no evidence that massage can permanently regrow lost hair," says Toby Mayer, M.D., co-director of the Beverly Hills Institute of Aesthetic and Reconstructive Surgery, clinical professor in the Division of Facial Plastic and Reconstructive Surgery at the University of Southern California in Los Angeles and co-author of *The Everyman's Guide to Hair Replacement.*

Here's the rub, says Dr. Mayer: "Stimulation of the scalp may produce some temporary growth of vellus hair, but no bald person I've seen has had cosmetically significant regrowth." Vellus hair is the thin, short, colorless hair known as peach fuzz.

But gentle massaging is not likely to do any harm, Dr. Mayer says. And it feels good, so why not?

Massaging Your Scalp

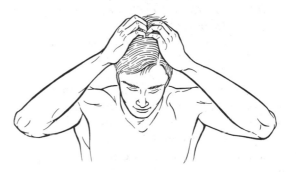

1. Curl your fingers and place the tips at the center of your scalp, close to your forehead.

2. Pull your hands slightly in opposite directions, applying moderate to deep pressure. Bring your fingers back together and repeat, creeping back along your scalp with each return. Work your way back to the base of your skull.

3. Repeat from front to back, starting about one-quarter inch to the side of the previous position. Do over and over, each time starting at a new spot along your hairline until you've covered your entire scalp.

4. If you discover a sensitive point, linger there before moving on. Return to it often until it is no longer sensitive.

Here's a more legitimate incentive. Your scalp, just like the rest of your body, discards old skin constantly. Massaging your scalp while shampooing helps the old sebum—essentially, old skin and dried-up scalp oil—rinse away instead of falling like snow on your jacket shoulders.

So the basics of scalp maintenance: Cleanse your scalp regularly with a mild, pH-balanced shampoo, removing excess and discarded sebum and hair product buildup, Dr. Mayer suggests. If your scalp is oily, shampoo daily; if it's dry, every other day may be okay.

Keeping Your Cool

The scalp's main job has little to do with hair. The scalp is one of your body's radiators—an amazing cooling system, notes

Dominic A. Brandy, M.D., clinical instructor of dermatology at the University of Pittsburgh School of Medicine and author of *A New Headstart! Doctor's Complete Guide to the Latest Advances in Hair Replacement.*

A tremendous amount of blood is drawn through the scalp's many blood vessels. They open wide when the body is overheated, increasing blood flow. About 80 percent of your body heat dissipates through your scalp, says Dr. Brandy. The blood vessels constrict when exposed to cold, but not enough to stop all heat loss. That's why we need to wear hats in frigid weather.

Itching to Scratch

"Skwatching, skwatching, skwatching. What have I told you about skwatching?" implores Elmer Fudd of his dog in the old Warner Brothers cartoon *An Itch in Time.* What does scratching tell you? Possibly that you have dandruff or seborrhea, both of which cause scaly white flakes to fall. Or you might have an excessively dry scalp or, less likely but still possible, a more serious infection.

Mild dandruff is simply the normal or slightly accelerated sloughing of dead skin cells. It's exacerbated by stress, illness, hair product buildup and allergy or reaction to ingredients in hair products. The first line of attack is to lighten up on the hair sprays and gels, shampoo more frequently with a gentle shampoo and use a nonallergenic conditioner, says Dr. Mayer.

If that doesn't help, switch to a dandruff shampoo for a while. Dandruff shampoo needs to be left on the scalp for three to five minutes in order for it to work. A number of dandruff shampoos are available with a variety of active ingredients: zinc, selenium, tar, salicylic acid and sulfur. Each works a little differently. Doctors suggest that if you don't get quick results with one type, try another.

Seborrhea is more serious dandruff caused by inflammation of oil glands. You'll see red bumps on your scalp. A dandruff shampoo usually clears it up quickly.

Shins

- Stretch them.
- Stretch them some more.

The thighbone's connected to the knee bone. The knee bone's connected to the shinbone.

And the shinbone's connected to whatever part of the brain it is that sends 10,000-gigawatt jolts of pain up and down your entire nervous system. If you've ever been kicked in the shin, you know. And if you've ever suffered from shinsplints or a stress fracture, you know double.

"Few things can hurt worse than your shins," says William L. Van Pelt, D.P.M., a Houston podiatrist and past president of the American Academy of Podiatric Sports Medicine. "Nobody thinks too much about them until they're injured. And then you can't stop thinking about them."

Anatomically speaking, there's not too much to the shin. You have a shinbone, called the tibia (you also have a smaller bone, called the fibula, in your lower leg). You have a group of muscles, the most prominent of which is called the anterior tibial muscle. And each muscle has a tendon, which connects to a bone and lets you move your lower leg.

Problems arise when you overwork the muscles and tendons and they become irritated or develop small tears. The throbbing pain you then feel is called shinsplints. Anyone who walks or runs can get them. But people who overpronate, which means rolling your feet too far inward as you walk, are at higher risk.

The best way to avoid shinsplints is to stretch before you exercise, says Dr. Van Pelt. If you already have shinsplints, he recommends icing your shins for about 20 minutes and taking a pain reliever such as aspirin or ibuprofen. (Keep a towel or some sort of cloth between the ice and your skin to prevent frostbite.) You'll probably need to rest for a couple of days before getting back to your exercise routine. And when you do start walking or running, take it easy for a couple of days.

Sometimes it's hard to tell the difference between a bad case of shinsplints and a stress fracture. "Both hurt like crazy when you're exercising," Dr. Van Pelt says. "But generally speaking, shinsplints hurt less as the exercise wears on, while a stress fracture hurts more and more."

In either case, don't mess around. If you think you may have a stress fracture, see your doctor, advises Dr. Van Pelt. Left untreated, a small crack in the bone could turn into a major, screws-in-the-bone-and-a-cast-for-two-months problem.

Stretching Your Shins

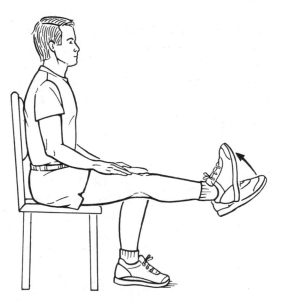

Sit in a comfortable chair, with both feet flat on the floor in front of you. Straighten your right leg and point your toes as far forward as comfortable. Hold for ten seconds. Then slowly bend your ankle so that your toes point toward your forehead. Don't stretch past the point of comfort. Hold for ten seconds. Repeat five times, then switch to your left leg.

Shoulders

- **Keep them limber.**
- **Keep them strong.**
- **Be smart about what you throw, lift and carry.**

If you ever get a chance to meet Bobby Bonilla, the star third baseman for the Baltimore Orioles, don't ask him about his shoulders. We doubt he'll have nice comments. Cumulative muscle and tendon tears in Bonilla's right shoulder forced him to leave the 1992 season early. Surgery took care of those problems. But one year later, a ligament in his other shoulder ruptured when he tripped rounding second base, ending that season early, too. Two for two.

The shoulder is an elegant joint, allowing men to hurl small balls at speeds approaching 100 miles per hour—and, of course, to hit those same balls 500 feet in the opposite direction. It is also one of the joints most vulnerable to sprains, strains, dislocations and damage. And you needn't be an athlete to encounter trouble.

Your Shoulders Made Simple

The shoulder's incredible maneuverability and strength are made possible by a unique variation of the ball-and-socket joint. Unlike the hip joint, where a neatly formed sphere fits tightly into a contoured bone cavity, the shoulder joint has the ball-shaped head of the humerus, the bone of the upper arm, resting against the shallow socket of the glenoid cavity. It's the glenoid cavity, which is formed by the shoulder blade, that gives the shoulder its distinct unhindered freedom of movement, but not without a price.

"The shoulder is unique because of its enormous range of motion," says David Altchek, M.D., team physician for the New York Mets and the orthopedic surgeon who operated on Bobby Bonilla's multimillion-dollar shoulder. "Unfortunately, because the joint is protected by a complex network of soft tissue rather than by rigid bone, the area is very vulnerable to injury."

The Science of Shoulder Pain

When Dr. Altchek talks about soft tissue, he is referring to a dense weave of ligaments, tendons and muscles that supports the shoulder joint. The most important part of this network is the four muscles and their tendons that doctors term the rotator cuff.

Encircling the joint, the rotator cuff maintains the shoulder's proper alignment and keeps the ball of the arm bone safely centered in its shallow socket, says Dr. Altchek. Problems can arise, however, when the shoulder is stretched or strained past its normal range. When that happens, the precious tendons can tear and the cartilage supporting the joint can become damaged or inflamed, a condition known as tendinitis.

Cumulative soft-tissue damage of this nature is precisely what sidelined Bonilla late in the 1992 season. With this type of damage,

which is usually caused by repetitive movement that puts constant stress on the shoulder, such as pitching or swimming, the joint's soft-tissue support becomes vulnerably weak. In this weakened condition, the tissue is susceptible to tearing. These tears can cause pain, tenderness, clicking noises and deep aching in the shoulder. A weak joint may also cause the shoulder's tendons to be pinched between the arm bone and the shoulder blade, a painful condition known as impingement.

Shoulder Health

No surprises here: If you want strong, injury-free shoulders, you have to exercise. "The key to maintaining a healthy shoulder is to keep muscles strong and balanced throughout the joint. You need muscle balance to stabilize the joint and prevent overstressing one area," says Dr. Altchek.

The second preventive measure is thoroughly easy or brutally hard, depending on your personality: It's called common sense. Do the same shoulder motion over and over, such as sawing wood for six hours, and it's all but guaranteed that you'll hurt. Try to remove an 80-

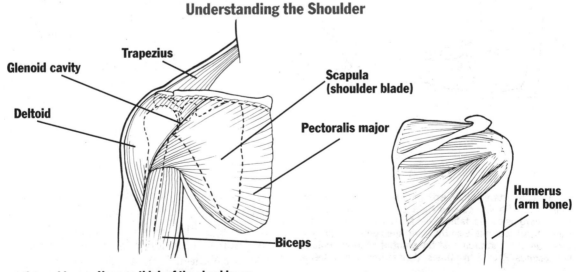

Understanding the Shoulder

Trapezius

Glenoid cavity

Deltoid

Scapula (shoulder blade)

Pectoralis major

Biceps

Humerus (arm bone)

The muscles and bones: You can think of the shoulder as having three layers: a powerful mix of muscles that stretch off into the arm, back and neck; beneath that, a set of four smaller muscles and their tendons that make up the rotator cuff; and an unusually flexible bone joint.

The rotator cuff: These four muscles lie below the deltoid muscle and encircle the shoulder joint. Their job is to hold the joint together.

pound box from an overhead compartment, and chances are you'll yank your shoulders silly. If you must put unusual strain on your shoulders, be sure to stretch them thoroughly before, during and after the work, suggests Dr. Altchek.

The final preventive measure is simply to pay close attention to pain, stiffness and other symptoms. The complexity of the shoulder joint makes it hard for a common Joe to diagnose these tweaks accurately. So if something seems at all wrong, give your doc a call, recommends Dr. Altchek. Remember: A bum shoulder means a bum arm, and who wants that?

You'll find several exercises and a good stretch for your shoulders starting on page 360 of our special workout guide. In addition, here's a simple, effective stretch for the rotator cuff: Hold a towel across your back, grasped in both hands. Slowly pull on each end two or three times, then switch hand positions and repeat.

Rotator Remedies

If your shoulder is troubling you, relax. Health care is getting smarter about these things. "The vast majority of shoulder problems, nearly 90 percent, can be resolved by eliminating the stressing behavior or with rehabilitation of the injured tissue," says James G. Garrick, M.D., an orthopedic surgeon and director of the Center for Sports Medicine at St. Francis Memorial Hospital in San Francisco. Here are a few ways for you to start the healing process on your own.

Accept an ache's advice. If your shoulder begins to ache while you're doing an uncommon activity, listen to the signal and stop, according to Dr. Altchek. Pain means that damage is being done.

Ease inflammation with ice. Wrap an ice pack in a light towel and apply it to your shoulder for 10 to 20 minutes, suggests Dr. Altchek. It will reduce painful swelling. Never apply ice directly to your skin; it may damage the tissue.

Then help with heat. Once you've beaten back the swelling, switch strategies. Heat will flush the injured area with blood and promote healing, explains Dr. Altchek.

Use medicinal methods. Anti-inflammatories and painkillers such as aspirin, acetaminophen and ibuprofen won't solve the underlying problem but can provide temporary relief. Be sure to follow the recommended dosage. But be wise about what's happening, cautions Dr. Altchek: Don't think that if aspirin kills the pain, the problem is solved.

When a Shoulder Goes Pop

Bobby Bonilla's first shoulder breakdown was several years in the making. His second took less than a second. He tripped, smashing his shoulder hard into the ground. That knocked the head of his arm bone clear out of the shoulder socket, an injury called a dislocated shoulder.

A less serious form of dislocation is called subluxation. This is when the ball pops out of the socket for a moment, then slips back in.

Rotator Cuff Stretch

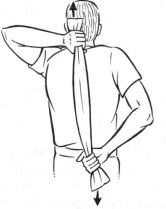

Hold a towel across your back, grasping an end with each hand. Pull slowly on each end two or three times. Switch hand positions, then repeat.

The third major type of shoulder trauma is separation. Shoulder separation occurs where the shoulder blade attaches to the collarbone. Crash your shoulder hard enough to tear the ligament that connects the two, and you have a separated shoulder accompanied by a whole world of hurt.

There's only one tip to give for any of these three injuries: Get to your doctor fast. Not only do all three hurt like mad, but they take professional help to fix.

Sinuses

- **Keep them moist.**
- **No viruses, no clogs.**

Empty spaces quickly get filled with useless stuff. It's one of those unwritten rules of life. It's true for car trunks, desk drawers, basements, computer hard drives. It's also true for your sinuses.

The sinuses are eight air-filled cavities located behind and around the nose and eyes. Their primary job is to filter out viruses, dirt, dust, allergens and other airborne particles that aren't welcome in the lungs. They also moisten dry air, cool hot air and warm cold air on behalf of the lungs, which prefer their air moist and temperate.

Other special duties: Sinuses give the voice resonance, and because they're actually cavities carved out of solid bone, they make the skull lighter than it would otherwise be. All of those caves in your skull make it easier for you to hold up your head.

They're also mucus factories. The membrane-lined cavities of the respiratory system create a pint to a quart of mucus a day. This sticky secretion traps particles that enter the nasal passages, while the cilia, which are microscopic hairlike filaments, sweep those particles toward the back of the nose.

Sinus Maintenance

Maybe superheroes don't have sinus problems. The rest of us mortals? Forget about it. Sinus trouble is a part of life. But if you want to make it a far smaller part of your life, you probably can. Here's how, according to Charles P. Kimmelman, M.D., professor of otolaryngology at New York Medical College and attending physician at the Manhattan Eye, Ear and Throat Hospital, both in New York City.

Just add water. Your nose and sinuses produce up to a quart of mucus a day, which flows down the back of your throat. Here's one more reason to drink lots of water each day: It ensures that the mucus isn't too thick or viscous to flow normally.

Choose the A list. Pick red and yellow fruits and vegetables for their high concentrations of vitamin A. Vitamin A helps keep your nasal lining healthy. Aim for the Daily Value of 5,000 international units.

Avoid bad air. To the extent that it's in your control, avoid exposure to heavily polluted or poorly ventilated air. Airborne particles and chemicals can irritate your sinuses.

Do the obvious. Why are we men so willing to silently tolerate our tortures? Don't be a hero, Bubba. If you're allergic to cats, don't move in with one. If you know your nose gets stuffy after eating pickles, don't eat pickles. Isn't the ability to breathe more important than a pickle?

Drink moderately. Alcohol, especially red wine, causes the nose to swell. This impairs the flow of mucus out of and air into the nose.

Fix it. If your nose is dry, moisturize it—especially during cold, dry winter months, when the front part of your nose dries excessively. Apply an ointment, petroleum jelly or a saltwater nasal spray at least several times a day.

All about Sinusitis

Sinusitis is when the membrane in one or more of your sinuses gets inflamed. (Inflammation, if you aren't clear, is your body's protective response to isolate an injured or infected body part and/or destroy the invader. The classic signs of inflammation are heat, redness, swelling, loss of function and pain.) When membranes inflame, sinuses can't drain. Sinusitis hurts your face, turns your snot greenish yellow, makes you tired and disrupts your breathing.

Infection is most often the cause of sinusitis; of these cases, 80 percent are bacterial, and 20 percent are viral. Often the infection creeps into the sinuses from another area of the body. That's why you might get sinusitis during or after a cold or the flu. Your lungs have finally expelled the germs, so some travel north to find a new home in your sinuses. Sometimes air pollution, underwater swimming and even temperature extremes cause some sinus membranes to inflame. This plethora of causes makes the sinuses rival the lower back for producing the most pain and discomfort of any body part.

Cases like those above are called acute because they are onetime affairs. Chronic sinusitis is when you have sinusitis for three months straight or longer or you have three or more sinus infections in a six-month period, says Robert Ivker, D.O., clinical instructor in the Departments of Otolaryngology and Family Medicine at the University of Colorado School of Medicine in Denver.

Roughly 32 million Americans have chronic sinus problems, and the number is climbing, in part because of increasing numbers of pollutants both indoors and outdoors, says Dr. Ivker. In fact, sinusitis is the number one chronic condition in men ages 30 to 45.

"The nose and sinuses are the body's primary air filters, and the air that they filter is getting dirtier and more toxic," Dr. Ivker says. "Try rubbing sandpaper over the back of your hand 23,000 times a day. Can you imagine the quality of that skin? The same thing happens to the membranes of your nose and sinuses."

A bout with sinusitis leaves a mucous membrane, especially its cilia, damaged and weakened. Sometimes, particularly when it's exposed to polluted and dry air, the membrane never completely recovers, leaving it much more susceptible to future infection.

Coping with the Clog

Although a bout with sinusitis can be a roadblock to comfortable living, there are many ways for you to pull the plug on congestion

Locating the Sinuses

If you've ever had a sinus headache, you probably have a good idea of where your mucus-producing sinuses are located. The frontal sinuses are above the eyes and nose and behind the forehead.

You also have maxillaries, which are pyramid-shaped sinuses located inside the cheekbones. And the ethmoids are multicompartmental sinuses lying above the maxillaries and between the bony orbits of the eyes. About 1 in 25 people doesn't even have frontal sinuses.

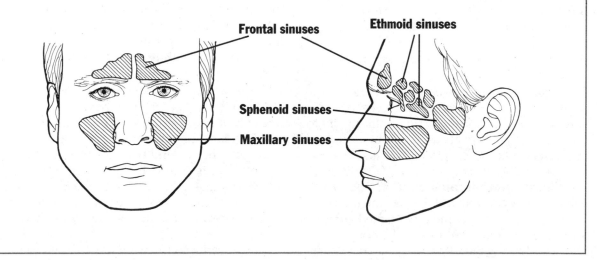

Frontal sinuses • Ethmoid sinuses • Sphenoid sinuses • Maxillary sinuses

Mucus Revelations

Trying to read your mucus isn't as interesting as reading, say, *Sports Illustrated*, but it could help you find out what's wrong with you.

With the common cold or an allergy, the mucus is thin, clear or white. But a sinus infection's nasal secretion is unmistakably thick and greenish yellow.

And how do you distinguish a cold from an allergy? There's no difference in mucus color, but other symptoms can tell you. With an allergy, the symptoms are likely to be sporadic rather than constant, often involving sneezing and itching. A cold is more likely to be accompanied by a headache, sore throat and low-grade fever.

---

and breathe easier. Here are some hints from doctors.

Get all steamed up. Steam is just what the doctor ordered to loosen up a mucus-packed nose and help drain the sinuses, says Anthony Yonkers, M.D., professor and chairman of the Department of Otolaryngology–Head and Neck Surgery at the University of Nebraska Medical Center in Omaha. "You should go into a steamy shower and just sit there for a while," he suggests.

Bow over vapor. Another way to get steamed is by leaning over a pot of piping-hot water with a towel over your head. Do this for five to ten minutes four times a day, says Alexander C. Chester, M.D., clinical professor of medicine at Georgetown University Medical Center in Washington, D.C. Adding a few drops of eucalyptus oil can add some decongesting punch as well, he says.

Note: A rush of rising steam can give you a severe burn. Before you lean over the pot, be sure to take it off the stove and to lift the lid to release any built-up steam. And whatever you do, don't drink the eucalyptus oil; it's poisonous if ingested.

Ax the antihistamines. Don't use antihistamines; they thicken and dry the mucus, says Dr. Ivker. "The thicker the mucus, the harder it is for it to drain from the sinuses," he notes.

Do decongest. Take single-action tablets

that contain only a decongestant such as pseudoephedrine, as in Sudafed, says David Zwillenberg, M.D., an otolaryngologist at Thomas Jefferson University Hospital in Philadelphia. Decongestants constrict the blood vessels, put air through the nose and alleviate pressure.

Don't overdo. Using a decongestant nasal spray for more than three days can make you stuffier than you already are, says Dr. Yonkers. "Any long-term use of a decongestant spray causes a chemical rebound problem with the lining of the nose," he notes. It becomes a vicious circle: You spray, which causes congestion, which means you spray again, and so on.

Take a hike. Getting at least 20 minutes of aerobic exercise three times a week could help you breathe easier, notes Dr. Yonkers. "One of the problems with sinusitis is that you have a decreased oxygen level in the tissue, which helps certain bacteria grow better," he says. "By increasing your metabolic rate, you might change that."

Spice it up. Spicy foods make your nose run, which helps loosen mucus and moisten the lining of your nose, says Dr. Yonkers. Try eating spicy Mexican food or a spoonful of horseradish, he suggests.

Salt your schnozz. To help flush your sinuses, Dr. Ivker recommends irrigating them with salt water. Mix one-third teaspoon of non-iodized table salt, a pinch of baking soda and one cup of lukewarm water (bottled water without chlorine is best, says Dr. Ivker). Stir well, until the salt and baking soda are completely dissolved, then pour the solution into a shot glass. Tilt your head back, close one nostril with your thumb and sniff the solution into the open nostril. Repeat with the other nostril.

You can also try a commercial saltwater

mist spray such as Ocean Mist or Ayr for a similar effect.

Stop smoking. Cigarette smoke contains irritants that are hard on your nasal lining, says Dr. Yonkers. "If you smoke at home, the smoke sits around your house, and you rebreathe it. If you must smoke, smoke outside and keep your home air sacred. The same goes for your car," he says.

Pop out of bed. Getting too much shut-eye can exacerbate congestion, says Dr. Chester. The lying position increases nasal congestion because drainage is slowed. Sleeping with several pillows or raising the head of your bed may help.

Don't make a spectacle of your sinuses. Eyeglasses sometimes pinch the nasal bridge and aggravate nasal congestion, says Dr. Chester. He suggests trying contacts or looser-fitting glasses.

Call for reinforcements. If all else fails, your doctor can help cut short a sinus infection with antibiotics. For an acute sinus infection, first-line therapy is usually amoxicillin (Amoxil) or erythromycin (E-Mycin) for ten days. For a chronic case, you may be given antibiotics and decongestants for at least a month, advises Dr. Yonkers.

But be careful not to overuse antibiotics. That could end up creating resistant bacteria that aren't killed by antibiotics. As a last resort, surgical drainage may be used to widen your sinus openings.

How to Deal with Colds

Chances are that this year, you'll be struck by cold viruses and succumb to humanity's most prevalent sickness at least twice and as often as four times. Why? There are hundreds of viruses that cause colds. It is im-

possible for your body to grow immunities to all of these strains, says Dr. Kimmelman.

At least you have it better than children, whose immune systems aren't yet fully developed. Kids can catch colds up to 12 times a year. Since colds are such a prevalent cause of sinus trouble, we offer these anti-cold strategies.

Wash up. Since colds are transmitted by hand-to-face contact, it's a good idea to wash your hands frequently and to try not to touch things that you know someone with a cold has touched, says Dr. Yonkers. "Everyone worries about people sneezing around them in the office because they think they'll breathe in germs and get infected," he notes. "But if you touch a doorknob that someone with a cold has just touched and then put your hand to your eye or nasal chamber, it's much more likely that you'll be infected."

Be extra-aware in the air. One of the more common places to pick up a cold virus is *(continued on page 288)*

Endoscopic Surgery: For a Grander Entrance

If you've been having sinus problems steadily, you can have your sinus passages surgically widened. This outpatient procedure, in which some or all of the ten passages linking the sinuses to the nose are widened, is performed on about 500,000 people a year.

After the doctor detects the infected sinuses by using a CAT scan, he performs the one- to two-hour operation with the aid of a tiny telescope that shows the inside of the nose, explains Thomas Pasic, M.D., assistant professor of otolaryngology at the University of Wisconsin–Madison. During surgery, the doctor removes the mucous membrane and thin bone in the sinus cavity, then widens the natural opening where the sinus connects to the nose from about two millimeters to a centimeter, says Dr. Pasic. The result: drainage tubes that won't clog as easily, which means bacteria won't back up into mucus-clogged sinuses.

What's the pain-to-gain ratio with this operation? "You'd think it would hurt, but when it comes down to it, it's less painful than people think," says Dr. Pasic. "Afterward, people say they're glad they did it."

Skeletal System

- **Number of bones in the adult body: 206**
- **Length of the stapes, the smallest bone in the body (located in the middle ear): 0.1 inch**
- **Number of cycles that the joints in the lower extremities rotate in a year solely from walking: 2 million**

Understanding Your Framework

The skeletal system isn't just bones. It's also cartilage, joints and connecting cords called ligaments and tendons. Together they provide a scaffolding for all of your meat, plus a strong but flexible frame that lets you run, throw and change television channels.

Cartilage is a clear, strong, somewhat elastic tissue that shows up in just a handful of spots: the nose, the joints and parts of the ribs.

Joints are where bones meet. They can be complex mechanical structures, as in the shoulders, or simple connections with just a few parts.

Ligaments are tough, flexible cords that connect bone to bone.

Tendons, which connect muscle to bone, and anti-friction sacs called bursae are found in joints that bend a lot, such as fingers, elbows and knees.

As the adult skeleton ages, bone loses mass, increasing the risk of fractures, especially in the spine and thighbones. Because you are your body's chief maintenance engineer, your chief goal for your skeletal system is to prevent loss of bone mass. ■

How to Keep Your Bones Strong Forever

Here's how to be a tough guy, at least in a skeletal kind of way, according to Harold Rosen, M.D., assistant professor of medicine at Harvard Medical School.

Keep 'em nutrified. The right nutrients for bones are calcium (1,000 milligrams a day) and vitamin D (400 international units a day). Your body maintains a certain blood level of calcium to keep muscles and nerves healthy. If you don't consume enough calcium, your body pulls the mineral from the calcium reserves in your bones, weakening them. But adequate calcium consumption isn't enough without the right amount of vitamin D, too. This key vitamin enables your gut to absorb calcium into your bloodstream.

Apply pressure. Weight-bearing exercise helps to strengthen your bones. Walking, for example, strengthens leg bones, and bench presses strengthen arm bones. Don't exercise, and your bones can get brittle.

Watch your alignment. Good posture does more than please your mother and impress people walking in the opposite direction. It keeps your skeleton aligned, removes unneeded pressure caused by slouching and decreases backache.

Stay limber. Babies can bend in ungodly ways. Forty years later, the same people can barely scratch mosquito bites on their calves without falling over. Range of motion is a terrible thing to waste. Flexibility reduces your chances of injury. It is a great tool for healthy, active living. It also keeps you young. So make stretching a key part of your exercise routine.

Use smart chemistry. The usual lineup of vices—alcohol, tobacco, fatty foods, drugs—is also bad for your bones. So is that other grand vice of adult males: couch potatoing. Yet one more reason to trade in your vices. ■

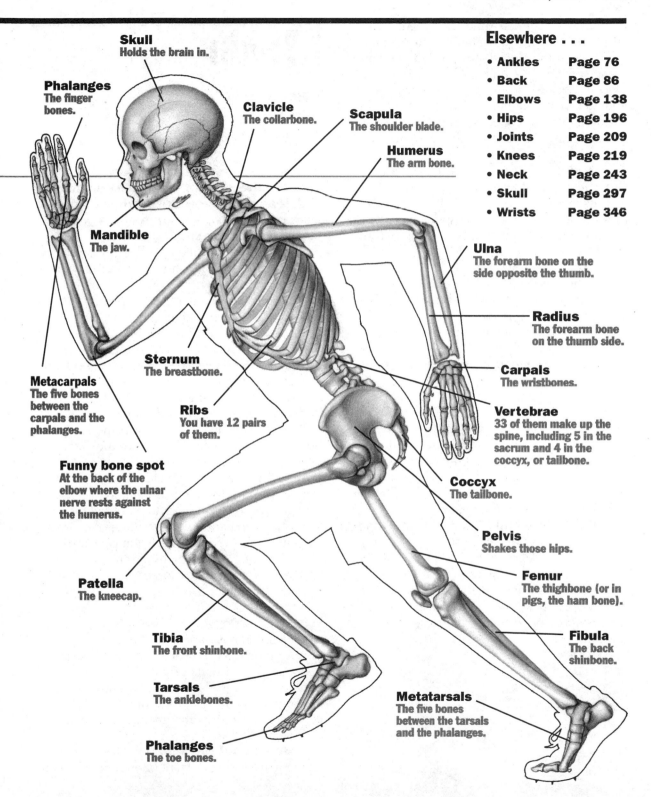

Skull
Holds the brain in.

Phalanges
The finger bones.

Clavicle
The collarbone.

Scapula
The shoulder blade.

Humerus
The arm bone.

Mandible
The jaw.

Metacarpals
The five bones between the carpals and the phalanges.

Sternum
The breastbone.

Ribs
You have 12 pairs of them.

Funny bone spot
At the back of the elbow where the ulnar nerve rests against the humerus.

Patella
The kneecap.

Tibia
The front shinbone.

Tarsals
The anklebones.

Phalanges
The toe bones.

Ulna
The forearm bone on the side opposite the thumb.

Radius
The forearm bone on the thumb side.

Carpals
The wristbones.

Vertebrae
33 of them make up the spine, including 5 in the sacrum and 4 in the coccyx, or tailbone.

Coccyx
The tailbone.

Pelvis
Shakes those hips.

Femur
The thighbone (or in pigs, the ham bone).

Fibula
The back shinbone.

Metatarsals
The five bones between the tarsals and the phalanges.

Elsewhere . . .

- Ankles   **Page 76**
- Back   **Page 86**
- Elbows   **Page 138**
- Hips   **Page 196**
- Joints   **Page 209**
- Knees   **Page 219**
- Neck   **Page 243**
- Skull   **Page 297**
- Wrists   **Page 346**

in an airplane, notes Anne Simons, M.D., assistant clinical professor of family and community medicine at the University of California, San Francisco, and co-author of *Before You Call the Doctor*. Because so many people are packed together in a plane and the flight attendant is handing out and collecting cups and utensils, be especially careful about hand-to-face contact when you're flying.

And don't forget that flying with a cold can cause a short-term blockage between your sinuses and nose, says Dr. Yonkers. If you have to fly with a cold, use nasal spray and take decongestants to shrink the nasal lining before you take off.

"C's" the day. Vitamin C can be a sure cold-fighter, notes Dr. Chester. "The theory is that it has a decongesting effect, and that's why it aborts a cold," he notes. Dr. Chester recommends 2,000 milligrams a day, in doses of 500 milligrams four times a day. Be aware that taking more than 1,200 milligrams a day could cause diarrhea.

One recent study showed that vitamin C also helps get rid of colds because of the way the nutrient assists immune function. Fifty-seven patients with bronchitis and broncho-pneumonia were given 200 milligrams of vitamin C a day. After four weeks, they showed significant increases in their plasma and white cell vitamin C concentrations.

Get souped up. You might have thought it to be an old wives' tale, but chicken soup really does work on colds, says Dr. Zwillenberg. Having a steaming bowl of chicken soup every day cuts down on the amount of time that people show cold symptoms. One theory suggests that breathing in the steam is what does it.

Skin

- **Stay out of the sun.**
- **Keep moist.**
- **Wash, don't scrape.**

Some guys feel pretty darn good about their skin. But few are as enamored with it as an Oregon writer whose dying wish was to have a volume of his poetry bound with his flesh.

"He was very fond of his skin," his widow explained. "He felt like it was one of his better attributes."

And with good reason. Despite occasional nicks and scratches, skin is extraordinary. The average man is covered by about 20 square feet of skin that weighs almost ten pounds, making it the largest and heaviest organ of the body. In a single square inch of skin, there are about 600 sweat glands, 100 fat glands, 65 hairs, 20 small blood vessels and thousands of nerve endings.

Skin varies in thickness over the entire body; it is thickest on the soles of the feet and thinnest on the eyelids. Yet everywhere it is a waterproof barrier that shields inner organs from chemicals and damaging ultraviolet sunlight and acts as the first line of defense against bacteria and other invading organisms. Skin also helps regulate body temperature, blood pressure and body fluids and is important in the production of vitamin D, an essential nutrient.

Getting Down to Basics

Because it is exposed to the world, your skin is more vulnerable to injury and disease than many other parts of your body. For the same reason, it is also more resilient. But keeping it looking good still requires some diligence. Here are the fundamentals for keeping your skin healthy.

Screen out the sun. "I've never seen anybody frolicking in front of an x-ray machine all day. But the sun basically produces the same type of low-level radiation, and people expose themselves to massive amounts of it," says Lawrence Gaughan, M.D., a dermatologist in Durango, Colorado. In addition to thinning the skin, which hastens premature aging, sun damage increases your risk of skin cancer.

And sorry, but there isn't such a thing as a safe tan, says Paul Lazar, M.D., a Highland Park, Illinois, dermatologist and co-author of *The Look You Like: Medical Answers to 400 Questions on Skin and Hair Care.* Tanning is really part of your skin's defense mechanism. Sun exposure triggers the production of

pigments that darken the skin and protect it from additional sun damage. But the tan itself is a sign that harm has already been done.

Now let's be real. It is a rare and odd man who never exposes his body to sunlight. Warm rays on wet skin, a cool ocean breeze and a frozen margarita: This is the moment we live for. But be smart about it. Don't expose unprotected skin when it's not necessary. If you are going to be outside for a while, wear a hat, long pants and shirt. And cover your skin with a waterproof sunscreen that has a sun protection factor (SPF) of at least 15 about 30

(continued on page 292)

The Skin's Layers

Your skin is layered like an onion into hundreds of tiers. Here's a look at the three main sections.

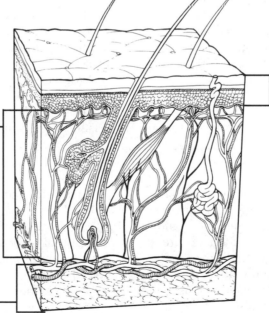

Dermis: Made of collagen, a tough protein, and other elastic fibers, the dermis is essentially the steel and concrete that support the skin. Within this structure are sweat glands and blood vessels, which help regulate body temperature. It also contains sebaceous (oil) glands, which help keep the epidermis smooth and soft, and nerve endings that sense touch, heat, cold, pressure and pain.

Subcutaneous fat: Sometimes called the subdermis, subcutaneous fat is an energy reserve that also provides insulation for the body and serves as a buffer between the skin and muscles.

Epidermis: Topped by a paper-thin layer of flattened dead cells that are bound together by natural oils, the epidermis is your body's tough outer covering. Just below the surface are layers of living cells that are moving toward the top to replace the dead cells, which are constantly being shed. It's estimated that the average man sheds nearly 40 pounds of skin in his lifetime.

In a young man, it takes about 21 days for a skin cell to migrate to the surface and die. By the time a man is age 35, it may take twice as long. As this turnover rate slows, the skin becomes dryer and develops a rougher, more aged appearance. Healing also takes longer.

Some cells in the epidermis produce melanin, a pigment that determines skin color.

🏠 Skin Repair

All about Scarring

In the Middle Ages, soldiers proudly displayed their battle scars. Some even let down their guard during warfare in hopes of receiving superficial disfiguring wounds.

Today, most of us view scars as ugly, unwanted reminders of accidents or surgery.

Any time your skin is deeply cut, there will be a scar. That's because as it heals, the wound is filled in with collagen, a tough, fibrous protein that forms the skin's underlying substructure. As new layers of skin grow, slight imperfections in the collagen develop, and a scar forms. How prominent the scar will be depends on the depth and width of the wound. Infection, poor blood supply, anatomical location, tension on the wound, age (the younger you are, the worse you scar), oily or dark skin type and sunlight also have an impact.

Although lasers and dermabrasion can make scars less noticeable, doctors can't eliminate them entirely. Here are a few tips about scars from Alan Matarasso, M.D., a plastic surgeon and clinical assistant professor of plastic surgery at Albert Einstein College of Medicine in New York City.

• If the wound is near a joint such as your knuckle, wear a splint for a couple of weeks. The splint will immobilize the area, relieve tension on the surrounding skin and make the scar smaller.

• Sun exposure will redden a scar and make it more visible. Wear sunscreen with a sun protection factor (SPF) of 15 or cover the scar with an adhesive strip.

• Massaging a new scar with your fingertips for five minutes three times a day can increase blood flow to the area and make the scar less noticeable.

• Avoid tension on the scar. This will prevent spreading.

• Consult your doctor to be sure that the scar is healing normally.■

The Skin Toolbox

Whether you jab a splinter into your finger or burn your arm while cooking burgers, you're probably going to need minor first-aid for your skin at some point. First-aid kits are available in most drugstores and from your local chapter of the American Red Cross. Some are designed for specific activities such as hiking and boating. You can also create your own. Here are a few suggested items for home skin repair.

• Adhesive bandages (assorted sizes)
• Adhesive tape
• Antiseptic ointment
• Blanket
• Cold packs
• Disposable gloves
• Gauze pads and gauze roller bandages (assorted sizes)
• Hand cleaner
• Plastic bags for ice and disposable materials
• Scissors and tweezers
• Small flashlight with extra batteries
• Triangular bandages.■

Elsewhere . . .
- **Sports Injuries   Page 62**
- **Feet   Page 154**
- **Fingernails   Page 160**
- **Hands   Page 179**

How to Fix It

Here are the initial first-aid treatments for four common skin emergencies, as suggested by the American Red Cross and Robert Adams, M.D., a dermatologist in Menlo Park, California.

Burns

Stop the burning. Put out the flames and remove the victim from the source of the burn.

Cool it. Use tepid water to cool a burn. Avoid using ice or cold water, except on small, minor burns, because cold water causes loss of body heat and shock. Use the nearest water source, whether it is a tub, a shower or a garden hose.

Cover it. Pat the wound dry, then loosely place a dry, sterile nonadhesive dressing over the burn to prevent infection and relieve pain. Avoid using antiseptic cream or ointment if the burn is severe or extensive, because it may interfere with proper healing.

Cuts and Scrapes

Think sterile. Put on sterile gloves, if available, before treating an injury. After treatment, wash your hands. Cleanse a minor cut or scrape with mild soap and water. Do not assume that it is clean just because you can't see any debris. Wash it anyway.

Press on it. To control severe bleeding, place a sterile dressing over the cut, apply direct pressure and elevate the wound. If the dressing gets soaked with blood, don't remove it from the cut. Instead, put clean gauze on top of it.

Dress it. Blot the cut or scrape dry with sterile gauze, then apply an antiseptic ointment and bandage the wound. If the edges of the cut can be brought together, use a butterfly bandage. If the cut is ragged, bandage it and seek medical help.

Poison Ivy

Shed those threads. Your clothes are probably covered with plant residue. So carefully remove your clothing, including your shoes, to minimize contact with your skin. Then wash everything in hot water.

Hit the shower. Scrub from head to toe with mild soap and warm water to remove any irritating oils.

Reach for lotion. If you develop a rash, use an over-the-counter remedy such as calamine lotion or a 1 percent hydrocortisone cream to reduce discomfort. Use as directed by the manufacturer.

Splinters

Boil water. Sterilize a pair of tweezers and a needle in boiling water or immerse them in antiseptic lotion.

Grab hold. Use the tweezers to pull the splinter out at the same angle that it went in. If the splinter is wood, avoid getting it wet, because it will swell and make removal difficult. If the splinter is under a fingernail, you may have to seek medical attention.

Coax it out. If the splinter is embedded under your skin, use the tip of the needle to gently lift it out. After you've removed the splinter, wash and bandage the area. ■

minutes before you go out into the sun, re-applying it every two to three hours, advises Dr. Gaughan. Take these precautions even on overcast days, he adds, because the sun's damaging ultraviolet rays can penetrate cloud cover.

Honor the siesta hours. In particular, stay out of the sun between 10:00 A.M. and 3:00 P.M. That's when sunlight is most intense and damaging to your skin, according to John E. Wolf, Jr., M.D., chairman of the Department of Dermatology at Baylor College of Medicine in Houston. If you don't have a watch with you, remember this rule of thumb: If your shadow is shorter than you are tall, that means the sun is high in the sky and is more likely to harm your skin.

Wash softly. Wash with a mild cream soap such as Dove or a glycerin bar such as Neutrogena once or twice a day and pat dry, suggests Timothy Flynn, M.D., assistant professor of dermatology at Tulane University School of Medicine in New Orleans. Mild soap cleanses your skin, and the soap residue washes off easily. Harsh soap dries your skin, washes off protective layers that act as barriers to disease and leaves behind a damaging residue.

Excessively hot or cold water can also harm your skin, so wash with tepid water that is skin temperature—95° to 100°F, Dr. Gaughan says.

Lather sparsely. "There's really no need to use a harsh soap all over your body. Most areas of your skin aren't producing anything that needs to be removed with a detergent," Dr. Flynn says. If you are sensitive to soap when you shower, wash your face, armpits and genitals with a mild soap and just rinse the rest of you with warm water, he suggests.

Take a hike. "There's no doubt that regular exercise will help keep your skin healthy," says Albert M. Kligman, M.D., Ph.D., professor of dermatology at the University of Pennsylvania School of Medicine and attending physician at the Hospital of the University of Pennsylvania, both in Philadelphia. "A nonexerciser's skin is thinner, and thinner skin is more fragile." Just walking for 20 minutes a day

three times a week can make a difference in your skin's durability, he says.

Corral stress. Stress can aggravate or even trigger skin problems, Dr. Gaughan says. Practicing a relaxation technique such as yoga or meditation for 10 to 15 minutes a day can help keep your skin in tip-top shape.

Eat right. No single food or vitamin will improve the appearance of your skin, doctors say. But eating a balanced diet that includes ample servings of fruits, vegetables, breads and pastas may lead to healthier skin, says Dr. Wolf.

Sunburn: Don't Get Baked

You thought you were a bit pink. Your wife said you were a little red. But when you got back to your hotel room and looked in a mirror, you were downright well-done.

Adios, vacation. *Hola,* agony.

A sunburn is caused by overexposure to ultraviolet light. These rays penetrate deep into the skin and injure several layers of cells. In response, blood vessels dilate, causing redness, and chemicals are released in the skin, causing inflammation. After a few days of pain and itching, the dead skin peels and the burn fades. In severe cases, sunburn can trigger vomiting and fever. Men who have fair skin, blond or red hair and freckles are more prone to burn than darker-skinned guys.

A sunburn is more than an annoyance. It reduces the skin's elasticity, making it more prone to premature wrinkling, and scrambles the genetic structure of the skin, increasing the risk of skin cancer.

Time will heal a sunburn—at least the part you can see. (Even though a sunburn looks healed, it always leaves its "fingerprint" in the form of damage at the molecular level.) In severe cases, healing time can be shortened with steroids; ask your doctor. In lesser cases, there are strategies to temporarily relieve your symptoms, doctors say.

Don't overglop. "You should minimize what you put on your sunburn, because some over-the-counter creams and lotions can cause allergic reactions or interact with other products and additionally irritate your skin," Dr. Wolf says. "I usually recommend just taking tepid baths or showers and applying moisturizer as needed. It works as well as anything else."

Make like a pickle. Pour a cup of white cider vinegar into a tepid bath and soak in it as needed, suggests Dr. Wolf. The vinegar can reduce inflammation and pain. A bath in colloidal oatmeal, such as Aveeno, is also soothing if you follow the manufacturer's directions.

Pop an aspirin. Taking aspirin or acetaminophen every four to six hours can help relieve most of the symptoms of sunburn, according to Dr. Wolf.

Skin Cancer: Be on Guard

Skin cancer is the most common type of cancer in the United States. Nearly 1 million men and women get some form of it every year, including 17,000 men who develop malignant melanoma. This is the most serious form of skin cancer, killing 4,300 men annually. Fortunately, melanoma and the two less deadly forms of skin cancer, basal cell and squamous cell, are highly curable if detected early.

Cumulative sun damage is the primary cause of skin cancer. But family history, repeated exposure to x-rays and industrial chemicals such as coal and arsenic may also increase your susceptibility. In many cases, it can take 10 to 20 years for skin cancer to develop. Fair-skinned men are ten times more likely than African-Americans and other dark-skinned men to develop skin cancer.

You can slash your risk of skin cancer significantly if you follow the guidelines suggested for basic skin care, such as limiting sun exposure and wearing a sunscreen. Here are couple of other things you can do.

Slash the fat. Cutting dietary fat to 20 percent of your calorie intake can reduce your risk of precancerous skin lesions and may also prevent skin cancer, according to researchers at Baylor College of Medicine. In their study, the researchers found that people who continued eating a normal American diet, which gets about 35 percent of its calories from fat, developed three times as many precancerous lesions as those who ate a low-fat diet. Try to eat a bal-

anced diet that includes plenty of fruits and vegetables and that derives 30 percent or less of its calories from fat.

Become an inspector. Do a head-to-toe self-exam of your skin once a month and see a dermatologist for a professional evaluation once a year, Dr. Wolf suggests.

During your self-exam, look for any new growths and for any changes in the size, shape, color, texture or thickness of existing moles, freckles and birthmarks. If you do find a suspicious spot, have it checked out promptly.

"Don't be afraid that you're going to look foolish. I can't tell you how many times men have come in and apologetically asked me to look at skin growths," Dr. Wolf says. "It's better to have it checked out so that if it is cancer, it can be treated and cured."

Wrinkles: Keep Them in Check

Take a piece of paper and crumple it up. Then smooth it out as best you can. Then do that again and again and again.

The creases that form become harder and harder to remove. That, in essence, is what happens to your skin as you age.

Wrinkles are a natural part of aging as the skin thins and loses elasticity. Despite claims, no product can permanently rejuvenate skin. Tretinoin (Retin-A), a prescription vitamin A–derivative cream, can help temporarily fade some light wrinkles. Cosmetic surgery can smooth out deeper furrows, but often the effect fades after about five years.

Most premature wrinkles are caused by excessive sun exposure, so the best way to fight wrinkles is to protect yourself from the sun. In addition, try these tips.

Don't smoke. Smoking decreases blood flow to the skin and triggers premature aging, Dr. Kligman says. In fact, heavy smokers are nearly five times as likely to have premature wrinkles as nonsmokers, according to researchers at the University of Utah in Salt Lake City.

Keep an eye on your looks. Everyday gestures such as smiling, squinting and arching your eyebrows can cause facial wrinkles. To some, these creases make you look wise and experienced. To others, they make you look old. In any case, they pose no medical harm. The issue boils down to personal image.

If you do wish to prevent these facial furrows, one trick is to look into a handheld mirror while you're talking on the telephone and notice your facial expressions as you speak. Then try not to do them. After a while, you should be able to suppress these facial expressions without using the mirror, says Melvin L. Elson, M.D., a Nashville dermatologist and president of the Cosmeceutical Research Institute in New York City.

Sleep on your back. Burrowing your face into a pillow in the same position night after night can cause wrinkling on your forehead and cheeks. "It's like folding up a napkin the same way and putting it in a drawer every night. Eventually, it will crease," Dr. Elson says.

To keep your skin looking more youthful, he suggests sleeping on your back. If you insist on sleeping on your side, however, try satin pillowcases, because they're less likely to cause wrinkles.

Dry Skin: You Can Brush It Off

Winter is the cruelest season for your skin. Wind, cold air and arid heating systems siphon moisture from your flesh.

"When you turn on the heat in an American house, the air actually becomes drier than in the Sahara," Dr. Elson says. "The air saps water right out of your skin and dries it out."

Your skin needs moisture to maintain a healthy outer layer of cells. Without it, these cells, which normally flake off

easily, clump together and cling to your body.

Aging also contributes to dry skin. As you get older, you produce less natural oils to combat dryness and to keep your skin smooth and healthy looking. Excessive bathing can aggravate the problem.

To give those dry, scaly cells the brush-off, the best thing you can do is moisturize your skin and the air surrounding you. Here are some suggestions.

Shorten your showers. Frequent long showers can strip protective oils from your skin and dry it out. Limit your showers to ten

Skin Art: It's More Than a Fad

Few men are as gung ho about tattoos as Bernie Moeller, the world's ultimate illustrated man with 14,000 individual designs embedded in his skin.

But tattoos do adorn many male bodies these days, including a surprising group of the rich and famous. This eclectic gang includes John F. Kennedy, Jr. (a shamrock), former Secretary of State George Shultz (a tiger on his rump), former Senator and presidential candidate Barry Goldwater (an Indian tribal symbol), Glen Campbell (a dagger on his arm), Tony Danza ("Keep on Truckin' "), Ringo Starr (a shooting star and a half-moon) and Michael Jordan (a horseshoe-shaped fraternity tattoo), according to Amy Krakow, author of *The Total Tattoo Book*.

While skin illustrations are experiencing a renaissance these days, men from all walks of life have been decorating themselves with tattoos for religious, artistic and sexual reasons since prehistoric times. Until the early twentieth century, for example, some Cambodian women wouldn't sleep with a man who didn't have a particular tattoo on his penis. They believed that without it, he wouldn't be guided by a "good spirit."

Serpents, buxom women, black panthers and hearts wrapped around the word "mother" are perennially favorite tattoos, says Lyle Tuttle, founder of the Tattoo Arts Museum in San Francisco.

"Some tattooists are creating true skin art. These are great masterpieces. It's hard to believe that someone could draw something that beautiful onto the skin. They look like oil paintings," says Steven B. Snyder, M.D., a dermatologist

minutes and use moisturizer on your skin until it revives, suggests Michael Kaminer, M.D., director of cosmetic dermatologic surgery at New England Medical Center in Boston and assistant professor of dermatology at Tufts University in Medford, Massachusetts.

Rub it in. After you shower, pat dry, so you leave your skin slightly damp. Then rub in a moisturizer that contains alpha hydroxy acids, which will help exfoliate dead skin and relieve itching, says Nancy Silverberg, M.D., assistant clinical professor of dermatology at the University of California, Irvine, College of Medicine.

Petroleum jelly is also effective. "If I have a patient whose funds are limited, I tell him to apply a thin coating of petroleum jelly on his skin once a day and to rub it in very well," Dr. Silverberg says. "For the money, you can't buy a better moisturizer."

Crank up the humidifier. Humidifiers add moisture to households, particularly in the winter, when heating systems dry the air. A humidifier is most useful in the bedroom, since that's where most of us spend the majority of our time, Dr. Elson says.

Unplug the blanket. If you use an electric blanket, turn it on to warm the bed, then get in and turn it off. "An electric blanket is like getting into an oven every night. It just dries everything up," Dr. Elson says. Turning it off minimizes that.

and laser surgeon in Owings Mills, Maryland, who specializes in tattoo removal.

Tattoos are particularly popular among men in their twenties. But many men have misgivings about their tattoos as they get older. So before you get one, Dr. Snyder suggests that you keep these caveats in mind.

• Don't get a tattoo on impulse. Tattoo ink penetrates deep into the skin and permanently lodges there. So wait at least 24 hours before getting one, and never make the decision while you're under the influence of drugs or alcohol.

By using several of the most advanced lasers, it is now possible to safely and effectively remove virtually any color tattoo without the risk of scarring seen with surgical techniques. The laser light selectively destroys the tattoo ink without removing the surrounding skin tissue. The lasers feel like the snapping of rubber bands against the skin, but local anesthesia can be used, rendering the procedure itself painless. Depending on the size and type of tattoo, the cost of laser tattoo removal averages between several hundred and more than a thousand dollars.

• Get it done by a tattoo artist who is a member of the Alliance of Professional Tattooists. Alliance members have received medical training in preventing disease transmission.

• Put it in a discreet location. If you can cover it, you're less likely to have regrets about it and to spend big bucks to have it removed later in life.

• Black, navy blue and other dark colors are the easiest to remove. Avoid greens and yellows.

Acne: Taking the Zip out of Zits

When you were 15, a pimple was devastating. But when you're 35—an age when most men are more concerned about wrinkles and receding hairlines—it's perplexing.

"Acne can have a profound effect on your personality and your outlook on life," Dr. Lazar says. "When you're an adult, it might bother you to meet people, because you can imagine them looking at you and thinking 'Gee whiz. He still has acne at his age.' "

Acne is actually a fairly common problem among adult men. About 1 in 100 men has outbreaks in his forties.

A pimple forms when an excessive amount of sebum, an oily substance produced by sebaceous glands, clogs a hair follicle or pore. Bacteria feed on the plugged-up sebum, producing irritating acids that inflame the area. The result is either a whitehead, meaning the follicle or pore is closed off, or a blackhead, meaning some sebum has seeped out and darkened.

Heredity and stress both contribute to acne in adults. Severe cases should be treated by a dermatologist, who may prescribe antibiotics, isotretinoin (Accutane) or a topical treatment such as Retin-A, says Dr. Lazar. For an occasional outbreak, try these tips.

Leave it alone. Picking at pimples is habit-forming. It also increases your risk of infection and inflammation, Dr. Lazar says. Increased inflammation can lead to a red or brown spot at the site of the pimple after it has healed, he adds.

Wash gently. Regular washing will remove excess oils, bacteria and dead skin cells that can clog pores, Dr. Lazar says. But you can't scrub acne away. In fact, vigorous washing can actually worsen a breakout. Gently wash your face two or three times a day using a mild soap, warm water and your fingertips or a soft washcloth, patting dry each time.

Zap it. Over-the-counter acne preparations containing 5 percent benzoyl peroxide can corral most mild outbreaks, Dr. Lazar says. The chemical seeps into your pores and kills the bacteria that aggravate acne.

Check your diet. Contrary to popular belief, chocolate, cola, cheese, greasy snacks such as potato chips and other foods and drinks have little to do with acne, Dr. Lazar says. If you suspect that your acne may be aggravated by a particular food or beverage, eliminate the item from your diet for a month, then try a small amount of it to see if it has any effect on your skin. In most cases, it won't. But if it does, then banish it from your diet.

Rosacea: The Never-Ending Blush

In the film *You Can't Cheat an Honest Man*, a character asks W. C. Fields "Are you eating a tomato, or is that your nose?" Red and swollen, the comedian's distinct nose was always good for a laugh. But the reason it was disfigured isn't so funny.

Fields had rosacea, a chronic skin disorder that causes unusual redness and dryness in the face, nose and forehead. It affects men between the ages of 20 and 70, especially those who are fair-skinned and blush easily. Although the cause is unknown, some doctors suspect that some may inherit a genetic predisposition for rosacea, since the ailment is particularly common among men of northern European ancestry.

Rosacea often begins with persistent facial redness, caused by enlarged blood vessels under the skin. As the redness becomes more permanent and noticeable, small bumps resembling pimples may form. If the condition goes unchecked, knobby growths appear on the nose, making it look swollen, and blood vessels form visible streaky lines on the face.

Although there is no cure, early treatment with antibiotics may prevent disfiguring symptoms. Stress, excessive sunlight, certain foods and beverages and temperature fluctuations can cause flare-ups. Here's what you can do.

Keep it bland. Avoid chili, tacos and other spicy foods that can aggravate rosacea, Dr. Kaminer says.

Watch what you drink. Hot beverages, alcohol and spicy drinks such as Bloody Marys can also trigger flare-ups, Dr. Kaminer says.

Avoid the extremes. Bitter cold or sizzling heat can make rosacea worse. Avoid saunas and hot tubs, bundle up on chilly days and keep the temperature in your home hovering around 72°F, Dr. Kaminer suggests.

Dermatitis: Subduing the Itch

Itching. Scratching. Rubbing. Reddening. Dermatitis, a catchall term for a myriad of related skin problems, can be a true annoyance.

Dermatitis types range from small, onetime rashes to chronic eczema and psoriasis. What's common to all is that the skin dries, itches and scales, usually in reaction to some trigger. There are hundreds of such triggers, including allergies, toxic chemicals, stress, infections and direct contact with an irritating substance such as mud, soap, sunlight or a plant such as poison oak or poison ivy.

While the cause may vary, the short-term treatment for rashes, eczema and other forms of dermatitis is generally the same. Here are a couple of tips. But see your doctor if the rash persists for more than a week.

Get away. Although not all rashes have easily identifiable sources, if you suspect that something is causing your rash, get away from it as soon as you can. Wash all clothing that came in contact with the irritant, including your shoes, in hot water to prevent a recurrence, says Dr. Kaminer.

Clean up. Rinse the rash with tepid water (90° to 100°F) and gently pat dry, Dr. Gaughan says. Avoid using soap, because it will strip off natural oils that help soothe the rash. Apply an over-the-counter 1 percent hydrocortisone cream such as Cortizone-10 or Cortaid two or three times a day to relieve the itching.

Age Spots: A Solar Nuisance

Age spots aren't necessarily a sign that you're getting older. But they are certainly a warning that you should be wiser about the sun.

These harmless flat, brown growths are caused by overexposure to the sun, which triggers excessive production of pigment in certain spots on the skin. It can take decades for age spots, also known as sun spots or liver spots, to form. But a man in his twenties or thirties can get them if he has spent significant time outdoors without taking precautions such as wearing sunscreen.

Your dermatologist may prescribe Retin-A, a cream effective for wrinkles, to help fade age spots. Laser surgery and chemical peels can also remove them. As an alternative, try this.

Bleach them. An over-the-counter skin-bleaching cream containing 2 percent hydroquinone, such as Ambi, Porcelana or Esotérica, may help fade age spots if used as directed by the manufacturer, Dr. Kaminer says. It may take four to six months before you notice any results.

Skull

- **Wear your seat belt.**
- **Wear a helmet while riding your bike.**
- **Stay light on your feet.**

Watch a professional wrestling match or a grade-B action movie, and you'll see head-butts every which way. Why do they do that? The answer, gentlemen, is that they are acting. If a childhood fight hasn't already revealed this to you, the skull does not make a good weapon. Think about it: A head-butt is a thin sheet of bone smashing against another thin sheet of bone. Lose the battle, and you bang your brain, a rather valuable item. This does not sound like a good fighting strategy.

Some guys can get away with it, though. In general, the skull bone's strength is in proportion to the size of the rest of the body. A stocky, strong lineman may have a thicker skull than a tall, thin distance runner. And the distance runner may have a thicker skull than a smaller track runner.

Brain Protection

Even though the skull seems like a single unit, it's actually an amalgamation of 22 different bones.

There's the cranium, or the top part of your skull that surrounds your brain like a helmet. It's made up of eight immovable, connected bones. The cranium encloses and protects your brain, eyes and ears and also provides a place for the muscles of your head to latch on.

Then there's the facial skeleton, which is also considered part of the skull. It is made up of 14 bones, including the mandible, or jawbone. The facial bones determine the shape of your face. Their structure also includes the pockets that hold the organs responsible for sight, smell and taste. The sinuses, by the way, are membrane-lined air pockets within the skull. Because of this airspace, the skull is lightweight for its size. The bones of the face are also the anchoring place for the facial muscles that you use to express your feelings.

The skull is less than one-half-inch thick in most areas. It is thinnest at the base and near the temples. It's tough bone. But even so, your skull is susceptible to lumps and bumps as well as to more serious injuries such as concussions and fractures.

Head-Banging Basics

Have you ever knocked your head so hard that you became dizzy or blacked out? A concussion is actually an injury to the brain rather than to the skull bone. A concussion means you've shaken up your brain enough to disrupt its function, says Kim Edward LeBlanc, M.D., clinical assistant professor of family medicine at Louisiana State University School of Medicine in New Orleans.

Men are more susceptible than women to concussions, and don't blame the NFL for skewing the numbers. Even though men's skulls are slightly thicker than women's, we fall with greater force because of the greater mass of our bodies, explains Dr. LeBlanc. If a man and a woman experienced an identical fall, the man would have a greater chance of sustaining a concussion.

Then there's the "big palooka" issue: We men love to participate in activities that put our skulls at greater risk, such as playing contact sports, crawling under cars, roughhousing with the kids, even banging our heads on our desks

How to Buy a Helmet . . .

Forget how it makes you look. A helmet is plain smart for any sport that puts you at risk for banging your head hard. That includes bicycling, in-line skating, mountain climbing, hockey, whatever. Bicyclists, for example, reduce their risk of head injury by as much as 85 percent when they wear helmets, notes Jeffrey Sacks, M.D., a medical epidemiologist in the Division of Unintentional Injury Prevention at the National Center for Injury Prevention and Control in Atlanta.

What do you need to know about helmets? These guidelines are offered by Kim Edward LeBlanc, M.D., clinical assistant professor of family medicine at the Louisiana State University School of Medicine in New Orleans.

- Size does matter. A well-fitting helmet, secured with a snug chin strap, protects you better.
- Visibility is key to sports safety. Don't wear a helmet that restricts your line of vision.
- Quality counts. Wear only a helmet with a seal of approval from a reputable organization such as the Snell Memorial Foundation.
- Quality changes. Old shoes may be comfortable, but they no longer support your feet. The same holds true for an old helmet. Time and abuse can cause a helmet to deteriorate. Examine it before each use to ensure that your helmet can still protect you.

Here's how to ensure proper fit for a bike helmet.

after screwing up a sale. Case in point: football. "It's estimated 250,000 American men get concussions each year playing football," Dr. LeBlanc says.

But the most common cause of concussion in the home is independent of gender. It's falling, says Dr. LeBlanc: taking a header down the basement stairs or losing your footing on a wet bathroom floor. You may lose consciousness for a few minutes. Depending on the severity of the concussion, the knockout blow may be followed by nausea, dizziness, headache, ringing in the ears, disorientation and related symptoms that can last for as long as 24 hours.

So how do you know if you need medical attention? It's pretty simple: Any time you've

. . . and How to Make It Fit

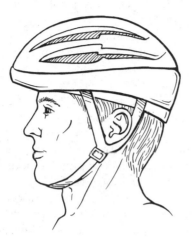

Make sure the helmet sits level on your head, covering your forehead. All straps should be tight when the chin strap is buckled. To verify the fit:

First, push up firmly on the front edge of the helmet with the heel of your hand. If the helmet moves backward, shorten the front straps, then tighten the chin strap so that you can feel the helmet top when you open your mouth. Repeat the process until the helmet can lift only slightly when you push it.

Next, grasp the helmet by its rear edge and try peeling it off to the front. If it covers your eyes, shorten the back straps without changing the front straps. Repeat until you are unable to tilt the helmet forward to cover your eyes.

Why be concerned? A broken skull can break open a blood vessel that runs through that area, causing a brain hemorrhage. A closed-head injury—one in which a fracture does not occur—can also cause bleeding. So just because nothing is broken doesn't mean that everything is all right inside your skull. For both a concussion and a skull fracture, your doctor will check for evidence of brain damage, which is the most important consideration with these types of head injuries.

Safety in the Car

Statistics show that in the general population, the number one cause of injury to the head is automobile accidents. And nearly half of these accidents involve the use of alcohol, according to Andrew Dannenberg, M.D., assistant professor in the Injury Prevention Center at Johns Hopkins University School of Hygiene and Public Health in Baltimore.

So you're helping to safeguard your noggin every time you buckle up, drive the speed limit and elect a designated driver. In addition:

Harness right. Don't ever put the shoulder harness behind you, says Dr. Dannenberg. When you're in an accident, the harness is what really holds you in place.

Buy bags. If you're in the market for a new automobile, get one with air bags on both the driver and the passenger sides, recommends Dr. Dannenberg. But don't give up your seat belt. "Some people say, 'Oh, I have an air bag, I don't need a seat belt.' But you really need both." The air bag won't prevent side-to-side motion, and it won't stop you from banging your head on the side window or door, he says.

been knocked unconscious, you should see your doctor, says Dr. LeBlanc. And even if you weren't out cold, call your doctor if you develop dizziness, nausea or a headache or if you feel disoriented after a knock on the head, he says.

More severe than concussions are skull fractures. When the bone actually breaks, the skull can mend, but the real danger is damage to the brain. Fractures happen more often to men than to women for the same reason that we have more concussions, but they're still relatively rare. The most vulnerable area is right around the temples, where the skull bone is thinnest, according to Bruce Janiak, M.D., director of the emergency center at Toledo Hospital.

⚠ Small Intestine

- **Don't wolf down meals.**
- **Lay off fatty and fried foods.**
- **Keep moving.**

Next time you can't close your luggage, ask your small intestine for advice. This vital organ is a master at cramming lots of stuff into a little space. Wrapped up tightly in your gut, your small intestine would stretch 20 feet long if uncoiled. Flatten out all of its surfaces, and it would cover 5,400 square yards. That's the equivalent of a doubles tennis court, with maybe enough gut left over to string your racket.

The small intestine's secret to space lies in the gazillions of fingerlike tentacles that carpet its surface. Called villi, these projections are each less than a millimeter in length. They, in turn, are covered with extensions known as microvilli. Combined, these millis and micros create 600 percent more surface area.

Why all of the space? Simple: It is along the walls of the small intestine that nutrients from food are passed into the bloodstream.

"In a sense, you have an oversupply of intestinal surface," says Marvin M. Schuster, M.D., professor of medicine at Johns Hopkins University School of Medicine in Baltimore. "You don't need that much, but it acts as a reserve. And the more surface space there is, the more it helps your digestive process."

Bigger Than the Rest

The stomach may get the attention of Madison Avenue, but the small intestine is the true star of the digestive system. In fact, you could say that the burrito that passed rather unceremoniously through your salivating lips several hours ago will not truly enter your body until it passes through your small intestine.

"You can do without a stomach, and you can do without a colon, but the small intestine is the only part of your intestinal system that is essential, the only part that can absorb nutrients," says Sidney Phillips, M.D., professor of medicine at the Mayo Clinic at St. Mary's Hospital in Rochester, Minnesota. Here's what happens.

Food, somewhat digested into a pasty chyme that is not dissimilar in appearance to the green effluence that came out of Linda Blair's mouth in *The Exorcist*, moves from the stomach into the duodenum, the first of three sections of the small intestine. The duodenum continues the digestive process, mixing and churning food by contracting both sideways and downward (imagine cement mixer meets washing machine). But it's not just the motion that digests; it's the solvent, too. The small intestine mixes five to ten quarts of food and digestive juices every day. Help is provided by the pancreas and the gallbladder, which pump, respectively, pancreatic enzymes and fat-emulsifying bile into this churning cauldron.

When the enzymes have broken down the complex molecules of food into substances that are simple enough and small enough to be passed into the bloodstream, that's exactly what happens in all of those villi: Nutrients, vitamins, minerals, fluids and other useful stuff transfer from the small intestine to the blood.

In the duodenum, carbohydrates and minerals such as iron, calcium and magnesium get absorbed. A longer middle section, the jejunum, absorbs most of the fat, protein and vitamins that you ingest as well as the carbohydrates that the stomach and duodenum miss. The ileum is the longest segment of the small intestine. It serves as a kind of backstop, catching any nutrients the other segments let by. But it also has a unique function as the only receptor of B-complex vitamins.

Small Wonders

"Unquiet meals make ill digestions," wrote William Shakespeare in 1593 in *The Comedy of Errors*. And to think, drive-through doughnut shops didn't even exist then. Today, a "quiet meal" means rolling up your car window or shutting your office door while you inhale lunch.

With mistreatment like that, it's a wonder

that your small intestine doesn't give you more trouble. Yet the care and maintenance of the small intestine is relatively easy. "It's a tough little organ, and it does well on its own," comments Dr. Schuster. Or put another way, "I know of nothing one can do to keep the small intestine healthy other than eating wisely and exercising regularly," says Debra Broadwell Jackson, R.N., Ph.D., chair of the Department of Public Health in the College of Health, Education and Human Development at Clemson University in South Carolina.

Here's the way to a happy small intestine.

Move for better motion. Nothing is better for your digestion than regular workouts. "Exercise increases motility," says Dr. Schuster, referring to the intestinal muscles' undulating motion, which keeps food moving through your system. Dr. Jackson explains that "healthy digestion depends on motility, motility requires a high concentration of blood flow, and exercise increases blood flow." Or put in simple language, "exercise helps keep you regular," says Peter McNally, D.O., a committee member of the American College of Gastroenterology who works in the gastroenterology clinic at Fitzsimmons Army Medical Center in Denver.

Break for meals. "These days, people don't dine. They refuel," says Kenneth Koch, M.D., professor of medicine in the gastroenterology division at Milton S. Hershey Medical Center of the Pennsylvania State University in Hershey, Pennsylvania. "Your small intestine does not respond well when you wolf things down. If you're rushing around doing 18 other things, you shortchange your digestive tract by distracting the flow of blood to other areas within your body."

So if you have the time, linger at the table. "Our bodies tell us that, but our culture demands other things," adds Dr. Koch. For those who can't make time to stop and smell the cappuccino, remember that food is getting passed on to your intestines for two to three hours after you've eaten, so slow down as much as you can.

Eat good stuff. Not surprisingly, your intake can affect the outcome of your small intestine. "Cut out fatty and fried foods," suggests Dr. Schuster. "Fat requires a lot of bile secretion. Bile itself tends to irritate the intestinal lining, and that leads to cramps and quite possibly to other complications, such as ulcers."

Dr. McNally adds that you should get plenty of water, fiber and fruits. Water keeps the mush soft and flowing through your system. Fiber is the undigestible part of fruits and vegetables. It gives bulk to the stool and helps bind the wastes and sweep your intestines clean.

What Can Go Wrong

For as much pleasure and sustenance as eating provides, it can also be the source of quite the opposite when the digestive system breaks down. Here's an overview of things that can go wrong with your intestines.

Lactose intolerance develops in people whose intestinal linings do not produce lactase, the enzyme that's in charge of breaking down milk sugar (lactose) into simpler forms that can be absorbed into the bloodstream. Levels vary: Some guys take a sip of milk and double over in pain, while others just get uncomfortable after eating a huge helping of, say, vanilla ice cream. Typically, symptoms include nausea, cramps, bloating, gas and diarrhea and occur between 30 minutes and two hours after consuming lactose.

This is not one of those obscure ailments specific to dwindling Amazonian tribal people. Between 30 million and 50 million Americans are lactose-intolerant, including as many as 75 percent of all African-Americans and 90 percent of Asian-Americans, according to the National Institute of Diabetes and Digestive and Kidney Diseases in Bethesda, Maryland.

With so many non-Westerners prone to it, Dr. Phillips suggests that lactose intolerance is the normal, rather than the abnormal, state. "Presumably, people of European descent are tolerant of milk because they have been milk drinkers for so much longer than Africans and Asians."

The first step with this problem is to figure out how badly you have it. Some people are fine if they eat dairy with other foods. Play with food combinations and amounts to get a feel for what your body can handle, says Dr. Phillips. Then you have a few choices. If you want to eat more dairy than your body can handle, buy lactase supplements, which digest the lactose for you, or seek out lactose-reduced dairy products. Or just swear off milk, cheese, ice cream or whatever it is that upsets you. In any case, if you sense that your body can't deal with dairy, talk to your doctor for more thorough advice.

Inflammatory bowel disease, or IBD, is a catchall for two relatively similar chronic conditions. Crohn's disease is an inflammation of the intestines. With ulcerative colitis, the colon becomes riddled with small sores. The symptoms of both are abdominal pain, rectal bleeding, cramps, diarrhea and sometimes fever. About 1 in every 100 men suffers from one of the two.

"We don't know what causes IBD or how to prevent it, as is the case with many inflammatory diseases," says Stephen B. Hanauer, M.D., director of clinical research and professor of medicine and clinical pharmacology in the Department of Medicine at the University of Chicago. "But we do know that you have a higher likelihood of contracting it if you have a blood relative with it."

Even if you are diagnosed with IBD, small changes in your diet and lifestyle can help make it less of a problem. Reducing the amount of raw nuts, seeds and popcorn that you eat helps

Food Poisoning

Throwing up is not anyone's idea of a good time. Nor is squinting, sweating and groaning on a toilet seat for an hour at a time. So tell us, please: Why aren't you cleaning your kitchen cutting board after each use?

Foodborne diseases, as illnesses derived from ingested foods are called, cause as many as 81 million illnesses and 9,000 deaths in the United States each year. And that's only the reported cases.

The culprits are bacteria, viruses, protozoans and toxins that deviously find their way—by catching rides on hands, butcher blocks, grills and serving platters—from food into your mouth, then through your stomach and into your small intestine. From there, the buggers are absorbed into your blood system. And that's when your whole system revolts, from both ends and the middle.

There are three levels of severity, according to Anne Simons, M.D., assistant clinical professor of family and community medicine at the University of California, San Francisco, and co-author of *Before You Call the Doctor.* She identifies them as "a mild case, accompanied by a short bout of queasiness and an upset stomach; a so-called real case, where you really feel like going to bed for a day or so; and a severe case that lasts for three to four days and leaves you swearing up and down that you'll never, ever eat potato salad at a picnic for the rest of your life." Here's how to avoid all three.

Follow the 40–140 rule. Microorganisms associated with food poisoning grow best between 40° and 140°F. So don't expose foods to temperatures in this range for longer than two hours. Refrigerate foods even after they've been cooked. "Don't thaw frozen meats and poultry on the kitchen counter," says Fred Angulo, Ph.D., medical epidemiologist in the Foodborne Disease Branch of the Centers for Disease Control and Prevention in Atlanta. "Even though it takes longer, let them defrost in the fridge." And check the refrigerator thermostat periodically to make sure it's at or below 40°F.

Be a human washing machine. Cleanliness may or may not be next to godliness, but it will absolutely reduce your risk of food poisoning, especially with chicken. "Wash anything that the raw bird has touched—the cutting board, the platter you've marinated it on, any utensils you've used with it—in hot, soapy water," Dr. Angulo says. Do not allow the cooked bird to touch any of the above before you wash them. Also, wash uncooked vegetables and any other produce with skin that grow close to the ground, he says.

Cook it well. Thorough cooking kills most cooties. So go buy a meat thermometer for a few bucks and keep it handy. The goal: to get the internal temperature of your meats up to about 160° to 165°F, says Sean Altekruse, D.V.M., an epidemiologist with the Food and Drug Administration.

Be a smart consumer. We doubt that you inspect the kitchens of the restaurants you eat in. So inspect your plate when it arrives. Hot foods should be really hot, cold foods should be really cold, and any fresh foods served at room temperature should make you think twice. Also, trust your instincts about the hygiene of a restaurant. If it seems grimy to you, don't take a chance, says Dr. Altekruse.

Preserve those preservatives. Temper your aversion to preservatives, says Dr. Altekruse. "People want foods that are fresh and contain no preservatives. To many people, preserved foods are unhealthy. But preservatives perform two important functions: They prevent spoilage, and they prevent the growth of hazardous bacteria," he says. Make sure that the label of any canned, sealed or processed food mentions a preservative. It is usually the last item in the list of ingredients and is accompanied by the words "as a preservative agent." Be wary of dips, olive oils with garlic cloves and similar foods that contain no preservatives as well as of unpasteurized fresh-squeezed orange juice.

Fear certain foods. Some things spoil faster than others. A small sampling of what to avoid:

- Anything with mayonnaise in it that has been left at room temperature for more than two hours
- Undercooked or raw eggs (as in hollandaise sauce, cookie dough and French toast)
- Undercooked or raw red meats (as in steak tartare), chicken, oysters and other shellfish
- Unpasteurized milk
- Fresh cider

If you do contract food poisoning, Dr. Simons suggests three things. First, drink lots of water, preferably by sipping continuously rather than by gulping down a glass every hour.

Second, when you are able to eat, go as bland as possible: unadorned white rice, a baked potato, toast. Meats are hard to digest, so stick with carbohydrates. Third, throw in the towel for a day or two. Read a book, watch movies, veg out. Let the bug win the battle but not the war.

ease symptoms. Reducing your stress level is a plus, too. "It happens to all of us, IBD or not: Stress increases the number of bowel movements that you have," says Dr. Hanauer. "But in people with IBD, this increase can aggravate symptoms." If you repeatedly suffer the symptoms listed above and the reasons aren't obvious, see your doctor.

Duodenal ulcers occur at the entrance to the small intestine, where gastric juices spill over from the stomach. These acidic juices eat at the lining of the intestinal wall. Typical scenario: nagging pain in your gut that comes and goes. Worst-case scenario: bleeding, obstruction, perforation, great pain and, if not addressed by a professional, maybe even the need for surgery. One way to tell if you have a duodenal ulcer, as opposed to a stomach ulcer, is if the pain recurs in the middle of the night, when the level of stomach acid reaches its peak. The pain wanes after you eat a small meal, says Dr. Hanauer.

For those suffering from these ulcers of the small intestine, Dr. Hanauer recommends cutting out cigarettes, cutting back on ibuprofen and aspirin-based drugs (better to use acetaminophen for pain relief) and eating more meals but less at each meal. And be smart: If you have chronic pain and you aren't sure what it is, see your doctor. It's pretty easy to diagnose an ulcer and not that hard to fix one.

Sperm

- **Quit smoking.**
- **Avoid groin injuries.**
- **Wear boxers.**

Oh, those silly scientists. In 1677, Johan Ham van Arnhem, peering through a microscope, discovered sperm. Biologists of the time argued the significance of the finding. Some concluded that the tiny, eel-like creatures observed in ejaculate were parasites. Others believed that they were the seeds that made babies. Still others insisted that they were babies—teeny-weeny, baby babies that, if they reached the proper place in the womb, would grow to become full-size human babes.

By the eighteenth century, scientists swore that they could see a tiny person curled up in each spermatozoon. (Scientists examining horse sperm swore they could see tiny horses galloping through the ejaculate.) In 1716, Anton van Leeuwenhoek, considered the greatest microscopist of his time, declared that he could see tiny males and tiny females in different sperm and that the sex of the baby depended solely upon the sex of the sperm that swam into the womb first.

Van Leeuwenhoek was mostly right. Although you can't see human forms in sperm, the sex of a baby is determined by whether a sperm carrying male chromosomes or a sperm carrying female chromosomes gets to the woman's womb and attaches to the egg first.

It's quite a race. Upward of 100 million sperm are expelled when a man ejaculates. Each sperm is so small it would take several thousand to cover the period at the end of this sentence. And they all have only one job to do: to swim like mad and to try to find and fertilize an egg. Whether this happens depends in part on you. Whether you produce Olympic-grade swimmers or sluggish, misshapen little rascals depends upon your environment, your health and your fitness, among other factors.

Quality Control

Something bad may be happening to sperm as we approach the end of the twentieth century. We have raised our standards as to what constitutes good sperm, notes Machelle Seibel, M.D., medical director of the Faulkner Center for Reproductivity in Boston. But aside from that, studies suggest that sperm counts and quality of sperm have dropped substantially in recent years. No one is sure why. Environmental toxins may play a role. Medications containing estrogen may also be involved; when taken by pregnant women, they may affect testicular function in male offspring.

Some studies show that the typical man nowadays produces only slightly more than half of the number of sperm of his 1940s counterpart. More than 25 percent of couples today have trouble conceiving, compared with 8 percent 30 years ago. In one-third of cases, the problem is with the male alone; in another one-third, the problem is with the woman alone; and in the remaining one-third, both the man and woman are having problems, says Dr. Seibel.

Testing often begins with a microscopic analysis of the man's sperm. It is checked primarily for how many sperm are present (normal these days is 50 million to 100 million per milliliter of semen, with anything below 20 million considered low); how many are swimming vigorously (ideally, 60 percent); and how many have well-shaped oval heads and nice straight tails (about 14 percent, according to strict criteria).

The doctor should examine the man to see if a physical problem exists that can be corrected. We'll look at some of these problems in a minute. For now, let's consider what we can do ourselves to improve the quality of our sperm and the chances of conception.

Pump Up Your Sperm

Our sperm reflect our general well-being, says Glen Hofmann, Ph.D., medical director of the Bethesda Center for Reproductive Health and Fertility in Cincinnati. When we're in peak health, we produce the healthiest sperm; when we're run-down, our sperm suffer. This can be bad news not only for achieving pregnancy but also for the health of our offspring when conception does occur.

Here are tips for keeping your sperm healthy and in the swim.

Don't tolerate toxins. Even modest exposure to poisons, heavy metals and so forth has been shown to adversely affect sperm, says Ken Goldberg, M.D., founder and director of the Male Health Center in Dallas. Whether you're spraying for bugs at home or surrounded by toxic chemicals at work, always take precautions. Wear the gear. Put on the gloves. Read the warning on the can. We're talking about not only your life but possibly your kid's life, too.

Watch your meds. If you're trying to conceive, be sure to ask your doctor about the possible sperm-damaging effects of any drug that you may be taking, including antibiotics, says Dr. Goldberg. Your pharmacist is also a good source of information and can probably provide you with a computer printout of side effects that may be caused by your medication.

Reduce stress. Doctors aren't sure why, but emotional stress is clearly detrimental to sperm health and production. Anything that you can do to reduce stress—deep breathing, listening to relaxation tapes or simply going for walks—can only help your sperm stay healthy.

Exercise regularly but moderately. Fitness helps sperm production, but highly demanding workouts, such as running more than 65 miles a week, hinders it. So if you and your partner are trying to conceive, you might want to keep your workouts to a moderate level, at least until the deed is done.

Arrest free radicals. Vitamins C and E, beta-carotene and the mineral selenium all act as antioxidants—that is, they scavenge potentially harmful unattached oxygen molecules called free radicals, which are known to interfere with sperm function, from the blood and semen, says Larry Lipshultz, M.D., professor of

urology at Baylor College of Medicine in Houston. Dr. Lipshultz recommends that infertility patients take a daily combination supplement containing 500 milligrams of vitamin C, 400 international units of vitamin E, 50 micrograms of selenium and 25,000 international units (15 milligrams) of beta-carotene.

Get your zinc. One study showed that when men's daily intake of the mineral zinc was cut from more than 10 milligrams to about 1 milligram, the amount of ejaculate they produced dropped by one-third, says Curtiss Hunt, M.D., of the U.S. Department of Agriculture Grand Forks Human Nutrition Center in North Dakota. He recommends getting the Daily Value of 15 milligrams of zinc. Some good sources of zinc are lean beef, crabmeat and oysters.

Come again? Your first squirt after a long period of abstinence (defined as a week or more without ejaculating) is simply not going to be your best, says Arthur L. Wisot, M.D., a fertility specialist at the Center for Advanced Reproductive Care in Redondo Beach, California. Sperm ejaculated after more than a four-day interval have impaired motility and may not function, says Dr. Wisot. Masturbating or having sex 48 hours before you actually aim to conceive will help improve sperm quality.

Keep cool. The testicles are designed to keep sperm several degrees cooler than the rest of the body. Spending long periods of time in hot baths, hot tubs and saunas can cause sperm to overheat, lowering their concentration and also their ability to swim vigorously.

Quit smoking. Studies suggest that men who smoke have a much greater chance of producing kids with birth defects, including hydrocephalus, a potentially fatal buildup of fluid on the brain. Since sperm production takes 70 to 100 days, you need to be smoke-free for a few months before you can expect your sperm to be free of harmful influences.

Drink lightly. Research also indicates that a man's heavy drinking can be a contributing factor in testicular failure. For most men, a drink a day is probably okay. More than that could cause problems, says Dr. Lipshultz.

Medical Problems and Solutions

Sometimes a man just doesn't produce good, healthy sperm and his doctor can't pinpoint the reason. Sometimes the doctor does find the problem but can do nothing to restore fertility. But usually, a urologist experienced in fertility problems can find the problem. And often the problem can be overcome.

Sperm begin their journey in the testicles. Eventually, they travel through the seminiferous tubules, the epididymis (all 20 feet of it) and the vas deferens and, if ejaculated, outward through the urethra.

A blocked tube—in the epididymis, for example—can sometimes be opened with microsurgery, although fertility is restored in less than 30 percent of cases, says Abraham Morgentaler, M.D., director of the male infertility and impotency program at Beth Israel Hospital in Boston and author of *The Male Body: A Physician's Guide to What Every Man Should Know about His Sexual Health*.

If good sperm are available but aren't being ejaculated effectively, a doctor may extract enough sperm to fertilize an egg in a glass dish. This process is called in vitro fertilization.

A correctable problem commonly found in men having trouble conceiving is a varicocele, a type of varicose vein in the testicles, says Dr. Seibel. Experts believe that a faulty valve in a vein sometimes allows warmer blood to back up, raising the temperature and inhibiting sperm production. The repair, which is considered quite simple, involves cutting and tying off the necessary vein so that blood flow—and temperature—return to normal.

Also treatable is a bacterial infection in the genital tract, which can create a sperm-killing environment. Antibiotics can kill the infection and restore fertility, says Dr. Morgentaler.

Some men, of course, want to be infertile and choose vasectomy as an easy, reliable form of birth control, says Dr. Lipshultz. The procedure, which is quite simple, involves cutting the vas deferens, a long, muscular tube running from the testicles to the prostate.

But while vasectomy is easy to perform, undoing it and restoring fertility years or even decades later is a lot more challenging. Doctors have found that by cutting the vas deferens higher in the scrotal sac and leaving a fairly long section of it in place, and by being particularly careful in sealing it off, they have a much better chance of successfully reversing the procedure, says Dr. Lipshultz.

Boxers Beat Briefs

It's one of those perpetuating pieces of male medical folklore: Tight underwear can make you infertile. That may overstate the case. But studies suggest that hanging loose is the safest stance in the boxers-versus-briefs controversy.

Briefly, the findings are this. Tight-fitting underwear seems to inhibit sperm production by keeping the testicles close to the body and thus warmer. Optimum sperm production takes place at a temperature that is 4° to 7° below the body's normal 98.6°F. The testicles are designed to hang away from the body to stay cooler. Boxers tend to facilitate nature; briefs frustrate it.

Polyester presents a different problem. When scrotal skin rubs against polyester underwear, a static electric charge tingles through the testicles. It's subtle. You don't feel it, but it zaps sperm production. Cotton does no such thing.

These studies show how wearing tight polyester briefs for a long time can harm fertility, says Sarah Brewer, M.D., author of *The Complete Book of Men's Health*.

Interestingly, Egyptian doctors have invented and successfully tested a male contraceptive device that combines the two sperm-killing factors, Dr. Brewer says. The device is basically a polyester jockstrap that hugs the testicles close to the body but gives the penis free reign. In tests, men who wore it for five months saw their sperm counts drop to zero, she says. Birth control of the future? Stay tuned.

Spinal Cord

- **Protect your neck; it's most vulnerable.**
- **Don't play tackle football.**
- **Watch where you're diving.**

One of the worst things you can say about a man is that he's spineless. That should tell you how important the spinal cord is. It's an information superhighway that conveys just about every sensation you have and every move you make to and from your brain. With a spinal cord, your body pulsates with the raw data of being alive. Without one, you're unplugged.

The spinal cord is white and rubbery and typically ranges from one-half to one inch in diameter. "If you could look at it microscopically, it's like a telephone cable. There are millions of individual nerve fibers," says Stephen Esses, M.D., professor of orthopedic surgery at Baylor College of Medicine in Houston.

Those millions of individual fibers are literally an extension of your brain. Together the spinal cord and the brain make up the central nervous system. The vast network of nerves throughout the rest of your body is called the peripheral nervous system because every nerve feeds into that central processing unit.

The spinal cord starts at the base of the brain and extends down the lower back, ending a few inches above the waist. From there it divides into a spray of nerve fibers called the cauda equina (Latin for "horse's tail," which is just what it looks like). Nerve impulses travel from the brain into the 31 pairs of nerves that branch off the spinal cord, then out to the rest of your body. It's a circular system: Nerve impulses carry information from the corporal hinterlands back to the brain by retracing the same route.

Protecting Yourself

Want to know the importance of your spinal cord? Look at how carefully your body

protects it. Openings in each of the spine's 33 vertebrae form a bony tunnel that surrounds the cord all the way down your back. In addition, around the spinal cord itself are several layers of membrane and liquid that insulate it even more.

All of this protection should signal you to take any threat to your spinal cord seriously. "If you start having a problem with your spinal cord, you can't mess around with it," says Alexander Vaccaro, M.D., an orthopedic surgeon and assistant professor of orthopedic surgery at Thomas Jefferson University in Philadelphia. "It's a dangerous situation that needs to be looked at."

By far the biggest threat to your spinal cord is a traumatic injury. Contact sports, cars and guns are among the usual causes. Damag-

The Spine's Structure

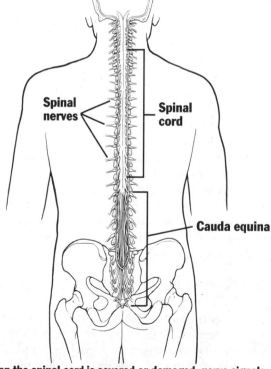

When the spinal cord is severed or damaged, nerve signals to and from everything below the injury get cut off. That's why you shouldn't move anyone showing signs of a neck or back injury—you risk making temporary damage permanent.

ing the spinal cord is one of life's worst nightmares. Recall the saga of actor Christopher Reeve: One minute he was enjoying a horseback-riding competition; the next he was paralyzed from the neck down. Like the majority of spinal cord injuries, Reeve's injury is in his neck, where the bones of the spinal column are most flexible and most prone to breaking.

When the spinal cord is damaged, information to and from everything below the location of the injury is cut off. That's why if you come upon an accident scene where someone shows any hint of having a neck or back injury, you should not move him. By turning the head of a person with a broken neck, you may drive bone shards into his spinal cord, turning what had been a temporary injury into a lifelong tragedy, says Peter Bruno, M.D., an internist for the New York Knicks basketball team and associate professor of medicine at New York University in New York City.

Other advice for preserving your spinal cord is pretty obvious but vital. Dr. Vaccaro, Dr. Bruno and Dr. Esses offer the following tips.

Suit up. Always wear a helmet when riding a motorcycle or bicycle.

Check it out. Don't dive into water until you know how deep it is.

Buckle up. Always use your seat belt and adjust your car's headrest so that it actually supports your head.

Designate a driver. Don't drive drunk and don't ride in a car with someone who is.

Dodge a bullet. Stay away from people who use guns unsafely. The same goes for people with knives.

Troubleshooting Other Problems

Most of the problems that we associate with back or neck pain develop because there are problems with the vertebrae themselves, with the disks between the vertebrae, with the nerves branching off the spinal cord or with the muscles and ligaments that support the whole complicated system. (For lots of information on the back and the neck, see pages 86 and 243, respectively.) Problems directly related to the spinal cord, by contrast, are relatively rare. The trouble is, how do you know for sure that your spinal cord is the source of your trouble?

According to Dr. Esses, the spinal cord does not register pain itself but rather sends out clues when it's in distress. "Pressure on or injury to the spinal cord will affect its ability to transmit the electrical signals that it carries to and from the body," he says. "Therefore, a spinal cord problem is going to manifest itself somewhere else, in the spot that those electrical signals had been going to or coming from."

If the problem is in the area of your neck, for example, you'll notice numbness, tingling or weakness in your arms, according to Dr. Vaccaro. If something is pressuring your spinal cord farther down, toward the middle of your back, the numbness, tingling or weakness will appear in your legs. If there is a stronger compression, you'll notice bowel and bladder problems, and you might lose the ability to have an erection. Finally, with severe pressure on your spinal cord, you'll begin losing your balance or the ability to feel in your hands or your legs.

A common source of pressure on the spinal cord is a ruptured, or herniated, disk. Other times, deposits can build up on the vertebrae, narrowing the channel through which the spinal cord passes. The medical name for this condition is spinal stenosis. Like arthritis, the growths usually don't develop until old age.

Some people, though, are born with unusually narrow spinal columns, which means that pressure can be put on their spinal cords more readily. Such people are prone to a sports injury called a stinger. According to Dr. Esses, a stinger results from the spinal cord being bruised, usually by a violent football tackle. In most cases, a player with a stinger will feel numbness, weakness or a burning sensation in his legs or arms for just 15 minutes or so.

But not always. Dr. Esses says several cases of stingers have led to paralysis among players with spinal stenosis. Dr. Bruno suggests that any time you feel pain or numbness in your arms, hands or legs while playing a sport, stop and get the condition assessed by your doctor.

Spleen

The spleen is your body's executioner, mortician, scavenger, blood bank director and sentry.

On a typical day, this multipurpose organ kills and disposes of decrepit red blood cells, filters out iron from the cells' carcasses so that it can be reused to make hemoglobin, stores up to a quart of blood that can quickly be released into your bloodstream in an emergency and produces disease-fighting antibodies and white blood cells called lymphocytes.

About the size of your fist and weighing six ounces, the spleen, the largest organ in the lymphatic system, is covered with a spongelike capsule of fibrous bands that cull damaged red blood cells as well as parasites and other invading microorganisms from your bloodstream so that they can be destroyed. In certain instances when the bone marrow is diseased and can't produce healthy red blood cells, the spleen can take over this important task as well.

The spleen itself is vulnerable to many diseases that cause it to enlarge and that disrupt its ability to work properly, including malaria, mononucleosis, anemia and leukemia. In addition, the spleen, which is located under the rib cage, can easily be injured in a fall, in a car accident or by some other severe blow to the abdomen.

An injured spleen is irreparable and must be surgically removed. Otherwise, it can rupture, which could cause severe bleeding and death.

Despite its hefty duties, the spleen isn't an essential organ. Once it is removed, most of its functions are taken over by other parts of the lymphatic system.

There is one serious risk that grows larger in its absence, however: the danger of getting certain infections. This is more a problem with children. Nonetheless, anybody who has had their spleen removed should be vaccinated against certain bacterias that can cause pneumonia or meningitis.

Stomach

- **Know your food reactions.**
- **Don't stuff yourself.**
- **Avoid excess stomach acid.**

The next time you eat so much that you wish you had a hole in your stomach to siphon out the excess, think about Alexis St. Martin. In 1822, the 18-year-old French Canadian accidentally shot himself with a musket, leaving a gaping hole in his left side and piercing his stomach wall.

St. Martin's adversity became medical science's advantage when Dr. William Beaumont, a U.S. Army surgeon, convinced the patient to become his human guinea pig. The doctor weighed small amounts of food, tied them with silk threads and lowered them through the hole into St. Martin's stomach. Like an ice fisherman, he pulled the food out every hour, noticing any changes. Macabre? Definitely. Revealing? Absolutely. It enabled Dr. Beaumont to identify hydrochloric acid as a gastric, or stomach, juice. He also found another juice, which was later identified as the enzyme pepsin.

It was the first time anyone could confirm that the stomach secretes digestive juices strong enough to corrode food and to potentially eat away at the stomach lining, paving the way for many a dramatic antacid commercial. By the way, don't pity St. Martin; he lived to the ripe old age of 76, siring 17 children before his death.

Inside the Belly of the Beast

Call it the gut, belly, breadbasket, gaster or ventriculus. As many names as it has, the stomach takes the rap for as many aches and pains for which it is not responsible.

"We blame all of the sensations in the abdomen on the stomach," says David Y. Graham, M.D., chief of gastroenterology at the Veterans Administration Medical Center in

Houston. "Any pain that people feel above or below the belly button they misperceive as coming from the stomach. Chances are that the problem is in the colon or the small intestine."

The stomach is an approximately 12-inch-long, J-shaped expandable bag located just below and to the left of the ribs. If the esophagus is the shipping department, then the stomach is the warehouse where foods and beverages are stored and processed before being passed along to the small intestine.

The stomach can expand to hold, on average, 1 to 1½ quarts at a time. After a typical meal, it takes carbohydrates two hours, high-protein foods four hours and high-fat foods six hours to travel through the stomach. The average American, by the way, consumes about 100,000 pounds of food in a lifetime.

While hanging out in the stomach, food gets pulverized by three layers of muscle that contract every 20 seconds. At the same time, glands in the stomach lining secrete hydrochloric acid, a chemical so powerful that even when diluted, it can dissolve mortar off bricks. This gastric juice destroys harmful bacteria in the food. Next, other glands produce the enzyme pepsin, which goes to work breaking down protein. The finished product, a creamy paste called chyme (pronounced *kime*), is then released into the small intestine.

Despite the incredibly corrosive potential of hydrochloric acid, the stomach does not eat itself from the inside out. For this, we should erect huge monuments in gratitude to the self-protective system called the mucosal barrier. It consists of a thick coating of alkaline mucus along the stomach wall and tightly joined cells that prevent gastric juices from leaking into the

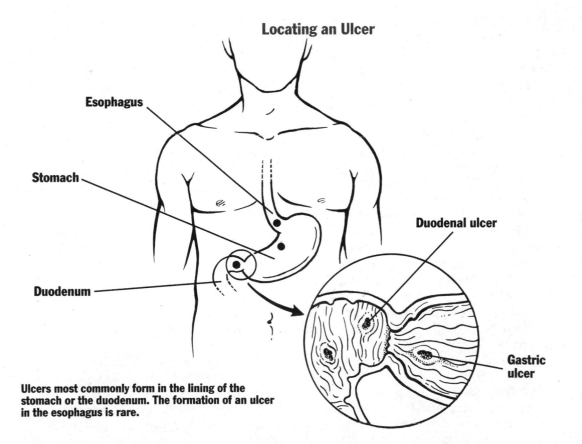

Locating an Ulcer

Esophagus

Stomach

Duodenum

Duodenal ulcer

Gastric ulcer

Ulcers most commonly form in the lining of the stomach or the duodenum. The formation of an ulcer in the esophagus is rare.

underlying tissue layers. A self-renewing process replaces damaged cells every three to six days.

If that barrier breaks down and those highly acidic juices penetrate your stomach wall, you can end up with a condition called gastritis, the fancy name for indigestion. Repeated inflammation can lead to a peptic ulcer. An ulcer is basically an erosion of the stomach wall—an open sore, like the canker sore you get in your mouth, that can cause a gnawing pain. It flares up one to three hours after eating and is often relieved by eating again. An untreated ulcer will eventually eat through the wall of the stomach, causing internal bleeding.

A Well-Fed Stomach

A couple of times a day, your stomach requires care and feeding. Be good to it, and it will be good to you. Here's how.

Learn your food biases. One man's poison can be another man's pleasure. So make no assumptions about foods; each person reacts differently. "Make yourself your own science fair project," suggests Ronald Hoffman, M.D., a physican in New York City, host of a radio show called *Health Talk* and author of *Seven Weeks to a Settled Stomach*. "In talking about the gastrointestinal tract, it's very individualized. People have to find what works for them. If certain foods don't seem to agree with you, cut down on them or cut them out."

Be anti-acid. If you experience stomach pain, the first step is to try an antacid, says David Peura, M.D., associate professor of medicine and acting chief of gastroenterology at the University of Virginia in Charlottesville. Antacids come in several forms, including tablets, liquids and caplets. For stomach problems, Dr. Peura finds the liquid form to be most effective. As their name suggests, antacids neutralize excess acid, which is usually what is causing your stomach to hurt. If your symptoms do not get better, or if stomach pain returns regularly, see your doctor.

Feed those grumbling sounds. It's your brain that gets hungry first. It sends signals to your stomach to start digesting even when there's nothing in there. That growling sound is air being forced through small openings in your digestive tract by stomach contractions, much like when air makes noise as it escapes through the neck of a balloon.

And why does your stomach always seem to growl at the most inopportune moments, such as in the midst of a romantic overture? "Blame the same brain-gut connection again," explains James George, M.D, a physician in the Division of Gastroenterology at Mount Sinai Medical Center in New York City. "When you're nervous, your brain sends signals to your gut to be on the alert." He suggests quieting your stomach with a little food.

Take a break after eating. If a big meal makes you want to take a nap, do so. Forcing yourself into lots of activity could hinder digestion. "Blood flows preferentially," explains Dr. George. "After you eat, your body's first priority is digestion. When you eat, blood gets taken away from your muscles and brain and directed to your intestinal area."

Know the mind-stomach connection. Though nausea and vomiting seem to emanate from your stomach, they begin in your mind and are stimulated by sights (blood and gore), smells (rotten food) and movement (roller-coaster rides) that are registered in your brain. "Vomiting goes far beyond the stomach," explains Thomas Gossel, R.Ph., Ph.D., professor of pharmacology and toxicology and dean of the College of Pharmacy at Ohio Northern University in Ada. "Most vomiting is caused in the central nervous system, in the brain." The violent convulsive reaction of the stomach muscles, he says, is merely the final step in a complex nervous reaction. So be aware of what pushes your nausea button and avoid it.

Take a lesson in swallowing. And you thought you had mastered this one in infancy. "Swallow while exhaling, not inhaling," says Marvin M. Schuster, M.D., profesor of medicine at Johns Hopkins University School of Medicine in Baltimore. Some men find that drinking liquids while eating causes bloating. "It's just that you tend to take in air when you drink, and the air gives you gas," Dr. Schuster says.

Ulcers: Curing the Cause

Back in the seventh century A.D., Byzantine physician Paul of Aegina wrote, "When there is an ulcer in the stomach or bowels, the patient must abstain from all acid food and drink." He wasn't too far off. Yet 1,300 years later, why ulcers occur is still a mystery. "We don't know the precise cause," confesses Dr. Gossel. "I wish I knew."

Until recently, ulcers were considered the worrier's disease, an occupational hazard for those in pressure-cooker positions, such as CEOs and stockbrokers. Experts now attribute ulcers to a tough little bacterium called *Helicobacter pylori*, or *H. pylori* for short. For many years, as it turns out, physicians have been treating the symptoms of ulcers; now, some believe, they can treat the cause. "You can heal an ulcer within two months if you take a drug such as cimetidine (Tagamet)," says Steven Peikin, M.D., professor of medicine at Robert Wood Johnson Medical School in Camden, New Jersey, and author of *Gastrointestinal Health*. "And you can prevent it from coming back with antibiotics such as tetracycline (Achromycin) and metronidazole (Flagyl)."

Here are some other things you can do about ulcers.

Know your family. "Ulcers do run in families," says Dr. Gossel. "If Mom or Dad has one, you may, too." If ulcers are hereditary, then the sensible thing to do, he adds, is to avoid those foods and substances that trigger them.

Avoid aspirin. If you are prone to ulcers, aspirin and other nonsteroidal anti-inflammatory drugs such as ibuprofen can make things worse. "These drugs inhibit the body's production of chemicals that protect the stomach's lining," says third-generation pharmacist John Gould of Emmaus, Pennsylvania. Instead, Dr. Peikin prescribes acetaminophen, a good short-term pain reliever.

There are hundreds of prescription drugs that warn you to take them with caution if you have a pre-existing condition, Dr. Gossel adds. Many such drugs are murder on your gut, so ask your doctor whether the medications in your life could be worsening your ulcer.

Try anti-ulcer meds. Now that Tagamet, one of the most popular anti-ulcer drugs on the market, has gone over-the-counter, sales may well go over the top. Why? "Because it works," says Dr. Graham. How? By blocking the production of a chemical that causes the release of acid in the stomach. Another new nonprescription drug, Pepcid AC, works in much the same way.

Fight fire with fire. Ironically, while eating certain foods may incite your ulcer, eating certain others might help alleviate discomfort—temporarily. "A late-night snack might be just what the doctor ordered," says Dr. Gossel. "Bread or crackers will serve as a good sponge for stomach acid."

Don't worry, be happy. He was your hero when you were eight years old. Why not now? So respond to stress like *Mad* magazine's Alfred E. Neuman: Shrug your shoulders and intone "What, me worry?" "Stress doesn't cause ulcers," says Dr. Peikin. "But stress can aggravate a pre-existing condition by enhancing the output of gastric acid." To minimize the effects of stress—short of retreating to a stressless cave in the Himalayan mountains—"treat your body with respect," Dr. Peikin suggests. "Also, eat and drink in moderation."

Stop smoking. Ulcers are more likely to occur, less likely to heal and more likely to cause death in smokers than in nonsmokers, according to Dr. Peikin.

Spice up your life. Go ahead; it's okay. Dr. Graham and two other researchers found that eating spicy foods causes no visible damage in people without histories of gastrointestinal disease. His advice: "If it doesn't cause you pain, eat it." And how's the following for license to spice? Two studies have shown that people who consume the largest amounts of chili powder have the lowest rates of peptic ulcers.

▣ Sweat Glands

- **Stay clean.**
- **Use a deodorant.**
- **Wash your clothes.**

In 1849, a German engineer named Charles Baunscheidt invented a device to create artificial pores. Baunscheidt thought that jabbing a cluster of 30 tiny needles into various parts of the skin 40 to 60 times and rubbing those areas with an irritating solution would help the body coax out "bad fluids."

Of course, like many half-baked ideas of early medicine, it was both popular and totally misguided. The sweat glands are perfectly capable of doing their main task—cooling the skin—without a lot of poking and prodding.

What Makes You Sweat?

The average man has about three million sweat glands scattered throughout his body. They are particularly abundant on the forehead, underarms, palms and soles of the feet. A typical sedentary guy will produce less than two quarts of sweat a day, but heat and physical activity can boost that output to nearly ten quarts. How much you sweat also depends on your age, race, sex, physical condition and sensitivity to heat. Most sweat is 99 percent water, with traces of salt and other dissolved substances. Each gland consists of a coiled tube, where the sweat is secreted, and a narrow passageway that carries the sweat to the surface of the skin.

There are two types of sweat glands. Eccrine glands, the most common, are embedded in every inch of your skin. These glands are considered a vital part of your body's temperature control system, because as eccrine sweat evaporates, it cools your skin.

Apocrine glands are concentrated around your underarms, navel, anus and pubic area. They have no known physiological role,
although some doctors suspect that in prehistoric times, apocrine glands may have released sexually arousing scents. Apocrines develop at puberty and are best known for interacting with bacteria to produce body odor.

Sweating is controlled by the nervous system, and certain situations trigger sweat in different parts of your body. Exercise, for example, usually produces sweat on your forehead, upper lip, neck and chest. On the other hand, fear or anxiety causes heavy sweating, sometimes called flop sweat, in your armpits and palms and on the soles of your feet. Jack Ramsay, one of the most successful coaches in the NBA, was notorious for his bouts of anxiety sweat during games. As he kneeled on the sidelines, sweat would soak through his shirt, his jacket and even his shoes. At times, he futilely tried taping sweat socks or cut-up disposable diapers to his armpits to control the problem.

Prickly heat, also called heat rash, is the most common problem affecting the sweat glands. In some rare cases, men have hyperhidrosis (excessive sweating all of the time) or hypohidrosis (inhibited sweating). Both of these disorders can be treated by a doctor.

No Stink Allowed

Sweating is both good and necessary. Smelling foul is neither. Here's how to battle body odor.

Stay clean. Remember that it is the sweat glands and the bacteria feeding on the sweat that cause the stink, not the sweat itself. So wash away the bacteria in your armpits and groin with a deodorant soap, says Michael Kaminer, M.D., director of cosmetic dermatologic surgery at New England Medical Center in Boston and assistant professor of dermatology at Tufts University in Medford, Massachusetts.

Forgo garlic. Spicy foods, particularly those made with garlic, can increase body odor, says Dr. Kaminer. Eliminate the food or spice from your diet if you suspect that it is causing a problem.

Choose your weapon. Antiperspirants can reduce sweating by up to 50 percent but do little to mask odor. Deodorants can help reduce body odor but have virtually no effect on sweating. If you sweat heavily, you're better off getting an antiperspirant containing aluminum chloride rather than a deodorant, because reducing the amount of sweat is more effective than trying to mask the odor, Dr. Kaminer says.

Clean your clothes. How does a guy tell if a shirt is clean? Easy: He smells the armpits. Dirty clothes reek of sweat even if the pits behind them are scrubbed. Know the limit on how long your clothes can last before cleaning.

Relax. If stressful situations cause you to sweat excessively, try practicing a relaxation technique such as meditation, yoga or progressive relaxation for 10 to 20 minutes a day to see if it makes a difference, says Lenise Banse, M.D., a dermatologist at Northeast Family Dermatology Center in Clinton Township, Michigan.

Taking On the Itch

To combat prickly heat, a rash that occurs when sweat ducts become plugged and sweat leaks into the surrounding skin and irritates it, try these simple techniques.

Chill out. Since hot, humid weather usually triggers prickly heat, your best bet is to get out of the sun and cool off, says dermatologist Anita Highton, M.D., medical director of clinical research at Westwood-Squibb Pharmaceuticals in Buffalo, New York. Take a tepid shower or bath or apply lukewarm (80° to 90°F) compresses to soothe the itching. Stay in air-conditioned rooms as much possible for at least one day after the rash subsides.

Shed tight clothes. Tight clothing sets you up for prickly heat because it traps sweat next to your skin and prevents it from evaporating, Dr. Highton says. Wear loose-fitting cotton or polypropylene garments instead.

Take a vinegar plunge. To relieve itching, pour a cup of white vinegar into a tepid bath and soak in it until you feel comfortable, Dr. Highton says.

Moisturize for relief. An over-the-counter moisturizer that contains dimethicone, such as Moisturel, can help relieve the itching, Dr. Highton says.

Tailbone

- **Fall properly: Curl and roll.**

Evolution continues to shape us. That is the best explanation for why we have body parts that no longer serve much purpose: the appendix, wisdom teeth and sometimes a tiny tail. Rarely, but occasionally, a baby greets this brave new world with a tail peeping up from his tailbone.

"It's a pretty rudimentary tail, a funny little appendage of skin, fat and occasionally some bone. It's just a disorganized hunk of tissue on the bottom of the butt," says John D. Loeser, M.D., director of the pain center and professor of neurologic surgery at the University of Washington School of Medicine in Seattle.

Dr. Loeser snips off about one tail a year—a "trivial operation," he says. And that's probably the only case in the state of Washington, he adds. "They really are quite rare."

Even if you weren't born with a tail, you were born with a vestigial tailbone. "It doesn't seem to do very much, except form an attachment for the pelvic ligaments," says Scott Haldeman, M.D., Ph.D., D.C., associate clinical professor of neurology at the University of California, Irvine, and adjunct professor in the research department at the Los Angeles Chiropractic College. Ligaments connect bone to bone.

The coccyx, the tailbone's proper name, is actually a little triangle of bone made up of four fused vertebrae. It got its name from the Greek word for *cuckoo*; apparently, the bone reminded someone of a cuckoo's beak. The coccyx sits below the sacrum, a much larger and more useful triangle of five fused spinal bones that supports the base of the spine.

You'd have to take a hard fall to actually injure your tailbone, since it curls under. So fall backward, and your buttocks take the shock instead, says Dr. Haldeman. "Some people have protruding tailbones, which are a little more vulnerable. But usually, an injury requires a direct blow."

Tailbone injury is rare for everyone, but it is more likely to happen to men than to women for two reasons. First, a woman's pelvis flares up, offering a slight measure of protection that a man doesn't have, according to Dr. Haldeman. Second, men tend to have less protective padding on their buttocks. As actor Michael Douglas reportedly remarked upon seeing himself naked on film: "Whew, what a bony butt."

If you do land just so and happen to crack, displace or bruise your coccyx, the injury is called coccydynia. "But that just means pain in the tailbone," says Dr. Loeser.

"A fracture hurts like hell, but it heals relatively painlessly," he says. "Permanent pain in the tailbone is hard to explain."

"For a while, doctors used to cut out fractured tailbones if there was chronic pain. But that wasn't successful," says Dr. Haldeman. "If there is pain, a doughnut pillow can be used for sitting. Luckily, coccydynia resolves itself for the majority of people."

Better not to fall. But if you do start to tumble and you have time to react, you can protect your tailbone. "Clearly, the way to fall is by using the martial arts technique," says Dr. Haldeman. "You want to curl and roll rather than plop. You don't want to take all of the force on any one part of your body. If you bend your legs and roll, that takes the force of the fall through multiple body parts and dissipates some of the shock."

Tear Ducts

- **Try a humidifier.**
- **Use the right eyedrops.**
- **Apply the drops properly.**

One-question quiz: Men cry less than women because (A) their tear ducts are smaller, (B) they are not subject to the same hormonal fluctuations, (C) they were raised differently or (D) all of the above.

Don't flatter yourself, you big oaf. It's C. "I've never heard of a single biological or hormonal explanation for why men cry less than women. There's absolutely no difference in the tear ducts or how they operate," says W. Steven Pray, R.Ph., Ph.D., professor of nonprescription drug products at Southwestern Oklahoma State University College of Pharmacy in Weatherford.

Okay. No lectures here on the glories of crying. If you want to play the stoic warrior, that's fine with us. This book covers ulcers, too. (Seriously, for help in expressing yourself more effectively, see page 21.) We'll just say here that crying is an all-purpose tool, good for expressing joy, releasing despair, protecting your eyes, watering beer.

Tears are salty secretions that keep two parts of the eye constantly moist. They flow over the cornea, the transparent coating of the eye, and they lubricate the conjunctiva, the membrane covering the white of the eye and lining the inside of the eyelid. Tears also wash away stray bits of dust and grit and help keep the eye infection-free with a natural antiseptic called lysozyme.

But even though one tear is as good as another, they come from different sources. The tears that keep your eyes constantly moist are produced on the conjunctiva and also in the eyelid. The tears you cry over a lost love, squandered savings or a sentimental movie are reflex tears, generated from a gland in the upper, outer corner of the upper eyelid. These tears also spring into action when you get something in your eye.

The Crying Mechanism

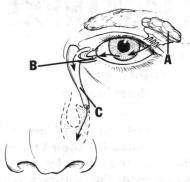

Emotional tears and tears to wash away dirt and such are secreted by the lacrimal gland, above the outer edge of each
eye (A). Overflow tears are channeled out of the eyes through
the lacrimal puncta, better known as tear ducts (B). This
overflow gets dumped into the nasal passages (C). This is
why you blow your nose so much when you cry.

Some of this overflow ends up in your
tear ducts, the pinpoint-size holes located in
the inside corners of your lower and upper
eyelids. Rather than producing tears, tear ducts
act as the drainage ducts through which tears
get washed into your nasal passages. That's
right: When you blow your nose after crying,
it's tears that you are blasting into your tissue.

Dry Times

You're not likely to pay much attention to
everyday tear activity until the wells go dry. But
when your eyes are dry, they'll feel scratchy or
irritated or they'll burn. There are many causes
of dry eyes, says Dr. Pray; winter winds, air-
conditioning and indoor heating are all potential culprits. You can also get dry eyes if you
have an allergy to contact lens products.
Chronic cases often result from rheumatoid
arthritis or Sjögren's syndrome, a gland condition that also causes dry mouth.

If you have dry eyes and none of these
causes is the culprit, maybe you can blame
your medication. A few of the drugs known to
have this effect are antihistamines and tricyclic
antidepressants. There are other medications as
well, so check with your doctor or pharmacist.

So what, if anything, can you do about
dry eyes? Here are some tear tips.

Steam up the air. Using a humidifier set
at about 80 percent humidity helps moisturize
the air, says Thomas Gossel, R.Ph., Ph.D.,
professor of pharmacology and toxicology and
dean of the College of Pharmacy at Ohio
Northern University in Ada. If your humidifier
does not mark off percentages, set it at the maximum steaming level. Since your corneas are always exposed to the air, you're putting moisture
on them when you humidify the air, he notes.

Drop in. Over-the-counter artificial tears are
the best remedy for dry eyes, Dr. Pray says. He
suggests using them two or three times a day.

Keep some drops out. Avoid eye care
products that "get the red out" by constricting the
eyes' blood vessels the way Visine does, advises
Dr. Pray. These drops only aggravate dry eyes.

Drip the drops correctly. The best way
to apply eyedrops is to pull your lower eyelid
down, says Dr. Pray. Then tilt back your head
until you're looking up and drop in the artificial
tears without touching your eye or eyelid with
the applicator. Close your eyes and cover the
inside corner of one eye with your thumb and
the inside corner of the other eye with your
index finger for a few seconds. This keeps the
drops from draining off through the tear ducts.

Applying Eyedrops

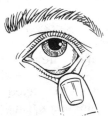

Pull your lower eyelid
down.

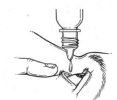

Tilt your head back and drop in the
solution.

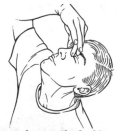

Close your eye and cover the inside corner of
your eye to prevent draining.

🦷 Teeth

- **Learn proper brushing and flossing techniques.**
- **Use these techniques many times a day.**
- **Fear no dentist.**

In a world full of Freddy Krueger movies, Mortal Kombat video games and John Travolta career comebacks, it's getting tougher and tougher to scare kids these days. So the next time you have to tell the ghost story at Junior's Cub Scout camp-a-thon, you'll have to break out the truly horrifying stuff.

You'll have to tell them about the dentist.

Tell them about the days before novocaine. Tell them about the slow drill and the fast drill. Tell them about that sinking feeling you got when that pointy metal prod stuck in one of your molars and the dentist said, "Well, Johnny, there's another one we'll have to fill."

Then watch them run screaming to their knapsacks for a toothbrush and a canteen.

Actually, the little tykes have it easy. Thanks to fluoridated water and better toothbrushes, toothpastes and dental techniques, cavities are becoming a rarity. Almost half of American children between ages 5 and 17 have no cavities in their permanent teeth. They'll never know the fun of "rinse, spit and open wide."

Then, sad to say, there's you. If you're a typical American adult between the ages of 18 and 64, you have 22.8 fillings in your bony little head. Only 4 percent of us made it through childhood without a cavity. Only one in three of us has all of his teeth.

But before you run screaming for a toothbrush, understand that it doesn't have to happen. There's a lot you can do to keep the teeth you have forever. Ten minutes of work each day, using the right tools and techniques, should keep your teeth in your head and out of a jar until the Grim Reaper himself wipes the smile off your face.

The Roots of the Problem

Teeth have many side benefits. They help you form words (try saying "thalassocracy" without touching your tongue to the inside of your teeth). They fill out your face, eliminating that unappealing caved-in-cheek look. They hold things such as pens and car keys when you have no other handy place to put them.

But mostly, they chew. Without teeth, you'd still be bellying up to the edge of the local pond and slurping down algae. Teeth cut, rip and grind your meal until it's thoroughly mixed with saliva (to aid digestion) and ready to swallow.

Adult humans have 32 teeth, divided into four main groups. The front teeth (4 upper, 4 lower) are called incisors. They are chisel-shaped, designed to bite through food. Then come the canines (2 upper, 2 lower), sharp teeth with very long roots. These are for tearing food and, if you have a fancy for caskets and black capes, for piercing the necks of beautiful women and drinking their blood. Next are the premolars, or bicuspids (4 upper, 4 lower). These are designed for grinding food that the incisors or canines have already bitten through or torn off. Finally come the molars (6 upper, 6 lower), flat-topped teeth that finish the grinding job and prepare food for swallowing. The molars include the wisdom teeth, the last in each row. These are the final teeth to appear, not emerging until late adolescence or early adulthood.

Although they are very hard, teeth are very much alive. (Fingernails, by contrast, are hard but not alive, which is why you don't need a shot of novocaine to trim them.) The outermost layer of a tooth is called the enamel. This protective covering, which shields the tooth from chicken bones and ice cubes, ends at the gumline. Underneath the enamel lies the dentin. This is a hard casing that surrounds the pulp, which is the mass of blood vessels and nerves that feed the tooth.

The root of the tooth fits neatly into a socket in the jawbone. The root is covered by a bony material called cementum, which is connected to the gum and the jaw by periodontal ligaments.

As strong as teeth can be, they're no match for many of mankind's more fiendish inventions. Take refined sugar. When sugar sits in your mouth, it combines with saliva to form a powerful acid. And this acid goes to work on the enamel. Once the enamel wears away, you have a cavity. Let the cavity go long enough, and the dentin erodes. Then bacteria invade the pulp, and you're looking at a root canal procedure to save your tooth.

You have plenty of other things to worry about, too. When food particles get between your teeth or wedged under your gums, they mix with saliva and bacteria. The result is a sticky, awful mixture called plaque. Unless removed, plaque turns into a hard, cementlike substance called tartar or calculus. Tartar grows between your teeth and gums and causes erosion at the roots of your teeth.

Maintaining Your Teeth

The world's greatest monument to tooth decay resides in Rome. It is there that between 1868 and 1904, a dentist, Brother Giovanni Battista Orsenigo, extracted and kept 2,000,744 of his patients' teeth. That's an average of 185 teeth per day—almost six full sets of choppers. No wonder Romans learned to slurp their spaghetti.

You have two major methods of avoiding the curse of Brother Orsenigo. You can brush your teeth three to five times a day—the right way. And you can floss your teeth at least once, and preferably twice, a day. These things, combined with a visit to your dentist every six months for routine maintenance, can keep the teeth thieves at bay.

"These are your best lines of defense," says Howard S. Glazer, D.D.S., president of the Academy of General Dentistry. "Everything else, from fluoride rinses to mouthwashes to antiseptic rinses, is purely secondary."

Truth is, you are probably brushing your teeth incorrectly: too short, too hard, wrong angle, wrong grip. To help you learn the perfect technique, we've put together the ultimate guide to mouth maintenance. Turn to "Cleaning Your Mouth" on page 320 to learn the right ways to brush and floss.

After you've taken care of the basics, consider some of this advice from Dr. Glazer.

Don't wait—fluoridate. Fluoride in tap water has gone a long way toward eliminating tooth decay, Dr. Glazer says. Fluoride builds resistance to the acid that erodes tooth enamel. You can get an extra level of protection by using an over-the-counter fluoride rinse every day. "This is especially important if your water supply isn't fluoridated," Dr. Glazer says. "It's the third most important thing you can do for your teeth, after brushing and flossing."

To get them white, do it right. Several things can discolor your teeth. Medicines, especially tetracycline, and iron supplements can

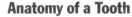

Anatomy of a Tooth

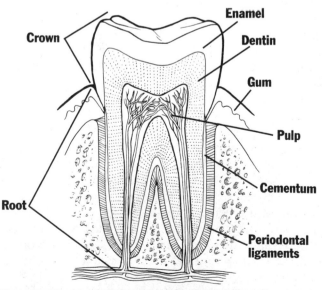

If you don't brush and floss often, acid can wear away the enamel of your teeth. If left untreated, the dentin can also erode.

leave stains. So can years of coffee and tea drinking. Smoking turns teeth yellow, too.

But if you want to whiten your teeth, resist the urge to do it yourself. Visit your dentist instead. Over-the-counter whitening agents aren't really strong enough to do the job, and some whitening toothpastes can be too abrasive for your enamel, says Dr. Glazer.

Don't miss a swish. If you are eating out and can't brush your teeth right after a meal, rinse your mouth out with water. It's not enough to just drink the water; you have to swish it around in your mouth for about ten seconds to reach all of your teeth, says Dr. Glazer. Do this two or three times.

Use a mouth guard. There's nothing like a hockey puck to ruin a perfect smile. If you play any sport where there's a chance of falling down or taking a flying object or elbow in your face—and we're talking everything from in-line skating to Roller Derby—buy a mouth guard. Your dentist can custom-fit one for you, or you can go to almost any sporting goods store and buy one. With most brands, you run hot water over the mouth guard until it's soft, then stick it in your mouth and let it mold to your teeth, says Dr. Glazer.

What That Pain Is Telling You

Breaking up with your girlfriend hurts. Shattering your
(continued on page 322)

Pain and Agony? No and Way

Put some words together, and they make your skin crawl. "Tax" and "audit." "You're" and "fired." "Mother" and "in-law." But no combination has the same exquisite effect as "root" and "canal." And that bothers Richard C. Burns, D.D.S.

"Johnny Carson joked about it all of the time," says Dr. Burns, past president of the American Association of Endodontists. "But it's not the root canal procedure that hurts so bad. It's the pain beforehand. If we didn't do root canals, a lot more people would lose their teeth."

Root canal surgery involves removing diseased tissue from the inside of a tooth and replacing it with gutta-percha, a rubberlike substance found in a Malaysian tree. The process eliminates the bacteria that eventually infect a tooth and the surrounding bone.

Here's how a root canal works.

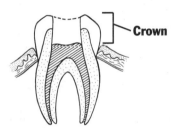

An opening is made in the crown of the tooth.

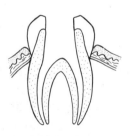

The diseased pulp is removed from the pulp chamber and the root canals. Instruments are used to clean the canals, and if the tooth is infected, medication is placed inside.

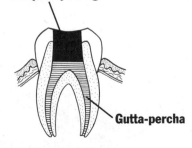

When the tooth has been disinfected, the canals and the pulp chamber are filled with gutta-percha. The opening of the crown is sealed with a temporary filling.

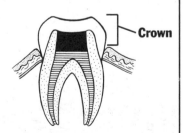

Your regular dentist will usually replace the temporary filling with a permanent filling or a crown during a follow-up visit.

▯ Cleaning Your Mouth

- **Brush three to five times a day. Minimum: after breakfast and before bedtime.**
- **Floss morning and night. Minimum: before your bedtime brushing.**
- **Eat foods that are good for your teeth.**
- **Drink lots of water to keep saliva flowing.**

How to Brush Your Teeth

You've been brushing your teeth for decades, so you pretty much have it all figured out, right? Guess again, bristle-breath. Here are some essential truths you should know about toothbrushing.

Brush longer. If you're the average toothbrushing American male, you're not coming anywhere close to the three-minutes-per-session minimum that most dentists recommend. Of course, 180 seconds of round and round and round and round can seem like an eternity, so try passing the time by watching television, listening to the radio for the duration of one song, soft-boiling an egg, petting the dog or reading the boss's latest memo.

Brush more often. Once after breakfast and once before bed is the absolute minimum. You should try to brush after each snack and meal, states Howard S. Glazer, D.D.S., president of the Academy of General Dentistry. The first 20 minutes or so is critical. If you don't remove the excess food, it can break down into harmful acid or contribute to plaque formation.

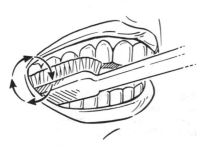

Brush in circles at an angle. Don't ever brush from side to side. This wears away your gums. Brush in an elliptical pattern, with the bristles turned at a 45-degree angle toward your gumline.

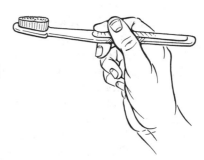

Brush softer. You're supposed to clean your teeth, not declare a holy war on them. Brushing too hard is counterproductive, says Dr. Glazer; you'll wear away your gums, exposing tooth roots. This can make your teeth more sensitive to hot and cold foods and can make it easier for bacteria to start wrecking teeth under the gumline.

Dr. Glazer recommends switching your brush grip from the usual deep-in-the-palm choke hold to a more delicate grip, as if holding a pen. Hold the brush between your thumb and index finger.

Brush with fluoride. Choosing a toothpaste is largely a matter of personal preference. As long as it contains fluoride, pretty much any paste or gel is acceptable. Dr. Glazer says a tartar control formula is a good idea. Baking soda toothpastes are fine, as well. But don't brush with just plain baking soda. It's too abrasive.

Brush your gums. Brushing is great for your gums. But too much can actually hurt. Be gentle when you brush, or you'll erode your gums, says Dr. Glazer.

Brush your tongue. Many dentists believe that you should brush your tongue. The tongue harbors bacteria, which can encourage bad breath. ■

How to Floss Your Teeth

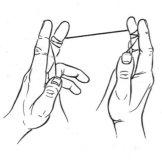

1. Break off about 18 inches of floss. Wrap the ends around the middle fingers on both hands until you have 6 to 8 inches of floss between them.

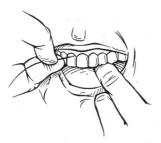

2. Pinch the floss with the thumb and index finger of one hand. With the index finger of your other hand, gently guide about one inch of the floss between your two front teeth. Create a C with the floss by bending it around one of the teeth.

3. Slide the floss between the teeth toward the gumline. When you feel resistance at the gumline, stop. Now slide the floss up and down between the tooth and the gumline to remove plaque. Don't use a sawing motion; this can damage the tooth. Repeat on the other tooth.

4. Remove the floss from between your two front teeth and unwind a short, clean piece from one of your fingers. Place the floss between one of your front teeth and the tooth next to it, then repeat the third step. Continue until you have worked between all of your teeth.

Note: It's okay to use tools that hold floss instead of wrapping floss around your fingers. Just be careful not to push too far under the gumline, and never use a sawing motion.■

Good Foods for Teeth . . .

1. ***Apples.*** They're crunchy and full of fiber, which helps scrape plaque off your teeth. Other crunchy raw vegetables do the same job.

2. ***Hot peppers.*** They make your mouth water, and the extra saliva helps neutralize acid in your mouth, cutting back on tooth decay.

3. ***Yogurt.*** Lots of calcium, which keeps your teeth and jawbone strong. Make sure you eat nonfat plain yogurt. The stuff with fruit on the bottom has lots of tooth-killing sugar. Mix in fresh fruit for better taste.

4. ***Low-fat cheese.*** Again, calcium. But the cheese also neutralizes acid. So eat an ounce or so after eating a sugar-laden food.

5. ***Carrots.*** They have loads of the nutrient beta-carotene, which studies show may lower the risk of oral cancer. Cantaloupe is another excellent source of beta-carotene.

. . . and Bad Foods

1. ***Soft drinks.*** Tons of sugar, which does to your teeth what acid rain does to your car's paint job.

2. ***Fruit juices.*** Healthy, yes. But also sugary, syrupy and acidic. Drink them—but swish water in your mouth when you're done.

3. ***Popcorn.*** The hard, unpopped kernels at the bottom of the bag can crack teeth. And unless you brush and floss when you're done, little pieces can wedge between your teeth and gums and create plaque.

4. ***Vinegar.*** Again, acid. Acid is bad.

5. ***Gumballs.*** Rock-hard balls of sugar. Need we say more? ■

thighbone in seven places hurts. Jumping from the 27th floor of a burning building into a Dumpster full of rusty roofing nails hurts.

But a toothache? Now we're talking pain.

"God, teeth can really hurt," says Richard C. Burns, D.D.S., past president of the American Association of Endodontists. "A person can live with a lot of pain if it's a sprained ankle or something. But tooth pain . . . nobody can take that for long."

Unfortunately, it's often hard to tell from the throbbing whether you have a major or a minor problem. Sometimes a loose filling feels like a dagger in your tongue, and sometimes a serious infection can cause just a minor, dull ache while it erodes your tooth or jawbone. If you have a toothache, Dr. Burns suggests taking 60 milligrams of ibuprofen every four to six hours for swelling and pain. Then take a peek at the list below to see what could be ailing you.

Cold or heat sensitivity. When eating a hot or cold food causes temporary pain, it's probably not a big deal. A filling may have come loose. Or your gum may have receded a little, exposing a sensitive tooth root. Try a toothpaste designed for sensitive teeth; components in the toothpaste can dull nerve receptors and help ease the pain, says Dr. Burns. At your next visit to the dentist, tell him about the sensitivity and let him take a look.

If the pain lingers for more than a few seconds after you've eaten, however, you may have a bigger problem. Dr. Burns says it's likely that you have sustained damage to the pulp of your tooth. You may need a root canal treatment to remove the pulp and preserve your tooth. See your dentist immediately.

Sharp pain and swollen gums. You may have an abscess. This little pocket of pus

---

Pop Goes the Molar: How to Save a Dislodged Tooth

Sometimes you're Larry, and sometimes you're Moe. Life is unpredictable like that. So on those occasions when you receive a frying pan in your chops instead of giving it, you'd better know what to do.

When a tooth pops out of your head, pick it up and drop it in a glass of water. Milk is fine, too. Just resist the urge to sterilize it, says Howard S. Glazer, D.D.S., president of the Academy of General Dentistry. "Don't put it in alcohol, because that will dry it out. And that's the worst thing you could do."

Also resist the urge to wipe it off with a tissue. Again, this will dry it out, which could damage the fibrous attachments still present on the root surface. If you can't find a glass of water or milk, just pop the tooth in your cheek and drive to your dentist. Although you have about one hour before the tooth becomes difficult to save, there's a 90 percent chance of success if it's implanted within 15 to 30 minutes.

---

is your body's natural response to bacteria growing in the root canal. Left untreated, an abscess can cause severe bone loss. You should see your dentist immediately; he may refer you to an endodontist, who specializes in diagnosing tooth pain and performing root canal work, says Dr. Burns.

Biting pain. If chewing on a carrot or another hard food causes sharp pain, you could have a cavity, a loose filling or even a cracked tooth, says Dr. Burns. The pain could also be a sign of advanced decay and pulp damage. See your dentist within a few days.

Dull ache in the upper teeth. If this is the first time you've felt the pain, it may just be caused by a bad sinus headache, says Dr. Burns. But if the pain occurs regularly, the problem could be bruxism, or tooth grinding. (See page 208 for more details about this condition.)

Constant pain in the head, ears or neck. Pulp damage from nerve exposure or trauma can cause generalized head pain, says Dr. Burns. So can dozens of other nondental conditions. See your physician or dentist immediately.

Testicles

- **Protect them dearly.**
- **Inspect often for lumps.**

You can lose the family jewels and still sparkle at sex.

"Balls!" you say? Consider this.

"The testicles have two functions. One is to produce sperm, which makes a man fertile. The other is to provide testosterone, which gives a man his sex drive," says Perry Nadig, M.D., clinical professor of urologic surgery at the University of Texas Health Science Center at San Antonio. "The testosterone can be replaced, and there will be no decline in sexual function. Testosterone, rather than causing an erection, only provides the desire for one."

So in the highly unlikely event that both of your testicles would be removed—by whatever means, for whatever reason—you could get by, says Dr. Nadig. Your doctor would drop prosthetic testicles into your scrotum. And he'd prescribe a testosterone patch or biweekly injections. You couldn't make babies, but you'd have no trouble making love. True story.

Nutty Information

Your testicles hang, side by side, in the bumpy, gnarly bag beneath your penis called the scrotum. The scrotum gets its unique texture from a muscle layer just beneath the skin. The muscle allows the bag to retract for warmth or protection. Usually, though, testicles hang away from the body to keep their cool, since overheated sperm don't perform well.

A normal testicle is a compressed ball of spaghetti-like tubes sealed in a tough casing. In size, it's somewhere between a Ping-Pong ball and an egg.

Your testicles started pumping testosterone into your bloodstream while you were still forming in your mother's womb. That con-

vinced various organs to develop in a manly way. Your testicles began manufacturing sperm after receiving a chemical wake-up call from your brain at puberty.

Keeping Your Testicles in Shape

Caring for and maintaining your testicles boils down to keeping them free of injury and monitoring them for unusual bumps or growths. Here are the details on how to keep your balls in play.

Avoid injury. Wear a protective cup during rough-and-tumble sports. That'll keep the jewels from dangling in the way of a rushing defensive lineman.

If your testicles do get hit, wrap an ice pack in a towel and cradle your scrotum with it to reduce swelling and tissue damage, says Wolfram E. Nolten, M.D., male infertility expert at the University of Wisconsin–Madison.

Work out. General fitness counts. Research shows that those who are sedentary or who sit at their desks for more than ten hours a day are more likely to develop testicular cancer.

Check 'em out. While showering, feel for lumps and abnormalities and report any to your doctor, says Paul Gleich, M.D., chief of urology at St. Paul–Ramsey Medical Center in St. Paul, Minnesota. This is how cancer is caught in time to be cured. (For further details, see "How to Do a Testicular Self-Exam" on page 48.)

Trim the fat. A fatty diet may interfere with testosterone production, and a lowered testosterone level may leave you feeling less than manly.

Hang loose. Loose underwear, such as boxer shorts, helps keep things cool in hot climates. Bikini briefs may overheat your delicate sperm.

Hurts So Bad

We may gasp, then chuckle when it happens to someone else. But a direct hit to the testicles is no laughing matter. Besides the fact that it hurts like nothing else, the lack of protective bone or muscle makes lasting damage more feasible. The situation requires immediate treatment. Dr. Nolten recommends ice packs, rest and anti-inflammatory medication to bring down swelling and lessen the tissue damage that can result in infertility. If the swelling doesn't subside quickly, your doctor may need to cut the casing to relieve pressure and prevent damage.

Why do we roll on the ground in agony when our testicles are crunched?

Look at it like this, says Dr. Gleich: The testicle responds to impact by swelling. The tough casing around the testicle immediately resists the swelling. The fight between testicle and casing creates enormous pressure inside the casing, inflaming nerves in the testicle and angering similar nerves in organs throughout the abdomen. When that happens, we're down for the count.

Here's a different view of the same issue, this one from Durwood Neal, Jr., M.D., associate professor of urology at the University of Texas Medical Branch at Galveston. Dr. Neal notes that the testicle, being an internal or visceral organ, feels pain differently than skin and muscle. When the latter get hurt, the pain is sharp and location-specific. But when a visceral organ gets hurt, the pain spreads widely—in the case of the testicle, throughout the abdomen. "That's why it feels like there's a fire in your abdomen and it's all-engulfing, making you keel over," Dr. Neal says.

What Goes Wrong

You don't have to be smacked to feel pain in the testicles. And not all lumps mean cancer. Other possibilities are:

Inflammation. The tangled mass of duct-work behind the testicles known as the epididymis can become inflamed or infected

The Testosterone Myth

Testosterone, the hormone that turns boys into men, has been unfairly blamed for nearly all obnoxious, vicious and unseemly male behavior. Now science is finding that the male hormone doesn't make most of us rough, tough and mean or callous and aggressive. In some ways, it's the opposite: High levels of testosterone seem to make us friendly and easygoing, energetic and sexy. Low levels make us testy and frigid.

The testicles pump copious amounts of testosterone into our bloodstreams during puberty. This fuels incredible fantasies, matures our genitals and signals chest and facial hair that it's time to sprout. By the time we hit middle age, however, our testosterone levels drop by about one-third. With this decline, we begin to feel differently. We think about sex less. We may also think less clearly.

What doesn't change is our ability to make babies. This is in contrast to women, whose hormonal dive in middle age ends their fertility and thus signals a major physiological milestone. For most men, "male menopause" is not nearly as dramatic, physiologically or psychologically.

But for 7 percent of us, testosterone levels drop too low by age 40. Twenty percent of us have too-low levels by age 60. But you can sling the zing back into your step with supplementation, by injection or patch, if a blood test shows that your testosterone level has drained too much.

Supplementation boosts sex drive, builds muscle, protects the heart by raising levels of HDL, the good cholesterol, and appears to increase bone density. But supplementation can increase the risk of stroke, shut down the body's ability to produce its own testosterone and cause prostate problems. So at this point, regular testosterone supplementation is recommended only for men whose levels are especially low.

for any number of reasons, including heavy lifting and chlamydia, a sexually transmitted bacterial infection. "The epididymis enlarges to a mass that's half of the size of a fist and is very painful," says Dr. Nadig. "Usually, you'll run a fever. It's treated with rest, hot baths and antibiotics."

Torsion. A testicle hangs like a pendulum, suspended from a cord that supplies its blood. While this doesn't happen often, a testicle can turn, twist and kink the cord. You'll feel enough pain that you'll want to go to your doctor. And you should. If the cord doesn't unwind, the testicle can atrophy and die in a matter of hours. Even if the testicle and cord untwist by themselves, surgery might be needed to stitch both testicles to the scrotum wall, says Dr. Gleich. Why? Because like Chubby Checker, a testicle that twists once is likely to twist again. And if one twists, the other may get ideas.

Fluid buildup. Sperm or water sometimes collects in sacs, called seals, inside the scrotum. "They're completely harmless. We don't do anything about them unless they're large enough to be bothersome. Then we remove them surgically," says Dr. Gleich.

Catching and Killing Cancer

Modern treatment of testicular cancer is a success story. The cancer is rare, but of the two types that hit the testicles, radiation zaps one, and a special blend of chemotherapy, radiation and surgery gets the other. The cure rate is greater than 90 percent. Cure, though, depends upon early detection. And that's where you come in. It's your job to detect testicular cancer.

"I don't think I've ever discovered a testicular cancer that the patient didn't know about," says Dr. Gleich. "Just washing yourself in the shower is usually enough contact to detect something abnormal."

What would you detect? "The only thing you'll feel is a painless lump or hardness or swelling of the testicle," says Dr. Nadig.

Eighty-five percent of testicular cancers are in men under age 50. The disease is most common between ages 15 and 39. It strikes 3 in 100,000 men annually and, for reasons undetermined, has doubled in incidence in the past 40 years.

When cancer is diagnosed, the testicle is usually removed. "If you lose one, you can still get along pretty well with the other," says Dr. Nadig. You'll need a few rounds of follow-up radiation or chemotherapy and, most important, close monitoring for a year or so.

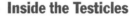

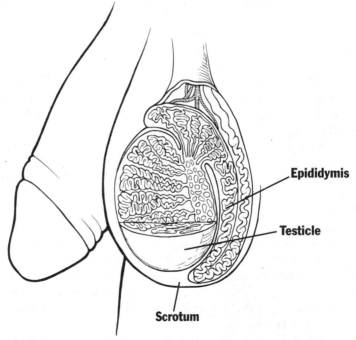

Chronic pain felt in the testicle is most often caused by an infection or inflammation of the epididymis.

Throat

- **Keep it moist.**
- **Breathe through your nose.**
- **Don't shout.**

John Stuart's career involves swallowing two-thirds of a three-foot sword. The Minnesota amusement park amuser simply tips back his head, exhales lightly, relaxes and slides in the sword.

"The person who taught me handed me a chrome-plated sword with no handle. I swore up and down that it folded up somehow," says Stuart, now in his mid-forties, who has been swallowing swords of various shapes and sizes since he was a teenager. "It took me four tries in 15 minutes. And on the fourth try, I felt that cold steel go down my throat, and I said, 'Yep, it's done for real.'"

We do not recommend this trick at home. But if there's a lesson to be learned, it's that your throat can be pretty pliable and that if you just relax, you can stop yourself from gagging, even in extreme situations, such as when your dentist is playing in your mouth with loud tools.

Your throat is strong, too. The five-inch passageway moves food and air along to their destinations—the esophagus and the windpipe, respectively. This funnel-shaped tube also houses the vocal cords, tonsils and Adam's apple.

Newton's law applies only partially to your throat. It's easier to eat when you're upright, allowing gravity to aid the task. But you could also swallow while standing on your head because of the powerful muscles that your throat boasts.

While food is in your throat, your body does things to prevent choking and backwash. Your tongue rises to the top of your mouth, preventing food from getting back into your mouth or nose. At the other end, the lidlike epiglottis closes over your airway, preventing food and liquid from getting into your lungs. But when someone cracks a joke while you're swallowing soda, these protective features sometimes fail. And your laughter is accompanied by a soda sneeze or cough.

On the Front Line

Your throat is one of the internal body parts most exposed to the external world. This makes it a first place of attack for incoming germs. Though your throat has numerous germ-fighting weapons, germs are fairly successful at making your swallowing life miserable. Sore throat causes some 40 million doctors' visits a year by adults alone, making it one of the most common medical complaints in America.

Generally, the throat has three types of enemies: viruses, bacteria and allergens. While all have similar symptoms—redness, soreness, swelling—the remedy for each is different.

Viruses, usually the same ones that cause the common cold and flus, are the top cause of sore throat. Because there are so many strains of viruses, there isn't a one-size-fits-all medicine. Treatment is usually built around soothing the symptoms and making the throat a more inhospitable host. The body usually cures itself within a week.

The most common bacterial infection is strep throat. The one plus of strep and other bacterial infections is that they are usually treatable with antibiotics. The downside is that they are more dangerous if left untreated: One complication could be rheumatic fever.

Allergens are things that should be harmless to your body but that your body mistakes as harmful, such as pollen and cat dander. When you breathe in an allergen, it can get stuck in your throat. Your immune system attacks it there, generating mucus and soreness. Common sense prevails here. Stay away from those things you are allergic to, and your throat won't be attacked, says Jerome C. Goldstein, M.D., visiting professor at Johns Hopkins University in Baltimore and Georgetown University in Washington, D.C.

Prevention and Maintenance

There's not much you can do to protect your throat from the outside elements. Eating and breathing really aren't optional. But you can help your throat indirectly by strengthening your immune system, your body's defense equipment, says Eleonore Blaurock-Busch, Ph.D., president and laboratory director of Trace Minerals International in Boulder, Colorado. One way to do this is to take protective supplements: 5,000 international units of vitamin A, 60 milligrams of vitamin C and 70 micrograms of selenium per day.

Zinc is also important for a strong immune system, Dr. Blaurock-Busch adds. Men need about 15 milligrams a day. A diet rich in lean meats, chicken and beans will take care of your zinc needs.

Here are some other things you can do to keep your throat healthy.

Make a steam room. Your throat is healthiest when it's moist. And dry winter air parches it. So when you're running your heater, it's best to use a humidifier and to drink plenty of liquids, suggests Dr. Goldstein.

Chase the vampires. Garlic has natural antibacterial properties. So popping some garlic pills when you feel something coming on may be the trick to help you avoid a full-fledged sore throat, Dr. Blaurock-Busch says.

Purify. Avoid irritants such as smoke, alcohol and tobacco products, advises Dr. Goldstein. They tend to irritate the throat lining. Also, smoking suppresses zinc absorption.

Smell the roses. When possible, breathe through your nose. It acts as a natural air humidifier. When air goes through your mouth, it dries out your throat, says Dr. Goldstein.

Pipe down. Yelling at the ump can be bad for your health. Straining your voice can strain throat muscles and membranes. That doesn't mean you can never raise your voice. But you should learn to do so by taking deep breaths and using your chest and abdominal muscles rather than your throat muscles, says Dr. Goldstein.

When Your Throat Gets Sore

What to do when your throat starts to hurt? We'll tell you.

Go gargle. Try mixing a tablespoon of salt into a quart of warm or cold water and gargling, recommends George Simpson, M.D., professor and chairman of the Department of Otolaryngology at the State University of New York at Buffalo. Gargling removes pus from your throat and may help promote healing as well.

Squeeze a lemon. This sour citrus fruit helps stimulate saliva production, which is the natural moisturizer for your throat, says Michael S. Benninger, M.D., chairman of the Department of Otolaryngology–Head and Neck Surgery at Henry Ford Hospital in Detroit. "Have herbal tea with lemon. Both the tea and the lemon work to coat and soothe your throat," he notes. "Or even a sugarless lemon drop would be good."

Try real tea. Dr. Simpson recommends regular tea as a throat helper. It's effective because it has a combination of caffeine, which is a mild stimulant, and tannic acid, which has a soothing effect, he says.

Warm it up. "Just applying a hot-water bottle or a towel soaked in hot water to the front of your neck would be effective," says Dr. Benninger.

Suck a lozenge. Medicated lozenges such as Cēpacol have a numbing effect, says Dr. Simpson. They also work by stimulating saliva flow, which eases throat pain.

Eat early. Eating naturally causes your stomach to secrete more acid. If you eat and then lie down and go to sleep, acid in your stomach may gradually seep upstream. Suppose you wake up every morning with a mild sore throat that usually goes away about the time you're having your first glass of milk. The cause of this morning sore throat could be a little trickle of acid from your stomach that has backed up through your esophagus and into your larynx. "It makes you wake up with a mild sore throat or a sense of a lump in your throat," says Dr. Benninger.

◗Thyroid

- **Eat enough iodine.**
- **Take your vitamins.**

In *Stand by Me*, one of the great male-bonding movies of the 1980s, skinny kid Gordie tells the story of a fat kid who seeks revenge by provoking the "ultimate barf-o-rama" at his town's pie-eating contest.

That's when the subject of the thyroid gland comes up.

"He was fat. Reeeaaal fat," says Gordie, trying to create a picture for his fireside pals. "Yeah," replies Vern. "My cousin's like that. They say it's 'cause of his kyroid gland."

Vern has more than the word wrong. The notion that the thyroid gland is responsible for someone being overweight is a common misconception, says Martin Surks, M.D., director of the Division of Endocrinology at Montefiore Medical Center in Bronx, New York, and author of *The Thyroid Book: What Goes Wrong and How to Treat It.* "Big-time obesity is rarely from the thyroid," he says.

Your Regulator

The butterfly-shaped gland located at the base of your neck does play a role in your body's metabolism, says Dr. Surks. "It regulates how your body uses fuel," he explains.

Your body burns food much the way a car burns gas, and the thyroid basically regulates how your motor is set. The gland does this by releasing thyroid hormones. With the right amounts of hormones, your body burns fuel at the proper rate. These hormones help get other systems working properly, too, including your heart rate and body temperature. But when the thyroid produces too much or too little hormone, you run into trouble.

When the gland produces too much hormone, a condition called *hyper*thyroidism,

it's as if the gas peddle to your engine were pressed to the floor, says Dr. Surks. Your motor, including your metabolism, gets revved up, and you're basically thrown into overdrive. Someone who has hyperthyroidism may have a rapid heartbeat, increased body heat and perspiration, nervousness, weight loss and muscle weakness, among other things, says Kay McFarland, M.D., professor of medicine at the University of South Carolina School of Medicine in Columbia. Men may also experience impotence.

When the gland is underactive and produces too little hormone, a condition called *hypo*thyroidism, your engine runs too slowly. When your thyroid is underactive, everything is in low gear, says Dr. Surks. That's why people with hypothyroidism tend to experience fatigue, constipation, weight gain, chilliness and mental sluggishness. Other symptoms can include dry skin, coarse hair, hearing loss and puffiness. Men may also experience decreased sex drive, potency and sensitivity, according to Stephen E. Langer, M.D., co-author of *Solved: The Riddle of Illness*, a book about the thyroid gland's effects on the body.

A Gland Plan

Men get thyroid disease at one-tenth of the rate among women. But that still means more than 51,000 of us are newly diagnosed with either hyperthyroidism or hypothryroidism each year. You can give your thyroid gland a fighting chance against malfunction by feeding it properly and avoiding risk factors. Here's what Dr. Langer suggests.

Learn your ABCs. Vitamin A has a major role in determining how well the thyroid gland functions. Aim for 5,000 international units per day. The B vitamins—thiamin, riboflavin, niacin and vitamins B_6 and B_{12}—maintain the thyroid and enable it to use iodine to generate hormones. Shoot for 1.5 milligrams of thiamin, 1.7 milligrams of riboflavin, 20 milligrams of niacin, 2 milligrams of B_6 and six micrograms of B_{12} each day. Finally, the thyroid needs an adequate amount of vitamin C to function properly. Get 60 milligrams every day.

Get iodine. As many as 100 million people worldwide have goiters because of inadequate dietary iodine. A healthy person needs 150 micrograms a day. This is not a big issue in the United States, however. Iodine is found naturally in the soil (although the amount varies by geography), meaning that vegetables are good sources. So are lobster, shrimp and oysters. And roughly half of the salt consumed in America is iodized. The bottom line is that the typical American diet provides far more iodine than you'll ever need.

Ask your parents. Find out if goiters and hypothyroidism run in your family. If so, your thyroid may be hypersensitive, and you may need more iodine than most people.

Drink bottled pure springwater. Fluoride, found in most tap water throughout the United States, is one of the strongest suppressants of thyroid function. So while fluoride does wonders for your teeth, you might want to avoid it if you have thyroid trouble. Other substances in drinking water restrict thyroid function and cause goiters. The water in the so-called Goiter Belt—the valley of the St. Lawrence River, the Appalachian Mountains, the Great Lakes basin, the northwestern United States and British Columbia—is iodine-depleted, and consumption can lead to goiters.

Don't pick plastic. Beverages stored in plastic may contain high concentrations of leached phthalate esters, contaminants that may interfere with thyroid function.

Ask about aspirin. If your doctor has suggested that you take aspirin daily to prevent blood clotting and protect your heart, he may be unaware that it can contribute to an underactive thyroid. Ask him about it on your next visit.

Remember your ratio. Your dietary ratio of zinc to copper should be around 8:1. So if you up your zinc intake to treat impotence or infertility, Dr. Langer says, don't exceed 40 milligrams daily and be sure to take 5 milligrams of copper daily as well. The zinc-copper balance is directly related to the functioning of your thyroid.

Toenails

They're flecked with lint. Crusted with dirt. Laced with the unmistakable stench of gym socks. Mmmmm, toenails: They're not just for breakfast anymore.

If you can believe it, approximately 13 million Americans chew their toenails, according to one survey. Hey, it's a free country. We'll spare you the toenail-tasting-is-totally-gross-and-not-real-hygienic lecture.

Instead, here's some advice on proper toenail care from Paul Kechijian, M.D., chief of the nail section at New York University Medical Center in Great Neck.

Square them off. Toenails are made of keratin, which is the same protein that gives hair and skin their toughness. They grow out from the lunula, the white, half-moon-shaped piece at the base of each nail. Because toenails usually receive less blood flow, they tend to grow only one-third to one-half as fast as fingernails. That means you'll need to trim them only every two weeks or so to keep them the proper length.

Cut your nails straight across rather than in an arc. This helps eliminate ingrown toenails, which occur when sharp nail edges

Trimming the Toenails

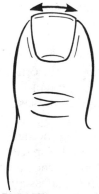 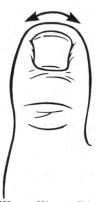

Right Way to Trim   **Wrong Way to Trim**

cut into the surrounding skin. Buy clippers or scissors designed for toenails; smaller fingernail clippers can leave little spikes that catch socks and damage nails.

Nail that fungus. About 5 percent of men are vulnerable to a nail fungus called a dermatophyte. You'll recognize the problem right away: Nails become thick and crumbly as the fungus eats the keratin.

Avoid fungus by washing and drying your feet every day. Since the fungus likes it warm and damp, use foot powder to help keep your feet dry. Gently clean under your nails a couple of times a week with a specially designed nail-brush.

Let your feet breathe outside of shoes whenever possible. But don't go walking barefoot through the grass. The fungus lurks in the lawn, always looking to grab a foothold.

Don't be tight-laced. Small shoes squeeze toes. That can lead to ingrown toenails, bruised nails and fungus growth. Shoes should give you enough room to wiggle your toes. Pointy-toed shoes are especially bad for your toenails, so opt for square- or round-toed models, if possible.

Coping with Ingrown Toenails

An ingrown toenail is a little spike of nail that pokes into the skin on either side of a nail. At best, it hurts like crazy. At worst, it hurts like crazy and then gets infected.

Here's some advice from Dr. Kechijian on how to deal with one.

1. Pull back the fold of skin from around the ingrown toenail. This should expose the piece of ingrown nail.

2. With a pair of good nail clippers or nail scissors, trim the ingrown spike at the corner of the nail. Also be sure to remove any nail fragments that may have broken off the last time you trimmed.

3. When you're done trimming the nail, apply an antibacterial ointment in the space between the skin and the nail. Repeat twice daily for a few days until the pain and redness are gone.

Tongue

- Watch for unusual patching or color.
- Keep sharp things, such as teeth, far away.

The three-horned chameleon of Madagascar can extend its tongue to close to 1½ times the length of its body, with enough accuracy to hit a moth larva and enough power to pull in a nestling mouse.

The forked tongue of the American rattlesnake can taste scents floating through the air up to 20 feet away. And the tongue of the anteater? You can imagine the accuracy and power.

But hold an election among men for the most powerful tongue in the wild kingdom, and there's no doubt who the winner would be: basketball giant Michael Jordan, of course, whose dangling, floppy tongue appears to add several feet of lift to his amazing midair maneuvers.

As for the rest of us, there's no reason to be humble, either. Whether it's used to humiliate professional athletes from the stands, swallow evening dinner or delight a bedroom partner, the tongue is one of the most multitalented muscles of men.

The Basics of Tongue Talk

This muscle-bound organ is essential to speaking and swallowing and is critical to the sense of taste. Attached to the floor of the mouth, the tongue is a thick slab of nimble muscle covered by a thin mucous membrane. This mucous membrane contains patches and clusters of highly specialized epithelial cells, commonly referred to as taste buds.

An extreme close-up of your tongue would reveal little nubs called papillae, which make your tongue resemble coarse sandpaper. On the front two-thirds of your tongue, these tiny projections take on conelike shapes, forming a sandpaper-like surface ideal for scouring a lollipop. They also give the tongue its whitish hue against the deep red background of blood-rich muscle tissue.

The mouth being a dirty place, more than 100 different bacteria might be sitting on each cell of your tongue even as you read this. And yet your tongue rarely gets sick because of its powerful defense system. "A normal, healthy tongue is very resistant to infection," explains Gerald Shklar, D.D.S., professor of oral pathology at the Harvard School of Dental Medicine. "Saliva contains enzymes to fight bacteria. Saliva also contains immune substances called immunoglobulins," which help your immune system fight disease.

Tongue Trouble

Your tongue pretty much takes care of itself. If something is wrong, it's usually something you've done to it, such as a cut, bite or burn that will heal itself. But occasionally, the tongue does have a medical problem. You should be aware of the following.

Geographic tongue. This does not mean that your tongue resembles South America. Rather, it is when the little nubs that normally cover your tongue disappear, leaving in their places smooth red patches. These bald spots begin to resemble a shifting pink map of healthy nub continents.

"Stress or emotion seems to help bring it out," says Dr. Shklar. "But it's not serious. It just sits around for a while, and then it heals."

The cause of geographic tongue remains undiscovered, and there is no specific treatment available. Normally, the problem resolves itself. But in the meantime, avoid alcohol, tobacco and hot and spicy foods, all of which may irritate your tongue.

Fissured tongue. More than 10 percent of men have this problem. Some tongues have grooves or pits that are unusually deep. Food can get lodged in the grooves, which can lead to a bad taste or odor. To keep your tongue clean, "mix one part hydrogen peroxide (make sure the label says it's 3 percent USP) and two parts warm water, then rinse out your mouth well with it. The rinse gets down into the grooves and fizzles and kills whatever bacteria are in them. It doesn't taste great, but it works," says Dr. Shklar.

Hairy tongue. Taking antibiotics will occasionally cause the nubs on the tongue to have a growth spurt. This can make the tongue appear to be covered with hair. Hairy tongue is usually more embarrassing than painful and disappears after the antibiotic treatment has ceased, says Dr. Shklar.

Glossitis. Imagine that the grasslike stubs on your tongue have been mowed to their roots, exposing the ground to the scorching sun. Glossitis has a similar effect. With it, your tongue becomes inflamed, tender, smooth and bright red.

"The problem could range from bacterial infection to vitamin deficiency to a traumatic injury," says Richard Price, D.M.D., clinical instructor of dentistry at Boston University's Henry Goldman School of Dentistry and consumer adviser for the American Dental Association. Once the cause has been figured out, glossitis is a fairly easy problem to resolve. Vitamin supplements can cure a deficiency, for example, and a simple antibacterial mouthwash can kill the guilty germs.

Mouth cancer. Although our tongues are well-equipped to battle off the organic nasties afloat in our mouths, they have little defense against the man-made agents of destruction that we choose to bombard them with: tobacco and alcohol. Each year, there are more than 30,000 new cases of oral cancer, which usually first appears as a small, off-white bump on the tongue. "It can be a raised tumorlike thing or an ulcer—an open sore—that doesn't heal," says Dr. Shklar.

These tumors are usually painless at first, but if you notice any strange changes in the soft tissue of your mouth that don't go away after two weeks, see your dentist immediately, says Dr. Shklar. Your dentist will usually take a small tissue sample of the affected area for testing. This is called a biopsy. Take heart: If detected early, oral cancer can often be cured completely.

🧂 Taste

- **Weight of the human tongue: 4 ounces**
- **Number of taste buds on the surface of the tongue: 10,000**
- **Ratio of sensitivity to taste between the nose and the tongue: 1,000:1**

The Science of Flavor

The tongue is a many-splendored thing, but you'd be wrong to think of it as the main player in detecting flavors. Yes, it's the home of taste buds. But taste buds can detect only four flavors: sweet, sour, bitter and salty. The rest of what we think of as taste is supplied by the sense of smell and by something called chemesthesis, a separate sensory system in the mouth that detects the flavors we identify as tangy, spicy and minty. This system tells us even more about food: It puts the zing in hot peppers and the bubbles in bubbly.

This team effort is a very good thing. When you were born, you had taste buds in almost every part of your mouth, as nature's way of encouraging you to eat to stay alive. Now that you are an adult, your taste buds are confined to your tongue. And as you age, you will inevitably continue to lose taste buds. By the age of 70, you will have roughly 36 percent of the taste buds you had at 30. In particular, the ability to taste salt declines, whereas sensitivity to sweet tastes is barely effected. Studies bear these points out: Seniors tended to find flavors less intense than younger subjects, and what flavors the two age groups found pleasant varied considerably.

But be grateful for memory. As you age, remembered tastes enable you to continue enjoying a wide range of flavors despite fewer and fewer taste buds. For example, you immediately stick your tongue out of your mouth when you taste something too bitter. That's because you unconsciously recall past experience in which the air improved the flavor.

Only a few things are known to affect your sense of taste. Obviously, anything that affects your sense of smell—colds, flus, congestion, exposure to toxic chemicals—will make eating less sensual. Those problems are usually short-term. One nutrient—zinc—also has been linked to taste disorders. A deficiency can impair your senses of small and taste. Zinc-depleting drugs, poor eating habits, alcoholism, kidney disease or even severe burns can contribute to a zinc shortage. Supplements can bring back your sense of taste within a few weeks. ■

How to Improve Your Sense of Taste

Although your diminishing number of taste buds is beyond your control, there is a lot you can do to fine-tune your ability to detect flavors. Follow these tips for a superior sense of taste.

Chew and sip slowly. You won't give your tongue enough time to sense flavors if you gulp your food and drink. The more you chew, the more flavors you'll unleash in your food, and the longer you'll have to enjoy them.

Cleanse your palate. Take a drink of water or nibble on bread or unsalted crackers between courses. This way, your tongue gets a clean slate before experiencing the next new flavor.

Tell a joke. Your taste buds can't receive flavors until they've been moistened by saliva. And you generate more saliva when you're happy or laughing. So if you remember a dish as having tasted better the last time you had it,

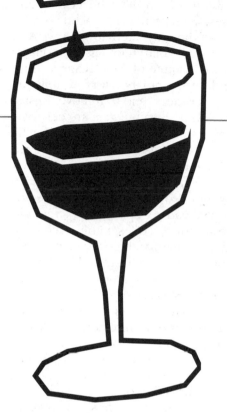

concoctions on the menu.

Get the right glass. The standard ten-ounce goblet with a round bowl is your best bet for maximizing the flavor of your drink. The roundness of the glass helps the liquid retain its flavor; in a larger glass, flavor dissipates, advises William DeWeese, director of beverages at the Waldorf-Astoria Hotel in New York City.

Choose variety. While you should be cautious about the amount of food you consume, you needn't be concerned about overtaxing your sense of taste. Your palate is primed for flavor for up to about ten courses. Only beyond that does your sense of taste begin to fatigue.

Warm up to leftovers. Cold pizza seemed like a fine meal in your college days, but if you really want to enjoy it, zap it in the microwave for 30 seconds. "The more you heat food, the more you agitate flavor molecules in the ingredients," says Charles Wysocki, Ph.D., a researcher at the Monell Chemical Senses Center in Philadelphia. ∎

there's a chance that the food is just as well-prepared this time around but your mouth isn't moist enough to detect it.

Discover other drinks. Alcohol is an astringent to your tongue and so dulls your sense of taste. Experiment with the newer nonalcoholic

How to Drink the Wine

Want to hold your own at the next wine-and-cheese gathering? Follow these tips from William DeWeese, director of beverages at the Waldorf-Astoria Hotel in New York City.

1. First, hold off on the cheese until after you've tasted the wine. The fat in cheese masks the flavor of wine. Serving cheese with wine is one of the oldest tricks in the wine business.

2. When you take a sip, draw in some air to help bring the wine to all of your taste buds and move it across your palate. The air also

allows your nose to smell the wine, and smell is the largest component of taste.

3. Next, allow some of the wine under your tongue. This area has plenty of sensitive nerve endings that allow chemesthesis and are responsive to chemicals found in foods, especially strong wines and cheeses. (You can use this same technique later with the cheese.) Swish the wine around the back of your tongue as well as the front, but hold off swallowing for a while. Be sure to garner all of the taste you can first. ∎

⌂ Tonsils

- **Don't eat germs.**
- **Treat infections with antibiotics.**

Think of all of the nasty things you breathe, eat and drink. Smoke inhaled at the nightclub. Patches of unseen green fur on five-day-old bread. Grime sucked from underneath your fingernails.

These are all dinner for your tonsils.

Part of the lymphatic system, your tonsils work with a few other small parts scattered throughout your airways, urinary tract and reproductive tract to protect your body from incoming germs. Your tonsils sit in a strategic location just behind your nose and mouth. It's the perfect spot to sample all of the gook that comes into your throat. When your tonsils sample something that they think the rest of your body won't like, they hold on to it. Then your immune system mobilizes for the kill.

Tonsils curve inward like slim half-moons on either side of the back of the throat. It's the tonsils' shape that can cause them trouble. Their anatomy allows bacteria to hide in the folds of the surface of the tonsil, making them susceptible to infections. Or sometimes so many irritants come in at once that the tonsils get overwhelmed. They swell up, sometimes so large that they prevent proper eating and breathing. That's called tonsillitis.

To Yank or Not to Yank

Tonsil removal isn't high on the list of things you need to worry about. Before the days of antibiotics, inflamed tonsils were routinely removed. But today, tonsils are rarely removed if the infection clears up with drug treatment.

And drug treatment is about the only way to guard yourself against tonsillitis. "If someone has just come up with recurrent attacks, we'll keep him on low-dose antibiotics to try to break the cycle. Or if a person knows a cold will trigger tonsillitis, he'll call in and have us prescribe antibiotics to head it off. But that's about the only alternative," says Austin King, M.D., an otolaryngologist and director of the Voice Institute of West Texas, a voice research and treatment laboratory in Abilene.

Doctors tend to remove tonsils only when the swelled-up buggers are destroying the patient's quality of life. For instance, the inflamed tonsils may disturb breathing. Or recurrent infections may cause you to miss a lot of work.

Here's a general guideline for when you might need to get your tonsils removed. If you've had six episodes of strep within one year, four episodes within each of two years or three a year for three years in a row, you're a good candidate for tonsillectomy.

If you have never suffered from recurrent infections, you probably won't get them now. Adults who get their tonsils removed have usually suffered from recurring bouts of tonsillitis throughout their lives. But it is possible to develop problematic tonsillitis after a severe bout of strep throat or another throat infection that causes the tonsils to swell.

Though your tonsils help keep you healthy, getting rid of them probably won't make you a sicker person. Your tonsils performed most of their work during your first few years of life. By the time you were three years old, they had become less important as germ-fighters. And they gradually shrink in size as you age, ending up the size of almonds.

"Nobody has ever proved that tonsil removal affects the immune system," says Dr. King. "We know that the function of the tonsils is to trap antigens and bacteria and to give the body a chance to produce antibodies against these substances. But nobody has ever proved that taking the tonsils out harms that function."

Underarms

- **Wash often.**
- **Use an antiperspirant-deodorant combo.**

There is only one crucial question when it comes to a man's armpits: Why do they stink so much? Believe it or not, science has not figured out the entire answer. If women could honestly say that they like the smell of a ripe man, then all of the pieces to the puzzle would fit. But women don't.

Sweat, of course, is the root cause of body odor. Your armpits are home to two different types of sweat glands, says Alan Schragger, M.D., a dermatologist with Advanced Dermatology Associates in Allentown, Pennsylavania. Eccrine glands, the first type, are much more numerous throughout your body and release the odorless secretion that men normally think of as sweat. Apocrine glands, the second type, are found mainly in the underarm and genital areas. These glands secrete a fluid that includes the basic components of regular sweat plus some fatty substances and proteins. On its own, apocrine sweat is odorless. But when bacteria on your hair and skin decompose it, you get that musky odor you know so well.

Why do apocrine glands exist? This is the piece of the puzzle that is missing. Apocrine glands play little role in keeping the body cool, as is the main function of body sweat. Rather, apocrine glands kick into high gear when they encounter other types of heat: work pressure, sexual stimulation, even pain. Some researchers believe apocrine sweat is a remnant of a time when a man's scent played a role in alluring sex partners, but this remains just theory.

Turning Down the Funk

Solutions for stinky pit syndrome are simple. Here are the details.

Pick the right pit product. The most popular solutions to pit pollution are antiperspirants and deodorants. Although both are used for essentially the same reason—to eliminate odor—they work in different ways.

Antiperspirants, according to Dr. Schragger, plug up the mouth of the glands, so perspiration doesn't come out. By preventing pits from becoming saturated with sweat, antiperspirants create an underarm environment that's inhospitable to bacteria, thereby eliminating odor.

Antiperspirants are considered drugs in the eyes of the Food and Drug Administration, since they affect how your body operates. Virtually all use an aluminum compound to clog pores, and they can reduce sweating by 15 to 50 percent. To get the most out of your antiperspirant dollar, Dr. Schragger recommends using a type that is applied directly to the skin, such as a stick or roll-on. Sprays are least effective.

Deodorants kill the offending bacteria or use perfumes to mask the odor, but they don't prevent sweating. The Food and Drug Administration considers them cosmetics.

Which is right for you? It's your choice. But for the best of both worlds, Dr. Schragger says, try using a product that combines an antiperspirant with a deodorant.

Scrub it away. Like we said: It's not just the sweat, it's the bacteria, too. So kill the odor-causing bacteria by washing your pits often with an antibacterial soap, says Dr. Schragger. Once a day is usually enough.

Be cool, man. If you like to squeeze a workout, a shower and some swipes of deodorant into your lunch hour, all of that rushing and stress may cause a torrent of sweat to flood your pits. Deodorants and antiperspirants work best when applied on dry skin. So make sure you take 10 to 15 minutes to cool down before dousing.

Wash smart. Clothes have this bad habit of hanging on to the bacteria and body oils that cause odor. So don't overstuff the washing machine and use an appropriate amount of soap to guarantee that a fresh shirt emerges.

🕳 Urinary System

- **Number of days marijuana remains identifiable in the urine: 35**
- **Fraction of the fluid you drink that leaves your body as urine: 2/3**
- **Number of gallons of blood that your kidneys filter each day: roughly 42**
- **Percent of people who admit to urinating in the shower: 59**

How to Have Healthy Urine

"Drinking water is the single most important thing you can do to keep your urinary system active," says Jack W. McAninch, M.D., chief of urology at San Francisco General Hospital and professor and vice-chairman of the Department of Urology at the University of California, San Francisco.

That's water—not soda and not juice, says Dr. McAninch. It's water that dilutes toxic substances excreted by your kidneys so that these substances are less toxic to surrounding tissue. "Compared with people with low fluid intakes, people who drink enough water have fewer kidney stones, urinary tract infections and overall bad side effects," he says.

Aim for about 68 ounces of water per day. And that's in addition to what you take with meals, adds Dr. McAninch.

Here are five more things you should do to keep your urinary system in peak condition, according to Dr. McAninch.

Test the waters. Each time you get a medical checkup, make sure a urine test is included. Consult your doctor if you find blood in your urine, feel pain when urinating or experience increased frequency or urgency.

Go with the flow. Give your bladder some creative control; don't rush urination or postpone it for too long. Take time to completely empty your bladder.

Urinate after sex. This will help you avoid urinary tract infections.

Read the smoke signals. Smokers are twice as likely as nonsmokers to develop bladder cancer.

Diversify your eating. Take some chances when strolling down your grocery store's fruit and vegetable aisle. Studies suggest a connection between eating a varied diet of fruits and vegetables and a reduced risk of bladder cancer. ∎

The Great Political Bladder Buster

The rules of most state and federal legislatures are specific when it comes to filibusters: If you move more than three feet from your desk, you lose control of the floor. Pee be damned.

This poses a dilemma for anyone conducting a filibuster, a political practice in which someone takes control of the floor during open debate and holds it for hours on end, preventing a vote or other action—specifically, urination—from being taken. For those lasting more than 12 hours, this is no dry matter.

Of course, where there is a need, there is a solution. Politicians in Texas have been known to strap on urinary leg bags before launching filibusters. But even these have their limits. Consider the 42-hour filibuster of Texas State Senator Mike McKool in 1972. After his bag filled up, colleagues gathered around him, providing a partial shield for him to place his leg into a plastic-lined wastebasket. One of his friends simply opened the spigot and drained the bag.

A record for filibustering was set in 1977 by Texas State Senator Bill Meier. He lasted 43 hours. But he should get an asterisk for the

Elsewhere . . .

- **Bladder**   Page 102
- **Kidneys**   Page 214
- **Penis**   Page 257
- **Urine**   Page 338

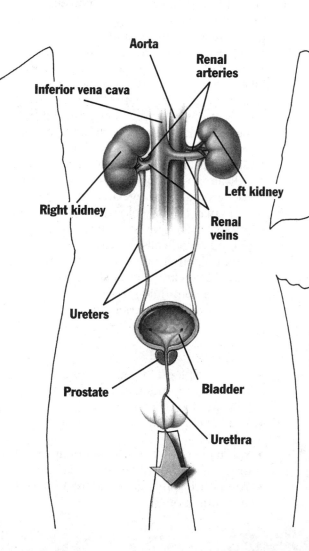

Aorta

Renal arteries

Inferior vena cava

Left kidney

Right kidney

Renal veins

Ureters

Prostate

Bladder

Urethra

record; his urine bag was strapped to his front, meaning that he would have had to drop his pants to empty it. The lieutenant governor instead let him go to the bathroom to empty it, according to an article written by James Petry, M.D., of Port Arthur, Texas, in the urology journal *AUA Today*.■

Water In, Water Out

3:00 P.M.: Fernando drinks an eight-ounce glass of water.

3:15 P.M.: The water rushes through to the small intestine, where most gets absorbed into the bloodstream.

3:20 P.M.: Blood is continuously piped through the kidneys, where excess water and unneeded ingredients, such as extra vitamins and dead blood cells, get filtered out. The clean blood circulates on. The impurities mix with water and get sent through tubes called ureters to the bladder.

3:15 P.M. to 7:15 P.M.: The bladder receives the full volume of eight ounces of water.

After 7:15 P.M.: Once the bladder fills (that varies by person, with the typical range being 6 to 16 ounces), Fernando feels the urge to urinate. The exact time depends on how much additional liquid he has drunk since 3:00 p.m., any medication he's taking and his level of hydration and salt intake.■

Urine

- **Keep the water flowing.**
- **Monitor for color.**

"Pee into the cup" may be the golden oldie of medical phrases. Because when ancient doctors weren't sticking their filthy fingers into battle wounds or conducting bloodlettings to extract evil "humours" from the body, they spent a lot of time contemplating urine.

Holding a flask up to the light and grimly scrutinizing its contents, these primitive healers believed they could diagnose many ailments simply based on the color, consistency, smell and (gag) taste of a patient's urine. More often than not, their diagnoses were way off target. But basically, they had the right idea.

Making a Pit Stop

Although it sometimes seems like beer and other fluids rush from your mouth to your bladder, urine is actually created through a complex process. It works like this: When you drink a glass of water, it is absorbed by the small intestine and goes into the bloodstream. The blood circulates through your body until it reaches the kidneys. The kidneys filter out waste products and form urine, which carries these contaminants into the bladder. There the fluid is stored until it is expelled. The average man produces up to two quarts of urine daily, depending on how much he eats, drinks and sweats.

Most men can reduce their risk of urinary tract problems if they drink at least six to eight glasses of water a day, says E. David Crawford, M.D., chairman of the Division of Urology at the University of Colorado Health Sciences Center and director of the Colorado Prostate Center, both in Denver. But avoid drinking excessive amounts of coffee, alcohol and cola, which are mild diuretics that can increase your urine output and cause dehydration.

Because fresh urine was thought to be sterile, doctors used to use it to cleanse wounds when other antiseptics weren't available. But more commonly, physicians use urine as a diagnostic tool, since telltale waste products from virtually every organ in the body are found in it.

Strive for Mellow Yellow

Urine is about 96 percent water and normally contains only small amounts of salt, potassium, sugar and other waste products. But minute changes in its chemical composition often help doctors detect heart disease, psoriasis, diabetes and other disorders. And as their ancient counterparts did, physicians consider the color and smell of urine as well.

Medications and foods such as red meats, fish, beets, brussels sprouts and asparagus can discolor urine or alter its aroma. But either change could also be a sign of disease. Here's a partial list of what urine colors could mean.

- Clear or pale yellow: the normal color of urine (the yellow pigment is caused by the breakdown of hemoglobin, the main component of red blood cells).
- Cloudy yellow: could be normal or could indicate pus, blood or fat droplets. Or if you're on a strict vegetarian diet, your urine may be this color most of the time.
- Smoky with a grayish cast: remnants of old red blood cells or yeast.
- Dark golden or orange: a symptom of dehydration and a clear signal to increase your fluid intake.
- Red: blood, which could indicate a kidney infection, bladder infection or bladder cancer.

See your doctor if:

- You have blood in your urine.
- You have a burning sensation or back pain when you urinate.
- You have trouble starting your urine stream.
- You have urine that is persistently cloudy or smells strongly like ammonia.
- You notice a change in the frequency of your urination.

Veins

- **Keep your legs busy.**
- **Take care of your heart.**
- **Keep cool for better blood flow.**

The commute home, big-city style: pothole-filled roads, stop-and-go traffic, highway construction, closed lanes, detours, bumps, pavement buckles. Just another day in the life of blood in the veins, particularly in men with varicose veins or phlebitis.

In your body's blood-flow system, the key is movement, the enemy is gravity, and all roads carry one-way traffic. For much of your body, the veins travel an uphill path, performing gravity-defying feats such as transporting blood from the tips of your toes to larger veins and, finally, to your heart and lungs. There, the blood expels carbon dioxide and stokes up on oxygen, then continues on its journey through the network of arteries and capillaries before returning once again to the veins for the trip back to your heart and lungs.

While the arteries are helped along by the pumping of your heart, the veins rely on a series of valves to keep the blood flowing onward and upward. Also, muscle contractions (particularly in your calves) cause veins to be compressed, which helps pump the blood in the right direction.

When Veins Are in Vain

Given all of the mechanics, there are several things that can cause blood flow through the veins, particularly those in the legs, to slow or halt: a misfunctioning valve, damage to a vein wall, the formation of a clot. If any of these happen, a vein can overfill with blood and expand under the pressure. The result can be a varicose vein—or worse.

A varicose vein isn't just cosmetic. Other symptoms include a feeling of heaviness in the limb, a dull ache and itching. The circulatory system is made for movement; over time, blood may clot when a vein fails to move it along. Sometimes swollen varicose veins may also prevent oxygen from reaching the skin, leading to skin ulcers and discoloration.

So the first tip for vein maintenance and care is to see your doctor if you notice any of the symptoms described in this chapter or if varicose veins are suddenly sprouting, advises Michael Silane, M.D., clinical associate professor of surgery at the New York Hospital–Cornell Medical Center in New York City.

Another condition that can plague your veins is phlebitis, or inflammation of a vein. Phlebitis is often accompanied by the formation of a blood clot in the vein, a condition that doctors refer to as thrombophlebitis. (A thrombus is a blood clot.) When the problem occurs in a vein near the surface, it's called superficial thrombophlebitis.

Superficial thrombophlebitis often occurs in people who have varicose veins, although it can be caused by an infection or injury. Symptoms include redness, pain, itching and swelling along the length of the vein, says David Green, M.D., a dermatologist and vein specialist at the Varicose Vein Center in Bethesda, Maryland.

Superficial thrombophlebitis generally goes away on its own, but you could be facing weeks of discomfort. To relieve the discomfort, doctors recommend treating the problem with rest, elevation of the limb, warm compresses and nonsteroidal anti-inflammatory drugs such as aspirin, he says. If your doctor suspects that an infection caused the problem, you'll get antibiotics as well.

Much more serious is when a blood clot forms inside one of the body's deep veins. Called, logically, deep-vein thrombophlebitis, this is a life-threatening condition. The most frightening risk is that a blood clot could break free from the vein and lodge in a main vessel supplying the heart or lungs.

With deep-vein thrombophlebitis, the

whole leg is swollen and painful; otherwise, there may be few, if any, symptoms. Your doctor can readily detect it with ultrasound. The condition requires immediate treatment with a blood-thinning medication such as heparin or warfarin, says Alan Kanter, M.D., medical director of the Vein Center of Orange County in Irvine, California.

Keeping Veins Healthy

Many experts feel that vein problems are genetic. That doesn't mean you have no control over their health, however. "As you get older, more veins go bad," according to Dr. Kanter. "But you can slow the process." Here's how you can keep vitality in your veins.

Stretch out. When you sit for hours at a time—on a long drive, for instance, or during an airplane flight—blood flow in your veins slows. So when you fly, ask for an aisle seat on the plane and stretch your legs, walking around every 30 minutes or so. On a long auto trip, pull over, stop your car and walk around. Give your veins some added benefit by flexing and then extending at your ankles, suggests Dr. Silane. This allows your calf muscles to aid your veins, propelling the blood upward.

Give yourself a leg up. When your feet are higher than your heart, the veins in your legs get a rest because the valves don't have to work against gravity. If you sit for hours at a time, put your feet up on your desk. When you watch television or read, lie down on the sofa with your feet on the armrest or a pillow. Avoid sitting cross-legged, with the ankle of one leg resting on the knee of the other, cautions Dr. Silane.

Prime your pump. Aerobic exercise improves blood flow through your veins. It also builds up uninjured veins, which can take the load off weak ones. Not to mention all of the things exercise does for your heart, lungs, muscles, digestion, sex life . . . . So take long, energetic walks at least three times a week. Take up bicycling, swimming, jogging on a soft surface or low-weight/high-rep weight lifting, suggests Dr. Kanter.

But exercise right. Not all workouts are good for leg veins. Jogging on a hard surface adds to the downward pressure on the valves and walls in your veins. So does weight lifting aimed at building muscle mass, says Dr. Kanter.

Stock up on support. Support stockings use pressure to help push the blood upward. They're also tight enough in the right places to constrict your veins, which helps partially defective valves to close properly. Support stockings temporarily relieve the discomfort of varicose veins and help keep varicose veins from turning into phlebitis, says Dr. Kanter.

Although you can buy support stockings in most pharmacies, those available by

Healthy versus Unhealthy Veins

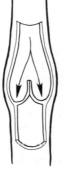

Normal Vein

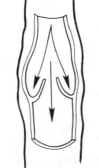

Functioning Valve

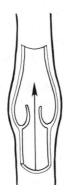

Varicose Vein

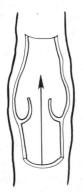

Faulty Valve

Valves in healthy veins help blood move back toward the heart. When valves are faulty, blood can pool up, causing varicose veins.

prescription work better and are less likely to cause problems. So check with your doctor first.

Stay cool. Heat causes your veins to dilate, which makes poorly functioning valves even less efficient. That's why many people have more vein pain during the summer, says Dr. Kanter. Use cold, not hot, compresses to relieve symptoms. Avoid hot showers and Jacuzzis.

Feed your veins right. A high-fiber diet helps substances pass through your gut more rapidly. You'll be less subject to constipation, which, because of the increase in pressure it creates, is a common cause of vein damage, says Glenn Geelhoed, M.D., professor of surgery and international medical education at George Washington University Medical Center in Washington, D.C.

Trim the fat. Experts theorize that weight loss helps prevent or reduce vein problems. When you carry around extra weight, your muscles can't help pump blood very effectively.

Get a handle on stress. When you're stressed, your body releases epinephrine, a hormone that sparks your heart rate. Reducing stress has many benefits, of which helping your veins is just a small one. Dr. Geelhoed has smart advice here. He advises patients to reduce stress by treating the unknown with fascination, not horror.

Vocal Cords

- **Speak from your belly, not your throat.**
- **Quit hollerin'.**

Reverend James M. Johnson's voice has the soothing quality one might expect from a preacher. It's not natural. He works at it. As he preaches, he consciously feels where his voice resonates. He makes sure to breathe. And he monitors his pitch.

Any other preacher might not be so concerned about his voice. But for years, Reverend Johnson's voice faltered as he preached. A lifetime of what doctors call spasmodic dysphonia, or strangled voice, threatened his career. "I think I probably misused my voice all of my life. I didn't use the right pitch. I put too much stress on the vocal cords rather than on the diaphragm. And after some years in the public ministry, it became more evident," says Reverend Johnson of Poplar Grove, Illinois, who formerly preached at the 800-member Jefferson Prairie Lutheran Church in Los Angeles.

Once he learned how to speak correctly, however, his voice became a powerful instrument of communication. It's an important lesson. We can grunt any old sound from our throats without much coaching. But turning those grunts into an ear-pleasing rhapsody often takes work.

The Sax in Your Throat

Your voice starts with two wishbone-shaped ligaments, each less than an inch long, inside the tunnel-like larynx, located just behind your Adam's apple. These strong, elastic vocal cords work much like the reed on a wind instrument. When a sax player blows air over the reed, it vibrates to make sound. When your lungs push air through your larynx, your vocal cords vibrate. The greater the puff, the faster the air moves, and the louder the sound.

Part of your voice is hereditary. The sound waves that your vocal cords create resonate in your nose, mouth and throat, so the shapes of these structures give your voice a unique sound. The length and thickness of your cords control some of the pitch. Men tend to have larger larynxes than women; this is what makes our voices deeper. Also, your ability to hit particular notes depends in part on how well your ears can hear different sound frequencies. Some ears are better than others.

But that's no excuse for singing off-key or talking like a squeak box. You do have some control. "A portion of it is training. Anybody can be trained to sing. But not anybody can be trained to sing like Pavarotti," said Austin King, M.D., an otolaryngologist and director of the Voice Institute of West Texas, a voice research and treatment laboratory in Abilene.

Learning the Basics

It seems natural. But according to some doctors, a lot of us are like Reverend Johnson. We still need to learn how to talk.

About half of us use our noses way too much when we speak. The nose creates a whiny, annoying by-product. It doesn't hurt your vocal cords. But it does make others wince when they hear your voice.

And about one-quarter of the talking public speaks from the lower throat rather than using the voice from the mask—that is, from the lips and tongue. In men, this creates an impressive, authoritative growl. In women, this emits that raspy, sexy tone.

"We are taken with the sexy voice. But you see, when you do that, you may have a sound that you like, but you can wind up with very serious problems," said Morton Cooper, Ph.D., known as the voice coach to the stars and author of *Stop Committing Voice Suicide*.

It's possible that voice abuse won't directly affect your vocal cords. You may be able to get through much of life growling vowels and consonants from the depths of your throat. But an allergy attack, a cold or a night of cheering on your favorite sports team will most likely make you feel like someone is choking you. You'll sound raspy. It may hurt to talk. And you'll feel like you've never had so much gunk in your throat.

Getting Good Vibrations

For the moment, we'll put the gunk threats aside and just talk about sounding good. Creating an impressive voice involves the mastery of three techniques: sound placement, breath control and posture.

Sound placement. You want your voice to come out of your mouth. Seems like common sense. But many of us let it resonate in the nose or the lower throat. If you tend to

What Makes a Voice

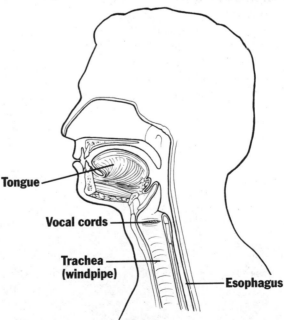

Tongue

Vocal cords

Trachea (windpipe)

Esophagus

Your vocal cords are at the top of your windpipe for a reason. To have a strong, firm voice, you need to power up your breath from your abdomen.

be nasal, you can learn to bring your voice away from your nose and into your mouth by saying energy words such as "right" and "do." These words have to resonate in your mouth. Even if you try to, you cannot say them nasally. Memorize that feeling and try to say other words the same way, Dr. Cooper says.

People who tend to talk from their throats can try a method called the instant voice press. You stick your finger between your breastbone and belly button, then pump your finger while humming. It makes your voice resonate through your nose and mouth, letting you know what correct talking feels like, Dr. Cooper says.

"You'll feel a buzz around your lips and nose. And that's where all good and great voices come from," Dr. Cooper says.

Breath control. The sound needs something to carry it out of your body; air works just fine. So talk while breathing out. Many people hold their breath while they talk, squeezing their vocal cords and choking their voices. To understand why this is bad, blow out all of your air and then count to 50. You'll be lucky if your voice makes it to 11. "The voice is like a rider, and the breath is a horse. You want the rider to go for a horseback ride with his horse. So you want the breath to be underneath whatever sound is produced. In this way, power for the voice comes from the breathing mechanism and not from the throat," says Bonnie Raphael, Ph.D., voice and speech coach at the American Repertory Theatre in Watertown, Massachusetts.

Posture. Think of your body as a tunnel and your voice

as a car. The car can get through the tunnel more efficiently if it doesn't have to navigate curves. Same with your voice. Keep your head aligned with your body. This allows your voice to travel a more direct route out of your mouth. Keep your voice from hitting a barrier before reaching the listener by opening your throat and your mouth.

Vocal Maintenance

Here are some other things you can do to ensure a long-lasting, better-sounding voice.

The Man with the Deep Voice

Shadoe Stevens has a manly voice. It's low. It's rich. It's deep. If he were a musical instrument, he'd be a tuba.

But this deep talker will tell you that speaking is not like dancing the limbo. Lower isn't necessarily better. For years, the former *American Top 40* radio host and *Hollywood Squares* celebrity attempted to make his voice even deeper. But with that quest, he swallowed his voice. Instead of letting it come out of his mouth, he rumbled and forced the sound from his throat. And he got one severe throat infection after another.

"I was lost in the idea that everything has to be low," says Stevens, who has more recently been a star in the television comedy *Dave's World*. "A lot of people who are voice-conscious, who grew up in radio, have the idea that lower is better. You get into that conditioned arena believing that only the lowest is the best."

But Stevens learned an enduring lesson through a Hollywood voice doctor. He could obtain that low, manly voice while projecting it from the mask area of his face—his lips and tongue—and not from his throat. Once he began speaking correctly, his voice became even deeper. His throat infections ceased. And he could concentrate on singing musical scales in his car.

"Your mind tells you that the voice is high and weak and that it doesn't sound good," Stevens says. "One of the things the doctor pointed out is that the highest I could get is baritone. When you start discovering that you're not going to get higher than that fairly low tone anyway, your mind relaxes and goes 'Okay, I can go anywhere within that range, and I'll still get the effect I want while gaining new range and freedom.' "

Listen up. Hearing yourself on a tape recorder allows you to check your progress as you move on to a better voice. You may think you sound strange, says Dr. Raphael. You may even think the tape recorder is misrepresenting your voice. That's because when you talk, you hear your voice through the bones in your head. Everyone else hears your voice through air. And the recorder records your voice through air, not through bone.

Be unique. When the surrounding sound is loud, such as at a football or basketball game, don't try to shout over the sound. Try to distinguish your voice from it instead. "The way to make yourself heard is to be different from the surrounding sound. We are capable of hearing lots and lots of different sounds at the same time. It's like a singer singing over the orchestra. The orchestra is very loud. But you hear the singer because the voice is different," Dr. Raphael says.

Talk over a cold. You can use the same technique when you have a cold, according to Dr. Cooper: Talk over it. When your nose is stuffed up and your energy is sapped, your natural tendency is to lower the pitch of your voice. That just makes your vocal cords work harder, however. A way to make people hear you when you can't breathe is to raise the pitch.

Sing in the shower. Your throat likes moisture. So when you're starting to feel scratchy, entertain yourself by singing in the shower. You'll inhale moist air, which will soothe your cords. At the same time, you'll boost your self-esteem. Your voice will bounce off the shower tiles, creating a richer sound. If you absolutely can't stand hanging out in the shower, try some cool-mist inhalation to soothe your vocal cords, says Dr. Raphael. Cool-mist humidifiers are widely available.

Blow, don't grind. Instead of clearing your throat, try softly blowing out the air, says Dr. King. This will clear the mucus from your cords without irritating them.

Eat earlier. When you lie down after eating or drinking, you allow acid to creep back up your esophagus into your throat. So if you have a habit of snacking before bedtime, you may awake with morning sore throat and hoarseness. To avoid this, try not eating for at least two hours before bedtime, recommends Dr. King.

Mum's the Word

People who make a habit of abusing their voices may do much more than irritate their vocal cords. They can actually change the shape of them. Unless there's excessive scarring, the body will naturally correct the condition once the voice abuse stops, Dr. King says.

Voice problems can be caused by anything from colds to drinking too much alcohol. Or they may be hereditary. They include laryngitis, polyps and nodules.

Laryngitis is a fancy term for a swollen larynx. Your larynx, one of two passageways inside your neck, houses your vocal cords. So when it swells, it distorts sound, and you lose your voice. It can be caused by anything from infections to allergies to crying fits to drinking really hot coffee to talking too much. When you get it, you should use a humidifier and try not to talk. It should go away within a few days. If the laryngitis is caused by a bacterial infection, you'll need to take antibiotics, says Dr. King.

Polyps are overgrowths of tissue that form on the vocal cords. They are usually caused by voice abuse or smoking. They give you a breathy, harsh-sounding voice. When the trauma stops—after you quit smoking, for example—the tissue returns to its normal size. But if the problem continues, the polyps grow larger and may have to be removed surgically.

Nodules are most often seen in singers and other people who use their voices a lot. They grow on the surface of the cord, much like a corn grows on a toe. They shrink with voice rest. And they can also be removed surgically. But they will grow back if the voice abuse continues.

Warts

- **Don't pick at them!**
- **Apply a wart removal acid.**
- **Consider natural remedies.**

Forget the folklore; dismiss the myths. Warts have nothing to do with frogs, toads or masturbation. They can't be cured by incantations or the light of a full moon.

"Some people actually urinate on their warts to get rid of them. But that's just an old folktale remedy that probably has little basis in fact. I certainly wouldn't recommend it to anybody," says Michael Kaminer, M.D., director of cosmetic dermatologic surgery at New England Medical Center in Boston and assistant professor of dermatology at Tufts University in Medford, Massachusetts.

Warts are harmless growths caused by any of more than 50 different strains of the human papillomavirus. They are highly contagious and can be spread by direct contact, such as a handshake. Warts are most common among children and teenagers but can appear at any age. Some men, however, may develop a stronger ability to resist the virus as they get older.

A wart usually develops within three to four months after you've been exposed to the virus, but it can take up to two years before a growth appears. Common warts—usually found on the face, hands, knees and feet—are firm, pale, skin-colored growths with rough surfaces. They are often about the size of a pencil eraser, but some, such as genital warts, are much smaller.

Although warts affect only the topmost layer of skin and do not have roots, they can be difficult to destroy. At least half of all warts disappear within two years without treatment. But the remaining 50 percent often are removed many times, and recur many times, before being subdued.

If you've never had a wart before and something wartlike develops on your skin, Dr. Kaminer recommends that you see your doctor to make sure that it's not something else, such as skin cancer. If it is a wart, your doctor can remove it by cutting, burning or freezing it. Or if you prefer, here are a few home treatments you can try.

Attack it with acid. An over-the-counter wart remedy that contains 17 percent salicylic acid, such as Compound W, can be effective, Dr. Kaminer says. You can boost the wallop of the product if you wet the wart about five minutes before applying the solution. This will help your skin soak in the medicine better. Apply the medicine at bedtime and cover the wart with a piece of adhesive tape or a bandage. Leave it uncovered during the day.

After two to three days, the wart will turn white. That's dead skin. Take a nail file and gently rub off this skin, so the medicine can penetrate deeper into the wart, Dr. Kaminer says. You do need to be patient, however, because it can take more than two months for a wart to disappear.

Patch it up. Some over-the-counter preparations come in patch form. Trim the patch to the size of the wart, wear it while sleeping and remove it during the day until the wart is gone.

Consider the alternatives. A long list of alternative remedies may help some people. They include squeezing the contents of a vitamin A capsule onto the wart once a day; applying a paste of crushed vitamin C tablets and water; wrapping the wart snugly with medical or first-aid tape and leaving it there around the clock for at least three weeks, with changes only for cleanliness; and even using your imagination to picture the wart shrinking. Ask your doctor for his recommendation.

Don't spread it around. Pick at a wart, and you risk spreading the virus that caused it to other parts of your body, says Dr. Kaminer. So keep your hands off, he advises, and if the wart has opened, wash your hands every time you touch it. Treat it like a contagious disease.

Wrists

- **Flex and stretch often.**
- **Sit right while typing.**
- **Give them frequent breaks.**

In 1786, Thomas Jefferson, author of the Declaration of Independence and future American president, was in Paris and in love. And like many men in love, Jefferson did something really stupid.

While rushing to meet his paramour, Jefferson attempted to leap over a small fountain. He tripped, landed hard on his right hand and fractured his wrist so badly that bone pierced his skin.

Few of us suffer such a devastating injury, one that left Jefferson's wrist permanently weak and stiff. But most men know all too well how susceptible the wrist is to pratfalls and the rigors of daily life.

A Guided Tour of the Wrist

The wrist consists of eight bones that allow the hand to bend nearly 150 degrees up and down and about 70 degrees from side to side. Across this complex joint run all of the vital nerves, blood vessels, tendons and ligaments that keep the hand clapping, grasping and holding.

Because of the wrist's strategic location, even a minor injury can make eating, writing or driving downright impossible for a few days. More serious injuries, such as a fracture of the scaphoid bone (the most vulnerable bone in the wrist, located at the base of the thumb), often never heal.

Although accidents account for a large percentage of wrist problems, repetitive strain injuries such as carpal tunnel syndrome, caused by typing, strumming a guitar and other repetitious motions, are increasingly common. That's because these tasks over and over again put pressure on the wrist that it isn't designed to withstand. In some cases, the amount of pressure on your wrist can be up to ten times more than you feel in your fingers. So if it takes 2 ounces of pressure for your thumb to press the space bar on your computer, the pressure on your wrist at that moment is about 20 ounces.

Over time, this increased pressure can cause swelling of the nine tendons that pass through the carpal tunnel in the wrist. As they swell, these tendons, which control finger movement, press against the median nerve, causing a tingling sensation and pain in the thumb and index, middle and ring fingers. It's like nine people trying to get through a narrow doorway all at once without bumping into a tenth person standing in the door frame. Eventually, the guy standing in the way will emerge bruised and battered, says Robert Markison, M.D., a hand surgeon and associate clinical professor of surgery at the University of California, San Francisco, School of Medicine.

Keeping Your Wrist Right

Stretching and proper wrist position are the best ways to prevent injuries from either accidents or repetitive strain, Dr. Markison says. Here are some tips and exercises that can help.

Give yourself a break. Take a 1-minute break every 15 to 20 minutes when you're doing a repetitive activity such as typing or tightening screws. Shake your wrists back and forth, close and open your fingers three or four times and move your hands from side to side. These simple movements will loosen up tense muscles and may prevent wrist pain, says Thomas Rizzo, Jr., M.D., a consultant in physical medicine and rehabilitation at the Mayo Clinic Jacksonville in Florida.

Straighten up. Poor posture, particularly if you work at a computer terminal all day, can put pressure on nerves in your neck that run down into your arms and cause numbness and tingling in your wrists and hands, says David Lichtman, M.D., professor of orthopedics and head of the Division of Hand Surgery at Baylor College of Medicine in Houston. To improve your stance, adjust your chair so that you can sit with both feet on the floor and with your back straight up against the back of the chair.

Holding a Tool

Wrong Way

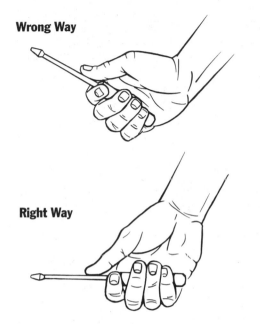

Right Way

To lessen strain, keep your forearm, wrist and thumb aligned.

In this position, you should be able to reach out and comfortably place your hands on the keyboard so that your wrists are straight and your elbows are bent at 45-degree angles.

Handle tools right. Holding a tool such as a screwdriver or a paintbrush with your hand in a twisted or bent position may pinch the median nerve in your wrist and cause pain or tingling, says Steven Bogard, hand therapy supervisor at the Mayo Clinic in Rochester, Minnesota. Try to keep your wrist in its natural position so that your forearm, wrist and thumb are in alignment.

To lessen the strain more, try using electric tools or tools with bent handles that are made especially for doing awkward jobs. Both are available in most hardware stores.

Sportsmen, start slowly. You'll be a lot less likely to be sidelined with a sports injury if you slowly limber up your wrist muscles before you toss a softball, lift weights or even fling a Frisbee, says Bogard. Begin doing the following exercises at least three to five times a week for a few weeks before you throw out your first pitch, whack your first golf ball or smash that first serve of the season, he says.

• Bounce a ball: If you play a racquet sport, gently bouncing a ball an inch or two off the racket for three to five minutes will not only improve your hand-eye coordination but also tone your wrist muscles, Bogard says.

• Grab a newspaper: Remove a two-page spread from a newspaper. Holding your palm up, grasp one corner with your thumb and index finger and let the open paper dangle away from you. Slowly crumple the paper so that it forms a tight ball inside your palm. And no, you can't use your other hand to help. Do this three to five times a day with each hand, and you should notice a dramatic increase the stamina of your wrists, Bogard says.

• Push hard: Pressing your fist against a table is a terrific isometric exercise that can strengthen your wrist, Bogard says. Make a fist and place it under a table ledge. Then press your fist against the bottom of the table for a count of five. Do this five times. Then put your fist on the tabletop and follow the same routine to exercise the opposite side of your wrist. Gradually work up so that you can do 15 repetitions of each exercise with each hand twice a day.

• Try soup lifts: Put your hand over the edge of a table, with your palm down and your wrist straight. Hold a bag containing a one-pound soup can while supporting the bag's weight with your other hand. Then let the supporting hand drop so that the hand on the

Soup Lift

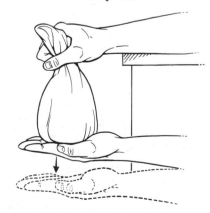

Side Wrist Stretch

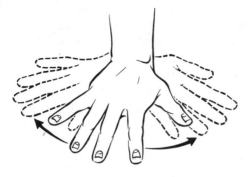

table is bearing all of the bag's weight. Try to keep your wrist straight as you hold for a count of ten. Do three repetitions, then turn your palm up and repeat the sequence. Then switch hands.

• Go from side to side: You can stretch the wrist muscles if you place your palm on a table and, without moving your arm, pivot your hand toward the thumb side as far as possible, according to Dr. Rizzo. Hold that position for a count of five. Then pivot your hand again, using only your wrist, toward the pinkie side. Do this stretch five to ten times with each hand.

• Do the twist: To improve flexibility, put your wrist on a table, thumb side up, and slowly bend your wrist forward toward the palm side as far as possible, Dr. Rizzo says. Be sure to keep your fingers straight. Hold for a count of five. Then slowly bend your wrist the opposite way as you curl your fingers. Hold for

Side Wrist Twist

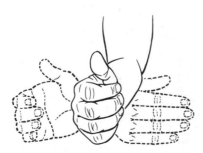

another count of five. Do this exercise five to ten times with each hand.

And If It Hurts . . .

Here are two important do's and one emphatic don't that can help you cope with a minor wrist injury.

Take the pain out of a sprain. To reduce swelling, wrap an ice pack in a towel and apply it to the injury in a 20-minutes-on, 20-minutes-off cycle for the first two hours. Then decrease the applications to 8 to 10 minutes of every waking hour for the next day or two. After a day or so, begin exercising your wrist to restore circulation, Dr. Lichtman says.

For pain, take 650 milligrams of aspirin (two regular tablets) or 400 milligrams of ibuprofen every four hours or according to the manufacturer's directions, says Dr. Lichtman. Elevate your wrist as much as possible to drain away fluids that cause swelling. If the injury is still sore after three days, apply a warm heating pad to the area for 10 to 15 minutes of every hour as needed. If the pain and swelling persist for more than four days, see your doctor.

Be a B$_6$ believer. Vitamin B$_6$ may help relieve symptoms caused by occasional overuse of the wrist. "B$_6$ will help cut down on pain and speed up healing, particularly if you have acute symptoms after doing something you don't normally do, such as cutting up firewood on a weekend," says Allan L. Bernstein, M.D., co-chief of neurology at Kaiser-Permanente Medical Center in Santa Rosa, California. Rest your wrist as much as possible and take 100 milligrams of B$_6$ once a day for one to two weeks, he advises. If your wrist is still painful after 10 to 14 days, see your doctor.

Don't sprint for a splint. Wrist splints are fine for certain conditions, such as carpal tunnel syndrome, but they're not good for everyone. In fact, wearing the wrong splint for the wrong amount of time can actually aggravate an injury and weaken the wrist muscles, Dr. Lichtman says. So if you suspect that you need a splint, ask your doctor about it first.

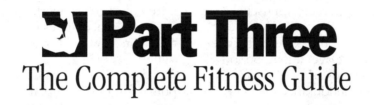

Part Three

The Complete Fitness Guide

¹³³ The Basics of Fitness

If your overall fitness regimen were a chair, what would it be?

If you answered a beanbag, a rocking chair or even a La-Z-Boy, then take a seat, friend, and read on. Because your fitness regimen, were it a chair, would ideally be a three-legged stool, with each leg representing one of three vital parts of the fitness equation: strength, endurance and flexibility.

Strength is the amount of force that a muscle group can exert in a onetime burst of effort. What's the most you can bench-press? That's how strong that particular muscle group is. Simple.

Endurance is the ability to resist fatigue and to exercise or work over a long period of time. There are two kinds of endurance.

• Cardiovascular endurance means your heart and lungs can efficiently deliver oxygen to your muscles, even when under the stress and strain of hard exertion. Exercise to make your heart and lungs more adept at delivering oxygen is called aerobic exercise and includes walking, running, bicycling and swimming. Of all of the elements of fitness, cardiovascular endurance is probably the most important to your long-term health and well-being, says Morris B. Mellion, M.D., clinical associate professor of family practice and orthopedic surgery at the University of Nebraska Medical Center and medical director of the Sports Medicine Center, both in Omaha.

• Muscular endurance is the ability of a muscle or a muscle group to keep exercising without rest—when you're riding a bike for hours on end, for example. It is related to how strong you are.

Flexibility means that your joints can move through their full range of motion, thanks to well-stretched muscles and tendons. Try to mimic the positions and movements of a one-year-old baby, and you'll quickly discover that your bones and muscles have just a fraction of the mobility they once had. Some of the motion can be regained, however, through the right types of stretching.

Put these three together, and you have the keys to vitality and fitness. Of course, there are an infinite number of ways of putting the three together. But at the core of any proper exercise program, experts now agree, are activities for each: aerobic exercise such as walking or biking for your heart and lungs, weight lifting for power and stretching for maximum muscle movement.

Because the activities used for aerobic conditioning, such as walking and biking, are so familiar, we don't need to teach you how to do them. We will give you tips on how to optimize your aerobic workout. But this section of the book concentrates on the other two legs of the chair: how to lift weights and do stretches safely.

Specifically, we'll take you through each primary muscle group and show you the best stretches and lifts. Then we'll offer workout programs for five different desired outcomes. Pick one and get started—after you finish this chapter. You can't exercise right without knowing what you're trying to achieve with all of that effort.

Endurance: Getting Winded

Your heart is a muscle, just like your biceps, and it needs exercise in much the same way. But since your heart is buried deep within your chest, it's a muscle that is easy to forget about—that is, until you're gasping for breath after three flights of stairs or huffing and puffing like a train while chasing your toddler down the block.

Aerobic conditioning is conditioning of the heart and lungs. When they are in shape, your entire body benefits by getting oxygen and nutrients delivered more efficiently. This

Five Essential Training Tips

It's one thing to work out; it's another to work out intelligently. We'll save you from learning the hard way at the Fitness School of Hard Knocks by giving you these insider tips on how to make the most of your muscles.

Warm up first. Most guys plunge into bench presses or leg curls with nary a warm-up. Do that, eager beaver, and you're courting trouble. Instead, first do five to ten minutes of light aerobic exercise, such as running in place or jumping rope, to get your blood moving. If you have time, turn your warm-up into a cardiovascular workout with 15 to 20 minutes of cycling, stair climbing or running. Make sure your warm-up is not too strenuous; you should still be able to breathe normally. This increases circulation, loosens muscles and primes your body for what is to come.

Stretch with style. Stretching does wonders for your health. It's also a good pre-workout ritual. To stretch properly: Stretch only to the point of resistance, not to the point of pain. Never stretch with a bouncing or jerking motion, or you could hurt yourself. And always hold a stretch for 20 to 30 seconds. Holding a stretch longer than 60 seconds isn't any better than holding it for 30 seconds.

Cool down when done. Just when you're ready to throw in the towel and call it a day, don't—at least not until you've cooled down. A cooldown complements a warm-up. It prevents your muscles from tightening up after a workout, which keeps you from walking around in knots the next day. To cool down, do ten minutes of light aerobic work such as jogging, followed by simple stretches for your arms, legs and back.

Learn to relax. The more you relax after a workout, the better you'll be. Relaxation speeds the elimination of metabolic waste products from your body, which makes it less likely that you'll be sore the next day. So take a few deep breaths, drink some water, congratulate yourself on a good workout. You'll be glad you did tomorrow.

Always go with the flow. Experts say most of us don't drink enough water. When it comes to working out, improper hydration means less power. And less power means you're not exercising as effectively as you could. Plus with all of the sweating you're doing, you run the risk of dehydration unless you top your tank. To keep your fluid level up, drink at least six to eight eight-ounce glasses of water a day, including sipping from a water bottle between sets, even if you don't feel thirsty.

can mean round-the-clock energy, faster fat-burning metabolism, long-distance stamina and protection against cardiovascular disease.

Most fitness authorities say that when you exercise aerobically, you should work hard enough to raise your heart rate to 70 to 85 percent of your maximum and then maintain that level for 30 minutes or more. Out-of-shape guys should aim for the 70 percent mark, while more fit individuals can shoot for 85 percent.

To estimate your maximum heart rate, subtract your age from 220. Then multiply that by the percentage you want in decimal form. So for a 40-year-old shooting for 70 percent of his maximum heart rate, it would be:

$$220 - 40 = 180 \times 0.7 = 126 \text{ beats per minute}$$

For best results, work out at least three times a week.

Just about any exercise that revs your heart and lungs can qualify as good aerobic conditioning. Running, cycling, swimming, a pickup game of basketball and a set of four-wall racquetball are all good choices. Even low-weight, high-repetition weight lifting can build aerobic power somewhat: Some studies show that a fast-paced low-weight workout can give your heart and lung power a 6 percent boost (although that pales compared with the 18 percent boost you get through traditional aerobic exercise, such as the activities mentioned above).

Of course, one of the surest, easiest ways to get into aerobic exercise is to do it gradually, one foot at a time, by walking.

"Walking is great exercise. It's fun, easy to do and effective, plus it's a fantastic way to ease into any aerobic program," says Bonnie Berk, R.N., a certified personal fitness trainer and exercise consultant in Carlisle, Pennsylvania. To start a walking routine, simply take a 10-minute stroll around the block after dinner tonight and for the next couple of nights. After a week or so, increase your walking time to 15 minutes, and so on until you're doing about an hour a day. That'll give you all of the aerobic conditioning you need, and then some. Or once you reach that point, increase the challenge by taking up jogging or cycling.

Strength: A Weighty Issue

Weight lifting is a crucial part of overall conditioning. But for years, it remained in the shadows of aerobic conditioning, which got the lion's share of attention from researchers and fitness buffs. Today, weight lifting is in the mainstream and no longer just a subculture of pumped-up muscleheads in smelly backstreet gyms.

The benefits of weight lifting make a strong argument in favor of joining the gym rats. For starters, there's the satisfaction of having a flatter belly, stronger-looking arms, a more defined chest. "Looking good can be a great motivator, and I would venture to say that most guys in the average gym are there to look good," says Berk.

But it doesn't end there.

"While weight lifting can be a real ego boost, you should still know the health benefits, because your muscles don't exist in a vacuum," Berk says. The benefits include increases in muscle strength, muscle mass, bone strength and your body's metabolism. This means that not only does your body look and feel harder, it is harder. Plus it torches fat faster.

When you lift weights, you have at your disposal more than 215 pairs of skeletal muscles—that is, muscles that are attached to bones and make the bones move. These muscles are made up of two kinds of microscopic fibers. Fast-twitch fibers provide explosive force, the kind you need for sprints or bench presses. Slow-twitch fibers provide endurance; they're the power source for aerobic efforts such as long-distance running or cycling.

Most guys have a 50-50 blend of fast-twitch and slow-twitch fibers, but genetics occasionally deals some of us a stronger hand one way or the other. Be aware of your own chemistry and play to its strengths.

Regardless of what mix of fibers you have, the important thing is how you use them. Weight lifting is tough and repetitive. The trick is to not get burned out or discouraged, even when results are coming slower than you'd like. If you don't enjoy it, you'll stop doing it.

"One of the things I stress a lot when training people is making them develop a positive mind-body connection," Berk says. "You want to push yourself, but not unrealistically. Always remember that you're in this for the long haul."

Once you have the motivation, you'll need the know-how to lift weights effectively. There's a lot of science to it, but you needn't concern yourself with much. The most important thing is to have a clear goal and to get the right program to achieve it. Want brute strength? Bulk? Stamina? Each of these outcomes is reached through a different type of weight-lifting technique. By varying the loads being lifted, the number of repetitions and the number of sets, you change the outcome for your body.

We'll show you several approaches later on, but the basics are this: For brute strength, lift heavy weights for 3 to 8 reps per set, with three to five minutes of rest between sets; for a muscular body, lift medium weights roughly 8 to 12 reps per set, with 60 to 90 seconds of rest between sets; for muscular and cardiovascular endurance and a lean appearance, lift light weights for 12 to 20 reps per set and only rest about 30 seconds between sets.

Weight-Lifting Lingo

Never be at a loss for words in the weight room. Here are common workout terms and what they mean.

Aerobic exercise: A repetitive exercise, such as running or bicycling, that causes your body's muscles to need more oxygen. Your heart and lungs work together to supply oxygen to your body. Aerobic exercise forces them to work harder and, in so doing, strengthens and conditions them.

Anaerobic exercise: An exercise that requires short bursts of power, such as weight lifting. This type of exercise strengthens muscles but does not particularly push the heart and lungs.

Atrophy: Loss of size and function of muscle tissue.

Hypertrophy: The opposite of atrophy; an increase in muscle fiber size.

Isokinetic exercise: A type of isotonic exercise in which resistance varies through the motion of the lift to match the muscle's strength. Nautilus and Cybex machines provide this kind of workout.

Isometric exercise: In these exercises, muscles contract, but joints don't move and muscle fibers keep a constant length. These exercises are typically performed against an immovable surface. An example is pressing your palm against a wall.

Isotonic exercise: Traditional dumbbell and barbell exercises are isotonic. These require a change in muscle fiber length and constant resistance.

Myositis: Also called delayed-onset muscle soreness; muscle soreness resulting from inflammation of the muscles, such as the pain that occurs a day or two after weight lifting.

Rep: Short for *repetition*; one complete movement of a particular exercise.

Set: A fixed number of reps.

Spotter: A training partner who watches you closely to lend help, if needed, during a specific exercise.

Flexibility: Taking Flex Time

Remember the chair analogy that was used to describe total fitness? Well, if one leg of that three-legged stool continually comes up short, it's the flexibility leg.

For most guys, stretching doesn't seem to be high on the list of fitness priorities. But without stretching your muscles, you're stretching your luck.

"Stretching for men is one of my pet peeves. Far too few men stretch as much as they should, and that's just asking for trouble," Berk says.

Good range of motion keeps injuries at bay. If you slip while running, for example, supple ankles might make the difference between continuing your run and limping to a doctor. Flexibility can give you an edge elsewhere, too. First, stretching is a great invigorator and stress reliever. Second, stretching can improve your weight lifting because it increases your range of motion, and full range of motion while lifting means your muscles are developing evenly and fully.

Flexibility comes from keeping the muscles and tendons surrounding each joint limber. Otherwise, the muscles become shorter, tighter and less likely to go with the flow when you move the wrong way. When you stretch, your nerves tell your muscles to contract as a defense mechanism. This keeps the muscles from overstretching. But if you hold a stretch for 20 to 30 seconds or more, the nerve impulses fade, and the stretch gets more comfortable. You should stretch to the point where you feel resistance, not pain.

And finally, let's forget the notion that you can't be flexible and muscular at the same time. If you devote enough time to each, you can be as big as Arnold but as limber as Gumby.

Workout: Forearms

Without forearm muscles, your hands wouldn't be able to make fists, hold a baseball bat, drive a nail, type a letter or grasp a bottle.

Unless you're a professional arm wrestler— or a shrimpy cartoon character named Popeye— you probably don't need monstrous forearm muscles. But taking the time to tone them up carries advantages.

First, forearms make a statement about your athleticism, since they're the only parts of your arms that most people see when you're wearing short sleeves.

Second, and more important, strong forearm muscles make your hands far more powerful. A study of college softball players at Pennsylvania State University in University Park found that the athletes increased their grip strength by as much as 15 percent after training their forearm muscles.

Anatomy of a Forearm

Your forearm is located between your elbow and your wrist. Also called the antebrachium, the forearm controls most of your gross gripping strength during activities that don't require fine motor skills. In other words, you call on your forearm muscles to swing a golf club, not to repair a watch.

Each forearm is made up of three main muscle groups: the brachioradialis, the flexors and the extensors. The brachioradialis runs from the humerus, the large bone in your upper arm, to the lower end of the radius, the bone on the thumb side of your forearm.

The flexors and extensors are numerous, plus they're all named in Latin, so there's little use in going into mind-numbing detail about them here. Suffice it to say that flexors move your palm toward your forearm; some also help move your fingers. The extensors move the back of your hand toward your forearm. They also help extend your fingers.

Nearly every exercise requiring a grip will work your forearms to some degree. "The forearms receive a lot of training even when you're not specifically performing forearm exercises," says Chip Harrison, a strength and conditioning coach at Pennsylvania State University. Yet as the study of softball players at Harrison's university suggests, giving these muscles their own workout can be a boon to your overall fitness, not to mention preventive medicine in protecting you from repetitive strain injury.

Flexibility

Forearm Stretch

Place your wrist on a table. Your hand should be on its side, with your thumb facing up. Keeping your fingers straight, bend your wrist so that your palm is moving toward the inside of your forearm. Bend your wrist as far as you can and hold.

Then move your wrist in the opposite direction, except curl your fingers as you're bending.

Next, place your hand on the table, with your palm facing down. Without moving your arm, pivot your hand to the left as far as possible. Then move your hand in the opposite direction, again letting your wrist do all of the work.

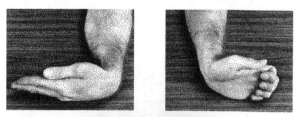

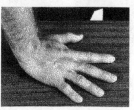

Do each exercise five to ten times, holding for five seconds each time. Then repeat with your other hand.

The Exercises

Forearm Curl

This is an excellent way to build the meaty section of your forearm on the palm side of your arm.

Start by sitting at the end of a bench, with your legs slightly more than hip-width apart. Place your right hand on your right knee and hold a dumbbell in your left hand in a palm up grip. Your left wrist should be over your left knee slightly, so you can bend your wrist

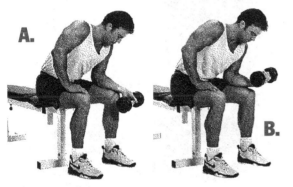

through its full range of motion. Your forearm should be resting against your thigh, and your upper body should be fairly upright.

Curl the dumbbell toward your body as far as you can. Don't let your arm rise up off your thigh. At the top of the curl, hold for a second, then lower to the starting position. Finish your reps, then switch hands.

Reverse Forearm Curl

This exercise works those sinewy muscles on the knuckle side of your forearm. Sit at the end of a bench with your legs slightly more than hip-width apart. Rest your left hand above your left knee and hold a dumbbell in your right hand in a palm-down grip. Your right wrist should be slightly over your right knee. The bottom, meaty part of your forearm should be resting against your thigh, and your upper body should be fairly upright.

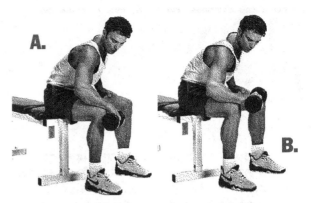

Curl the dumbbell toward your body as far as you can. Don't let your arm rise up off your thigh. At the top of the curl, hold for a second, then lower to the starting position. Finish your reps, then switch hands.

Wrist Roller

Stand upright, with your feet about shoulder-width apart. Hold a wrist roller (a weight hanging by a rope from the center of a bar, as shown) in both hands, with your palms facing down. Keep your arms extended in front of you and the weight dangling before you.

Slowly roll the weight up by curling your left hand over and down, then curling your right hand over and down. Use long, exaggerated up-and-down movements with your wrists to get their full range of motion. Don't sway your body or drop your arms. When the weight has reached the bar, slowly lower it, reversing the motion of your hands.

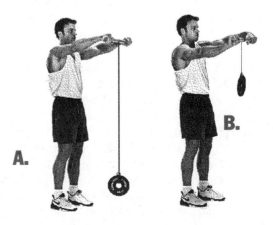

⚡ Workout: Biceps

Biceps are among the muscles that are the easiest to build and the fastest to respond to proper training. Even the leanest set of garter snakes can be pumped into a powerful pair of pythons in a relatively short time.

But you needn't have a goal of bigger arms to justify exercising them. Simply taking the time to tone your upper arms does wonders for your image and your health. And by increasing the strength of your biceps, you'll strengthen your grip and tone other arm muscles, such as your forearms, as well.

"I think a lot of us forget that when we work certain body parts, we're actually working other muscles at the same time," says Bonnie Berk, R.N., a certified personal fitness trainer and exercise consultant in Carlisle, Pennsylvania.

Strong-Arming Yourself

The biceps part of your arm includes the biceps brachii and the brachialis muscles. The biceps brachii has two heads—thus, the *bi-* part of its name (*bi* means "two"). It's responsible for the bulge you see when you "make a muscle" with your arm. The brachialis, on the other hand, is the larger of the two muscles. It runs underneath the biceps brachii. Both muscles are used whenever you flex your elbow; the biceps brachii is also used whenever you move your shoulder.

Arm strength is to your body what horse-power is to your car. In day-to-day life, you don't use the extra capacity much, but a stronger machine runs more efficiently, and it's great to have that instantaneous surge of power available when you need it. But a word of cau-

tion: Even though the rewards are quick and great, don't spend all of your time working your biceps, or you may overdevelop them at the expense of other body parts. And don't be tempted to rush the job by lifting more than you can handle, or you'll run the risk of hurting yourself. Proper form and technique are more important than lifting lots of weight.

Flexibility

Arm/Shoulder Stretch

Stand in a doorway, grasping the door frame on either side at about shoulder height. Lean forward while keeping your chest up and

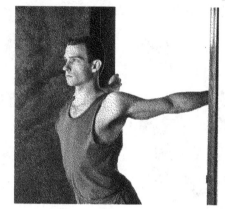

your chin in. Gradually straighten your arms as you lean farther into the stretch. Hold for 20 to 30 seconds.

The Exercises

Barbell Curl

This is the cornerstone of all biceps exercises. Start in a standing position and grip a barbell in an underhand grip (palms facing up). Your hands should be about shoulder-width apart, your arms should be extended downward, and the barbell should be around thigh level. Do not lock your knees.

Keeping your elbows close to your body, use your biceps to slowly curl the bar toward your chin. Be certain to keep your wrists straight throughout this curling motion; don't sway your back or rock your body for momentum. That's cheating, and it could pull

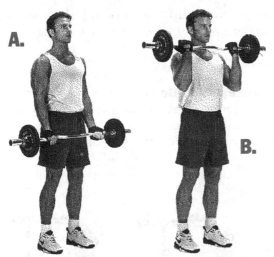

or strain another muscle. Lower the barbell to the starting position.

Concentration Curl

This is another tried-and-true biceps exercise, though it's even harder than a normal curl because it isolates the muscles and doesn't allow you to cheat. Start by straddling the end of a weight bench while holding a dumbbell in one hand. Your feet should be wider than shoulder-width apart, with your knees bent.

Bend forward and extend your arm between your legs so that your elbow and upper arm are braced against your thigh. The dumbbell should be held in a palm-up grip, and you should be leaning slightly toward that side. Rest your other hand on your other knee.

Curl the dumbbell toward your shoulder, bracing your elbow against your thigh and leaning on your other hand for support. Hold, then lower with control to the starting point. Finish your reps and switch hands.

Alternating Hammer Curl

Because of wrist positioning, this exercise works the brachialis more thoroughly. Start by sitting at the end of a bench with your feet slightly apart and your arms down at your sides. You should be holding a dumbbell in each hand, with your palms facing your body in an overhand grip. Your shoulders should be back, and your upper torso should be upright.

Now curl one dumbbell toward your biceps. Don't rock or sway to build momentum; that's not good technique, and you could hurt yourself. Your wrist should be locked, and your palm should continue to face in toward your body as you lift. Lower to the starting position, then repeat with the other arm.

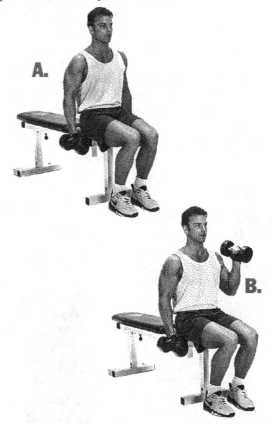

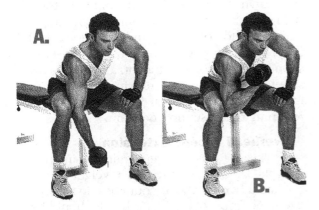

Workout: Triceps

The triceps are the underdogs of the muscle world, overshadowed by the more showy biceps. Yet the triceps aren't to be neglected. For starters, they're big, accounting for two-thirds of your upper-arm mass.

They're big for a reason: The triceps are responsible for much of your everyday arm movement. So if you really want impressive-looking upper arms, your triceps are worthy body parts to keep in shape.

Your triceps muscle is located along the back section of each upper arm. It has three heads, which accounts for the *tri-* in *triceps*. These include the long head, the medial head and the lateral head. When they're properly developed, the three heads combine to create an impressive horseshoe-shaped appearance.

The triceps have an important job in arm mobility. Without them, you wouldn't be able to straighten out your arms. They're also responsible for extending your arms after they have been bent at the elbow.

Flexibility

Upper Arm/Triceps Stretch

From a standing position, raise your arms overhead and cross them at your wrists. Place your palms together so that they face out, away from your body. Your arms should be straight, with only a slight bend at the elbows.

Breathe in and stretch upward and

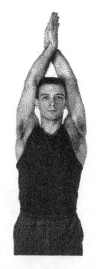

slightly backward. You should feel the stretch in your upper arms, shoulders and sides.

The Exercises

Triceps Pull-Down

Here's an easy-to-do exercise that can give quick results. It requires a triceps pull-down machine. Start by standing facing the machine and grasping the handle with both hands. Use a narrow grip, with your palms

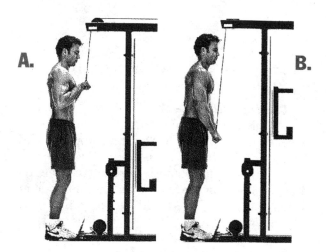

facing away from you. Grip the bar as high as you comfortably can while keeping your upper arms at your sides, with your elbows bent up.

From the starting position, pull down on the bar until you've straightened out both arms and they're pointing toward the floor. This pull-down should be smooth, with your triceps doing all of the work. Your elbows should remain close to your body, and you should feel the contraction in your triceps. Your wrists should be locked and straight, and you shouldn't be swaying or rocking your body for momentum. Raise the bar with control, returning to the starting position.

Overhead Triceps Extension

This is a classic triceps trainer using free weights. Lie on your back on a weight bench, holding a barbell above your chest in a narrow overhand grip—that is, your hands should be

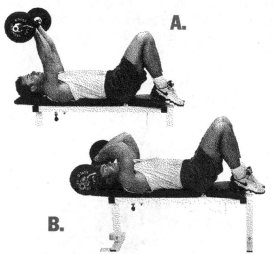

A.

B.

roughly four to six inches apart, palms facing up. Your feet should be up on the bench, with your feet together and your legs slightly parted.

Bend your elbows, slowly lowering the weight toward the top of your head. Don't sway your arms through the motion; keep them stationary and concentrate the effort in your triceps. Raise the barbell to the starting position.

Dumbbell Kickback

Kickbacks are an easy exercise to do, especially since you're using dumbbells, which can be lugged around just about anywhere.

Start with a dumbbell in your right hand, palm facing in toward your body. Rest your left

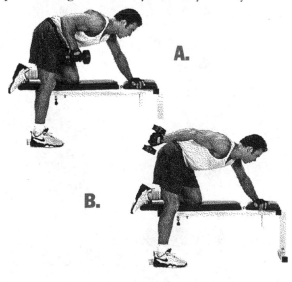

A.

B.

knee and left hand on a weight bench or on a low table for support. Bring the dumbbell up and in toward your body, close to your chest muscles. Your arm should be in close to your rib cage, and your elbow should be pointing up toward the ceiling. Your back should be straight and roughly parallel to the floor.

While resting on your left knee and hand, extend the dumbbell back by straightening your right elbow. You should feel the contraction in your triceps. Extend your arm until it's straight and your triceps are fully contracted. Don't lean, sway or arch your back for momentum; it's bad technique, and you'll only wind up pulling a muscle. Lower the dumbbell to the starting position.

Narrow-Grip Seated Overhead Triceps Extension

Start by sitting at the end of a bench with your feet firmly on the ground and a barbell held overhead in a narrow grip, palms facing

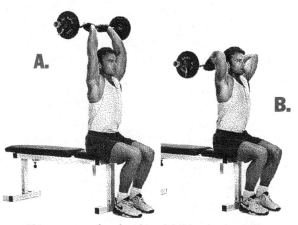

A.

B.

out. Your upper body should be erect and facing forward, with a natural slight forward lean in your lower back.

Holding your upper body in place, lower the barbell behind your head. Keep your upper arms close to your head and lower the bar until your forearms are as close to your biceps as possible. You might lean slightly forward to help offset the weight, but don't sway or arch your back. Your elbows should be facing forward or slightly to the sides. Raise the barbell to the starting position.

☷ Workout: Shoulders and Neck

Growing up, lots of men had a G.I. Joe doll, the kind with the kung fu grip. Joe weathered all sorts of adventures, but if you pulled too hard on his arms, his rubber-band joints snapped, turning the poor soldier into a disabled veteran.

Like G.I. Joe's shoulders, yours are extremely versatile, mobile and useful joints. But without shoulder muscles holding everything in place, you, like Joe, might end up disarmed.

Shoulder muscles contract every time you move your arms up or away from your body. They're also nice to look at: Cannonball shoulders fill out shirts, jackets and suits even better than big hangers.

The shoulder muscle is called the deltoid. The name comes from a Latin word meaning triangular, which describes its shape.

The deltoid is attached to various parts of your collarbone and shoulder blade. It's also connected to the humerus, that large bone in your upper arm. Functionally, the deltoid lifts, rotates and extends your arm.

The trapezius runs along the side of your neck, from the base of your skull to your mid-back. It helps lift your shoulder and rotate your shoulder blade.

Flexibility

Head Turn

With your head in an upright position, simply turn it to the left as far as you can and hold for about five seconds. Repeat on the right side.

Gently rotate your head back to the center in an upright position. Look down toward your chest and hold for about five seconds, then return to the starting position.

Whatever you do, don't tilt your head back, lift your chin toward the ceiling or rotate

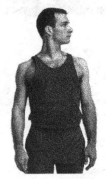

your head in a circular motion. This places too much stress on your neck's delicate vertebrae.

Overhead Shoulder Stretch

This is an excellent way to loosen up your shoulders and upper arms. Start in a standing position, with your shoulders back, your chest out and your feet about shoulder-width apart. Raise your right arm overhead, bending it at the elbow so that your right hand is resting between your shoulder blades.

Put your left hand on your right elbow and push your right arm down. Your right hand should be sliding farther down your back. When you're finished stretching, switch arms and repeat.

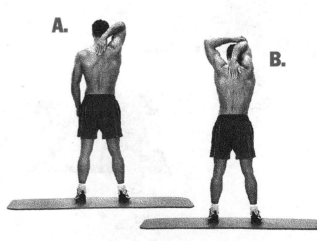

The Exercises

Shoulder Shrug

This exercise is a standard for building bigger traps. Start by standing upright and holding a lightly weighted barbell at upper-thigh level. Use a medium grip, with your palms facing in toward your body. Your feet should be shoulder-width apart, with your shoulders back but drooped. Your chest is out, and your lower back is straight, with a slight forward lean.

Lift the barbell up and out by raising both shoulders to the front of your body. At the

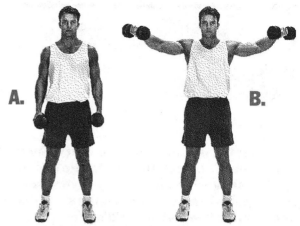

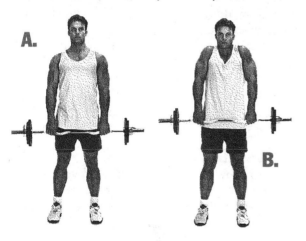

highest point, rotate your shoulders toward your ears, lifting them higher. Lower to the starting position.

Side Lateral Raise

This exercise is excellent for those hard-to-work lateral deltoids. Start by standing with your arms at your sides. Hold a dumbbell in each hand, with your palms facing in toward your body and your elbows slightly bent. Keep your feet shoulder-width apart, your shoulders back, your chest out and your lower back straight, with a slight forward lean.

In unison, raise both dumbbells in a straight line until they're shoulder level. Keep your elbows slightly bent and don't let your arms leave the same plane as your upper body. Slowly lower to the starting position.

Alternating Seated Dumbbell Press

To protect your back, it's a good idea to wear a weight belt when you do this exercise.

Straddle a bench, with your legs slightly parted and your feet firmly on the floor. Grasp a dumbbell in each hand. Bend your arms so that you are holding the dumbbells at shoulder level, with your palms facing in.

Raise one dumbbell until your arm is straight, but don't lock your elbow. Lower and repeat with your other arm. Continue alternating arms as you complete your reps.

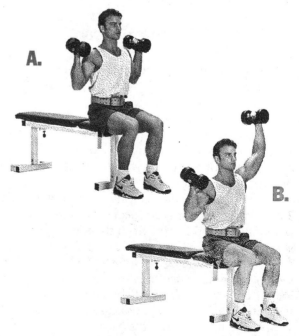

Workout: Chest

What body parts do men worry about most when it comes to their image? Guess again—skinny legs are easily covered by baggy pants. The correct answers are the chest and the waist, according to researchers in Canada who interviewed college-age men.

Why? For one thing, a muscular chest covers up other flaws, such as being a little thick around the middle. A strong chest also gives you the aura of power, a don't-mess-with-me physique that draws eyes and respect.

Yet a chiseled chest is a worthy goal for more than just vanity's sake. The chest is an important player in everything you do, from maintaining good posture and poise to reaching forward to grab the steering wheel while driving.

Building the Best Chest in the West

When you're talking chest muscles, you're talking about the "pecs" (short for *pectorals*). There are two of them.

The pectoralis major is the biggest chest muscle. It's a thick, fan-shaped muscle that spans your breastbone and collarbone and attaches to your upper arms. It makes up the bulk of your chest.

Then there's the pectoralis minor, which is a thin, triangular muscle located beneath the pectoralis major. It runs from the top of your shoulder blades to your middle ribs.

Chest muscles get a lot of attention in the weight room because they're very strong, and lots of guys try to show off by lifting heavy weights. While this may look macho, it's not in your best interest. Lifting too much too fast can

pull a muscle, strain your back or worse.

If you want to build your chest, keep in mind that endomorphs—people who are genetically predisposed to fleshiness—tend to have the largest chests. Of course, that doesn't mean their chests are all muscle. Muscle building takes time, but it does come. Just ask Isaac Nesser of Greensburg, Pennsylvania. He has the world's largest muscular chest: It measures 74¹⁄₁₆ inches.

Strength is one thing; flexibility is another. You've probably never thought about your chest being flexible. But if you've ever taken a really, really big breath or arched your back, you know that your chest muscles can stretch. Since chest muscles are the counterparts to your back muscles and both are critical in posture and everyday movement, a flexible chest means a healthier you. So be sure to do the following.

Flexibility

Chest Stretch

Start by standing upright, with your shoulders back, your chest out and your feet shoulder-width apart. Clasp your hands behind

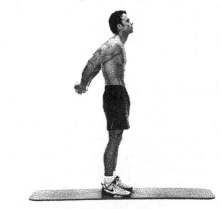

your back so that your fingers are interlaced and at about the same height as your butt.

Now lift your arms in unison up and away from your body until you feel your chest and shoulder muscles stretch. Don't hunch over. Keep your chest out and your chin in. Raise your hands as far as you can, then lower them.

The Exercises

Bench Press

Lie on a bench-press bench with the barbell above your chest. Grasp the bar with your hands about shoulder-width apart, palms facing your legs. Your feet should be resting on the ground, and your back should be straight and against the bench.

Lower the barbell until it touches your chest around the nipple line. Your elbows

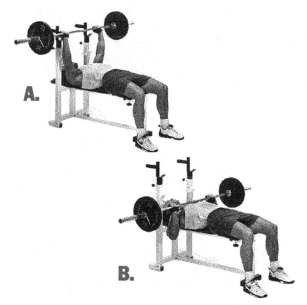

should be pointing out, but the rest of your body should remain in position. Don't arch your back or bounce the bar off your chest; you could hurt yourself. Raise the barbell to the starting position. For any bench press exercise, be sure to use a spotter.

Alternating Dumbbell Press

Grasping two dumbbells, lie back on a bench with your legs slightly parted, your feet firmly on the floor and your arms raised. Hold the dumbbells above you about shoulder-width apart, with your palms facing each other. Your arms should be extended, and your back should be straight and firm against the bench. Don't lock your elbows.

Lower the left dumbbell until it's even with your chest. Your elbow should be pointing

toward the ground, with your palm still facing in. Raise the dumbbell to the starting position, then alternate by lowering the other dumbbell.

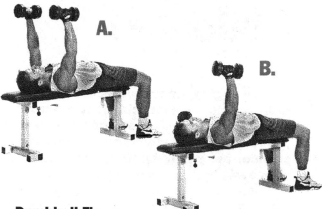

Dumbbell Fly

Lie on your back on a bench, with your legs slightly parted and your feet firmly on the floor. With your palms facing each other, hold two dumbbells above you so that they're nearly touching above your chest. Keep your back straight and firm against the bench and your elbows unlocked.

Slowly lower the dumbbells out and away from each other until they're at chest level, keeping your wrists locked. Your elbows should be bent slightly, and your back should be straight. Raise the dumbbells to the starting position.

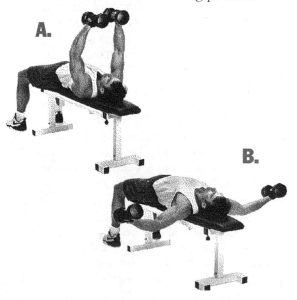

![icon] Workout: Abdomen

Let's play a game of word association. What's the first thing that comes to mind when you hear the word "crunch"? If you answered potato chips or car fenders, chances are you're sporting more flab than abs.

Physically powerful men know that the secret to a strong, chiseled belly and a healthy, well-supported back is exercises called crunches.

Now don't get mixed up about what crunches will do. Exercising your belly muscles won't get rid of belly flab. Spot reducing doesn't work; you're better off jogging or swimming to burn fat. But if you are relatively lean, well-exercised abdominal muscles will show through with the washboard look that both men and women seem to love.

Finding the Rock in Your Roll

More important, strong abs have big health benefits. The abdominal muscles work together with the muscles in your back to help support the spine, according to Morris B. Mellion, M.D., clinical associate professor of family practice and orthopedic surgery at the University of Nebraska Medical Center and medical director of the Sports Medicine Center, both in Omaha. Neglecting your abdominals may lead to a muscle imbalance that could result in back pain, so it's important to keep your abs well-toned, he says. Here are the four muscle groups that make up your abdominals.

• The rectus abdominis is the muscle you want to work for that washboard look. It covers the length of your abdomen, from the breastbone to the bottom of the pelvis. The rectus helps flex your trunk, such as when you sit up. It also helps keep your internal organs in place.

• The external obliques run down the sides of your body between the chest and the pelvis. Flexing one of these muscles while relaxing the other rotates the body away from the side that is being flexed. Contracting them in unison assists the rectus in flexing your trunk.

• The internal obliques lie beneath the external obliques, connecting the last four ribs with the pelvis. These muscles function similarly to the external obliques, only they pull in the opposite direction.

• The transversus abdominis is the deepest of the abdominal muscles. As its name suggests, its fibers are arranged horizontally across your middle, like a girdle. It functions a lot like a girdle, too, contracting inward to compress your abdomen and support the organs within.

The abdominal muscles are the only muscles in your body that can safely be exercised every day. Even so, some experts advise splitting your daily abdominal routine into two separate workouts. This will give you the time to do your exercises slowly, allowing you to concentrate on proper technique.

Flexibility

Belly Stretch

A tough workout can cause your abdominal muscles to get tight, but there is a very simple way to stretch them out. Lie flat on your back, with your legs straight and your arms on the floor above your head. Slowly

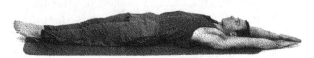

reach your arms and legs away from the center of your body as far as you can. Hold the stretch for five to eight seconds, then relax.

The Exercises

Crunch

Lie flat on your back, with your fingertips cupped behind your ears. Keep your feet together, flat on the floor and about six inches from your butt. Your knees should be bent at about 45-degree angles.

Without moving your lower body, curl your upper torso up and in toward your knees until your shoulder blades are as high off the

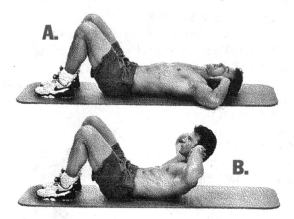

ground as you can get them. Lift only your shoulders, not your back. Feel your abs contract. Hold the raise for a second, then lower to the starting position. Continue with your next rep without relaxing in between.

Crossover Crunch

Lie flat on your back in the crunch position, with your feet flat and your knees up.

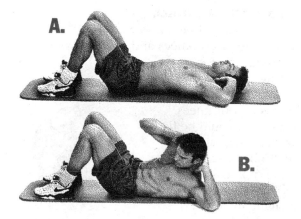

Keep your feet about hip-width apart and cup your fingertips behind your ears.

Raise your trunk, lifting your shoulders and shoulder blades off the ground. But instead of pausing at the top, slightly twist toward your left knee. Hold the contraction for a split second, then lower to the starting position. Repeat, but this time twist toward your right knee. Don't relax between reps.

Oblique Crunch

Lie flat on your back, with your knees bent and your fingertips cupped behind your ears. Let your legs fall as far as they can to your right side so that your upper body is flat on the floor and your lower body is on its side.

Keeping your shoulders as close to parallel to the floor as possible, lift your upper body until your shoulder blades clear the ground. Concentrate on the oblique contraction and hold the crunch for a second. Then lower to the starting position and do your next rep. Don't rest between crunches; keep your abs tight. After one set on your right side, switch to your left and continue.

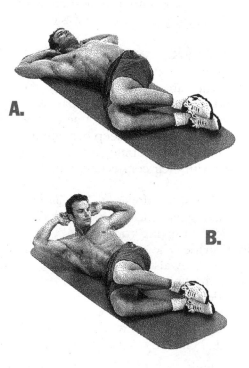

⚡ Workout: Back

The back is a many-splendored thing. It's a wheelbarrow for carrying heavy loads. It's a saddle for giving kids pony rides. It's a playground for the fingers of a talented masseuse.

The back is so impressive because it is awash in muscles large and small. These muscles work in harmony.

But with so many moving parts, the back is also fairly delicate. One wrong turn can pull a muscle, sprain a ligament or hurt a disk, one of those elastic shock absorbers between your vertebrae. General back pain is the leading cause of disability for men under age 45, and 80 percent of all people will eventually get it before they turn 50. Next to the common cold, back pain symptoms are the most common cause of visits to primary care physicians.

Building Blocks of the Back

Your back features several primary muscles. They are the latissimus dorsi, the rhomboideus and the erector spinae. Also important are the supporting structures, which include smaller muscles deep beneath the skin's surface, 33 vertebrae and the intervertebral disks with their connecting nerves and ligaments.

The latissimus dorsi, or "lats," are muscles that run along the sides of your back. They're responsible for giving your upper body that manly V shape. They extend, rotate and pull in your arms. They also help you cough.

The rhomboideus include the rhomboideus major and minor; most people call them rhomboids for short. These compact muscles are located a few inches down from your neck, between your spine and shoulder blades. They retract and rotate your shoulder blades.

The erector spinae run along your spine, and it's their job to help support and move your spine from side to side.

The key to back maintenance is to treat the region like any other muscle group. That means regular stretching and strengthening. Here's what to do.

Flexibility

Upper Back Stretch

Face a ledge that is roughly chest height or higher. The top of a refrigerator or filing cabinet will work just fine. You should be about arm's length from the ledge, and your feet should be shoulder-width apart. Now grasp the ledge with both hands and let your upper body drop down as you keep your knees slightly bent. Your hips should be above your feet. You'll feel the stretch throughout your shoulders and back. Hold for about 30 seconds. To change the area stretched, bend your knees or move your hands to a different height.

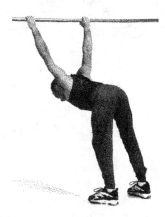

Lower Back Stretch

This easy stretch also works your groin, Achilles tendons, knees and ankles. From a standing position, simply squat down so that your elbows are between your knees. Your feet should be flat on the floor, with your heels about 4 to 12 inches apart. Your toes should be pointing out at slight angles, and

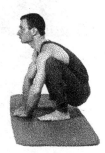

your knees should be positioned over your big toes. A slight forward lean will help you keep your balance. Hold the stretch comfortably for 30 seconds.

The Exercises

Lat Pull-Down

This, too, works your upper back, with a strong emphasis on the lats. Sit at a lat pull-down machine (unless it doesn't have a seat, in which case you should kneel underneath it).

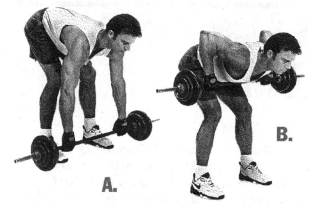

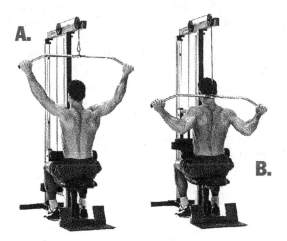

Grasp the handle overhead in as wide a grip as is comfortable, but make sure your hands are at least farther than shoulder-width apart. Your palms should be facing away from your body, and your upper body should be straight, eyes forward.

Pull the bar down to your body, behind your neck. Your upper body should stay upright, but your elbows should be pointing at the ground and slightly outward. Raise the bar to the starting position.

Bent-Over Row

Stand bent over at your waist, with your back straight. Grasp a barbell with your hands in a wide grip, palms down. Your feet should be shoulder-width apart, your neck straight and your face toward the floor. Keep your legs straight and your knees unlocked.

Pull the barbell in toward your body so that the bar is touching your lower chest. Keep

your back straight and your elbows pointing up toward the ceiling. Lower to the starting position.

Good Morning Exercise

This exercise works your lower back, primarily the erector spinae. Stand with your legs shoulder-width apart while holding a barbell with very light weights across your shoulders and behind your neck. Your hands should be a little wider than your shoulders, palms facing out. Make sure to keep your upper body upright, your shoulders back and your chest out, and maintain a slight forward lean in your lower back.

Slowly bend over at the waist until your body is at roughly a 90-degree angle and parallel to the floor. Keep your back straight and your head up. Keep your legs straight and your knees unlocked. Rise to the starting position.

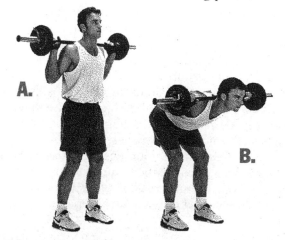

✗ Workout: Butt

Granted, this isn't something you'd bring up on a fishing trip with the guys. But if you walk, jump, cycle or do just about anything involving your lower body, you can't talk about muscles without talking about the butt.

Most of us don't spend a lot of time fretting about our butts. To us, the butt is just a built-in seat cushion that keeps our bones from bruising every time we sit down. But a strong butt is more than that: It gives your lower body explosive power for all sorts of activities.

"A strong butt also contributes to good posture, and it helps support your lower back," states Bonnie Berk, R.N., a certified personal fitness trainer and exercise consultant in Carlisle, Pennsylvania. In fact, some experts believe that strong butt muscles can actually help alleviate lower back pain. That's good news for the 80 percent of us who will suffer from aching lower backs at some point before we reach age 50.

Maximus Muscle

The butt is the bulkiest muscle in the body. It's made up of three muscles, collectively called the gluteals. The gluteals include the gluteus maximus, the gluteus medius and the gluteus minimus.

The gluteus maximus, as you probably guessed by its name, is the biggest of the butt muscles. Combined with the medius and the minimus, which is the smallest butt muscle, the maximus helps move your legs away from your body as well as rotate them and extend them behind you. The gluteals come into to play every time you sit down, take a step or lift your knee.

Here's how to make the most of your maximus.

Flexibility

Spinal Twist

A good butt and lower back stretch that Berk suggests is the spinal twist. Start by sitting on the floor with both of your legs extended in front of you. Bend your right leg over your left leg, keeping your right foot flat on the floor on the outside of your left knee. Place your left elbow on the outside of your right knee and extend your right arm behind you, with your palm flat on the floor for support.

Twist your upper body to the right by slowly looking over your right shoulder. As you twist, exhale and gently pull your right knee to the left with your left arm. Keep your abdominal muscles tight and your upper body straight. Hold, return to the starting position and repeat on the same side. Then switch sides and repeat the sequence.

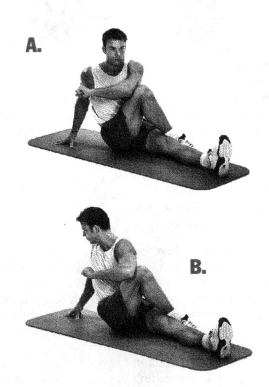

A.

B.

The Exercises

Bent-Kick Cross

Get down on the floor on your hands and knees and slightly raise one heel off the ground.

Push your leg up and back, reaching your

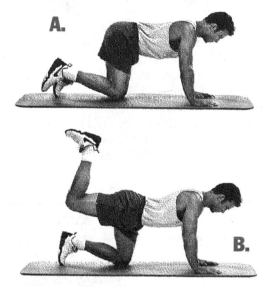

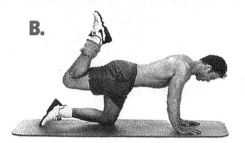

heel to the ceiling. You should feel your butt contract as you push up. Don't let your thigh go beyond parallel to the floor; your leg should stay bent at a 90-degree angle. Lower to the starting position, finish your reps and switch to the other leg.

ground. All of the movement comes from your knee. Don't move your thigh, and be careful not to sway your body or arch your back. When you are finished with your reps, switch the ankle weight to your other leg and repeat.

Raised Leg Curl

Get down on the floor on your hands and knees, wearing an ankle weight on one ankle. Raise the weighted foot to butt level and extend your leg straight out, away from your body and parallel to the floor.

Now curl your heel toward your butt, keeping your thigh level and parallel to the

Standing Kickback

Stand facing a wall, leaning against it with both hands for balance. You should be wearing an ankle weight on one leg. Lean forward slightly so that your whole body is in a straight line, with your weight shifted on the unweighted leg.

Move your weighted leg back as far as you can, until you feel the contraction in your butt. Your knee should be slightly bent, but be careful not to arch your back or overextend yourself. Hold, then lower your leg to the starting position. When you have finished your reps, place the ankle weight on the other leg and repeat.

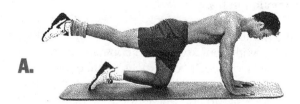

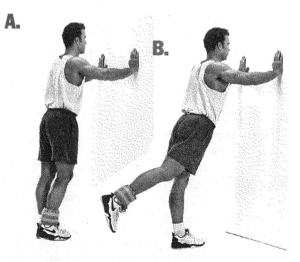

Workout: Thighs

A succulent ham. A grilled chicken leg. A juicy haunch of beef. When we want to eat a hunk of meat, nothing beats a leg.

Legs, and thighs in particular, are among the meatiest and most muscle-bound parts of most animals' bodies. Yours is no different.

Legs are power centers. You can push more pounds with your legs than with any other muscle group around. The stars of the legs are all found in the upper parts. The thighs play host to two major muscle groups: the quadriceps on the front of your thighs, and the hamstrings on the back.

The quadriceps, or "quads" for short, are a grouping of four muscles, the most prominent of which is the rectus femoris, which crosses the joints of both your hip and your knee. The rectus flexes your hip and, with the help of the other three muscles, extends your knee.

On the flip side of your quadriceps are your hamstrings. They're a group of three muscles that run along the back of your leg. Pulled hamstrings are among the most common sports injuries. For the most part, proper stretching, as we're about to show you, will help you avoid that. Moreover, working your hamstrings in the weight room is a good way to round out the shape of your legs and build explosive power.

Flexibility

Quadriceps Stretch

Stand a few inches away from a wall, with your feet about shoulder-width apart. Place your right hand against the wall for balance and bend your right knee, raising your right foot behind your body until you can grasp it with your left hand.

Your thigh should be perpendicular to the floor, and your heel should gently be pulled in

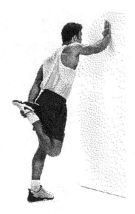

toward your butt until you feel a stretch in your right thigh. Hold. Return to the starting position and repeat with your left leg.

Hurdler's Stretch

Sit on the floor with both legs extended in front of you. Bend your right knee and draw your right leg in until the sole of your right foot is against the inside of your left thigh, somewhere around your knee. Your left knee should be unlocked and slightly flexed, and your upper body should be upright, with your back straight and your arms in front of your body.

Keeping your back straight, bend over at the hips and reach for the toes on your left foot. Gently pull your toes back slightly toward your upper body. Your legs should be kept on the ground, with your left knee unlocked, and you should feel the pull in your hamstrings. Hold the stretch, relax and return to the starting position. Then repeat with your other leg.

The Exercises

Leg Extension

Sit in a leg extension machine, with your legs behind the padded lifting bars and your hands grasping the machine's handles or the sides of the bench. Your knees should be bent at 90 degrees or slightly more, with your toes pointing in front of you.

Using the machine's handles or the sides of the bench for support, straighten your legs by lifting with your ankles and contracting your quads. Don't lock your knees at full extension; rather, keep them slightly bent. Your toes should be pointing up and out at about 45-degree angles. Lower to the starting position.

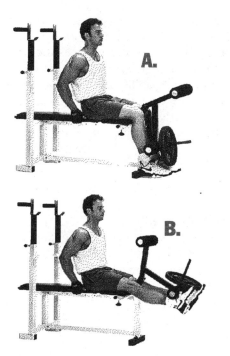

upper body should be upright but relaxed.

Push forward on the foot plates and straighten your legs until they're fully extended in front of you. Your knees should be kept slightly flexed, your upper body should remain upright, and your hands should be holding on to the machine's handlebars for support. Lower the weight to the starting position.

Leg Curl

Lie on your stomach on a leg curl machine, with your ankles hooked under the lifting pads and your knees hanging just over the bench's edge. Hold on to the machine's handle-

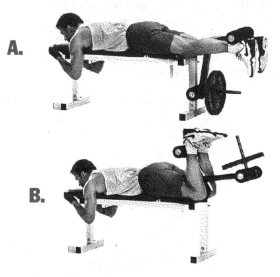

Leg Press

Sit in a leg press machine with your feet on the pedals in front of you. The seat should be adjusted so that your knees are bent at about 90-degree angles. You should be grasping the handlebars at your sides, and your

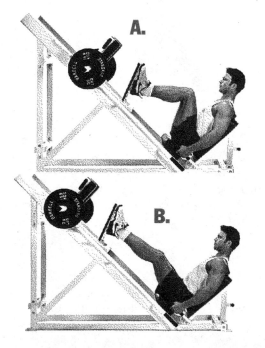

bars, if any, for support. Your legs should be fully extended, with some natural flex at the knees, and your toes should be pointing down in a natural position. Some leg curl machines are slightly bent at the end to relieve pressure on your pelvis. If your machine is not, place a small pillow under your pelvis. The hamstrings are weaker than the quads, so use less weight for leg curls than for leg extensions.

Keeping your pelvis flush against the bench, raise your heels up toward your butt so that your legs bend to about 90-degree angles. Use the machine's handlebars or the sides of the bench for support and keep your feet pointing away from your body. You should feel the contraction in your hamstrings. Lower to the starting position.

⚡ Workout: Calves and Lower Legs

Imagine that you were doing 25 push-ups every day to build your upper body. Over time, those 25 push-ups would get easy, so you'd have to do 25 more. Then 25 more and so on, until the number of push-ups you were doing would exceed the population of Iowa.

The push-ups would grow easy because your muscles would strengthen to meet the demands that you were putting on them. But eventually, you'd reach a point of diminishing returns: You'd have to do far too many push-ups for them to be very effective at building muscle. What you'd need instead would be weight-lifting exercises to increase the demand on your muscles.

This same concept applies to your lower legs. You work those muscles with every step you take and every stair you climb. Generally speaking, this keeps your legs so toned that in order to make progress muscle-wise, you need more than just more walking. You need to up the ante with weights. After all, your feet and ankles carry around the equivalent of 200 tons of weight on an average day. It's going to take a little weight-room magic to give your lower legs the challenge they need.

The muscles of the lower leg center around the gastrocnemius, or calf muscle. It's the fleshy muscle on the back of your leg, below your knee. Together the gastrocnemius and the soleus, which is near the gastrocnemius, flex your foot downward, which helps you walk, jump and sprint.

On the front part of your lower leg is the oft-neglected anterior tibial muscle. It runs along your shin area and works very much like the calf muscle, except it flexes the foot upward, which also helps you walk.

Just as flexibility of the upper legs is important to prevent hamstring pulls, flexibility of the lower legs, particularly in the gastrocs, is important to prevent injuries such as Achilles tendon tears. Here is how to stretch and exercise your lower legs.

Flexibility

Calf Stretch

Start by standing a few feet away from a wall, with your feet shoulder-width apart. Step forward with your left foot and bend your torso at a slight angle so that your hands are resting against the wall. Bend your left knee and extend your right leg behind you, keeping your knee straight and your heel flat on the floor.

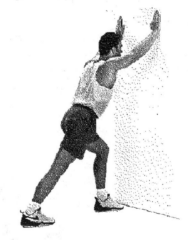

Keeping your back straight and your toes forward, push your hips in toward the wall. Keep the heel of your extended leg firmly on the ground. You should feel the stretch in the lower portion of your right leg, particularly in the calf. Hold, then repeat with your other leg.

The Exercises

Heel Raise

This is a classic exercise for the gastrocs. Start by standing with a dumbbell in each

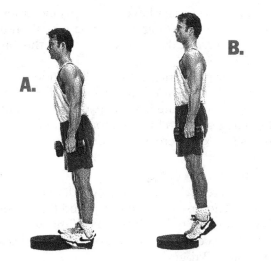

hand. Your feet should be hip-width apart, and your toes should be on a weight plate or a platform that is raised a couple of inches off the ground. Your heels should be on the floor, with your arms and the dumbbells at your sides.

Rise all the way up onto your toes. You'll feel the contraction in your calves. Pause briefly at the top. Your body will probably be a little more upright. Lower to the starting position.

Standing Jump and Reach

This works your calves and quadriceps and uses your body weight for resistance.

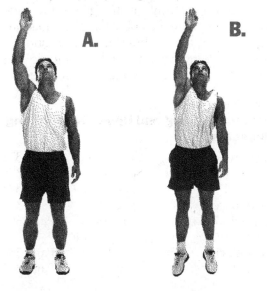

While it won't build huge muscles, it will enhance your legs' explosive power. Start easy by doing no more than 60 ground contacts. Eventually, as your legs strengthen, increase your workout to 180 ground contacts.

Start by standing upright, with your feet shoulder-width apart. Your left arm should be at your side, and your right arm should be raised above your head, pointing to the ceiling. Your knees should be slightly bent, but you should not be bending over at the waist.

Jump explosively upward, reaching for the ceiling with your right hand. Jump as high as you can, then land in the starting position and repeat, this time reaching with your left hand.

Weighted Foot Flex

This exercise builds the tibs, those muscles near your shins. Sit on a table so that your feet are dangling in the air. You should have ankle weights wrapped around your feet, near the base of your toes. Your upper body should be upright, with your arms resting at your sides and your toes pointing down toward the floor in an unflexed position.

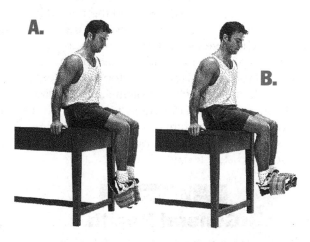

Raise your toes up toward your shins as high as possible. The rest of your body should stay in place, but your weighted toes should be lifted up and in, so you feel the contraction along your shins. Lower and return to the starting position.

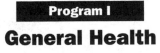 Workout Programs for Every Occasion

Going to a gym can be intimidating. We're not talking about all of the Davids and Goliaths there; forget them. We're referring to all of those exercise choices. So many weights, so many machines, so little time. Which ones to use? And when you pick, how much and how often do you lift?

Relax. Figuring out how to spend your workout time is simpler than you think. It all comes down to one thing: achieving your own fitness goals.

But what are those? Do you know?

Answer that, and we'll take care of the rest.

We talked to pros and read the research; we studied the surveys and surveyed the studies. Then we asked John Graham, a certified strength and conditioning specialist and director of the Human Performance Center at the Allentown Sports Medicine and Human Performance Center in Pennsylvania, to help us build the ideal programs for five different fitness goals. Just find the program that's right for you and start today.

Program I
General Health

No exercise program will apply to a broader audience than this one. That's because a lot of people are in that gray area of health: They're neither in fantastic shape nor completely out of shape.

Throughout this book, we've explained how fitness helps your mental and physical health. If you don't have more specific fitness goals, such as getting ready for a marathon run or a summer of daily basketball, then this program is for you.

Our program offers a well-rounded routine that has you lifting weights three times a week and getting aerobic exercise (walking, bicycling or stair climbing, for example) three times a week. Here are the details.

Weight Lifting

There are two routines you'll need to know. The first works the legs and the upper-body muscles that pull (we'll call this Program A). The second works the upper-body muscles that push (Program B).

The idea is to alternate between the two workouts. For example, in the first week, do Program A on Monday and Program B on Wednesday, then go back to Program A on Friday. The following week, reverse the order: Start with Program B on Monday, then do Program A on Wednesday and Program B again on Friday.

Here are the exercises in each program, followed by the pages where you can learn how to do them. We've also provided a key bit of information about each exercise: whether it is compound (meaning it works several muscle groups at once), specific (it works a single muscle group) or trunk (it strengthens the midbody). These categories play into the equation when it comes time to hurry up your routine or to start adding weight. You'll want to do these exercises in the order in which they're listed.

The Routines
Program A: Leg and Upper-Body Pulling Muscles

• Leg press	Compound	Page 371
• Leg extension	Specific	Page 370
• Leg curl	Specific	Page 371
• Heel raise	Specific	Page 372
• Lat pull-down	Compound	Page 367
• Seated pulley row	Compound	
• Barbell curl	Specific	Page 356
• Crunch	Trunk	Page 365

Program B: Upper-Body Pushing Muscles

- Bench press   Compound   Page 363
- Incline bench press Compound
- Alternating   Specific   Page 361
  seated dumbbell
  press
- Shoulder shrug   Compound   Page 361
- Triceps pull-down   Specific   Page 358
- Back extension   Trunk

Repetitions

The number of lifts per exercise should increase over time. Here's how many lifts to do each time you work out.

- Month 1: one set of 12 reps
- Month 2: two sets of 12 reps
- Months 3 through 6: three sets of ten reps
- Month 7: three sets of eight reps
- Month 8: one set of ten reps and three sets of six reps
- Month 9: three sets of ten reps

How Much to Lift

On your first gym visit, determine the most weight you can lift and still complete 12 repetitions. This is known as your 12-repetition maximum. You'll start your workouts at 60 percent of that amount. Use that weight for four to six workouts with compound exercises such as the leg press and bench press and for eight workouts with specific exercises such as the leg curl and barbell curl before you increase the weight. As for the trunk exercises, you can increase the number of reps you do after just three workouts.

Never increase the weight by more than 5 percent at a time. So if you start with 100 pounds, for example, you would increase to 105 pounds after the required number of workouts.

The Next Level

Once you get to month 10 and you're ready to continue, congratulations! Time to vary things. Ask a fitness expert at your gym to develop an alternate set of exercises for the muscles that you have been working. Or if you don't have an expert, consider some of the alternate exercises that this and other books provide. Then for the next three months, follow the set and rep pattern for months 7, 8 and 9. Switch exercise routines every three months, rotating the one described above and the one planned by your fitness expert or presented in a book.

This program is based somewhat on the principle of periodization. This approach regularly changes the training variables—exercises, number of sets and number of reps—to help prevent burnout and injury from overtraining.

Other Suggestions

Get checked first. If you have a history of medical problems, or if you are getting to or are past middle age and haven't exercised in years, you should see a physician before you start a program, cautions Graham. And if the doctor gives you a green light, consult a fitness professional who is certified by the American College of Sports Medicine or is a certified strength and conditioning specialist. He'll have the knowledge to teach higher-risk exercisers proper lifting and breathing techniques.

Rest properly. Graham suggests that you use a 1:2 or 1:3 work-to-rest ratio between sets. So if it take a minute to do a set, you should rest for two or three minutes before starting the next set.

Structure your workout. If you've read the chapters on the basics of fitness (page 350) and sports injuries (page 62), you know the importance of warming up and stretching before and after a workout. We'll reiterate here the proper sequence of a complete workout.

- Active warm-up: Start with five minutes of light activity—stationary cycling, walking, jogging, rowing—to get your blood flowing and warm your muscles.
- Stretching: Continue with five to ten minutes of upper- and lower-body stretches.
- Weight lifting: The above routines should take 30 to 45 minutes.
- Aerobics: If you want to combine weight

lifting and aerobic exercise into the same workout session, this is when you do your 30 minutes' worth.

- Cooldown: Five minutes of light activity gradually brings your body to close to its normal resting state.
- Stretching (again): Five minutes of the same routine helps prevent soreness and tightening.

Want to do your cardiovascular exercise on other days? No problem. Focus on weight lifting one day and your running or biking the next. Spend about 45 minutes on your workout each day instead of about 75 minutes. Still warm up, stretch and cool down each day.

Get compound benefits. If you're pressed for time, alter your workout plan to focus on the compound exercises. These are the exercises that strengthen multiple muscle groups at the same time. If you can't do the leg curl and leg extension, for example, do the leg press. It works all of the leg muscles at once, suggests Graham.

The bench press is another example of a compound exercise. This exercise, while primarily working the chest, also hits the triceps and the front of your shoulders. If you finish your compound exercises and still have a little time left, consider doing some muscle-specific exercises, such as the barbell curl, triceps pull-down and side lateral raise, suggests Graham.

Aerobics

While it's true that you get some aerobic benefit from fast-paced weight lifting, you still need to incorporate a cardiovascular program into your fitness plan to truly get your heart and lungs into shape. For general health, augment your weight-lifting regimen with a good 20- to 30-minute cardiovascular workout at least three times a week, according to the American College of Sports Medicine.

Intensity Level

With aerobic exercise, you measure intensity via your heart rate. You'll need to do some math to determine your training heart rate range. Then you'll need to become familiar with taking your pulse (we teach you how on page 191), unless you want to buy a heart rate monitor (not a bad idea).

In the chapter on the basics of fitness, we teach you how to figure out your target heart rate. But to recap, here's the formula: Subtract your age from 220. Then multiply that figure by the percentage of your maximum heart rate (in decimal form) that you want to work at. So for a 40-year-old trying to keep his heart rate at 70 to 85 percent of his maximum, his bottom level would be:

$$220 - 40 = 180 \times 0.7 = 126 \text{ beats per minute}$$

And his top level would be:

$$220 - 40 = 180 \times 0.85 = 153 \text{ beats per minute}$$

Exercise Choices

Exactly what you do is your choice. Taste in aerobic exercises varies as much as taste in ties. To help you choose, here's a list of a few activities that burn the most calories. The number given is the calories burned per hour and is based on a 154-pound man.

- Cross-country skiing, five miles per hour — 700
- Running, eight minutes per mile — 700
- Cycling (stationary bike), 15 miles per hour — 655
- Walking, five miles per hour — 555
- Swimming (crawl), 45 yards per minute — 540
- Hiking (with a 20-pound pack), four miles per hour — 450
- Aerobic dance, moderate intensity — 350

Program II

Muscle Building

For some guys, bigger always seems better. It's these guys who want an intense strength-building program like this. But first this caveat: Genetically, we're all different, and no matter how much iron pumping you do, your muscles will eventually reach their maximum development. Don't strive for some unrealistic ideal. The most important thing is reaching your maximum potential.

Why try a muscle-building routine? Done correctly, it's a really satisfying accomplishment. And since the average guy's muscle fibers can increase in size by up to 40 percent, there's plenty of opportunity to see improvement.

The price of entry is steep, however: four weight-lifting sessions, plus three cardiovascular sessions, per week. If you're serious about building your muscles, here's what to do.

Weight Lifting

The hints from the general health workout apply here as well: See your doctor, get professional assistance, progress gradually. This workout follows the same pattern of warm-up, stretching, weight lifting, cardiovascular training, cooldown and stretching that is described for the general health program. But since you are concentrating on muscle development, the cardiovascular portion has been shortened to 20 minutes.

The Routines

Surprise! You'll be doing the exact same lifts as the guys following the general health program. You'll need to learn two routines. The exercises should be done in the order shown.

Program A: Leg and Upper-Body Pulling Muscles

- Leg press   Page 371
- Leg extension   Page 370
- Leg curl   Page 371
- Heel raise   Page 372
- Lat pull-down   Page 367
- Seated pulley row
- Barbell curl   Page 356
- Crunch   Page 365

Program B: Upper-Body Pushing Muscles

- Bench press   Page 363

- Incline bench press
- Alternating seated   Page 361
  dumbbell press
- Shoulder shrug   Page 361
- Triceps pull-down   Page 358
- Back extension

The difference here is that you'll be doing four sessions a week, not three, and as you'll see in a moment, you'll follow a much different pattern of lifting.

Again, you'll rotate the two programs. One approach: Work on the leg and upper-body pulling muscles (Program A) Monday and Thursday and on the upper-body pushing muscles (Program B) Tuesday and Friday. That's the model we've used below to describe what to do.

A final note: This program initially appears complicated. That's because the directions change each and every workout day. We suggest that you take a few minutes to sit down and pencil out a month or two of program details. Then take that sheet with you on a clipboard when you work out. Keeping track of the program and your progress will make this much easier to adhere to—and enjoy.

Repetitions

You'll do three sets of each exercise in every workout, but you'll change the number of reps per set on a weekly basis. The first week, you'll do 12 reps per set; the next week, 10; the next week, 8. Then repeat.

How Much to Lift

You'll change your intensity from workout to workout by rotating through three levels of lifting: light, medium and heavy. For example, if you start with a light routine on Monday, you'll go medium on Tuesday, heavy on Thursday and back to light on Friday. The next week, you'll continue the cycle with a medium-weight routine.

After three weeks, start the rotation over, but at the next level up. For example, if you start your first three-week rotation at the light-weight level, then you'll start the next three-week rotation with a medium routine on the first day. This way, you're guaranteed a different workout every exercise day for nine weeks.

Why bother with the changes? Because you don't want to train at your all-out maximum at each and every workout. If you do, your body doesn't have time to recover, and you become prone to injury.

Finally, you'll need to know how much to lift each workout. The method: Over the first three weeks, determine the maximum number of lifts you can do at each rep level. For example, on the first day of the first week, you might determine that the most you can bench-press 12 times straight is 110 pounds. The next week, you might determine that you can bench-press no more than 120 pounds 10 times straight. The third week, you might lift a maximum of 140 pounds for 8 straight reps. Write these numbers down, because they'll be your starting points from here on.

So how do you calculate how much weight to lift each workout? Here's the formula.

Twelve-Rep Weeks

- Light: 60 to 65 percent of your 12-rep maximum
- Medium: 75 to 85 percent of your 12-rep maximum
- Heavy: 90 to 100 percent of your 12-rep maximum

Ten-Rep Weeks

- Light: 70 to 75 percent of your ten-rep maximum
- Medium: 80 to 90 percent of your ten-rep maximum
- Heavy: 95 to 105 percent of your ten-rep maximum

Eight-Rep Weeks

- Light: 80 to 85 percent of your eight-rep maximum
- Medium: 90 to 95 percent of your eight-rep maximum
- Heavy: 105 to 110 percent of your eight-rep maximum

So here's what nine weeks of workouts might look like for just one of the exercises, the bench press, along with the amount of weight to use based on the maximums mentioned above. You'll discover that the routine cycles back to its beginning spot every nine weeks.

Week 1

Monday	Light	12 reps	
Tuesday	Medium	12 reps	85 pounds
Thursday	Heavy	12 reps	
Friday	Light	12 reps	70 pounds

Week 2

Monday	Medium	10 reps	
Tuesday	Heavy	10 reps	115 pounds
Thursday	Light	10 reps	
Friday	Medium	10 reps	100 pounds

Week 3

Monday	Heavy	8 reps	
Tuesday	Light	8 reps	115 pounds
Thursday	Medium	8 reps	
Friday	Heavy	8 reps	150 pounds

Week 4

Monday	Medium	12 reps	
Tuesday	Heavy	12 reps	100 pounds
Thursday	Light	12 reps	
Friday	Medium	12 reps	85 pounds

Week 5

Monday	Heavy	10 reps	
Tuesday	Light	10 reps	85 pounds
Thursday	Medium	10 reps	
Friday	Heavy	10 reps	115 pounds

Week 6

Monday	Light	8 reps	
Tuesday	Medium	8 reps	125 pounds
Thursday	Heavy	8 reps	
Friday	Light	8 reps	115 pounds

Week 7

Monday	Heavy	12 reps	
Tuesday	Light	12 reps	70 pounds
Thursday	Medium	12 reps	
Friday	Heavy	12 reps	100 pounds

Week 8

Monday	Light	10 reps	
Tuesday	Medium	10 reps	100 pounds
Thursday	Heavy	10 reps	
Friday	Light	10 reps	85 pounds

Week 9

Monday	Medium	8 reps	
Tuesday	Heavy	8 reps	150 pounds
Thursday	Light	8 reps	
Friday	Medium	8 reps	125 pounds

Stress recovery time. Your muscles need rest after a hard workout, just as you do after a hard day's work. "The most important part of your workout schedule is penciling in time for rest," says Bonnie Berk, R.N., a certified personal fitness trainer and exercise consultant in Carlisle, Pennsylvania.

Graham suggests 48 to 96 hours of rest between high-intensity workouts of the same muscle group. The four-day-a-week schedule, where you have 72 hours between workouts of the same muscle groups, has this rest period built in.

Lift with a friend. Lifting for muscle development requires high-intensity workouts. Having a workout partner has two big benefits: You can spot for each other, which is crucial for safety; and you can motivate each other. It's harder to miss a workout or even to glide through one if a friend is there to goad you on.

Equip yourself properly. Use safety equipment in the gym, especially when you're working with heavy weights. Any time that you're doing fewer than eight reps per set of the compound exercises, the technique for developing truly brute strength, strap on a weight belt to stabilize your lower back. Or use a weight belt when you're hefting barbells or dumbbells above your head or when you're doing squats, suggests Graham.

Alter your diet. If you are going to put yourself through an intense weight-lifting regimen, you'll need to alter your diet some to accommodate the effort. There's a whole science of eating right for exercise. But we'll boil it down to some essentials.

• Increase your overall calorie consumption. As for an exact calorie count, there's no secret formula. A rule of thumb is to eat enough to keep your weight stable, suggests Wayne W. Campbell, Ph.D., an applied physiologist at Noll Physiological Research Center at Pennsylvania State University in University Park. Given that you'll be burning more calories by exercising four times a week and that it takes extra calories merely to build muscle, it's all but guaranteed that you'll be eating more.

• Increase your intake of carbohydrates. Carbs give you energy for training. Shoot for 11 to 13 grams for every five pounds of body weight, suggests Peter Lemon, Ph.D., professor of applied physiology at Kent State University in Ohio.

• Get enough protein. Protein provides the raw material that your muscles need to grow. Shoot for four grams of protein for every five pounds of body weight, says Dr. Lemon.

• Spread the extra eating throughout the day rather than eating bigger meals. Do this by eating healthy snacks such as a banana or pumpernickel bread, suggests Dr. Campbell.

Program III

Weight Loss

Why is it that shedding a few pounds seems more daunting than the 12 labors of Hercules? You say you'd rather clean the Augean stables with a toothbrush than rein in your appetite?

Well, keep the toothbrush clean, buddy, because losing weight doesn't have to be such hardship. It boils down to one thing: burning more calories than you take in. And that boils down to two things: proper diet and more exercise. Many exercise regimens can do the trick; here are some broad guidelines to follow.

Exercise

Fat-fighting exercise programs almost always emphasize aerobic conditioning.

Aerobic exercise is best because it literally burns fat for energy. Studies have shown that during the first hour of moderately paced exercise, about 50 percent of your energy comes from fat. By the third hour, assuming you're still hanging in there, up to 70 percent of your energy comes from fat. Plus doing aerobic exercise stimulates your metabolism, meaning that your body burns calories even after your workout is over, Graham says. Classic examples of aerobic exercise include running, cycling, rowing, cross-country skiing, tennis and racquetball.

But just because aerobic exercise is the A-bomb in the fight against fat doesn't mean you should retire the weight plates. One study, by Wayne Westcott, Ph.D., strength-training consultant for the YMCA and other national organizations, followed 313 people who combined a low-fat diet with a program of strength training and aerobic exercise. After eight weeks, they had lost eight pounds of fat and gained three pounds of muscle, for a net loss of five pounds. But those three pounds of muscle were lean muscle, and lean muscle burns more calories day in and day out, making future weight loss more attainable. So supplement your aerobic exercise with two or three weight-lifting sessions a week, modeled after the general health program above.

Here are some other exercise tips to help you clobber corpulence.

Get at least your bare minimum. If you are overweight, chances are you are not a gym rat. Yet when it comes to fighting fat, the simple truth is that it takes a balanced exercise and fitness program to effectively burn away the pounds. Dietary changes won't do it alone. So aim for the bare minimum of 20 to 30 minutes of cardiovascular exercise three times a week and do your best to stick to a weight-lifting program, says Graham. Once you're comfortable with that, and as your fitness level rises, move on to four times or more a week for maximum fat burning.

Get the 85 percent solution. To make the most of your fat-burning aerobic efforts, you need to work at 70 to 85 percent of your heart rate reserve, suggests Graham. Beginners should aim for the 70 percent mark, while more fit guys should aim for 85 percent. (For details on how to determine your maximum heart rate and workout range, see Program I earlier in this chapter.)

Give it three months. Three months is about the break-off point for most exercise programs, says Wayne C. Miller, Ph.D., assistant professor of kinesiology at Indiana University in Bloomington and director of the university's weight-loss clinic. If you make it past that, maintaining the program becomes easier.

Diet

Enemy number one is fat; that much seems obvious. But we're not talking about the fat on your sides or stomach. We're talking about the fat in your food. Most men between ages 20 and 70 get about 35 percent of their calories from fat, which is more than the government-recommended 30 percent.

Here are some food tips for weight fights.

Follow the fat-fighting four. Researchers at Indiana University developed four simple steps that are guaranteed to cut fat from the worst of diets. If you follow these tips faithfully, your diet should be well within the healthy range.

- Don't cook in oil or fry in grease.
- Don't add butter or oil-based products to your foods.
- Make all of the dairy products you eat and drink low-fat.
- Eat only lean red meats, fish and poultry without the skin.

Watch the protein. High-protein foods, especially meats, are often rich in calories and loaded with fat. The protein your body doesn't use as fuel it stores as fat. Nutrition experts suggest limiting protein to no more than 10 percent of your total calories. Most guys, however, are already in this range.

Crack down with carbs. Eating lots of carbohydrates stuffs your gut, so you won't crave fat as much. They also are the body's fastest-burning form of energy and aren't easily converted to fat. This means that upping your carb intake leaves you less appetite for fat and more energy for exercise.

Experts recommend that we get at least 60 percent of our calories from carbohydrates. Most of us, however, get only about 46 percent. Good sources: fruits, vegetables and whole grains.

Program IV

Endurance

There are two kinds of endurance: muscular endurance and cardiovascular endurance. Muscular endurance means that you can paint the ceiling all day without feeling like your arms are going to fall off. Cardiovascular endurance means that you can walk up six flights of stairs and not have your heart thumping and lungs huffing when you reach the top.

Both types of endurance can be bolstered with a workout regimen called circuit training. Circuit training is a blessing because it's two workouts in one: one for your muscles and one for your cardiovascular system. The concept of circuit training is simple: You go through a high number of lifts at a fast pace, so you challenge your muscles as well as your heart and lungs.

While aerobic exercise is key to all of the previous programs, it is particularly important in achieving endurance. So don't slack on this part of the program. Each week, get at least three 30-minute aerobic workouts.

And for all of your workouts, be they in the weight room or on a bicycle seat, follow the basic workout pattern. When combining weights with aerobic exercise, this is the order: active warm-up, stretching, weight lifting, aerobic exercise, cooldown, light stretching.

Weight Lifting

The key to building endurance with circuit training is to keep the pace brisk. A study at the University of Idaho in Moscow found that 15 seconds of rest between sets seems optimum, but in general, take no more than 30 seconds.

The Routine

Many of the exercises that you'll be doing are the same as in the other programs. The difference here is that you'll be doing the same exercises every time you work out, and at first, you'll be doing just one set of each exercise. ("Doing one circuit" means doing one set of each exercise on the list in rapid succession.)

Do these ten lifts in the order in which they're listed.

- Back extension
- Leg press   Page 371
- Leg extension   Page 370
- Leg curl   Page 371
- Bench press   Page 363
- Lat pull-down   Page 367
- Alternating seated   Page 361
  dumbbell press
- Barbell curl   Page 356
- Triceps pull-down   Page 358
- Crunch   Page 365

Repetitions

As mentioned above, do just one set of 8 to 12 reps of each exercise, with two exceptions. For the back extension and the crunch, do one set of 15 to 25 reps. And remember: Immediately move from one exercise to the next, with just a 15- to 30-second rest in between. If you are doing this right, your heart and lungs will be getting a workout along with your muscles.

Do this circuit three times a week; a Monday-Wednesday-Friday program works fine. How should you progress?

- For the first month, do just one circuit per workout.
- In the second and third months, go through the circuit twice per workout.
- From the fourth month on, do three repetitions of the circuit per workout.
- After seven months, ask your fitness professional to help you design an alternate circuit. Then switch between the two programs every three months.

Other Tips

Take a 48-hour break. Wait at least 48 hours between workout sessions for your muscles to recuperate, says Carlos DeJesus, a world-champion bodybuilder and fitness trainer in Richmond, Virginia. This recovery period is vital for making sure that your muscles are ready for the next workout.

Pace yourself. For each rep, take two or three seconds to complete the lift. Then take another three or four seconds to return the weight to the starting position, suggests Graham. Sure, we've all seen speed lifters blasting out reps as fast as they can, grunting furiously along the way, their forehead veins ready to burst. That's wrong. The goal is to lift smoothly, evenly and at a medium pace, with good breathing habits (that usually means exhaling on each lift and inhaling on each return).

Program V

Flexibility

Flexibility is critical and often overlooked. But it's something that you should incorporate into every fitness regimen you ever have. Here's a full-body stretching routine, the body part each addresses and then some advice on the finer points of flexibility. Follow the order in which the stretches are listed.

The Routine

* Head turn — Neck — Page 360
* Overhead shoulder stretch — Shoulders — Page 360
* Chest stretch — Shoulders and chest — Page 362
* Spinal twist — Back and butt — Page 368
* Calf stretch — Calves and Achilles tendons — Page 372
* Quadriceps stretch — Upper thighs — Page 370
* Hurdler's stretch — Lower back and hamstrings — Page 370

If greater flexibility is your fitness goal, it helps to view stretching as the workout, not as the warm-up. This means that you should start each stretching workout with a brief warm-up to get your muscles ready for action. To warm up, do five to ten minutes of light aerobic exercise, such as jogging in place or jumping rope, says Wade A. Lillegard, M.D., of the Uniformed Services University of the Health Sciences in Bethesda, Maryland. Then stretch lightly just to get the motion.

Now you're ready. Launch into your stretching exercises with vim and vigor, keeping these tips from Dr. Lillegard in mind.

Don't cross the pain threshold. Most of us reach a point where stretching hurts like the dickens. The stretching pros—dancers, physiologists, aerobics instructors—know that you should never reach that point. Instead, stretch to the point of resistance, not to the point of pain. And never stretch with a bouncing or jerking motion, or you won't be stretching your muscles—you'll be stretching your chances of injury.

Hold it right. Fitness experts recommend holding a stretch for 20 to 30 seconds or more. In fact, researchers at the University of Central Arkansas in Conway found that a 30-second stretch is ideal for improving hamstring flexibility. They divided 57 people into groups and assigned them to do stretches five days a week for six weeks. One group stretched for 15 seconds, another group for 30 seconds and the third group for 60 seconds. The people who stretched for 30 seconds acquired substantially more flexibility than those who stretched for 15 seconds. Those who stretched for 60 seconds improved no more than the 30-second bunch.

Start slowly, then build up. Stretching is a lot like weight lifting in that you won't see miraculous results overnight. If you're just starting out, begin slowly and gradually, and increase the length of your workout sessions as you progress. Perform each stretch four times per session, with short rest periods in between. Stretch daily, including weekends. It may take months before you notice any improvement, and you may never reach the point where you can quit your day job and join a carnival as Pretzel Man. But you will see improvement. Better yet, you'll feel it.

✕ Index

Note: <u>Underscored</u> page references indicate boxed text. **Boldface** references indicate primary discussion of topic. *Italicized* references indicate tables, illustrations and photos. Prescription drug names are denoted with Rx.

C

G

S

Tools, how to hold, 347, *347*
Toothaches, 319, 322
Tooth brushing, 168, 318, 320
   to eliminate bad breath, 239, 242
Tooth flossing, 168, 320–21
Tooth grinding, 208
Toothpaste, allergic reaction to, 224
Tooth whitening, 318–19
Touch, sense of, **180–81**
Transfusions, blood. *See* Blood transfusions
Treadmill test, 53
Tretinoin (Rx), for fading
   age spots, 297
   freckles, 162
   wrinkles, 293
Triceps, workout for, **358–59**, *358*, *359*
Triceps extension
   narrow-grip seated overhead, 359, *359*
   overhead, 358–59, *359*
Triceps pull-down, 358, *358*
Trigger points, pain in, 55, 60
Triglyceride test, 52
Tropical oils, fat content of, 4
Tuberculin skin test, 51
Tuberculosis, 51
Tylenol, as pain reliever, *56*
Type A personality, 192–94

U

Ulcerative colitis, 126–27, 302
Ulcers, 312
   duodenal, 303
   peptic, 311
   types of, *310*
Underarms, **335**
Underwear, tight, infertility and, <u>306</u>
Upper arm/triceps stretch, 358, *358*
Uric acid, gout and, 157, 158, 214
Urinalysis, 51, <u>51</u>, 217
Urinary system, **336–37**, *337*
Urinary tract infections. *See* Bladder infections
Urination, 336–37
   and preventing prostate trouble, 265

problems with, 102–3, 268–69
   in public rest rooms, <u>103</u>
Urine, **338**
   protein in, 216, 217

V

Vaccination, hepatitis, 227
Varicocele, 306
Varicose veins, 339
Vasectomy, 306
Vegetables
   buying fresh, <u>8</u>
   fiber in, 6
   guidelines for eating, <u>4</u>, 8–9
Veins, **339–41**
   healthy versus unhealthy, *340*
Ventricular fibrillation, 187
Vision, 146–47, **148–49**, 150–53
Vision tests, 51–52, <u>51</u>, 152
Vitamin A, for promoting health of
   immune system, 205, 327
   nasal lining, 251, 282
   reproductive system, 270
   respiratory system, 272
   salivary glands, 276
   thyroid gland, 328
Vitamin B$_6$
   for immune system strengthening, 205
   for memory improvement, 112–13
   for nervous system health, 246
   for wrist pain relief, 348
Vitamin B$_{12}$
   deficiency of, 104–5
   for hearing loss prevention, 134
   for nervous system health, 246
Vitamin C
   for promoting health of
      blood, 105
      gums, 169
      immune system, 205–6, 327
      lungs, 233, 234
      reproductive system, 270, 271
      respiratory system, 272

An Easy Guide to Writing

An Easy Guide to Writing

PAMELA D. DYKSTRA
South Suburban College

PEARSON
Prentice
Hall

UPPER SADDLE RIVER, NEW JERSEY 07458

Library of Congress Cataloging-in-Publication Data
Dykstra, Pamela D.
    An Easy Guide to Writing / Pamela D. Dykstra.— 1st ed.
        p. cm.
    ISBN 0-13-184954-9 (alk. paper)
    1. English language—Rhetoric—Handbooks, manuals, etc. 2. English language—Grammar—
    Handbooks, manuals, etc. 3. Report writing—Handbooks, manuals, etc. I. Title.
PE1408.D95 2005
808'.042—dc22   2005006489

AVP/Publisher: *Leah Jewell*
VP, Director of Production and Manufacturing:
    Barbara Kittle
Executive Acquisitions Editor: *Craig Campanella*
Managing Editor: *Ann Marie McCarthy*
Production Editor: *Fran Russello*
Full Service Project Management:
    Katie Ostler and Sue Katkus, Schawk, Inc.;
    Publishing Solutions for Retail, Book, and Catalog
Prepress and Manufacturing Manager: *Nick Sklitsis*
Prepress and Manufacturing Buyer: *Ben Smith*

Director of Marketing: *Brandy Dawson*
Marketing Manager: *Kate Stewart*
Marketing Assistant: *Kara Pottle*
Editorial Assistant: *Joan Polk*
Cover Design: *Bruce Kenselaar*
Line Art Illustrations: *Schawk, Inc;*
    Publishing Solutions for Retail, Book,
    and Catalog
Cover Photo: *Kiwi Design*
Media Editor: *Christy Schaack*

This book was set in 10/12 Janson by Schawk, Inc.; Publishing Solutions for Retail, Book, and Catalog, and was printed and bound by Courier. The cover was printed by Phoenix Color.

Credits and acknowledgments borrowed from other sources and reproduced, with permission, in this textbook appear on page 293.

Pearson Education LTD., London
Pearson Education Australia PTY, Limited, Sydney
Pearson Education Singapore, Pte. Ltd
Pearson Education North Asia Ltd, Hong Kong
Pearson Education Canada, Ltd., Toronto

Pearson Educación de México, S.A. de C.V.
Pearson Education-Japan, Tokyo
Pearson Education Malaysia, Pte. Ltd
Pearson Education, Upper Saddle River, New Jersey

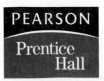

10 9 8 7 6 5 4 3 2 1
ISBN: 0-13-1849549

CONTENTS

PREFACE

Easy Guide to Writing is a basic skills handbook for students who struggle with sentence structure and the conventions of standard written English. During the five years that it has been class tested, students' responses have been consistent: For the first time, grammar makes sense. Students particularly like the examples, the clear explanations, and the nonintimidating tone. Above all, they like the bike, the image used in the book to describe how sentences work.

The bike analogy will help your students see the sentence as a carrier of meaning. The subject is one wheel, telling us *who or what*. The predicate is the other wheel, telling us *what about it*. These two parts connect to form a stable structure, which can then carry additions. Through this concrete image, students see how the whole communicates meaning, how the parts relate to the whole, and how punctuation signals these connections.

Easy Guide gives students a systematic understanding of how sentences work. Understanding, of course, is key because what students understand, they can remember and apply. This book also includes instruction on writing paragraphs and essays so that students can work on grammar, punctuation, and usage in the context of writing papers.

• •

Features

1. CLEAR, STRAIGHTFORWARD INFORMATION

Short, easy-to-understand explanations help students retain an overview of the material, remember what they have read, and find what they are looking for when using the book as a reference tool.

2. ABUNDANT EXAMPLES

Throughout the book, examples support the instruction, making the abstract concrete.

3. STUDENT MODELS

The chapters on paragraphs and essays include student models, helping students see what they are aiming for.

4. CHARTS AND *HOW TO* BOXES

Visuals highlight the instruction, making it easily accessible.

5. VARIETY OF EXERCISES

Sentence combining, sentence completion, original-sentence generation, and paragraphs for editing reinforce the instruction.

6. SELF TESTS

The first exercise in each section (the Self Test) has answers and explanations for those answers at the back of the book. Students can check their comprehension, catch their errors, and through the explanations correct any misunderstandings before moving on to subsequent exercises.

7. CHAPTERS ON PARAGRAPHS AND ESSAYS

Simple analogies help students understand and use the writing process to present their ideas in paragraphs (Chapter 18) or essays (Chapter 19). The presentation of essay writing in a separate chapter gives you the option of including essays during the course.

8. NUMEROUS WRITING PROMPTS

Over one hundred thought-provoking topics give students a variety of choices for developing ideas.

9. GLOSSARY OF GRAMMATICAL TERMS

Grammatical terms used in the book are defined in the glossary. These definitions, often with examples, reinforce the instruction. Students can turn to this resource for a quick review of grammatical terms—in both this course and future English courses.

• •

Organization

Part 1

Sentence Essentials covers the essentials of writing effective sentences, presenting students with clear explanations of what a basic sentence is, what dependent clauses are and how they function, how certain punctuation marks (i.e., period, comma, semicolon) function to set sentence boundaries, and how fragments and run-on sentences can be recognized. Beginning the course with a comprehensive overview of sentence structure maximizes the amount of time students have to improve their sentences. In addition, you and the students will have, early in the course, a common vocabulary for discussing the strengths and weaknesses of the sentences in their papers.

Part 2

Word Choice concentrates on the words that often cause problems for basic writers: verbs, subject and verb agreement, irregular verbs, easily confused words, and pronouns.

Part 3

Fine-Tuning Sentences returns to sentence-level concerns as it highlights clarity, parallel structures, and sentence variety. The chapter on sentence variety expands the overview of additions given in Part 1, thus reinforcing the varying sentence patterns essential for mature writing.

Part 4

Punctuation and Mechanics covers capitalization, as well as the punctuation marks not covered in Part 1. Particular attention is given to apostrophes and quotation marks.

Part 5

Writing Paragraphs and Essays gives students the instruction they need to write one- and two-paragraph papers and, if assigned, short essays. The section gives you the option of using whole writings as the context for the course.

Part 6

Basics for Nonnative Speakers highlights some of the English-language patterns that can be confusing for nonnative speakers.

Appendix: Answers to Self Tests

Glossary of Grammatical Terms

• •

Ancillaries

ONLINE INSTRUCTOR'S MANUAL

Written by the author, this Instructor's Manual includes three parts to use as you plan and implement your course. The first part, "Using Easy Guide," includes a chapter overview and suggestions for teaching sentence structure and whole writings, followed by guidelines for creating a writing community, planning your course, and a sample syllabus. The second part, "Answers to Chapter Exercises," contains the answers to the exercises in the book. The third part, "Additional Exercises," provides supplemental materials to use as exercises or quizzes. Visit www.prenhall.com to request access to the Instructor's Manual.

COMPANION WEBSITE www.prenhall.com/dykstra

Free to students, this Companion Website will include chapter objectives, a total of 40 self-grading quizzes (two per chapter), writing prompts, Internet writing assignments, and more!

ACKNOWLEDGMENTS

I would like to thank the students at South Suburban College, whose questions inspired this book and whose feedback informed it. I also thank my colleague Steve Springer for designing the bike graphics. At Prentice Hall, I thank Craig Campanella for enthusiastically supporting this book and Joan Polk for answering my questions so promptly—and at Schawk, Inc., thanks to Katie Ostler for skillfully managing the editing process. In addition, thanks to the following reviewers for their valuable feedback: Roy Bond, *Richland Community College*; Bill Crandall, *Fullerton College*; Jill Lahnstein, *Cape Fear Community College*; Jean Gorgie, *Santa Monica College*; Marybeth Ruscica, *St. John's University*; Richard W. Rawnsley, *College of the Desert*; Nancy Brown, *Davidson Community College*; Patricia Plaskett, *Palm Beach Community College*; Janet Cutshall, *Sussex County Community College*; C. Ann Ritter, *Baltimore City Community College*.

I am especially grateful to Martha Kolln—author, linguist, educator, and friend. Martha's suggestions guided my revisions and helped me see additional teaching strategies. For years, Martha has inspired me. Participating in her workshops, studying her textbooks, and talking with her have taught me the value of grammar. I am indebted to her.

Above all, I thank my mother, Patricia Dykstra, for her steadfast lifetime support and encouragement.

INTRODUCTION

$\bullet \bullet$

Differences between Talking and Writing

Which is easier for you: talking or writing? Once you have answered that question, ask yourself why. Why is one easier than the other? Thinking about the reasons will help you recognize some of the differences between writing and talking.

One of those differences involves the audience—the people you are talking or writing to. When you talk, the listeners are right there with you. They can see your facial expressions and body language, which communicate all kinds of information. They can also hear what you say and how you say it. Pauses tell them where your ideas begin and end. The pitch of your voice tells them whether you are making a statement or asking a question. The tone of your voice tells them how to interpret your words. For example, you could say, "It's my fault," and the tone of your voice could mean it really is your fault, or your tone could convey the opposite—"No way!"

It works the other way, too. You can also see and hear your audience. You can see from their reactions whether or not they understand and whether or not they agree. If they do understand, you often don't have to finish what you were going to say. If you sense that they don't agree or that you may have offended them, you can explain further. Above all, because the listeners are present, you're not alone. You create the conversation together.

Writing is a different situation: The readers can't see you or hear you. They get no information from facial expressions or body language—and neither do you. As you write, you have to anticipate your readers' questions and make sure you answer them. Readers also can't hear you pause, so you have to use punctuation to tell them where your ideas begin and end. If you forget the punctuation, readers will see nothing but non-stop words, and they may even quit reading. Finally, because readers are not there to help you create the conversation, you may find yourself rambling. If you ramble when you write the way you sometimes do when you talk, readers will think you are disorganized and confused.

The readers' absence, however, does give you a valuable advantage: time. You have probably had the experience of saying something you shouldn't have said—and realizing it only after the words escaped your lips. Although you can say you're sorry, you can't erase those words from the listener's mind. When writing, however, you can delete those words or throw out the paper. You have time to decide what to say and how best to say it. You have time to keep writing—and rewriting—until you get it right.

There is another difference between writing and talking: They have different structures. When writing, you put your ideas into sentences that have both a subject and a verb. But when talking, you communicate in chunks of information, saying things such as "In a minute," "Because I was busy," or "Sometime tomorrow night." People listening to you do not reply, "That's not a sentence" or "You left out the verb." People do not expect sentences when you talk.

Understanding the differences between writing and talking will help you recognize the importance of punctuation and spelling. It will also help you understand errors in writing. If you are writing fragments, you are writing the way you talk: in chunks of information. If you are writing run-on sentences, you are also writing the way you talk: stringing along ideas. For example, you might say something like, "Johnny was bored last night so that's when he decided to call us and we weren't home so he left a message and then he called Tiffany." When you have said what is on your mind, your voice goes down in pitch and you stop. If you are writing run-on sentences, you are stringing along your ideas and using a period to mark the place where your voice lowers and stops.

Talking and writing are like football and basketball. One sport is not better than the other sport; they are just different.

Ways to Improve Your Writing

In addition to taking your current English course, there are three ways to improve your writing: read, write, and increase your vocabulary.

READ

Have you ever listened to one of your favorite CDs and found yourself humming the next song before it even begins? How did you know what the next song would be? You didn't sit down and try to memorize the notes; you learned the song because you heard it over and over again. Learning language involves a similar process. We learned to talk when we were babies by listening to others talk. We picked up (internalized) how words are put together—learning, for example, to say "down the street," not "street the down." If we were read to as children, we also heard how ideas are put together in sentences. We learned the patterns of writing, the sounds of sentences.

As an adult, if you want to improve your writing, you must read. When you read, you unconsciously pick up the sound of sentences, just as if you were listening to music on a CD. When experienced writers write, they hear their ideas flow in sentence form. If you read often, you will begin to hear your ideas flow smoothly into sentences when you write. You will hear the rhythm—the sound of your sentences. The more you read, the better writer you will become.

When you are reading, also pay attention to the words that writers use and how they put those words together. Learning to write well is similar to learning how to play a sport or an instrument. The game of tennis is a good example. If people are casually watching a game on television, they will probably watch the ball and check the score. However, if they want to improve their own game, they notice where the players place their feet and how they move. They pay careful attention to how the players do what they do. The same process—that same careful attention—applies to writing.

WRITE

The second way to improve your writing is by writing. Start a journal that you write in daily. Write about your experiences that day; write about what you are thinking or feeling. The more you write, the more easily your thoughts will flow from your mind to your paper.

INCREASE YOUR VOCABULARY

Finally, your writing will improve as you increase your vocabulary. When you are reading, look up words you don't know and write down their definitions. You can also increase your vocabulary by listening. When you are in the car, listen to educational radio stations; when you are watching television, turn to the PBS channels. These programs include vocabulary that you will need to use and understand in college and the workplace. You don't have to look up the words people say; just hearing them will help you become familiar with their meanings.

• •

Welcome to This Book

Writing, like any skill, is learned by practicing. Watch musicians rehearsing or athletes training. They learn the basic movements and repeat them until the patterns are second nature. They know that playing well takes time. It involves making errors, discovering what those errors are, and going back to train until they get it right.

This book will help you write effectively. Each section includes examples so that you can see what you are aiming for. Exercises at the end of the sections give you a chance to practice what you have just learned. The first exercise in each section is called a *Self Test* because the answers are included in the back of the book. Checking your answers will let you know right away if you are on the right track.

Use this book to your advantage. Take time to review the chapters. Mark the pages that contain information you want to remember and return to these pages often. New information needs to be repeated until it becomes part of long-term memory, until the pathways in the brain are formed. The process is similar to walking through the woods. If you walk through the woods just once, your footsteps will not make a path—that is called short-term memory. You need to continue to walk that path until the pathway is formed—then it becomes part of long-term memory. Once the information is part of long-term memory, you will remember it. The neural (brain) pathways will have been formed.

The information and skills you gain will benefit you throughout life. In college, you will be writing papers, reports, and answers to short-essay questions. To enter the workplace, you will be writing letters of application. Writing, in fact, can make the difference in employment. Often the applicant who writes a letter thanking a company representative for an interview is the one who gets the job. Writing is power—not only in college and at work but also in your everyday life. Whether you're writing a note to friends or family, a complaint letter to a company, correspondence to an elected official, or a memo to a child's teacher, being able to write effectively and persuasively makes a difference. Good writing gets results.

PART 1

SENTENCE ESSENTIALS

THE BASIC SENTENCE

Section A: Subjects and Predicates

Let's begin with three **sentences**:*

> **Robert laughed.**
> **The sun will shine tomorrow.**
> **The small town's elderly doctor still makes house calls in emergencies.**

As the examples above show, length does not determine what is or is not a sentence. Regardless of how long or short a group of words is, it must have two parts—a **subject** and a **predicate**—in order to be a sentence. The subject tells us *who or what*. The predicate tells us *what about it*. These two parts connect to form the **basic sentence,** which is also known as an **independent clause.**
It's possible to have just one word in each part:

Subject	Predicate
Students	study.
Rivers	flow.
Wheels	squealed.

---

*Words in bold face are defined in the Glossary, beginning on page 289.

These two-word sentences are rare. Most of the time our ideas include more details. We expand the subject and predicate parts.

Subject	Predicate
Students in my algebra class	*study* each morning in the cafeteria.
Rivers on the west side of the mountain	*flow* toward the sea.
The train's metal *wheels*	*squealed* along the track.

We can have more than one subject (which is called a **compound subject**) and more than one predicate (a **compound predicate**).

Compound subject
Many doctors and *scientists* believe that laughter boosts the immune system.

Compound predicate
The mechanic *changed the oil* and *rotated the tires*.

Whether the subjects and predicates are long or short, they give the same kind of information. The subject gives the topic of the sentence, telling us *who or what*. The predicate answers the question, *What about it?*

Who or what (subject)	*What about it* (predicate)
Robert	laughed.
The sun	will shine tomorrow.
The small town's elderly doctor	still makes house calls in emergencies.
Apple pie and chocolate cake	are my favorite desserts.
Listening to music	calms my mind and helps me relax.

SENTENCES AND BICYCLES

We have been looking at the subject and predicate as the two parts of a sentence. Another way of describing a sentence is to compare it to a bicycle.

The subject is one wheel; the predicate is the other wheel.

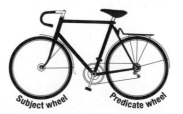

Subject wheel   Predicate wheel

These two wheels connect to form a stable structure.

The subject and predicate connect directly. When talking, we sometimes pause after the subject, but when writing, we need to make sure the subject and predicate connect without pause. Do not place a comma between them.

Example 1

> **Correct:** Jeanne and her family taught us the importance of loyalty.
> **Incorrect:** Jeanne and her family, taught us the importance of loyalty.

Example 2

> **Correct:** My determination to succeed has given me strength to face many obstacles.
> **Incorrect:** My determination to succeed, has given me strength to face many obstacles.

The most important part of the subject wheel is the **simple subject**—the essential word(s) that explain the *who or what*. The most important part of the predicate wheel is the **verb**—the essential word(s) that give the *what about it*. In the following examples, the simple subjects and verbs are in italics.

Subject wheel	Predicate wheel
Few *employees*	*spend* their entire career at any one company.
The antique *clock*	*chimes* on the hour and *keeps* perfect time.
All the *pictures* in this roll of film	*were taken* last summer in California.
Driving without sunglasses	*hurts* my eyes.
A new *theater* on Hilltop Road	*will open* on Tuesday.

IDENTIFYING SUBJECTS AND PREDICATES

Every sentence has a subject and predicate. The two parts can be long or short, and they can carry a variety of information. Yet, regardless of what kind of information these parts contain, you can find the subject and predicate by asking *Who or what?* and *What about it?*

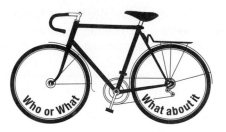

Subject	Predicate
Who or what?	*What about it?*
Cotton	keeps us warm in winter and cool in summer.
Athletes from all over the world	compete at the Olympic Games.
We	walked down the dusty road to Sandy's house.
Sleeping late on Saturday mornings	is a luxury.
Reporters with microphones and cameras	swarmed around the candidate.

There is another way to find the subject and predicate. You can see where the subject ends and the predicate begins by substituting the subject with a **pronoun.** When you do that, the *who or what* becomes *he, she, it, we,* or *they.*

Subject	Predicate
The man in the back row	looks like my uncle.
He	looks like my uncle.
The river at the north side of campus	freezes each winter.
It	freezes each winter.
Clothes labeled "Dry Clean Only"	can often be washed.
They	can often be washed.

• •

Exercises: Section A

◯ **Self Test A:** In each of the following sentences, place a slash between the subject and the predicate. To find these two parts, ask *Who or what?* and *What about it?* (You can also substitute a pronoun for the subject to help you find the dividing line.)

Example

> **Life expectancy / has increased thirty years in the past century.**

1. Tulips and daffodils are spring flowers.

2. The National Weather Service predicts above-normal temperatures over the Great Lakes.

3. Rescue workers carry global-positioning systems and radio equipment.

4. The team stopped for pizza after practice.

5. City planners encouraged development of apartments and condominiums near the train station.

6. Friends and family members packed the auditorium bleachers.

7. The youth organization emphasizes character building and community service.

8. Nearly sixty percent of the best-selling prescription drugs in America's pharmacies are based on compounds taken from nature.

9. The San Francisco French Bread Company produces approximately two million loaves of bread each week.

10. The local hospital is sponsoring a class to introduce young people to medical and hospital-related careers.

◯ **Exercise 1a:** In each of the following sentences, identify the subject (*who or what*) and the predicate (*what about it*). Then write your answers to the questions that follow.

Example

> **The glove compartment in our car is stuffed with old gas receipts and outdated coupons.**
>
> Who or what: *The glove compartment in our car*
>
> What about it: *is stuffed with old gas receipts and outdated coupons*

1. The company moved to a new facility on Jackson Boulevard.

   Who or what: _____

   What about it: _____

2. They paid the bills and balanced their checkbook.

   Who or what: _____

   What about them: _____

3. A path of moonlight glittered across the water.

   Who or what: _____

   What about it: _____

4. Many opportunities for part-time work are now available.

   Who or what: _____

   What about them: _____

5. Vegetable oil will remove wood stain or paint from your skin.

   Who or what: _____

   What about it: _____

6. Adults and teenagers from all walks of life volunteer each Saturday at the soup kitchen.

   Who or what: _____

   What about them: _____

7. The park's wide open spaces attract visitors each summer.

   Who or what: _____

   What about them: _____

8. Scientists measured the oil spill's impact on the environment.

   Who or what: _____

   What about them: _____

9. The aroma of freshly baked bread hangs in the air.

   Who or what: _____

   What about it: _____

10. More efficient train service will relieve traffic congestion.

    Who or what: _____

    What about it: _____

⬤ **Exercise 2a:** Place a slash between the subject and predicate.

Example

Our community firemen and paramedics / are dedicated volunteers.

1. The thunder rumbled slowly across the prairie.

2. Chris's sense of humor makes us laugh and helps us relax.

3. Students' grades will be processed on Tuesday and mailed on Friday.

4. The Head Start program teaches children math and reading.

5. Turning down the temperature on the water heater can decrease your electricity bill.

6. Everyone in the lab was trying to connect to the Internet.

7. Many trucking agencies use satellite technology to guide their delivery trucks.

8. Widespread flooding and mudslides displaced thousands of people from their homes.

9. Cookies with chocolate chips and macadamia nuts are delicious.

10. The company's financial records will be released tomorrow.

⬤ **Exercise 3a:** Read the following weather report, adapted from the *New York Times*, and place a slash between the subject and predicate in each sentence.

A few inches of snow and some sleet will accumulate early today in the higher elevations of North Carolina and Virginia. Rain will drench the eastern Carolinas and southern Virginia through midday. Rain and snow will end in the afternoon. Dry weather will cover the Northeast. Some sunshine will occur near the coast from New England to the northern Middle Atlantic. The interior will be mostly cloudy with a few flurries. Expansive high pressure will keep most of the West and Plains dry (C22).

• •

Section B: Expanding the Parts

We can write a sentence that has only two or three words, such as *The children yawned*, but most of the time we include more details. We add **adjectives, adverbs, and prepositional phrases.**

> The *sleepy* children yawned *continually throughout the movie.*

> • *Sleepy* is an adjective; *continually* is an adverb; *throughout the movie* is a prepositional phrase.

ADJECTIVES

An adjective is a word that describes a **noun** (a person, place, or thing). Adjectives are usually placed before nouns.

generous gift	*happy* people	*easy* exam	*homemade* muffins
foggy morning	*painful* tooth	*sincere* apology	*wise* decision
unfamiliar territory	*sweaty* shirt	*careful* driver	*comfortable* furniture

Notice the specific details that adjectives add to these sentences:

> An *honest* employee gave me *valuable* information about the *new* job.
> A *gentle* breeze drifted across the *quiet* streets.
> The *environmental* group will offer *free* tours and *inexpensive* classes.

Adjectives Ending in –*ed*

Some adjectives end in -*ed*. They are actually verb forms called **past participles,** which can be used as adjectives. (Verb forms are explained in Chapter 7.) When you use these words, remember to add the -*ed* ending.

excited fans	*confused* tourist	*distinguished* guests	*depressed* person
determined students	*bored* speaker	*embarrassed* child	*tired* employee

Adjectives in Comparisons

Adjectives change form when they are used to compare things. Most short adjectives end in *-er* to show *more* (**comparative**) and *-est* to show *most* (**superlative**).

Adjective	More	Most
sweet	sweeter	sweetest
fast	faster	fastest
tall	taller	tallest
soft	softer	softest

The adjectives *good* and *bad* change spelling rather than adding *-er* and *-est:*

Adjective	More	Most
good	better	best
bad	worse	worst

To compare two things, use the adjectives in the *more* column. To compare three or more things, use the adjectives in the *most* column.

More: My mom's chili is *hot,* but my grandmother's chili is *hotter.*

Most: My chili is the *hottest* chili anyone has ever tasted.

More: Traffic is *bad* on Monday, but *worse* on Friday.

Most: The *worst* traffic is on holiday weekends.

Longer Adjectives

For most adjectives with two or more syllables, the words *more* and *most* are used instead of the *-er* and *-est* endings:

Adjective	More	Most
peaceful	more peaceful	most peaceful
valuable	more valuable	most valuable
beautiful	more beautiful	most beautiful
comfortable	more comfortable	most comfortable

The living room chairs are *more comfortable* than the kitchen chairs.

My cousin is the *most curious* child I know.

Double Comparisons

The *-er* ending means *more;* the *-est* ending means *most.* Do not repeat the meaning by using both *-er* and *more,* or both *-est* and *most:*

The day is ~~more~~ warmer than we had expected.

Last week was the ~~most~~ happiest week of my life.

ADVERBS

We can also use adverbs to add details to a sentence. Adverbs are words that describe verbs. Most adverbs end in *-ly.*

eventually	quickly	actually	persistently	smoothly	obviously
silently	skillfully	evidently	unfortunately	nervously	quietly

Notice how the adverbs in the following sentences give additional information about the verbs:

The rain forced us to drive *slowly* and *carefully.*

Car dealerships are *currently* offering cash rebates and low financing.

Television commercials *continually* interrupt the programs.

You can turn many adjectives into adverbs by adding *-ly.*

Adjective	Adverb
slow	slowly
gentle	gently
patient	patiently
sudden	suddenly

Adjectives and adverbs perform different roles in a sentence. Adjectives describe nouns; adverbs describe verbs.

The *slow* turtle crawled along the road.

- *Slow* describes *turtle*, which is a noun. *Slow* is an adjective.

The turtle crawled *slowly* along the road.

- *Slowly* is not describing *turtle*. It is describing the verb *crawled*. We therefore add *-ly* to form the adverb *slowly*.

PREPOSITIONAL PHRASES

Most sentences include prepositional phrases. A prepositional phrase begins with a preposition (a word such as *in*, *on*, or *with*) and ends with a noun or pronoun (called the **object of the preposition**). Here are some examples of prepositional phrases:

on Monday night	with us	under the desk	in the morning
during dinner	for twenty minutes	around the corner	from the beginning

COMMON PREPOSITIONS

about	before	during	off	under
above	behind	except	on	underneath
across	below	for	outside	until
after	beneath	from	over	up
against	beside	in	past	with
along	between	inside	through	within
among	beyond	into	throughout	without
around	by	like	to	
at	down	of	toward	

Notice the detail that these phrases add to a sentence:

> **The actor sat *on an upside-down pail* and talked *to the audience*.**
> **People *throughout the city* gathered *for free summer concerts*.**
> **A group *of crows* met *on the telephone wires*.**

To find where a prepositional phrase ends, repeat the preposition and ask *What?* The answer will be the object of the preposition, which is where the phrase ends.

Example 1

> **The president *of the board* outlined the company's goals.**

- The preposition is *of*. To find where the phrase ends, repeat the preposition and ask the question: "*Of* what?" The answer to that question will identify the object of the preposition: *the board*.

Example 2

Nicole hurried *down the hall to the library*.

- Sentences sometimes have prepositional phrases next to each other. The question technique remains the same. The first preposition is *down*. Asking "*Down* what?" will give us the object of the preposition: *the hall*.

- The next preposition is *to*. Asking "*To* what?" will give us the object: *the library*.

• •

Exercises: Section B

Self Test B: Correct the sentences that have adjective or adverb errors. If a sentence is correct as is, mark it with a *C*.

1. The second test was more easier than the first, but the last test was the most easiest.

2. The children listened careful to the instructions.

3. The confuse and frighten tourist stopped at the gas station and asked for directions.

4. Yellowstone National Park is the oldest national park in the world.

5. The weather was worst on Friday than it was on Saturday.

Exercise 1b: Correct the sentences that have adjective or adverb errors. If a sentence is correct as is, mark it with a *C*.

1. John stood patient at the intersection and waited for the light to change.

2. Betty's ring is her valuablest piece of jewelry.

3. My faith has made me a more stronger person.

4. The exhaust student fell asleep in the middle of the lecture.

5. This is the heaviest suitcase I have ever lifted.

6. Our current mail carrier is more friendlier than our last one.

7. I ran as quick as I could.

8. Lester walked up to the microphone and introduced the distinguish guest.

9. I will do more better once I get some sleep.

10. We laughed as we shared stories of our best and worse teachers.

● **Exercise 2b:** Expand the following two-word sentences by adding adjectives, adverbs, and prepositional phrases. You may select words from those listed below or create your own.

Tourists walked.

<u>Curious</u> **tourists walked** <u>cautiously past the Keep Out sign to the open balcony.</u>

1. Students studied.

2. My neighbor stared.

3. The plants withered.

4. Children tiptoed.

5. Sunlight streamed.

Adjectives

warm	optimistic	easiest	intelligent	tiny	outdoor	clear
shy	sincere	curious	new	gentle	healthy	hazy

Adverbs

impatiently	suddenly	quickly	easily	slowly	silently
carefully	carelessly	patiently	gently	frantically	intently

Prepositional Phrases

outside the door	with cold hands and feet	for the final exam
in the hallway	up the creaky stairs	through the open window
at the scribbled message	behind the stadium bleachers	in the hot summer sun

● **Exercise 3b:** Studying the words and structures professional writers use will help you improve your writing. The following fill-in-the-blank exercise is one way of focusing attention on good writing. Below each quoted sentence is a similar sentence with blanks. Replace the italicised words in the models with your own words. Be creative; the words you choose can entirely change the meaning of the sentence.

Example

The house stood alone in a *city* of *rubble* and *ashes*. —Ray Bradbury, "There Will Come Soft Rains"

The house stood alone in a <u>forest</u> of <u>pine trees</u> and <u>flowers</u>.

1. Our shouts echoed in the *silent* streets. —James Joyce, "Araby"

   Our shouts echoed in the _____ streets.

2. The wind blew *mournfully*. —Bernard Malamud, "The Presence of Death"

   The wind blew _____.

3. He looked at David, standing quietly beside him, gazing not at *the jewels* but at *the people*. —Pearl S. Buck, *Come, My Beloved*

   He looked at David, standing quietly beside him, gazing not at _____ but at _____.

4. A *heavy* blanket of *red dust* settled over me. —Roger Hoffman, "The Dare"

   A _____ blanket of _____ settled over me.

5. They knew the women were haunted by the *starvation* of *the coming year*. —Bessie Head, "Looking for a Rain God"

   They knew the women were haunted by the _____ of _____.

6. A *soft* fall rain slips down through the *trees*, and the smell of *ocean* is so strong that it can almost be licked off the air. —Sebastian Junger, *The Perfect Storm*

   A _____ fall rain slips down through the _____, and the smell of _____ is so strong that it can almost be licked off the air.

7. Waves of *relief* ripple *down my spine*. —Jon Krakauer, "Straight up Ice"

   Waves of _____ ripple _____.

8. He blew the candle out *suddenly*, and we went outside. —Joseph Conrad, *Heart of Darkness*

   He blew the candle out _____, and we went outside.

9. A *faint* wind was prowling about the schoolhouse. —Albert Camus, "The Guest"

   A _____ wind was prowling about the schoolhouse.

10. We cannot fill up our emptiness with *objects*, *possessions*, or *people*. —John O'Donohue, *Anam Cara*

    We cannot fill up our emptiness with _____, _____, or _____.

CHAPTER 2

DEPENDENT CLAUSES

Section A: Subordinating Conjunctions

In the preceding chapter, we focused on the basic sentence. It is an independent clause—it can stand alone and make sense. In this chapter, we look at **clauses** that *cannot* stand alone because they begin with a word that makes them dependent.

Sentence: Ron bought a car.

- The subject is *Ron.* The predicate is *bought a car.* This is a sentence.

Not a sentence: *When* Ron bought a car.

- The minute we add *when*, we no longer have a sentence. The word *when* sets up a questionable situation. Readers wonder what happened when Ron bought a car.

- *When Ron bought a car* is a **dependent clause.** Dependent clauses cannot stand alone. They need to be connected to a basic sentence.

Dependent clause	basic sentence
When Ron bought a car,	he faced car payments for the first time.

The word *when* changes a sentence into a dependent clause. It is one of the **subordinating conjunctions.**

COMMON SUBORDINATING CONJUNCTIONS

after	because	unless
although	before	until
as	even though	when
as if	if	whenever
as soon as	since	wherever
as though	though	while

USING SUBORDINATING CONJUNCTIONS

A clause that begins with a subordinating conjunction is not a sentence; it is a dependent clause.

As soon as I type my paper   Before Maria left the house
Because I couldn't find my car keys   If it rains tomorrow

Dependent clauses are like baskets that need to be attached to a bike. We can put them on the front of a bike:

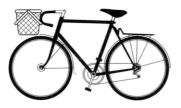

As soon as I type my paper, I am taking a break.

Because I couldn't find my car keys, I was late for class.

Before Maria left the house, she grabbed her cell phone.

If it rains tomorrow, we will reschedule the picnic.

We can also place them on the back of the bike:

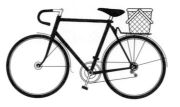

I am taking a break *as soon as I type my paper.*

I was late for class *because I couldn't find my car keys.*

Maria grabbed her cell phone *before she left the house.*

We will reschedule the picnic *if it rains tomorrow.*

- Notice that these sentences have the same dependent clauses (baskets) as the sentences in the previous group. The baskets have merely been flipped from the front to the back of the sentences.

USING COMMAS

Whenever you start a sentence with a dependent clause (basket), readers will be looking for a comma. Put the comma at the end of the basket so readers know where that idea ends and the basic sentence begins. It is easy to figure out where the dependent clause ends. Read your sentence out loud. You will hear yourself pause at the end of the clause.

If they leave before dawn, they will avoid rush hour traffic.

When he heard the question, the press secretary smiled.

As soon as we graduate, we are taking a cruise down the Mississippi.

Because technology has recently improved, solar electric systems are now more efficient.

When you place these clauses after a basic sentence, a comma is usually not used.

They will avoid rush hour traffic if they leave before dawn.

The press secretary smiled when he heard the question.

We are taking a cruise down the Mississippi as soon as we graduate.

Solar electric systems are now more efficient because technology has recently improved.

• •

Exercises: Section A

○ **Self Test A:** Read each sentence, and place a comma at the end of the dependent clause.

Before Joseph selected his classes he talked to his counselor.

Before Joseph selected his classes, he talked to his counselor.

- Notice that the comma goes after the whole idea (*before Joseph selected his classes*)—not just the word (*before*).

1. Since the beginning of the year life has gone smoothly for us.

2. Because I forgot to set my alarm I was late for class.

3. Even though the price of gas has increased commuters continue to crowd the expressways.

4. Unless we hear from you we will meet for dinner at seven.

5. Although the electricity went out for only a split second everything we had not saved on the computer was lost.

○ **Exercise 1a:** Use each of the following dependent clauses to start a sentence. Complete the thought by adding your own basic sentence. Be creative!

If the weather forecast is correct, _____.

If the weather forecast is correct, next week will be hot and humid.

1. Wherever Henrietta goes, _____.

2. Whenever I hear my favorite song, _____.

3. Although everyone else panicked, _____.

4. As soon as class is over, _____.

5. While we were on vacation, _____.

● **Exercise 2a:** In most sentences, we can move the dependent clause. The following sentences begin with a dependent clause. For each sentence, flip the dependent clause from the beginning to the end of the sentence.

Example

> **Whenever Mary calls, Mom smiles.**
> *Mom smiles whenever Mary calls.*

Example

> **Because we studied, we did well.**
> *We did well because we studied.*

1. After the deli lowered its prices, sales dramatically increased.

_____

2. If you'll cook, I'll do the dishes.

_____

3. Because we needed a quiet place to study, we went to the library.

_____

4. As soon as they gather the research, the committee members will meet.

_____

5. Unless the temperature dips below zero, the pond will not freeze.

_____

● **Exercise 3a:** Create your own sentences that begin with *when, because,* and *if.*

Sentences that begin with *when:*

1. _____

2. _____

Sentences that begin with *because:*

3. _____

4. _____

A sentence that begins with *if:*

5. _____

⬤ **Exercise 4a:** Read the following paragraph adapted from "Chicago Marathon Weather" and look for the three sentences that begin with a dependent clause. The commas marking the end of those clauses have been deleted. Replace those commas.

> Weather is a critical factor in determining a runner's success. Temperatures in the upper forties and lower fifties provide optimum conditions for marathon runners. If it's too warm a runner can overheat and develop heat exhaustion. If it is too cold hypothermia and frostbite can set in. Because marathon organizers want the most ideal running temperatures they schedule many of the large marathons in spring and fall (12).

Section B: Sentence Combining

Dependent clauses help us show how our ideas are related. They also help us change short, choppy sentences into smoothly flowing **complex sentences.** In your papers, look for sentences that sound choppy and see whether you can combine them by adding a subordinating conjunction. The process involves changing one sentence into a dependent clause and attaching that clause to the other sentence.

Example 1

Choppy: I walked across campus yesterday. I saw Jerry talking to Jan.

- Change one sentence to a dependent clause by adding a subordinating conjunction, such as *when, because, if,* or *while.*
- Let's add *when* to the first sentence: *when I walked across campus yesterday.*
- Now, we'll attach that basket to the other sentence, either before or after it.

Connected: *When I walked across campus yesterday,* I saw Jerry talking to Jan.
Connected: I saw Jerry talking to Jan *when I walked across campus yesterday.*

Example 2

Choppy: The choir was popular. Their music inspired and uplifted the audience.

- Change one sentence to a dependent clause by adding a subordinating conjunction.

- Let's add *because* to the second sentence: *because their music inspired and uplifted the audience.*

- Now, we'll attach that basket to the other sentence, either before or after it.

Connected: *Because their music inspired and uplifted the audience*, the choir was popular.

Connected: The choir was popular *because their music inspired and uplifted the audience.*

· ·

Exercises: Section B

● **Self Test B:** In each pair of sentences, change the second sentence to a dependent clause by adding the subordinating conjunction in parentheses. Then place that basket in front of the first sentence. Once you have written that sentence, write another one by flipping the basket from the front to the back of the basic sentence.

Example

Charlie groaned. I ordered a crabmeat omelet for breakfast. (when)

a. *When I ordered a crabmeat omelet for breakfast, Charlie groaned.*

b. *Charlie groaned when I ordered a crabmeat omelet for breakfast.*

1. I make mistakes. I try to do things quickly. (whenever)

    a. _____

    b. _____

2. We moved to the middle of the auditorium. We could not see the stage clearly. (because)

    a. _____

    b. _____

3. We should leave now. We want to be on time. (if)

    a. _____

    b. _____

4. I have had little time for studying and no time for partying. I started my new job. (since)

    a. _____

    b. _____

5. We made our plane reservations. We heard that the airlines were raising their prices. (as soon as)

    a. _____

    b. _____

⬤ **Exercise 1b:** As in the previous exercise, change the second sentence to a dependent clause by adding the subordinating conjunction in parentheses. Then place that basket in front of the remaining sentence. Once you have written that sentence, write another sentence by flipping the basket from the front to the back.

Example

We are going to walk daily. We need to get in shape. (because)

a. *Because we need to get in shape, we are going to walk daily.*

b. *We are going to walk daily because we need to get in shape.*

1. The electricity went out. Students were working in the computer lab. (while)

    a. _____

    b. _____

2. He shuns the spotlight. He is shy and reserved. (because)

    a. _____

    b. _____

3. They will not get a seat in the auditorium. They arrive early. (unless)

    a. _____

    b. _____

4. I researched the company on the Internet. I scheduled the interview. (before)

    a. _____

    b. _____

5. The muddy river climbed to the top of its banks. The heavy rains continued. (as)

    a. _____

    b. _____

⬤ **Exercise 2b:** Combine each pair of sentences into three different sentences by using a different subordinating conjunction for each sentence. (Check the list of subordinating conjunctions on page 22.)

Example

    The game started. Steve grabbed a hamburger.

    a. *Before the game started, Steve grabbed a hamburger.*

    b. *After the game started, Steve grabbed a hamburger.*

    c. *As soon as the game started, Steve grabbed a hamburger.*

1. We finished dinner. We took a long walk.

    a. _____

    b. _____

    c. _____

2. The road was closed for repairs. The businesses in the area lost customers.

    a. _____

    b. _____

    c. _____

3. Henry realized that he would be late. He called home.

    a. _____

    b. _____

    c. _____

4. The sun goes down. The fireworks begin.

    a. _____

    b. _____

    c. _____

5. The college hired a new food manager. The cafeteria food improved.

    a. _____

    b. _____

    c. _____

⬤ **Exercise 3b:** Read the following paragraph for an overview of its meaning. Then focus on the four sets of sentences in italics. Each set consists of two sentences; combine those two sentences into one sentence by using a subordinating conjunction.

Example

We need to cancel the game. *The rain stopped an hour ago. The field is still muddy.*

Although the rain stopped an hour ago, the field is still muddy.

Money can't buy happiness. (1) *I know that now. I didn't know it when I was younger.* I grew up in a family that did not have much money. We bought used cars, used furniture, and often secondhand clothes. (2) *Other people with money looked happy. I thought money was the road to happiness.* In high school, I was only attracted to guys who had money. They bought me gifts and took me to expensive places, but I wasn't happy. (3) *I graduated from high school and met Brian. My life began to change.* (4) *Brian did not have much money. He made me happy.* Instead of buying me gifts, he gave me his love and attention. Instead of going to expensive restaurants, we had picnics in the park. We are still dating, and our relationship continues to grow. I know now that happiness does not have a price tag.

Student writer

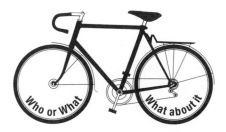

CHAPTER 3

MORE DEPENDENT CLAUSES

Section A: The Relative Pronouns *Who, Which,* and *That*

In Chapter 2, we looked at dependent clauses that begin with subordinating conjunctions, such as *if*, *when*, and *because*. In this chapter, we look at another kind of dependent clause. These clauses begin with the **relative pronouns** *who*, *which*, and *that*.

> *who have a positive attitude*
> *which she bought in 1990*
> *that are located on the beach*

These clauses are not sentences. They are baskets that need to be attached to a basic sentence. Here are three basic sentences that could carry the baskets:

People can usually laugh at themselves.
Grandma's car is a gas guzzler.
The hotels are now booked.

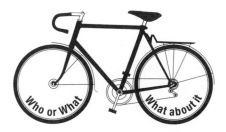

We can now attach the dependent clauses (baskets):

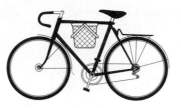

People *who have a positive attitude* **can usually laugh at themselves.**
Grandma's car, *which she bought in 1990,* **is a gas guzzler.**
The hotels *that are located on the beach* **are now booked.**

These clauses give extra information about another word, and they are placed after the word they describe. Depending on where that word is, the baskets will be in the middle or on the back of the bike. In the preceding examples, the baskets are in the middle of the bike. We can also write sentences that have baskets on the back:

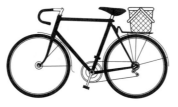

Many school-age children have parents *who work outside the home.*
I have ten dollars, *which I just found in my pocket.*
Jasmine likes movies *that have happy endings.*

PLACING CLAUSES CORRECTLY

When you use these dependent clauses, make sure you place them after the word they describe. You can see that placement in the sentences that follow. The clauses are in parentheses, and the words they describe are highlighted in bold.

People (who have a positive attitude) can usually laugh at themselves.
Grandma's **car,** (which she bought in 1990), is a gas guzzler.
The **hotels** (that are located on the beach) are now booked.
Many school-age children have **parents** (who work outside the home).
I have ten **dollars,** (which I just found in my pocket).
Jasmine likes **movies** (that have happy endings).

USING *WHO, WHICH,* AND *THAT*

The words *who, which,* and *that* are used differently:

Use *who* to describe people.
Use *which* to describe things. Do not use *which* to describe people.
Use *that* to describe things and sometimes people.

Shannon, *who lives across the street*, **will help us move.**

- The clause describes *Shannon.* Because *Shannon* is a person, we use *who.*

I had one hour, *which was enough time to proofread and print my paper.*

- The clause describes *hour.* Because *hour* is a thing, we use *which.*

The program *that we want to attend* **focuses on developing leadership skills.**

- The clause describes *program.* Because *program* is a thing, we use *that.*

Sometimes, you can omit the word *that* if the meaning of the sentence remains the same.

Example 1

Sentence with *that:* The song that I heard last night keeps playing in my mind.
Sentence without *that:* The song I heard last night keeps playing in my mind.

Example 2

Sentence with *that:* Everything that Jeremy said was true.
Sentence without *that:* Everything Jeremy said was true.

Exercises: Section A

◉ **Self Test A:** In each of the following sentences, the dependent clause is highlighted in italics. Draw an arrow to the word(s) each one describes and underline that word(s).

Example

The book is about a <u>father and son</u> *who learn to forgive each other.*

1. The kids *who were snapping their gum* distracted us during the movie.
2. The college is remodeling the computer lab, *which will open in January.*
3. Participants *who arrive early* will receive free lunch tickets.
4. The companies *that upgraded their technology* increased their sales.
5. The U.S. Supreme Court, *which consists of nine men and women,* debates valuable issues and interprets the law.

◉ **Exercise 1a:** In each sentence, put parentheses around the dependent clause, underline the basic sentence, and then write the basic sentence. The dependent clauses are in italics for the first five sentences to help you get started.

Example

<u>The college cafeteria</u>, *(which is under new management)*, <u>has an excellent salad buffet</u>.
What is the basic sentence? *The college cafeteria has an excellent salad buffet.*

1. Senior citizens *who qualify for medical assistance* should fill out an application form.

   What is the basic sentence? _____

2. The back door, *which we entered cautiously,* had been pried open.

   What is the basic sentence? _____

3. The team *that won three state titles in the past four years* is going to state.

   What is the basic sentence? _____

4. The Federal Reserve, *which wants to stimulate the economy,* has lowered interest rates.

   What is the basic sentence? _____

5. The mayor wants a neighborhood park *that includes a zoo, a museum, and a golf course.*

   What is the basic sentence? _____

6. Solar storms, which occur every eleven years, affect earth's power supplies and satellite communication.

   What is the basic sentence? _____

7. Andrew, who lives one hour from work, spends five hundred hours a year commuting.

   What is the basic sentence? _____

8. All the refrigerators that are on sale are discontinued models.

   What is the basic sentence? _____

9. The director, who had a degree in childhood education, explained the program's goals.

   What is the basic sentence? _____

10. We studied for the midterm exam, which was easier than we had expected.

    What is the basic sentence? _____

● **Exercise 2a:** Read each sentence, paying attention to the dependent clause in italics. Then fill in the blanks with your own dependent clause. Be creative.

Example

The message on the postcard, *which had been smeared by rain*, was impossible to read.
The message on the postcard, <u>*which a two-year-old child had scribbled,*</u> **was impossible to read.**

1. The apple crisp *that I baked last night* is soggy.

   The apple crisp *that* _____ is soggy.

2. The stranger *who gave us directions* saved us a lot of time.

   The stranger *who* _____ saved us a lot of time.

3. We crossed the river, *which was dwindling down to a wobbly stream.*

   We crossed the river, *which* _____ .

4. The elderly gentleman, *who was leaning on his cane*, pointed the way to the old schoolhouse.

   The elderly gentleman, *who* _____ , pointed the way to the old schoolhouse.

5. The shoes *that I want to buy* cost too much money.

The shoes *that* _____ cost too much money.

⬤ **Exercise 3a:** Fill in the blanks with your own dependent clauses. Be creative.

Employees usually respect employers *who are fair and consistent.*

1. The person who _____ will find happiness.

2. I admire people who _____ .

3. Alicia, who _____ , is allergic to dairy products.

4. Vernon, who _____ , gave me directions to the airport.

5. My car, which _____ , is for sale.

6. The new office, which _____ , overlooks the lake.

7. The college parking lot, which _____ , is being expanded.

8. The tour director showed us scenery that _____ .

9. The movie that _____ was exciting.

10. The night course that _____ will not be offered until spring.

. . . .

Section B: Sentence Combining

One quality of effective writing is saying as much as possible in as few words as possible. Readers often become bored if our sentences are choppy and we take too long to get to our point. Using the dependent words *who, which,* and *that* helps us omit unnecessary words and pack our sentences with information. Therefore, when you are working on your papers, follow these steps:

1. Look for places where two sentences could be combined by using the words *who, which,* or *that.*

2. Change one of these sentences to a dependent clause (basket). This involves adding *who, which,* or *that* and omitting other unnecessary words.

3. Attach this basket to the other sentence, placing it after the word it describes.

COMBINING SENTENCES WITH *THAT*

Let's begin with clauses beginning with the word *that*. We use *that* to describe things and sometimes people. These clauses connect directly to the basic sentence. Do not add commas.

> The bookshelves *that we ordered last month* have still not arrived.
> We are avoiding roads *that are under construction*.
> The scent of apples *that had been crushed for cider* filled the air.

Example 1

Choppy: The cell phone does not work. It's the one Curtis gave me.

- Change the second sentence to a dependent clause (basket): *that Curtis gave me*.

- Place this dependent clause after the word it describes.

Concise: The cell phone *that Curtis gave me* does not work.

Example 2

Choppy: We want to know more about the study-abroad programs. Our college is offering them.

- Change the second sentence to a dependent clause: *that our college is offering*.

- Place this clause after the word it describes.

Concise: We want to know more about the study-abroad programs *that our college is offering*.

COMBINING SENTENCES WITH *WHICH*

Use the word *which* to describe things—not people. These clauses usually need commas around them. When you read your sentence out loud, you will usually hear yourself pause when you get to the idea beginning with *which*. Adding commas around this idea will tell readers to pause also.

> The drugstore on the corner, *which still sells ice cream sodas*, has been in business for seventy-five years.
> An upbeat musical, *which has a talented new cast*, opens today at Storefront Theater.
> Video cameras, *which were mounted in each corner*, recorded activity in the bank.

Example 1

Choppy: The medical report includes the blood tests. The report came in the mail yesterday.

- Change the second sentence to a dependent clause (basket): *which came in the mail yesterday.*
- Place this dependent clause after the word it describes.

Concise: The medical report, *which came in the mail yesterday*, includes the blood tests.

Example 2

Choppy: I finally found an empty seat in the auditorium. It was crowded with high school students.

- Change the second sentence to a dependent clause: *which was crowded with high school students.*
- Place this clause after the word it describes.

Concise: I finally found an empty seat in the auditorium, *which was crowded with high school students.*

COMBINING SENTENCES WITH *WHO*

Use *who* to describe people.

Sam Johnson, *who was just here,* **left his credit card on the counter.**
Musicians *who practice daily* **have skills and confidence.**
The award was given to Elizabeth, *who deserves it.*

Sometimes these clauses are marked with commas; sometimes they are not. It all depends on whether the *who* idea is necessary information or extra information that could be left out.

Necessary information: This information is necessary because it identifies the person we are writing about. We do not use commas because we want this information to connect directly to the person.

All employees *who work overtime* **will get a raise.**

- This *who* information is necessary because it identifies who gets a raise. If we take this information out, we have *All employees will get a raise.* But that is not what the sentence said. The only employees who are getting a raise are those who work overtime. We need the *who* information to connect directly to *employees.* Therefore, we do not use commas.

Extra information: This is information that could be left out. If readers omitted it, the sentence would have the same basic meaning. We put commas around this *who* information so that readers know it is extra.

Janice and Chuck, *who live in the neighborhood,* will organize the block party.

- The *who* information is extra. If we took it out, the basic meaning of the sentence would remain the same: *Janice and Chuck will organize the block party.* We use commas so that readers can see where the extra *who* information begins and ends.

HOW TO DECIDE: COMMA OR NO COMMA

Look at the *who* information. Is it extra information?

If the information is necessary, do not use commas.

If the information is extra, use commas to separate it from the sentence.

No commas: All the people who work in the bookstore are my friends.

Who work in the bookstore identifies what people are friends. If we delete this information, the sentence will read *All the people are my friends.* That is not what the writer meant; all the people are not friends. We do not use commas because the *who* information is necessary and must be directly connected to *people.*

Commas: Kelly Samson, who works in the bookstore, is my friend.

The person is identified by her name, so we do not need *who works in the bookstore* to identify her. If we delete this information, the meaning of the sentence is the same: *Kelly Samson is my friend.* The commas are like handles that allow the reader to lift out the extra *who* information.

• •

Exercises: Section B

◉ **Self Test B:** In each pair of sentences, change the second sentence to a dependent clause (basket) beginning with *that*. Then place this clause after the word it describes in the first sentence. (Remember: Clauses beginning with the word *that* are not marked with commas.)

Example

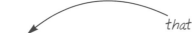

The walls need to be painted. ~~These walls~~ have smoke damage.

The walls that have smoke damage need to be painted.

- The word *that* has been added, and the unnecessary words *these walls* have been deleted.

- Notice that the clause goes after *walls*, not *painted.* Make sure you place the clause after the word it describes.

1. The two disks need to be formatted. I bought them yesterday.

   _____

2. The clothes need to be washed and ironed. They are stuffed in the suitcase.

   _____

3. All of the books were on sale. Frederick bought them.

   _____

4. The workshop is free to the public. The workshop explains the new Medicare rules.

   _____

5. I can't read the notes. I wrote them in class yesterday.

   _____

◉ **Exercise 1b:** In each pair of sentences, change the second sentence to a dependent clause (basket) beginning with *which*. Then place this clause after the word it describes in the first sentence.

Example

which

The beach glistened in the sun. ~~The beach~~ was covered with seashells.

The beach, which was covered with seashells, glistened in the sun.

- Notice that the clause goes after *beach*, not *sun*. The beach is covered in seashells, not the sun. Make sure you place the clause after the word it describes.

- Notice that commas are placed on both sides of the clause. Commas let readers know where the clause begins and ends.

1. Hurricanes are approaching Florida's coastline. Hurricanes form over warm ocean water.

   _____

2. My old car is causing me nothing but trouble. It has been in the family for fifteen years.

   _____

3. The local bank continues to support small businesses. It was established in 1921.

   _____

4. Haze clouded the skies. Haze consists of tiny particles of smoke and pollution.

   _____

5. I'll meet you at the basketball game. It begins at noon in Center Park.

   _____

Exercise 2b: Change the second sentence to a dependent clause (basket) beginning with *who* and place it after the word it describes in the preceding sentence. The dependent clauses in this exercise are extra information. Therefore, place commas on both sides of each clause.

Example

                                    who
Ned covered his ears. ~~He~~ was distracted by the siren.

Ned, who was distracted by the siren, covered his ears.

1. Our upstairs neighbors have become close friends. The neighbors were once strangers.

   _____

2. Jackie and Marcus Anderson are moving to New York City. They have lived all over the world.

   _____

3. My parents are taking night classes at the community college. They want to start a new business.

_____

4. Shantae faces each day with a positive attitude. She takes responsibility for her actions.

_____

5. The president will present the budget at the annual meeting. He has spent months analyzing the company's financial problems.

_____

● **Exercise 3b:** Read the following paragraph for an overview of its meaning. Then focus on the two sets of sentences in italics. In each set, combine the two sentences into one by changing the second sentence to a clause beginning with the word *who*, *which*, or *that*. Then attach the clause to the end of the preceding sentence.

When I was a child, I didn't pay attention to my parents' rules. *I thought parents were just nervous adults. They had rules for everything.* My mom had warned me countless times, "Never go outside without your shoes," but I did anyway. One day, I began walking to the store without my shoes. On the way, not paying much attention to where I was walking, I stepped on a piece of glass. As blood gushed out of my foot, I panicked. I was afraid my mother would scream at me, yet I was also afraid of bleeding to death. I didn't know which was worse, but I decided I'd rather face my mother than die. As I ran into the house screaming for my mom, she walked into the room asking, "What's wrong?" Before I could answer, she saw blood all over the floor and knew what had happened. "No shoes," she huffed, and off we drove to the doctor. Two shots and fifteen stitches later, we returned home. *My mother said nothing but looked at me with a smile. Her smile said she understood.* I smiled back. I had learned my lesson well: Never go outside without shoes, and Mom knows best.

Student writer

SENTENCE FRAGMENTS

A sentence can stand alone and make sense by itself. A **fragment,** however, is just part of a sentence. It may lack a subject (*who or what*) or a predicate (*what about it*), or it may not make sense by itself. In this chapter, we focus on the most common fragments. Understanding what fragments are and knowing how to fix them will improve your writing.

People often write fragments as they move to a more mature style of writing. If you are writing fragments, this could be a sign that you are entering a new stage of writing where you will improve your sentence style by creating sentences in a wider variety of patterns.

● ●

Missing-Subject Fragments

Every sentence must include a subject. We can correct a missing-subject fragment by adding the necessary words or by attaching it to the preceding sentence.

Example 1

Fragment: They spent twenty dollars on lunch. Then turned around and spent forty-four dollars on dinner.

● The second "sentence" is a fragment. We can correct it by adding a subject.

Sentence: They spent twenty dollars on lunch. Then *they* turned around and spent forty-four dollars on dinner.

Example 2

Fragment: Leslie listens to my problems. And understands my point of view.

- The second "sentence" is missing a subject. We can correct it by attaching it to the preceding sentence.

Sentence: Leslie listens to my problems and understands my point of view.

• •

Missing-Verb Fragments

One of the most common fragments involves verbs that end in *-ing*. A verb that ends in *-ing* is not a complete verb. It needs a **helping verb** such as *is*, *are*, *was*, or *were* to complete it. (See Chapter 7 for more information about verbs.)

Example 1

Fragment: Dave working weekends to get the job done.

- This is not a sentence because an *-ing* verb needs a helping verb to complete it.

Sentence: Dave *is* working weekends to get the job done.

- There are other helping verb options, such as *was* working, *should be* working, *will be* working, and *could be* working.

Example 2

Fragment: I knew it was time to get off the treadmill. My heart pumping really fast.

- The second group of words is not a sentence because *pumping* is not a complete verb.

Sentence: I knew it was time to get off the treadmill. My heart *was* pumping really fast.

• •

Dependent Clause Fragments

In Chapters 2 and 3, we looked at dependent clauses that begin with subordinating conjunctions and the relative pronouns *who, which*, and *that*. These words introduce dependent clauses, which cannot stand alone.

COMMON SUBORDINATING CONJUNCTIONS		
after	because	unless
although	before	until
as	even though	when
as if	if	whenever
as soon as	since	wherever
as though	though	while

COMMON RELATIVE PRONOUNS		
who	which	that

Dependent clauses give only part of a thought. They need to be attached to a sentence that completes the thought. When we write dependent clauses, the sentence is usually nearby.

Example 1

> **Fragment:** If Norma and Rick work hard. They will finish the project by midnight.
>
> • *If Norma and Rick work hard* is a fragment. It needs to be connected to a sentence to complete the thought.
>
> **Sentence:** If Norma and Rick work hard, they will finish the project by midnight.

Example 2

Fragment: We must pay our bills. Which have been piling up for a month.

- *Which have been piling up for a month* is not a sentence. It belongs next to the word it describes in the preceding sentence.

Sentence: We must pay our bills, which have been piling up for a month.

. . . .

Added-Description Fragments

Added-description fragments lack a subject and verb. We can correct these fragments by placing them after the word they describe or by adding the necessary words.

Example 1

Fragment: Lydia introduced me to her boyfriend. A gentle man with a shy smile.

- *A gentle man with a shy smile* is a fragment. Because these words describe *boyfriend*, we can attach them to the end of the preceding sentence.

Sentence: Lydia introduced me to her boyfriend, a gentle man with a shy smile.

Example 2

Fragment: Ramon is different from my other friends. Easy-going and open-minded.

- *Easy-going and open-minded* is a fragment. We cannot place the words after *friends* because they describe *Ramon*, not *friends*. We can correct the fragment by adding a subject (*he*) and a verb (*is*).

Sentence: Ramon is different from my other friends. *He is* easy-going and open-minded.

Added-Detail Fragments

Some fragments consist of details that have been disconnected from the preceding sentence. These fragments often begin with *especially*, *except*, *such as*, and *like*. We can correct these fragments by attaching them to the sentence they explain.

Example 1

> **Fragment:** Mary Beth likes to sleep late on Saturdays. Especially in the winter.
>
> - *Especially in the winter* is a fragment that has been disconnected from the preceding sentence. We need to attach it.
>
> **Sentence:** Mary Beth likes to sleep late on Saturdays, especially in the winter.

Example 2

> **Fragment:** Jack enjoys all of his courses. Except chemistry.
>
> - *Except chemistry* has been disconnected from the preceding sentence. We need to attach it.
>
> **Sentence:** Jack enjoys all of his courses, except chemistry.

Example 3

> **Fragment:** Javier will bring the snacks. Such as popcorn, pretzels, and peanuts.
>
> **Sentence:** Javier will bring the snacks, such as popcorn, pretzels, and peanuts.

Example 4

> **Fragment:** The restaurant is known for its unusual sandwiches. Like buffalo burgers with barbeque chips.
>
> **Sentence:** The restaurant is known for its unusual sandwiches, like buffalo burgers with barbeque chips.

• •

-ing Fragments

Ideas that begin with *-ing* words are a common cause of fragments. We can correct them by attaching them to the preceding sentence or by adding the necessary words.

Example 1

Fragment: William sprinted down the street. Hoping to catch the train.

- *Hoping to catch the train* is a fragment. We can attach an *-ing* fragment to the end of a sentence if it describes the subject of that sentence. In the example above, the *-ing* idea describes William, so we can attach it to that sentence.

Sentence: William sprinted down the street, hoping to catch the train.

Example 2

Fragment: Rachael stood patiently at the intersection. Waiting for the light to change.

- *Waiting for the light to change* is a fragment. We can correct it by adding a subject and a helping verb.

Sentence: Rachael stood patiently at the intersection. She was waiting for the light to change.

• •

To Fragments

Ideas that begin with the word *to* are often mistaken as sentences. These fragments need to be connected to the sentence that comes before or after them.

Example 1

Fragment: George's family will be here on Friday. To celebrate his birthday.

- *To celebrate his birthday* is a fragment. We can connect it to the preceding sentence.

Sentence: George's family will be here on Friday to celebrate his birthday.

Example 2

Fragment: To graduate in May. Linda is taking five courses.

- *To graduate in May* is not a sentence. We can connect it to the sentence that follows.

Sentence: To graduate in May, Linda is taking five courses.

. . . .

Finding Fragments

As you check your writing, be on the lookout for the specific fragments we have just studied. In addition, use the following general guidelines for finding fragments.

HOW TO FIND FRAGMENTS

◉ Test 1

Does the group of words tell *who or what* and explain *what about it?* If so, chances are you have a sentence.

◉ Test 2

Does the group of words answer one of these questions: *Who is doing what?* or *What is happening?* If so, chances are you have a sentence.

◉ Test 3

Does the group of words make sense when you insert it after the words *I am convinced that . . .* ? If so, you have a sentence.

Here is how to use this fill-in-the-blank test. Insert the words you have written in this blank: *I am convinced that* _____. If your words make sense in this new sentence, your words themselves are a sentence.

Example 1

Sentence or fragment? A good friend with a positive attitude.

Test: I am convinced that <u>a good friend with a positive attitude</u>.

Answer: This does not make sense. Therefore, *A good friend with a positive attitude* is not a sentence.

Example 2

Sentence or fragment? Today will be a good day.

Test: I am convinced that <u>today will be a good day</u>.
Answer: This makes sense. Therefore, *Today will be a good day* is a sentence.

• •

Exercises

● **Self Test:** Read each item and decide whether it is a sentence or a fragment. If you think it's a sentence, mark it with a *C*. If you think it's a fragment, mark it with a ✓.

1. If the weather changes.

2. Students studying in the cafeteria.

3. People who love to fish.

4. I understand.

5. To find out which phone companies were offering the best promotions.

6. Because we didn't watch the news.

7. Looking beyond the present moment.

8. Choosing a career is often difficult.

9. Which is the best decision we could have made.

10. The hubcap that fell off my car.

● **Exercise 1:** Some of the following items are correct sentences; others are fragments. If the item is correct, place *C* next to it. If it is a fragment, add your own words to make it a complete sentence.

Example

Thinking about my long-term goals.
Thinking about my long-term goals keeps me focused on today.
or
I am thinking about my long-term goals.

1. Always smiling and cracking jokes.

   _____

2. Which was easy.

   _____

3. Because he is a good listener and has been a friend for years.

   _____

4. The storm arrived.

   _____

5. Parents need to help their children handle peer pressure.

   _____

6. Saturday nights with friends and Sunday mornings with family members.

   _____

7. Someone that I have learned to trust and respect.

   _____

8. Such as washing the car or changing the oil.

   _____

9. The most influential person in my childhood.

   _____

10. Learning to stand up for what is right.

    _____

● **Exercise 2:** Read each item to see whether it contains a fragment. If the item is correct, place *C* next to it. If it contains a fragment, change the fragment to a sentence by attaching it to a nearby sentence or by adding the necessary words.

Example

> **The campers had difficulty living without modern conveniences. Such as heat and electric lights.**
>
> *The campers had difficulty living without modern conveniences, such as heat and electric lights.*

1. I have two dollars. Which is enough to buy a cup of coffee.

   _____

2. We stood at the water's edge. Watching the waves come ashore.

   _____

3. Ralph wants pizza with pepperoni. Not anchovies.

   _____

4. The movie lifted our spirits and helped us relax. We could finally laugh.

_____

5. All our cousins are coming for Thanksgiving. Even those who live out of state.

_____

6. If no dishes are in the sink and no wet laundry is in the washing machine. Jeff thinks the house is clean.

_____

7. Most car accidents are due to irresponsible behavior. Like speeding, drinking, and reckless driving.

_____

8. Everyone in my family loves Aunt Betty's desserts. Especially me.

_____

9. To celebrate the new year. We waited for the morning sun to creep over the horizon.

_____

10. He leaned against the car door. Chatting with his friends and smiling at us.

_____

● **Exercise 3:** Each set of sentences contains at least one dependent clause fragment. Correct each fragment by attaching it to the sentence that comes before it or after it, whichever makes more sense.

Example

The shy second grader was given a perfect attendance award. As soon as the audience applauded. She blushed.

The shy second grader was given a perfect attendance award. As soon as the audience applauded, she blushed.

1. I knew I should have worn a raincoat. As soon as I left the house. The thunderstorm began.

_____

_____

2. When my parents told me to choose my friends wisely. I wish I had listened. Because I was only sixteen. I thought I knew more than they did.

_____

_____

3. Stanley talked to every car dealer in town. He finally decided to buy a car from Shaver's Cars Unlimited. Because the company has a reputation for giving good service.

_____

_____

4. Although the restaurant's menu changes daily. Local people know they can count on homemade breads and muffins. Because people are used to home cooking. Fast-food restaurants are not popular here.

_____

_____

5. California has been plagued for months with above-normal temperatures. Unless the heat wave ends soon. State officials expect forest fires.

_____

_____

● **Exercise 4:** Find and correct the fragments.

When I was a child. I was terribly shy. First grade was painful. Because so many kids made fun of me. They harassed me and called me names. Such as fat boy and sissy girl. I was an easy target for them. I was defenseless. A kid with no friends. My goal was to retreat into a world by myself. I did everything I could to avoid school. Like telling my mother I was sick. On weekends, I spent my free time in my backyard. Playing alone with sticks and ants. As I look back on those years now. I wish that I had stood up for myself. I also realize that I have grown through that childhood loneliness into a self-confident adult.

Student writer

● **Exercise 5:** Take a paper you are currently writing and read it carefully, looking for fragments. Use the tests provided in *How to Find Fragments* on page 53.

CHAPTER 5

PUNCTUATING SENTENCES

Punctuation is a system of signs, similar to the road signs and traffic lights we use to navigate the road. The author Pico Iyer says it well: "Punctuation marks are the road signs placed along the highways of our communication—to control speeds, provide directions, and prevent head-on collisions (80)." In this chapter, we review the road signs that signal the end of a sentence and concentrate on a common writing problem: **run-on sentences.**

• •

Periods and Semicolons

Although periods and semicolons are both used to signal the end of a complete thought, they each have a unique purpose.

PERIODS

A period (.) marks the end of a sentence. It is like a red light, a full stop, telling readers that one idea is over. A period is a sign to take a breath before moving on. If you forget to add a period, you will have a run-on sentence.

> **Run-on:** Edward understands and accepts my shortcomings he has been a
> loyal friend for years.
>
> **Correct:** Edward understands and accepts my shortcomings. He has been a
> loyal friend for years.

SEMICOLONS

A semicolon (;) is like a flashing red light, telling readers to come to a quick stop. A semicolon is a combination of a period and a comma, so it is a little of both. It is weaker than a period and stronger than a comma. You can use a semicolon to separate two sentences if those sentences are closely related. When using a semicolon, do not capitalize the second sentence. (Keep in mind that you don't have to use a semicolon. A period works just as well.)

Example 1

> **My sister works Friday nights; my brother works Saturday nights.**
> **My sister works Friday nights. My brother works Saturday nights.**

Example 2

> **Fran's interview went well; she thinks she will get the job.**
> **Fran's interview went well. She thinks she will get the job.**

A semicolon is also used between two sentences linked with a transitional expression such as *furthermore, in fact, in other words, however, instead, likewise, nevertheless, then, therefore,* or *thus.* Again, you don't have to use a semicolon. A period works just as well.

Example 1

> **I recognized everyone there; however, I forgot most people's names.**
> **I recognized everyone there. However, I forgot most people's names.**

Example 2

> **We studied for four hours straight; then, we took a break.**
> **We studied for four hours straight. Then, we took a break.**

Run-on Sentences

When we talk, we string together our ideas, often connecting them with *and* or *so.* As soon as we have completed what is on our mind, our voice goes down in pitch and we stop. If you are writing run-on sentences, you are probably writing the way you talk. You are stringing along your ideas and when you are done, marking that spot with a period.

When we talk, we do not say, "I need a break from studying period what are you doing this weekend question mark." We don't say the punctuation marks because our voice tells readers where one thought ends and the next begins. When we write, however, readers cannot hear us. If we don't mark the end of a sentence, that sentence will run into the next one.

Sentence: A sentence consists of two parts: a subject (*who or what*) and a predicate (*what about it*). When that information has been given, we mark the end of that thought with a period.

Sentence: *Who or what / what about it.*

Run-on: A *run-on* sentence is two sentences that run into each other.

Run-on: *Who or what / what about it / who or what / what about it.*

If we forget to use any punctuation at all to mark the end of a sentence, we will be writing one kind of run-on: a **fused sentence.** If we use a comma rather than a period, we will be writing another kind of run-on: a **comma splice.** Both kinds of run-ons are problems for readers who will keep reading and become confused.

Example 1

Run-on: My job is now enjoyable the new manager is relaxed and supportive.

Run-on: My job is now enjoyable, the new manager is relaxed and supportive.

Correct: My job is now enjoyable. The new manager is relaxed and supportive.

Correct: My job is now enjoyable; the new manager is relaxed and supportive.

Example 2

Run-on: Dr. Richards postponed our midterm exam everyone in the class was relieved.

Run-on: Dr. Richards postponed our midterm exam, everyone in the class was relieved.

Correct: Dr. Richards postponed our midterm exam. Everyone in the class was relieved.

Correct: Dr. Richards postponed our midterm exam; everyone in the class was relieved.

CORRECTING RUN-ON SENTENCES

The most common way of correcting a run-on sentence is to use a period and a capital letter.

Example 1

Run-on: Sandra prepared for the concert she practiced daily and put her social life on hold.

Correct: Sandra prepared for the concert. She practiced daily and put her social life on hold.

Example 2

Run-on: The waiting room in the doctor's office is noisy, it is filled with children who don't want to be there.

Correct: The waiting room in the doctor's office is noisy. It is filled with children who don't want to be there.

FINDING RUN-ON SENTENCES

A few simple tasks can help you find run-on sentences.

HOW TO FIND RUN-ONS

1. **Read out loud.**
   One of the easiest ways to find run-on sentences is to read your writing out loud. Notice where your voice goes down in pitch and where you stop. These two signs usually indicate the end of a sentence. Then check to see whether the words you just read are a complete thought with two parts: a *who or what* (subject) and a *what about it* (predicate). If so, you have a sentence, and you need to punctuate it as a sentence. Make sure you read out loud; reading silently does not work.

2. **Check pronouns.**
   Watch for the pronouns *he, she, it, they, I,* and *we*.

3. **Look for unnecessary *and*s and *so*s.**
   Check to see whether you are stringing sentences together with unnecessary *and*s and *so*s.

Check Pronouns

If you are writing run-on sentences, be on the lookout for the pronouns *he, she, it, they, I,* and *we.* These pronouns are often subjects that begin a new sentence.

Example 1

Run-on: I applied for the job last month I will begin working in a few weeks.

Asking *who or what* and *what about it* shows we have two sentences:

Who or what: *I*
What about it: *applied for the job last month*

Who or what: *I*
What about it: *will begin working in a few weeks*

Correct: I applied for the job last month. I will begin working in a few weeks.

Example 2

Run-on: My uncle wants to lose weight, he is exercising every day.

Who or what: *My uncle*
What about it: *wants to lose weight*

Who or what: *he*
What about it: *is exercising every day*

Correct: My uncle wants to lose weight. He is exercising every day.

Look for *And*s and *So*s

Check to see whether you are stringing sentences together with unnecessary *and*s and *so*s. If you are, delete these words and punctuate each sentence individually.

Run-on: My car needed a new oil filter and I knew that I had to do something about it so I called the auto mechanic last Saturday and he told me he had nothing open for the rest of the month so I decided to fix it myself.

Correct: My car needed a new oil filter. I knew that I had to do something about it. I called the auto mechanic last Saturday. He told me he had nothing open for the rest of the month. I decided to fix it myself.

- The run-on sentences are corrected, revealing a series of short, choppy sentences. Adding dependent words will help create smoothly connected sentences.

Improved: My car needed a new oil filter. Because I knew that I had to do something about it, I called the auto mechanic last Saturday. When he told me he had nothing open for the rest of the month, I decided to fix it myself.

Exercises

○ **Self Test.** Read each sentence and decide whether it is a correct sentence or a run-on sentence. If it's correct, mark it with a *C*. If it's a run-on, mark it with a ✓.

1. Ann's boss is supportive he gave her a day off.

2. Our neighbors just moved from Texas, they seem friendly.

3. When we made plans for the weekend, we did not know that Marcus would have to work.

4. My grandmother didn't let disappointment bother her she just kept living day by day.

5. I can trust Serena and Valerie they don't gossip about others.

○ **Exercise 1:** If the sentence is correct, place *C* next to it. If it is a run-on sentence, use a period to punctuate it correctly.

1. The construction workers hit a gas line, the houses on the block had to be evacuated.

2. The roads are covered with ice it is too dangerous to drive.

3. The woman at the tollbooth told us to take the next exit she knew the area well.

4. Regular physical activity and a strong social support system benefit people of all ages.

5. The discount store has been closed for repair, it has lost money daily.

6. My father attended all of my basketball games he was my inspiration and support.

7. My job has been boring people are not buying major appliances.

8. Community residents are concerned about the proposed mall because they believe it will increase noise and traffic in the neighborhood.

9. I put on my uniform, which included my good-luck shorts they were an old pair of University of North Carolina basketball shorts that I have worn since sixth grade.

10. The father listened carefully to his daughter he knew that something important had happened.

⬤ **Exercise 2:** Read the following paragraph out loud to find where the sentences end. Then mark the end of each sentence with a period and capitalize the first word of the following sentence.

My biggest accomplishment was learning to play the drums I started studying classical music at the age of ten and then moved to religious music many years of practice made playing progressively easier and gave me confidence audiences began to give me smiles and nods of encouragement their approval inspired me to continue practicing and perfecting my performance I am now playing with the professionals and performing in large concert halls I never dreamed that a little ten-year-old child would one day grow into a confident musician.

Student writer

● **Exercise 3:** Read the following paragraph out loud to find where the sentences end. Then mark the end of each sentence with a period and capitalize the first word of the following sentence.

> Moving into my own apartment was an exciting event in my life I gained my freedom and was finally independent the relief of being on my own lasted until the bills started to arrive I was prepared for my car and insurance payments because I had been responsible for these bills I was not prepared for the living expenses electricity, gas, water, and phone bills kept arriving I also had to pay the rent and buy my food all the expenses that my parents had once covered were now mine I soon realized that more money was going out than was coming in it took me months to readjust my lifestyle living on my own taught me that freedom and independence have a price tag.
>
> Student writer

● **Exercise 4:** If our sentences are closely related, we can use semicolons to separate them. Correct each of the following run-on sentences by inserting a semicolon.

Example

> **The hurricane was the worst disaster in centuries it produced raging floods and mudslides.**
>
> *The hurricane was the worst disaster in centuries; it produced raging floods and mudslides.*

1. E-mail messages are casual, letters are more formal.

2. Republicans blame the country's problems on the Democrats, the Democrats blame the Republicans.

3. Registration ends on the twelfth late registration ends on the fifteenth.

4. Janette is taking morning classes I am taking night classes.

5. Mario is an excellent student, he studies daily.

● **Exercise 5:** Take the paper you are currently writing and read it carefully, looking for run-on sentences. Use the guidelines provided in *How to Find Run-ons* on page 62.

USING COMMAS

Punctuation marks help readers navigate your sentences. One of the most important signs is the comma, which we explore in this chapter. (Additional uses are discussed in Chapter 16.)

SUMMARY OF COMMAS

Use a comma to

1. Separate three or more items in a series
   - I will bring fried chicken, potato salad, hamburgers, and paper plates.

2. Connect two sentences with the words *and, but, or, so, yet, for,* or *nor* (**coordinating conjunctions**)
   - We can arrive at seven to set up picnic tables, or we can show up at six to start the grill.

3. Set off an addition at the beginning of a sentence
   - If it rains, we will have the picnic indoors.

4. Set off an addition in the middle of a sentence
   - Marvin, who lives down the street, will grill the chicken.

5. Set off an addition at the end of a sentence
   - We need someone to send out invitations, which is an easy job.

· ·

Section A: Rules 1 and 2

COMMAS WITH ITEMS IN A SERIES

We use commas to separate three or more items in a series. The items may be single words or groups of words. Place a comma after each item except the last.

Single Words

Nutritionists claim that broccoli, pears, apples, and bananas have high fiber content.

- Commas have been placed after *broccoli*, *pears*, and *apples*. No comma follows *bananas* because it is the last item.

- Also notice that no comma precedes *broccoli*. The comma goes after the item—not before it.

Groups of Words

Gary will assemble my computer, load the software, and make sure the programs work.

- Commas have been placed after *assemble my computer* and *load the software*. The same rule applies: Place commas after each item except the last.

COMMAS WITH COORDINATING CONJUNCTIONS

We also use a comma with *and, but, or, so, yet, for,* and *nor* when these words connect two sentences.

COORDINATING CONJUNCTIONS

and	means	*in addition*
but and *yet*	mean	*in contrast, just the opposite*
for	means	*because*
or	means	*either*
nor	means	*not either* (It is the negative form of or.)
so	means	*as a result*

To remember the coordinating conjunctions, think of FANBOYS: *for, and, nor, but, or, yet, so.*

These conjunctions link two sentences together to create a **compound sentence.**

> **They shopped all day Saturday, *and* they bought nothing.**
> **They shopped all day Saturday, *but* they bought nothing.**

- Notice that the comma is placed before the coordinating conjunction. One way to remember where the comma goes is to say the word *comma* out loud, calling these connectors "comma *and*," "comma *but*," "comma *or*," and so on. For example, saying "comma *but*" out loud will help you remember that the comma goes first, the word *but* second.

HOW TO DECIDE: COMMA OR NO COMMA

Use a comma with a coordinating conjunction when it connects two sentences, not two things. You can tell the difference by using the pencil test.

Pencil test

Place your pencil on the word *and, but, or, so, yet, for,* or *nor*. Read the words to the left and ask yourself *who or what* and *what about it*. If you have both a *who or what* (subject) and a *what about it* (predicate), you have a sentence. Then read the words to the right, asking again *who or what* and *what about it*. If both sides have a subject and predicate, use a comma.

Use a Comma

In the following examples, the pencil test explains why commas are necessary.

Example 1

> **Bill is working the night shift, and Kathy is working the day shift.**

Place your pencil on *and*. Read the words to the left. Ask *who or what* and *what about him*.

- Bill / is working the night shift. (This is a sentence.)

Read the words to the right. Ask *who or what* and *what about her*.

- Kathy / is working the day shift. (This is a sentence.)
- Because a sentence is on each side of *and*, a comma has been added.

Example 2

We can study in the library before class, or we can meet in the cafeteria after class.

Read the words to the left of *or.* Ask *who or what* and *what about them.*

- We / can study in the library before class. (This is a sentence.)

Read the words to the right of *or.* Ask *who or what* and *what about them.*

- We / can meet in the cafeteria after class. (This is a sentence.)
- Because a sentence is on each side, a comma has been added.

Do Not Use a Comma

When the coordinating conjunction connects two words or **phrases** (groups of words), we do not use a comma. The most common error is made with the word *and.* Do not use a comma when *and* connects two words or phrases.

Example 1

Michelle wants ice cream and cake for dessert.

Read the words to the left of *and.* Ask *who or what* and *what about her.*

- Michelle / wants ice cream. (This is a sentence.)

Read the words to the right of *and.* Ask *who or what* and *what about it.*

- Cake for dessert. (*What about it?* This is not a sentence.)
- A comma has not been added. The *and* connects *ice cream* and *cake*, not two sentences.

Example 2

The twins held their mother's hand and walked toward their kindergarten teacher.

Read the words to the left of *and.* Ask *who or what* and *what about them.*

- The twins / held their mother's hand. (This is a sentence.)

Read the words to the right of *and*. Ask *who or what* and *what about it*.

- Walked toward their kindergarten teacher. (There is no *who or what* here—the *twins* are in the other sentence. This is not a sentence.)

- A comma has not been added because the *and* does not connect two sentences. It connects *held their mother's hand* and *walked toward their kindergarten teacher*.

. . . .

Exercises: Section A

● **Self Test A:** Use the pencil test to decide whether to place a comma in the following sentences. If there is a subject and predicate on both sides of the *and*, use a comma. If not, do not use a comma.

1. The dog grabbed the ham bone and dashed out the back door.

2. The mechanic changed the oil and rotated the tires on my car.

3. The stores will be closed on Friday and Saturday for inventory.

4. Terry works in the garden on Saturdays and his children help him.

5. We bought a couch last week and will pick it up next week.

● **Exercise 1a:** Use the pencil test to decide whether to place a comma in the following sentences. If there is a subject and predicate on both sides of the *and*, use a comma. If not, do not use a comma.

1. Friends from Cincinnati and Columbus surprised Henrietta and her husband on their anniversary.

2. The sun slowly inched up the horizon and the sky was layered in pinks and reds.

3. Nick hopes that his new job will increase his free time and decrease his tension.

4. The performing arts center will have a theater on the first floor and dance studios on the second floor.

5. The altos will practice on Wednesday and the sopranos will practice on Thursday.

● **Exercise 2a:** In the following sentences, use commas to separate the items in each series. Remember: Place a comma after each item except the last.

Example

> **The ceiling walls baseboards and closets need to be painted.**
> *The ceiling, walls, baseboards, and closets need to be painted.*

Example

> **We need to know whether we should cook dinner pick up fast food or go to a restaurant.**
> *We need to know whether we should cook dinner, pick up fast food, or go to a restaurant.*

1. The Amish are known to be kind gentle modest and patient people.

2. The meat was undercooked tasteless and tough.

3. Her hat was decorated with gold silver blue and red sequins.

4. Vanessa is a caring sensitive and responsible friend.

5. Washing the dishes doing the laundry shopping for food and paying the bills take time.

6. We can use the Internet to register for a course check our tuition balance access our current schedule and check the availability of a course.

7. The Johnsons are looking for a home with a family room three bedrooms a small yard and a two-car attached garage.

8. Few Americans would give up the modern conveniences of the automobile television and telephone.

9. Their emergency kit included a flashlight first-aid supplies canned goods blankets and a three-day supply of drinking water.

10. Summer tourists enjoy flea markets on Tuesdays weekly auctions on Wednesdays music festivals on Fridays and art fairs on Saturdays.

● **Exercise 3a:** In the following paragraph, the commas that separate items in a series are missing. Place them where they belong.

Almost everyone in America faces stress. School jobs families and friends can be demanding. One method of relieving stress involves music. Many therapists encourage people to listen to soothing music. Music can help us relax relieve anger avoid depression and gain energy. Soothing sounds calm the mind and heal the body. Music can also improve memory boost the immune system and reduce pain. Turning on the radio or popping a favorite CD into the stereo is a healthy way to relax and cope with everyday tensions.

Section B: Rules 3, 4, and 5

We also use commas to mark additions (baskets) to a basic sentence. As explained in Chapter 1, a basic sentence is like a bike. The subject and predicate connect to form a stable structure.

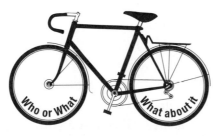

Subject wheel	Predicate wheel
Michael	smiled.
Kevin	called last night.
The restaurant	has delicious seafood.

Once we have a stable bike, we can add extra information to it. We can place baskets on the front, in the middle, or on the back of the bike. We usually use commas to mark these additions so that readers can see what is an addition and what is the basic sentence.

COMMAS WITH ADDITIONS ON THE FRONT

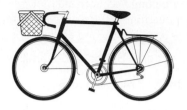

In the middle of our conversation, Michael smiled.

To confuse the opposing team, Michael smiled.

As soon as he saw us, Michael smiled.

An optimistic person, Michael smiled.

Asked about his future plans, Michael smiled.

Waving to his neighbor, Michael smiled.

- Notice that a comma separates the basket from the basic sentence. Readers expect the subject to come first. When you begin with an addition instead of the subject, use a comma to let readers know that something different is happening.

COMMAS WITH ADDITIONS IN THE MIDDLE

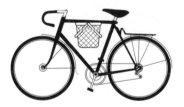

Kevin, *who is carefully considering his options,* called last night.

Kevin, *a good friend since high school,* called last night.

Kevin, *needing advice about which job to take,* called last night.

Kevin, *determined to make the best decision,* called last night.

- These baskets are called interrupters because they interrupt the flow of ideas in a sentence. Notice that commas are placed on both sides of the interrupter. The first comma says to readers, "Something different is happening. Hold on—the basic sentence will return soon." The second comma tells them, "The extra information is now over. We're back to the basic sentence." Readers are always looking for the basic sentence so that they can understand the main idea. These two commas help readers see the main idea.

COMMAS WITH ADDITIONS ON THE BACK

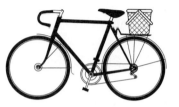

The restaurant has delicious seafood, *which is not too expensive.*
The restaurant has delicious seafood, *especially its broiled salmon.*
The restaurant has delicious seafood, *the finest food in town.*
The restaurant has delicious seafood, *ranging from perch to prawns.*

- Notice that a comma separates the basket from the basic sentence.

Helpful hint: Keep the bike in mind not only when writing but also when reading. When you read, look for the *who or what* and the *what about it*. When you come across a comma, remember that it often marks where an addition begins and ends.

. . . .

Exercises: Section B

⬤ **Self Test B:** In the following sentences, the same basic sentence is used to support a variety of additions. Underline the basic sentence.

Example

As soon as she heard about it, <u>Debra enrolled her children in the after-school program</u>.

1. Debra enrolled her children in the after-school program, which runs throughout the year.

2. Debra, my neighbor across the street, enrolled her children in the after-school program.

3. Debra enrolled her children in the after-school program, a series of enrichment opportunities that include art and drama.

4. Debra, wanting to give her children a safe and nurturing environment, enrolled her children in the after-school program.

5. At the beginning of the year, Debra enrolled her children in the after-school program.

⬤ **Exercise 1b:** In each sentence, put parentheses around the addition and then answer the question that follows.

Example

(After the flood), swarms of mosquitoes took flight.
What is the basic sentence? *Swarms of mosquitoes took flight.*

1. Inside and outside, the car is well designed.

   What is the basic sentence? _____

2. The day, overcast with light breezes, began slowly.

   What is the basic sentence? _____

3. Everyone hung around the buffet table, munching on ham sandwiches and potato chips.

What is the basic sentence? _____

4. The artist, after spending ten to twelve hours a day at the drawing board, was exhausted.

What is the basic sentence? _____

5. The elderly woman depends on the telephone, her lifeline to the outside world.

What is the basic sentence? _____

6. To meet the increasing demand for electricity, the state will build three new power plants.

What is the basic sentence? _____

7. Taking matters into their own hands, residents created an organization to attract new businesses to their community.

What is the basic sentence? _____

8. The small town, despite its increasing popularity with tourists, maintained its simplicity.

What is the basic sentence? _____

9. Some herbal medicines may be dangerous, especially if they are taken before surgery.

What is the basic sentence? _____

10. Hiking in the Canadian Rockies, we saw a chain of glaciers that separate Alberta from British Columbia.

What is the basic sentence? _____

⬤ **Exercise 2b:** The writer did not mark the additions with commas, so the following sentences are confusing. Read each sentence, find the addition, and set it off with a comma or commas.

> **Before we make plane reservations we should check out the prices on the Internet.**
>
> *Before we make plane reservations, we should check out the prices on the Internet.*

1. Gazing out the window Andrea daydreamed about summer vacation.

2. Patrick and Kay our new neighbors just moved from Atlanta.

3. Peaking out from his blanket the shy toddler greeted me with a smile.

4. Because Jenny often runs ten miles a day is an easy workout.

5. Mr. Sanchez my high school history teacher encouraged me to go to college.

6. Without warning the lights went out.

7. Tara the student in the back row is struggling to stay awake.

8. To get to my house you need to turn left on Eighty-third Street and right on Ridgelawn Avenue.

9. With his hands in constant motion the director described the scenes in the movie.

10. Pizza Depot our favorite restaurant will close in January for renovations.

⬤ **Exercise 3b:** The *Summary of Commas* chart on page 69 lists five ways we use commas. Write a sentence for each one.

Example

   (with items in a series)
   My favorite sports are baseball, football, and soccer.

1. (with items in a series)

   _____

2. (with a coordinating conjunction)

   _____

3. (with an addition at the beginning of a sentence)

   _____

4. (with an addition in the middle of a sentence)

   _____

5. (with an addition at the end of a sentence)

   _____

PART 2

WORD CHOICE

CHAPTER 7

VERBS

Say to yourself, "I like to . . ." Any word that makes sense in that slot is a verb. Verbs are powerful words. They can create vivid pictures in readers' minds. For example, when we write a sentence such as *They walked down the stairs*, the verb *walked* provides a particular image. When we choose another verb, we change that image. *They tiptoed down the stairs*—or *staggered, limped, charged, skipped down the stairs*.

Verbs are also powerful because they can change tense, showing different time situations. For example, *I paid the bills* is different from *I will pay the bills* or *I should pay the bills*. We change **tense** (time) by selecting the verb form we want. Verbs have five forms (principal parts): the **base form, -s form, past tense, past participle,** and **present participle.** We use these forms to create a variety of tenses.

REGULAR VERB FORMS

Base form	-S form	Past tense	Past participle	Present participle (-*ing* form)
work	works	worked	worked	working
play	plays	played	played	playing
listen	listens	listened	listened	listening

Present Tense

Present tense refers to events that occur in the present or on a regular basis. It can also be used to explain general truths. It uses the base form and the *-s* form.

PRESENT TENSE			
Singular		**Plural**	
I	*talk*	we	*talk*
you	*talk*	you	*talk*
he, she, it	*talks*	they	*talk*

We use the *-s* form (sometimes spelled *-es*) when the subject is *he, she,* or *it.* This means not only *he* but any male, not only *she* but any female, and not only *it* but anything that is an *it.**

> **My brother** *reads* **the newspaper every morning.**
>
> **My sister** *takes* **the bus.**
>
> **The bus** *runs* **daily.**

We usually use the *-ing* form along with *am, is,* and *are* to describe events that are happening right now.

> **I** *am writing* **a paper.**
>
> **Ken** *is studying*.
>
> **They** *are watching* **television.**

Future Tense

Future tense refers to events that have not yet happened; they will occur in the future. We form the future tense by adding *will* to the base form: *will see, will listen, will eat.*

> **We** *will work* **tomorrow.**

---

* Matching the correct form of a verb with the subject is called **subject-verb agreement.** We will focus on this in Chapter 8.

We can indicate future time in other ways also:

> **We *will be working* for the next two weeks.**
> - This action will continue in the future.

> **In January, we *will have worked* for a year.**
> - This action will be completed by a specified time in the future.

We can also indicate future time by adding a time phrase to the present tense:

> **I leave *tomorrow*.**
> **The bus leaves *at noon*.**

Another way to indicate future action is with the phrase *am (is, are) going to:*

> **I *am going to* graduate in May.**
> **My neighbor *is going to* take me out for dinner.**

• •

Past Tense

Past tense refers to events that have already happened. When we write in the past tense, we add *-d* or *-ed* to the base form of **regular verbs:** *danced, lived, whispered, laughed*. When we talk, we may not always pronounce the *-d* or *-ed* ending. Therefore, check to make sure you have included these endings when you are writing in the past tense.*

> **We *walked* to the park.**
> - The action occurred at a specific time in the past and is now over.

You can also indicate past tense with verb combinations:

> **We *were walking* in the park when the storm hit.**
> - This action continued over a period of time in the past.

---

* Some verbs are irregular: Their past tense is not formed by adding *-d or -ed*. We will study **irregular verbs** in Chapter 9.

We *have walked* in the park for many years.

- This verb form can have three different meanings, depending on the context:

  1. The action occurred in the past and continues in the present.
  2. The action occurred in the past and just recently ended.
  3. The action occurred at an unspecified time in the past.

We *walked* to the park because we *had arranged* to meet Mandy there.

- Both actions (walking and arranging) happened in the past, but one of them happened earlier. We use *had* to show which one happened first.

The Infinitive

Infinitives consist of the word *to* plus the base form: *to live, to wonder, to meet, to smile.* The infinitive does not change, regardless of what tense you are using. The verb in the sentence will show the time change.

Today, I want *to eat* dinner early.

Tomorrow, I will want *to eat* dinner early.

Yesterday, I wanted *to eat* dinner early.

- The verb *want* indicates present tense; *will want* indicates future tense; *wanted* indicates past tense. The infinitive *to eat* stays the same. Therefore, when you are writing in the past tense, do not add *-d* or *-ed* to the infinitive.

Helping Verbs

We can change the tense of a verb by adding **helping verbs.** Helping verbs include the various forms of *be, do,* and *have* and the words *may, might, must, can, could, will, would, shall, should,* and *ought to.* These verbs are added to the base form, the past participle, and the *-ing* form.

The following sentences show some of the helping-verb combinations. The first sentence uses the verb *order* by itself; the remaining sentences include helping verbs. The verbs are in italics.

ACTIVE VOICE

These sentences are in **active voice,** which means the subject does the action.

We *order* pizza.   We *have been ordering* pizza.
We *will order* pizza.   We *have ordered* pizza.
We *did order* pizza.   We *had ordered* pizza.
We *could order* pizza.   We *should have ordered* pizza.
We *are ordering* pizza.   We *would have ordered* pizza.
We *were ordering* pizza.   We *could have ordered* pizza.

PASSIVE VOICE

These sentences are in **passive voice,** which means the subject receives the action. Verbs in the passive voice use the past participle and a form of *be* as a helping verb: *am, are, is, was, were, been, being.* Notice the *-ed* endings:

The pizza *is ordered.*   The pizza *had been ordered.*
The pizza *was ordered.*   The pizza *could have been ordered.*
The pizza *will be ordered.*   The pizza *should have been ordered.*
The pizza *should be ordered.*   The pizza *would have been ordered.*
The pizza *could be ordered.*   The pizza *must have been ordered.*
The pizza *has been ordered.*   The pizza *might have been ordered.*

Active voice is more direct and lively than passive voice because the subject does the action.

Active

The *dentist* pulled my tooth.

- The subject, the *dentist*, does the action.

Passive

My *tooth* was pulled by the dentist.

- The subject, *tooth*, doesn't perform the action. Instead, something happens to it.

We sometimes use the passive voice when we don't know or don't want to name the doer of the action or when the receiver of the action is the topic we are discussing.

Signs will be posted in the cafeteria.

- We don't know who will post the signs.

Mistakes were made.

- We don't want to name who made the mistakes.

President Lincoln was killed by John Wilkes Booth.

- We are discussing President Lincoln, rather than John Wilkes Booth, the doer of the action.

FIXED-FORM HELPING VERBS

The following helping verbs are called fixed-form because they do not change form.

FIXED-FORM HELPING VERBS		
may	can, could	ought to
might	will, would	
must	shall, should	

We have learned to add *-s* to present-tense verbs when the subject is *he*, *she*, or *it*.

He walks.

Fixed-form helping verbs, however, freeze the verb. Notice that *-s* is not added:

He may walk.	He can walk.	He could walk.	He ought to walk.
He might walk.	He will walk.	He would walk.	
He must walk.	He shall walk.	He should walk.	

Can and *Could*

Use *could* as the past tense of *can*.

Today, I *can laugh* about my mistake.
Yesterday, I *could laugh* about nothing.

- In the first sentence, *can* shows that the action is in the present.
- In the second sentence, *could* shows that the action is in the past.
- Notice that *could* carries the past-tense information. The correct verb is *could laugh*, not *could laughed*.

Could also indicates future possibility.

> **The weather *could* turn cold tonight.**

Will and *Would*

Use *would* as the past tense of *will*.

> **Today, I think it *will rain*.**
> **Yesterday, I thought it *would rain*.**

- In the first sentence, *will* shows that the action is in the present.
- In the second sentence, *would* shows that the action is in the past.
- Notice that *would* carries the past-tense information. The correct verb is *would rain*, not *would rained*.

Would also carries the meaning of possibility.

> **I *would* go with you if I could.**

• •

Exercises

⬤ **Self Test:** Many of the verbs in the following sentences are missing the *-d* or *-ed* ending. Find and correct them.

planned
We have ~~plan~~ this party for a long time.

1. The game was postpone because of weather.

2. I should have stay in high school and graduate with my class.

3. Their work schedule has been shorten to four days a week.

4. For the past two months, we have walk three miles every day.

5. Pat was hire in April as an orderly in the operating room.

6. Everyone in the class has practice these verb forms.

7. Technology has change how we live.

8. Our friends have encourage and help us in the past.

9. We learn yesterday that our medical benefits will be increase.

10. The soldiers have serve their country well.

● **Exercise 1:** Read the following excerpt adapted from Ted Conover's "Peru's Long Haul," and then change the verbs in italics from present tense to past tense.

> With a gasp of brakes, the truck *nears* the rickety, one-lane bridge on a hot Amazon afternoon. As it *slows,* the cloud of dust in its wake *rolls* toward the truck and then *washes* over it, enveloping the seventeen people riding on top with fine red dirt. The passengers, both tourists and locals, *close* their eyes and for a moment *stop* talking as the truck *continues* down the narrow dirt road that *curves* like an earthworm down into the humid rain forest (82).

● **Exercise 2:** Fill in each of the following blanks with the correct form of the verb in parentheses.

Example

   (will, would) **Today's newspaper predicts that it** _will_ **rain.**

1. (can, could) Dan lists every check he writes so that he _____ balance his checkbook.

2. (will, would) The jury hoped that the trial _____ not last long.

3. (can, could) When Crystal finally found her wallet, all she _____ feel was relief.

4. (rent, rented) We decided to _____ the apartment on Oak Street.

5. (change, changes) A kind word can _____ a bad day to a good day.

6. (begin, begins) The festival _____ October 22.

7. (flash, flashes) When lightning _____ across the sky, a crack of thunder is often heard several seconds later.

8. (get, gets) Marlin knows that he may _____ a raise.

9. (concentrate, concentrates) My little sister can do the work if she

_____.

10. (watch, watches) Every evening Trisha and Terry sit on the back steps and

_____ the sun set.

● **Exercise 3:** The following sentences are written in the passive voice. Rewrite each sentence in the active voice.

Example

The treaty was signed by both presidents.
Both presidents signed the treaty.

Example

Lunch will be provided by the park district.
The park district will provide lunch.

1. The whole dinner was prepared by my eighty-year-old grandmother.

_____

2. The rap stars will be surrounded by bodyguards.

_____

3. The calendar changes were approved by the college board.

_____

4. The door prizes will be donated by local merchants.

_____

5. I was encouraged by Jessica's comments.

_____

SUBJECT-VERB AGREEMENT

Subjects and Verbs

The subject of a sentence determines whether the present-tense verb ends in *-s*. A **singular** subject (one that can be substituted by *he*, *she*, or *it*) takes the *-s* form. A **plural** subject (more than one) does not. When the correct verb follows the subject, we have subject-verb agreement.

PRESENT TENSE			
Singular		**Plural**	
I	*understand*	we	*understand*
you	*understand*	you	*understand*
he, she, it	*understands*	they	*understand*

When the subject is *he*, *she*, or *it*, or anything that is a *he*, *she*, or *it*, the present-tense verb ends in *-s*.

My brother *understands*.

When the subject is plural, the verb does not end in *-s*.

My brothers *understand*.

You can check for subject-verb agreement by temporarily substituting the subject with a pronoun.

> **Joan (she) *wants* to cook dinner.**
> **Joan and Dylan (they) *want* to cook dinner.**
> **The car in the driveway (it) *runs* smoothly.**
> **The cars in the driveway (they) *run* smoothly.**

• •

The Verbs *Be, Do,* and *Have*

Subject-verb agreement is especially important when using the verbs *be*, *do*, and *have*. These verbs, which we use as both **main verbs** and helping verbs, have irregular forms.

THE VERB *BE*

Present tense		Past tense	
I *am*	we *are*	I *was*	we *were*
you *are*	you *are*	you *were*	you *were*
he, she, it *is*	they *are*	he, she, it *was*	they *were*

Present Tense

If the subject is *he*, *she*, or *it*, use *is*. If the subject is plural, use *are*.

> **Julie *is* happy. She *is smiling*.**
> **Julie and Andy *are* happy. They *are smiling*.**

Past Tense

If the subject is *he*, *she*, or *it*, use *was*. If the subject is plural, use *were*.

> **Julie *was* happy. She *was smiling*.**
> **Julie and Andy *were* happy. They *were smiling*.**

Using Contraction

We often use the word *not* or the **contraction** of *not* (*n't*) with a form of *be*. Make sure the form of *be* agrees with the subject.

> Ron *isn't* nervous. Ron and Evelyn *aren't* nervous.
> The tire *wasn't* flat. The tires *weren't* flat.

THE VERB *DO*

	Present tense		Past tense
I *do*	we *do*	I *did*	we *did*
you *do*	you *do*	you *did*	you *did*
he, she, it *does*	they *do*	he, she, it *did*	they *did*

Present Tense

If the subject is *he*, *she*, or *it*, use *does*. If the subject is plural, use *do*.

> Tracey *does* chores on Saturday. She *does wonder* where the time goes.
> Tracey and Nick *do* chores on Saturday. They *do wonder* where the time goes.

Using Contraction

We often use the word *not* or the contraction of *not* (*n't*) with a form of *do*. Make sure the form of *do* agrees with the subject.

> Dexter *does not* (*doesn't*) worry about tomorrow.
> The children *do not* (*don't*) worry about tomorrow.

Past Tense

When writing in the past tense, change the helping verb *do* to *did*, but do not change the form of the main verb.

> Present: I *do love* chocolate, and I eat it daily.
> Past: I *did love* chocolate when I was a child.

- In the first sentence, *do love* shows that the action is in the present.

- In the second sentence, *did love* shows that the action is in the past.

- Notice that *did* carries the past-tense information. The correct verb in the second sentence is *did love*, not *did loved*.

THE VERB *HAVE*

	Present tense		Past tense	
I *have*	we *have*	I *had*	we *had*
you *have*	you *have*	you *had*	you *had*
he, she, it *has*	they *have*	he, she, it *had*	we *had*

Present Tense

If the subject is *he*, *she*, or *it*, use *has*. If the subject is plural, use *have*.

> Ed *has* clear goals. He *has thought* about his future.
> Ed and Tammy *have* clear goals. They *have thought* about their future.

Using Contraction

We often use the word *not* or the contraction of *not* (*n't*) with a form of *have*. Make sure the form of *have* agrees with the subject.

> Lydia *has not* (*hasn't*) had time to relax.
> The packages *have not* (*haven't*) arrived.

Helpful hint: All present-tense verbs end in *-s* when the subject is *he*, *she*, or *it*. This means not only *he* but any male, not only *she* but any female, and not only *it* but anything that is an *it*. This rule applies to both regular verbs (*walks, talks, listens*) and irregular verbs (*is, does, has*).

• •

Singular Subjects

Words that end in *-ing*, collective nouns, and amounts are usually singular.

GERUNDS

Verbs that end in *-ing* can be used as nouns. These *-ing* nouns, which are called **gerunds,** are singular. Therefore, when the subject is an *-ing* word, the present-tense verb ends in *-s.*

> **Writing** *takes* **time.**
> **Exercising** *increases* **energy.**
> **Relaxing on weekends** *is* **important.**

COLLECTIVE NOUNS

When a group acts as one unit, it is usually considered singular.

GROUPS OFTEN TREATED AS SINGULAR				
audience	crowd	jury	class	team
family	choir	public	committee	society

> **The choir** *practices* **every Thursday night.**
> **Sharon's family** *is planning* **a vacation together.**
> **Our class** *wants* **to postpone the exam.**

AMOUNTS

Quantities of time, money, weight, and length are usually singular because they refer to one unit.

> **Six years** *was* **a long time to wait.**
> **Two hundred dollars** *is* **a lot of money.**
> **Fifteen pounds of luggage** *was* **easy to carry.**
> **Ten miles** *is* **not far if we drive.**

. . . .

Plural Subjects

Sometimes a sentence has more than one subject, which is called a **compound subject.** If the subjects are joined by *and,* the subject is plural. The verb does not end in *-s.*

Compound subject	Verb
Varnish and paint	*stain.*
Todd and his nephew	*paint* houses during the summer.
He and I	*drive* to work together.

As you check for subject-verb agreement, keep in mind that most nouns form the plural by adding *-s: streets, breakfasts, shoes, books.* Yet, the rule has some exceptions.

1. If the noun ends in *-y,* change the *-y* to *-i* and add *-es.*

Singular	Plural
body	bodies
party	parties
story	stories

2. If the noun ends in *-s, -sh, -ch,* or *-x,* add *-es.*

Singular	Plural
dress	dresses
dish	dishes
ditch	ditches
box	boxes

3. If the noun ends in *-fe* or *-f,* change the *-f* to *-v* and add *-es.*

Singular	Plural
knife	knives
life	lives
thief	thieves

4. A few nouns do not follow any consistent plural pattern:

Singular	Plural	Singular	Plural
child	children	goose	geese
man	men	foot	feet
woman	women	alumnus	alumni
ox	oxen	deer	deer
mouse	mice	moose	moose

Tricky Agreement Situations

Sometimes subject-verb agreement can be tricky. We will look at three of those situations: when prepositional phrases come after the subject, when sentences begin with *There is/are* or *Here is/are*, and when we ask questions.

PREPOSITIONAL PHRASES

Prepositional phrases often come after the subject. We need to find these phrases when checking for subject-verb agreement because the verb must agree with the subject—not with a word in the prepositional phrase. Putting parentheses around the phrase temporarily can help you see the subject more clearly. (See page 17 for a review of prepositional phrases.)

Example 1

> The *videos* (on the kitchen table) *are* overdue.

- The subject is *videos*. *Table* cannot be the subject because it is in a prepositional phrase. Because the word *videos* is plural, we use *are*.

Example 2

> *One* (of my courses) *is* easy.

- The subject of this sentence is *one*. *Courses* cannot be the subject because it is in a prepositional phrase. Because *one* is singular, we use *is*.

Example 3

> *Students* (at the college) *were studying* for finals.

- The subject is *students*. Because *students* is plural, we use *were studying*.

THERE IS / THERE ARE AND HERE IS / HERE ARE

We often begin sentences with *There is, There are, Here is,* or *Here are.* The words *there* and *here* are not the subjects of a sentence. They act as arrows that point to the subject. To find the subject of the sentence, you need to follow the arrow to see which word it points to.

Example 1

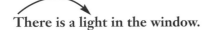

There is a light in the window.

- *There* points to *light.* Because *light* is singular, we use *is.*

There are many chores to do today.

- *There* points to *chores.* Because the word *chores* is plural, we use *are.*

Example 2

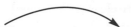

Here is my car.

- *Here* points to *car.* Because *car* is singular, we use *is.*

Here are the keys.

- *Here* points to *keys.* Because the word *keys* is plural, we use *are.*

QUESTIONS

In a question, the subject usually follows the verb. If you mentally rearrange the question as a statement, you will be able to identify the subject and verb. In the following examples, the subject is underlined once and the verb twice.

Example 1

<u>Is</u> <u>she</u> your sister?

- Restate this question as a statement: <u>She</u> <u>is</u> your sister.

Example 2

<u>Has</u> the <u>mail</u> <u>arrived</u>?

- Restate this question as a statement: The <u>mail</u> <u>has arrived</u>.

Example 3

Where <u>are</u> my <u>shoes</u>?

- Restate this question as a statement: My <u>shoes</u> <u>are</u> where.

• •

Exercises

● **Self Test:** Read each sentence, choose the correct verb, and write that verb in the blank.

1. (has, have) Both socks _____ holes in them.

2. (doesn't, don't) The lawnmower _____ work well because the blades need sharpening.

3. (has, have) The mechanic _____ replaced the brake drums.

4. (was, were) He _____ leaving when I arrived.

5. (has, have) If Carla _____ the answer, she will tell us.

6. (do, does) He _____ whatever he can to help our neighbors.

7. (was, were) The people _____ friendly and helpful.

8. (has, have) My uncle, who _____ been married for ten years, is planning an anniversary party.

9. (doesn't, don't) My friends _____ want to leave for vacation until Saturday.

10. (was, were) We heard the news while we _____ walking home.

● **Exercise 1:** In each pair of sentences, use the present tense in the first sentence and the past tense in the second.

Example

(do) Scott hopes he <u>does</u> his best today. Yesterday, he <u>did</u> his worst.

1. (have) Norma _____ two exams this week. Last week, she only _____ one.

2. (be) Antonio _____ now the manager. Last year, he _____ the assistant manager.

3. (do) I _____ my best work in the morning. Yesterday, I

_____ all the math assignments before dawn.

4. (have) That restaurant _____ inexpensive prices. Before the

owners hired a new manager, the restaurant _____ expensive

prices.

5. (be) The grandparents _____ always asleep by 8 p.m. They

_____ asleep when the smoke alarm rang.

● **Exercise 2:** Read each sentence, choose the correct verb, and write that verb in
the blank.

1. (want, wants) Betty and Brad _____ to be members of the

association.

2. (is, are) Both the computer and printer _____ now working.

3. (don't, doesn't) Worrying about a problem _____ solve the

problem.

4. (hasn't, haven't) Matthew _____ met my relatives.

5. (seem, seems) The employees _____ satisfied with the new

schedule.

6. (is, are) The group _____ planning a trip to New Orleans.

7. (go, goes) Every Halloween, the children _____ trick or treating.

8. (spend, spends) Cynthia _____ her free time reading about mutual

funds.

9. (is, are) The women in the class _____ smiling at me.

10. (take, takes) Writing papers _____ time.

● **Exercise 3:** Correct any present-tense verb errors by adding -*s* or -*es* where necessary.

> My neighbor Mr. Anderson is a trustworthy friend. Although he is seventy-five years old, he drive his car, mow his lawn, and cook for himself. But most importantly, he spend his afternoons sitting on the front porch or in his living room, watching the children in the neighborhood. He know when Jeffrey, my ten-year-old child, get off the bus. If I am not home, Jeffrey go to his house for snacks. My son enjoy Mr. Anderson because he listen quietly and laugh a lot. He never give harsh criticism; he give sound advice. Sometimes I think Jeffrey listen to him more than he do to me. Although Mr. Anderson says little, he know everything. He know who Jeffrey's friends are, and he know what kids are bothering him. If a situation look strange, he come down his porch steps and stands in the middle of the sidewalk. Children in the neighborhood call him "Mr. Watchdog." They say it kindly, for they know that they have a friend in the neighborhood they can trust.
>
> Student writer

● **Exercise 4:** In each sentence, put parentheses around the prepositional phrase(s) that come after the subject, underline the subject of the sentence, and then select the correct verb.

Example

   (is, are) The <u>clothes</u> (in the bottom drawer) *are* clean.

1. (show, shows) The movie theaters in our town _____ the exact same movies.

2. (need, needs) The wires inside the basement wall _____ to be replaced.

3. (is, are) Tickets for the annual banquet _____ now available.

4. (continue, continues) The number of cars and trucks on the road _____ to increase.

5. (is, are) A bag of groceries _____ sitting on the kitchen table.

6. (care, cares) The doctors in the clinic _____ about their patients.

7. (begin, begins) Registration for college courses _____ next week.

8. (is, are) The oatmeal cookies in the oven _____ for dessert.

9. (has, have) Musicians from New Orleans _____ entertained audiences since the dawn of jazz.

10. (has been, have been) Local farmers from Lincoln County _____ getting ready for the festival.

○ **Exercise 5:** Some of the following sentences have errors in subject-verb agreement. Correct each error by using the correct present-tense verb. If a sentence is correct as is, mark it with a *C.*

1. Six dollars are enough money if we go to the early movie.

2. People walks barefoot in the cool, moist sand.

3. Some airlines offers bonuses of one thousand frequent-flier miles to customers who book their flights online.

4. Here is my favorite jacket.

5. An increase in taxes are expected next year.

6. There is two important decisions to be made.

7. Few roads in the small village is wide enough for two lanes.

8. The weight of the boxes are listed on the receipt.

9. Where is my checkbook?

10. The crowd are excited.

● **Exercise 6:** Write five sentences about the weather today, using present tense. Then go back and underline the subject once and the verb twice.

_____

_____

_____

_____

_____

IRREGULAR VERBS

Irregular verbs do not follow the regular pattern for forming tenses. Their past tense and past participles do not end in *-ed*. These verbs are unpredictable; you must simply memorize them. In this chapter, we focus on using these forms as the main verbs in a sentence. Let's begin with the verb *eat*. We don't say, "Yesterday I eated . . ." or "Often I have eated . . ." Instead, we say the following:

Yesterday I *ate* in the cafeteria.

Often I *have eaten* in the cafeteria.

VERB FORMS		
Base form *(Today I . . .)*	**Past tense** *(Yesterday I . . .)* (Used alone)	**Past participle** *(Often I have . . .)* (Needs a helping verb)
eat	ate	eaten
fly	flew	flown
go	went	gone
see	saw	seen

The past tense is used alone. Do not add a helping verb.

> I *saw* a great film last night.
> Theresa *went* shopping on Saturday.
> Scott *flew* to Boston last weekend.

The past participle is *not* used alone. You need to add a helping verb, such as *have*, *could have*, or *should have*.

> I *have seen* that movie many times.
> Theresa *should have gone* shopping on Friday.
> Scott *would have flown* to Manchester, but the flight was cancelled.

A List of Irregular Verbs

As you review this list, keep in mind that the verbs in the middle column stand alone. The verbs in the right hand column, however, do not stand alone; they need a helping verb. Look over these verbs to see which ones you already know and which ones you need to study. Then, in the future, refer to this list to find the correct form of a particular verb. (In a few cases, you will see more than one form. The form listed first is the more common one.)

Base form (Today I . . .)	Past tense (Yesterday I . . .) (Used alone)	Past participle (Often I have . . .) (Needs a helping verb)
beat	beat	beaten, beat
become	became	become
begin	began	begun
bend	bent	bent
bite	bit	bitten, bit
bleed	bled	bled
blow	blew	blown
break	broke	broken
bring	brought	brought
build	built	built
buy	bought	bought
catch	caught	caught
choose	chose	chosen
come	came	come
cut	cut	cut
dig	dug	dug

Base form (Today I . . .)	Past tense (Yesterday I . . .) (Used alone)	Past participle (Often I have . . .) (Needs a helping verb)
do	did	done
draw	drew	drawn
drink	drank	drunk
drive	drove	driven
eat	ate	eaten
fall	fell	fallen
feed	fed	fed
feel	felt	felt
fight	fought	fought
find	found	found
fly	flew	flown
forget	forgot	forgotten
forgive	forgave	forgiven
freeze	froze	frozen
get	got	got, gotten
give	gave	given
go	went	gone
grow	grew	grown
hang (suspend)*	hung	hung
have	had	had
hear	heard	heard
hide	hid	hidden
hit	hit	hit
hold	held	held
hurt	hurt	hurt
keep	kept	kept
know	knew	known
lay (put)	laid	laid
lead	led	led
leave	left	left
lend	lent	lent
let	let	let
lie (recline)**	lay	lain
lose	lost	lost
make	made	made
meet	met	met
put	put	put
quit	quit	quit
read	read	read

*Hang meaning "execute by hanging" is a regular verb: *hang, hanged, hanged.*
**Lie meaning "tell a falsehood" is a regular verb: *lie, lied, lied.*

Base form (Today I . . .)	Past tense (Yesterday I . . .) (Used alone)	Past participle (Often I have . . .) (Needs a helping verb)
ride	rode	ridden
ring	rang	rung
rise	rose	risen
run	ran	run
say	said	said
see	saw	seen
sell	sold	sold
send	sent	sent
set (put)	set	set
shake	shook	shaken
shut	shut	shut
sing	sang	sung
sink	sank, sunk	sunk
sit (rest)	sat	sat
sleep	slept	slept
speak	spoke	spoken
spend	spent	spent
stand	stood	stood
steal	stole	stolen
stick	stuck	stuck
sting	stung	stung
swear	swore	sworn
sweep	swept	swept
swim	swam	swum
swing	swung	swung
take	took	taken
teach	taught	taught
tear	tore	torn
tell	told	told
think	thought	thought
throw	threw	thrown
understand	understood	understood
wake	woke, waked	waked, woken
wear	wore	worn
win	won	won
write	wrote	written

• •

Exercises

⬤ **Self Test:** Some of the sentences use irregular verbs correctly; others do not. If a sentence is correct, mark it with a *C*. If the sentence is incorrect, correct the verb error.

1. Last week, we buyed all our school supplies because they were on sale.

2. My phone has rang all morning.

3. After Henry had drove for three hours, he asked me to take over.

4. We have worn the same clothes for three days in a row.

5. We have came too far to turn back now.

6. I have a sore throat. I think I catched a cold from someone.

7. Our neighbors can't babysit because they have went shopping.

8. Have you seen that movie?

9. Joanna has brung the food for the picnic.

10. We have torn out the coupons.

⬤ **Exercise 1:** Fill in the blank with the correct verb form.

Example

(leave) Everyone had *left* the party by midnight.

1. (become) The new company has _____ a financial success.

2. (begin) After we finished the first paper, we immediately _____ the second paper.

3. (blow) The wind has _____ for three straight days.

4. (break) The child gasped when she _____ the china platter.

5. (bring) At last year's block party, everyone _____ food to share.

6. (buy) The parents _____ their children's school supplies last July.

7. (choose) Our friends _____ not to leave until they had helped us wash the dishes.

8. (come) They could have _____ to the party, but we forgot to invite them.

9. (do) Samantha has _____ her homework.

10. (drive) Last September, Kristina _____ from the East Coast to the West Coast.

11. (eat) The guests have _____ everything on the buffet table.

12. (fall) After the leaves had _____, we spent three days raking them into piles.

13. (forget) Once again, my cousin has _____ to shut the garage door.

14. (give) At the concert, the audience _____ the performers a standing ovation.

15. (freeze) When the temperature fell below zero, the water in the pipes _____ .

16. (go) We should have _____ food shopping yesterday.

17. (grow) The child's jacket was too short because he had _____ two inches.

18. (know) For a long time, employees have _____ about the company's plans to downsize.

19. (ring) I think my phone is broken because it has not _____ all day.

20. (run) Because the staff _____ an effective fund-raising campaign, it met the budget.

21. (see) Everyone who was outside last night _____ the shooting stars.

22. (sing) The choir has _____ an encore at every concert.

23. (sleep) After last night's storm, the campers pitched their tent and _____ until dawn.

24. (throw) We must have _____ out the receipt.

25. (write) I have _____ four papers this week.

● **Exercise 2:** Read the following paragraph and correct any errors you find in the italicized verbs. (The writer does not use past tense consistently and sometimes doesn't use the correct form of the past tense.)

> Graduating from high school *were* a huge relief. When I *begin* high
>
> school, I did not *want* to be there. I wanted a fast route to money, so I
>
> *selled* drugs and *hanged* out on the streets. But when everyone else in
>
> my class *graduates,* I *woked* up. Catching up *were* not easy. For a year
>
> and a half, I *attend* day and evening classes. During the summer, I *taked*
>
> courses for additional credits. When I finally walked across the stage at
>
> graduation, I *am* a proud man. I had finally *succeed,* and I realized that,
>
> with determination, I could become the man I wanted to be.
>
> Student writer

⬤ **Exercise 3:** In the following paragraph of *The Runaway Son*, Brent Staples
writes of one of his childhood memories, visiting his grandmother. Rewrite the
paragraph, changing the italicized verbs from present tense to past.

The log house *has* no running water, no electricity. At night I *bathe* in a
metal washtub set near the big, wood-burning stove. Once washed, I *get* into
my white dressing gown and *prepare* for the trip to the outhouse. My
grandmother *holds* a hurricane lamp out of the back door to light the way.
The path *is* long and dark and *goes* past the cornfield where all the monsters
are. I *can* tell they *are* there, hidden behind the first row, by the way the corn
squeaks and *rustles* as I *pass*. Most feared among them *are* the snakes that *turn*
themselves into hoops and *roll* after you at tremendous speed, thrashing
through the corn as they *come* (13).

_____
_____
_____
_____
_____
_____
_____
_____
_____

⬤ **Exercise 4:** Rewrite the following paragraph from Leo Buscaglia's *Personhood*, changing it from past tense to present.

> A young, anxious businessman helped me to find my way on a busy, smoggy and humid Tokyo afternoon. He went miles off his busy path to direct me to the address I was seeking. In the short period we were together we hardly spoke. We finally bowed in parting and he went quickly on his way. A part of me went with him (3).
>
> Leo Buscaglia, *Personhood*

_____

_____

_____

_____

_____

_____

⬤ **Exercise 5:** For each item that follows, write one sentence.

Example

Write a sentence that includes the word *given*.
I wish that they had given us a choice.

1. Write a sentence that includes the word *begun*.

_____

2. Write a sentence that includes the word *broke*.

_____

3. Write a sentence that includes the word *done*.

_____

4. Write a sentence that includes the word *forgave*.

_____

5. Write a sentence that includes the word *forgotten*.

_____

6. Write a sentence that includes the word *rang*.

_____

7. Write a sentence that includes the word *saw*.

_____

8. Write a sentence that includes the word *spoken*.

_____

9. Write a sentence that includes the word *went*.

_____

10. Write a sentence that includes the word *wrote*.

_____

CHAPTER 10

EASILY CONFUSED WORDS

Because many words look or sound alike, it's easy to make a mistake. Many of those words are listed here in alphabetical order so that you can use these pages as a reference when editing your writing.

a / an / and

A: one. Used generally before a word that begins with a consonant (all letters except vowels)

> *A* **kind man helped my grandmother cross the street.**

An: one. Used generally before a word that begins with a vowel sound (*a, e, i, o, u*)

> *An* **old friend stopped by to say hello.**

And: used to join words or ideas together

> **We hope to pack the car** *and* **leave before dawn.**

accept / except

Accept: to receive (verb)

> **We** *accepted* **the gift and were grateful.**

Except: but, other than. *Ex* means *out* as in *exit.*

> Erin will supply all the food *except* the appetizers.

advice / advise

Advice: an opinion (noun)

> Whenever I want good *advice*, I talk to Philip.

Advise: to give an opinion (verb)

> Philip *advised* me to return to school.

affect / effect

Affect: to influence something (verb)

> Her gentleness *affects* everyone around her.

Effect: a result (noun)

> The *effects* of the winter storm tangled traffic for hours.

a lot

A lot: much. Do not write this as one word. *A lot* is two words.

> We have *a lot* to do before morning.

are / our

Are: a form of the verb *be*

> Matthew and Vanisha *are* happy.

Our: a pronoun showing ownership

> They want to borrow *our* car for the weekend.

break / brake

Break: to smash (verb)

We were determined not to *break* the speed limit.

an interruption (noun)

Everyone is looking forward to spring *break*.

Brake: a device on a vehicle used to slow down or stop (noun)

The *brakes* on our car squeak.

breath / breathe

Breath: the air that goes in and out of lungs (noun)

We went outside for a fresh *breath* of air.

Breathe: to inhale and exhale (verb)

Fumes from the paint factory often make it difficult to *breathe*.

buy / by

Buy: to purchase (verb). Tip: The *u* in the middle can remind you of a U.S. dollar.

We will *buy* what we need and nothing more.

By: near, before (everything that is not *buy*)

We need to be at Chester's house *by* eight o'clock.

confident / confidence

Confident: sure of oneself (adjective). Someone *is* confident.

Joan is *confident* that she can do the job.

Confidence: a belief in one's own abilities (noun). Someone *has* confidence.

Everyone admires Joan's *confidence* and courage.

A number of words have these *-t* and *-ce* endings. One way of explaining the difference between these words is to compare them to the words *happy* and *happiness*.

Adjectives	Nouns
happy	**happiness**
arrogant	arrogance
confident	confidence
different	difference
patient	patience
tolerant	tolerance
violent	violence

Whenever you wonder which word to use, read your sentence and substitute the word *happy* and then *happiness*. If *happy* makes sense, use the word ending in *-t* (*arrogant, confident, different . . .*). If *happiness* makes sense, use the word ending in *-ce* (*arrogance, confidence, difference . . .*). For example, in the following sentences, which is correct: *patient* or *patience*?

Jake is a _____ person.

- Would we say "Jake is a *happy* person" or "Jake is a *happiness* person"? Because we would say *happy*, the correct word is *patient*.

His _____ helps me relax.

- Would we say "His *happy* helps me relax" or "His *happiness* helps me relax"? We would say *happiness*, so the correct word is *patience*.

conscience / conscious

Conscience: a person's sense of right and wrong; an inner voice (noun)

The parents counted on their children's *conscience* to guide them.

Conscious: awake, aware (adjective)

I was *conscious* of a strange tingling in my foot.

desert / dessert

Desert: a hot, dry place (noun)

During summer, wildflowers bloom in the *desert*.

to abandon, to leave (verb)

The birds *deserted* our feeder when natural food was available nearby.

Dessert: food eaten after a meal (noun). Tip: *Dessert* has two *s*'s. It is something we would like two of.

We skipped lunch and ordered *dessert*.

due / do

Due: owed as a debt

Many of our bills are *due* on the fourteenth of each month.

expected

Their baby is *due* in September.

Do: to perform (verb)

We *do* the chores on Saturday mornings.

a helping verb

They *do* like to eat.

find / fine

Find: to locate (verb)

We *find* satisfaction in a job well done.

Fine: good (adjective)

My sister-in-law said she had a *fine* time at the barbeque.

penalty (noun)

Because the meter ran out, we have to pay a seventy-five-dollar parking *fine*.

gonna

Gonna is incorrect. When people say *gonna*, they are simply saying *going to* quickly.

We are *going to* register for classes on Monday.

good / well

Good: adjective, describes a noun

Our neighbor across the street is a *good* woman.

Well: adverb, describes a verb

Calvin plays the drums *well*.

adjective: healthy

My grandmother looks and feels *well*, even at the age of eighty-seven.

hear / here

Hear: to pick up sound (verb). Tip: Notice the word *ear* in h*ear*.

I *hear* someone singing.

Here: in this place

How many people are planning to be *here* over the weekend?

hole / whole

Hole: a cavity, an opening (noun)

After a harsh winter, the expressway is filled with *holes*.

Whole: complete (adjective)

Their *whole* argument was brilliant.

it's / its

It's: a contraction of *it is*

If *it's* a nice day, we are heading for the beach.

a contraction of *it has*

***It's* been a long time since we have had a vacation.**

- It's always means *it is* or *it has*. If you do not mean *it is* or *it has*, write the word without the apostrophe: *its*.

Its: a pronoun showing ownership

The company is reviewing *its* health care benefits.

knew / new

Knew: to understand (past tense of the verb *know*)

Shandra *knew* that we would help.

New: unused, recent (adjective)

The *new* restaurant will open next month.

know / no / now

Know: to understand (verb)

Ernesto *knows* everything about computers.

No: used to form the negative

We will *no* longer postpone our decision.

Now: present time

We are ready to act *now*.

lose / loose

Lose: to misplace something (verb)

Did you *lose* your sunglasses?

Loose: not fixed in place (adjective)

The fan belt on the car is *loose* and must be replaced.

mind / mine

Mind: the brain (noun)

Grace will make up her *mind* as soon as she knows her options.

to object (verb)

We don't *mind* if it takes a long time.

Mine: pronoun showing ownership

Doug can borrow anything of *mine*.

of: could have / would have / should have

Could of, would of, and *should of* are incorrect. The way we say these words makes the *have* sound like *of*. When we say *would of*, we are really saying *would have* quickly.

I *should have* listened to the weather report.

pass / passed / past

Pass and *passed:* verbs showing action

We will *pass* this test easily.

He *passed* the ball to Marcos.

The past tense, *passed*, is also used to refer to death.

My friend *passed* away last week.

Past: beyond (preposition)

We walked *past* the theater.

what happened before the present moment (noun)

The *past* is gone; the future is before us.

- Notice that *pass* and *passed* are verbs, but *past* is not a verb. *Past* does not name any action. Another word in the sentence will name the action, and *past* will tell something about it.

peace / piece

Peace: calm, no disagreement

After leaving the past behind, a sense of *peace* came over us.

Piece: a portion

He ordered a *piece* of blueberry pie.

quiet / quit / quite

Quiet: not noisy (adjective)

Juanita studies in the library because it is *quiet*.

Quit: to stop (verb)

If people don't start smoking, they will not have to *quit*.

Quite: a bit, very (adverb)

The receptionist was *quite* helpful.

right / write

Right: correct (adjective)

Claude knew the *right* answer immediately.

Write: to put words on paper or another surface (verb)

If I don't *write* it down, I'll forget it.

sit / set

Sit: to be seated, usually in a chair

We arrived early so that we would have time to *sit* down and relax.

Set: to put

Please *set* the table.

- *Set* is always followed by something: set a record, a table, a goal.

suppose / supposed

When the word *to* follows the word *suppose*, add *-d* to *suppose* (*supposed*).

They were *supposed* to call before they left.

then / than

Then: next, at a certain time. *Then* refers to time.

They ran a mile and *then* walked three miles.

Than: a word used in a comparison

My aunt would rather cook *than* go out for dinner.

they're / their / there

They're: a contraction of *they are.* When writing, ask yourself, "Do I mean *they are?*" If you do, write either *they are* or *they're.*

All the cousins said that *they're* planning to be with us on Thanksgiving.

Their: a pronoun showing ownership

Their car is parked in our driveway.

There: a word used in two ways. It can refer to a location, or it can introduce an idea. Tip: Notice the word *here* in *there.*

a location

We went *there* early, hoping to find a seat in the front row.

introducing a thought

There are countless opportunities for volunteer work.

threw / through / though

Threw: a verb, the past tense of the verb *throw*

The child *threw* the ball across the fence.

Through: from one side to the other (preposition)

Commuters drive *through* the tunnel to reach New York City.

Though: although

Even *though* they don't agree with my decision, they understand and support me.

two / too / to

Two: the number 2

The restaurant coupon offers *two* dinners for the price of one.

Too: excess, also. Tip: the additional *o* can remind you of too much, as in *excess.*

The sleeves are *too* long, and the pants are *too* short. (excess)
My nephew wants to watch the movie *too.* (also)

To: used as part of an infinitive or as a preposition.

infinitive, such as *to see, to drive, to dance*
Alex is determined *to* succeed.

a preposition, such as *to the game, to Florida*
We drove *to* the concert on Saturday.

use / used

When the word *to* follows the word *use,* add -*d* to *use* (*used*).

Kathy *used* to write letters; now she sends e-mail.

weather / whether

Weather: climate (snow, rain, sunshine, clouds)

Warm *weather* is predicted for Saturday.

Whether: suggests a question

We have to decide *whether* to fly or drive.

we're / were

We're: a contraction of *we are*

We're relieved that the exam is over.

Were: past tense of the verb *be*

Julia and Vincent *were* best friends in high school.

where / wear

Where: a place or location

Where did the time go?

Wear: to put on clothes (verb)

The invitation said to *wear* casual clothes.

who's / whose

Who's: a contraction of *who is*

Who's planning to help clean up?

a contraction of *who has*

We do not know *who's* signed the petition.

- If you don't mean *who is* or *who has*, write *whose*.

Whose: a pronoun showing ownership.

The student *whose* book I borrowed was absent today.

worse / worst

Worse: a form of the word *bad*, meaning "badder." Use it to compare two things.

The weather on Saturday was *worse* than it was on Friday.

Worst: a form of the word *bad*, meaning "baddest." Use it to compare three or more things.

The weather on Sunday was the *worst* weather we had all week.

you're / your

You're: a contraction of *you are*. When writing, ask yourself, "Do I mean *you are*?" If you do, write either *you are* or *you're*.

You're a faithful friend.

- If you do not mean *you are*, write *your*.

Your: a pronoun showing ownership

Your lunch is ready.

• •

Exercises

⬤ **Self Test:** Find and correct the easily confused word errors in the following sentences. A sentence may have one to three errors or none at all. If a sentence is correct as is, mark it with a *C*.

1. Its not to late to change your mine.

2. I no now that we should of paid are bills on time.

3. Some people get angry when your right and there wrong.

4. John past the ball to Mark, who was suppose to grab it.

5. I can talk faster then I can right.

6. Who's bringing the dessert?

7. The angry customers announced that they would take there business elsewhere.

8. Kristin an Kelly were to surprised to say anything to they're boss.

9. Because I excepted responsibility an didn't quiet, I succeeded.

10. After the fire, we could not breath because the hole room was filled with smoke.

● **Exercise 1:** Find and correct the easily confused word errors in the following sentences. A sentence may have one to five errors or none at all. If a sentence is correct as is, mark it with a *C*.

1. I use to think that its better to win then to loose.

2. You should of adviced me not to by the worse car on the lot.

3. We have the patience and confidence we need to succeed.

4. After taking the medication, I am suppose to set down and rest for twenty minutes.

5. After working threw are problems, we were able to leave the passed behind and find piece.

6. I will have a clear conscious once I right a letter to apologize.

7. We hear that the whether will be warm and we should where comfortable clothes.

8. I thought know one could read my mine.

9. If he runs as good as he can in the three-mile race, he will brake the record.

10. My uncle told me yesterday, "Your foolish. You should of saved your money, but know its to late."

⬤ **Exercise 2:** Edit the following draft by correcting the easily confused word errors.

Change is a part of life, and adapting to different seasons is essential. When I was four years old, I had a knew roommate I did not want. I was use to getting all the attention, and all of a sudden my parents brought home a screaming newborn they called "your little baby brother." This little baby took over. That was my first experience of winter. I have known other winters. Grade school an high school we're not easy. Then soon after my high school graduation, my parents were divorced, leaving me with the responsibility of looking after my brother.

But I have also known springtime. Taking college courses at night has allowed me to keep my daytime job. Last month, my boss surprised me with a raise, saying, "Your the most responsible man I have hired in years." Most of all, I am now dating a wonderful woman. Knew possibilities are opening for me, and today feels as if its springtime. Although my future will not always be this green, I no that I can adapt too winter. When the whether changes, I can change with it.

Student writer

⬤ **Exercise 3:** For each item that follows, write one sentence that includes both words.

Example

    Write a sentence that includes the words *their* and *there*.
    My friends want to know whether they can park their car there overnight.

1. Write a sentence that includes the words *are* and *our*.

_____

2. Write a sentence that includes the words *confidence* and *patient*.

_____

3. Write a sentence that includes the words *due* and *do*.

_____

4. Write a sentence that includes the words *here* and *hear*.

_____

5. Write a sentence that includes the words *know* and *no*.

_____

6. Write a sentence that includes the words *then* and *than*.

_____

7. Write a sentence that includes the words *weather* and *whether*.

_____

8. Write a sentence that includes the words *we're* and *were*.

_____

9. Write a sentence that includes the words *worse* and *worst*.

_____

10. Write a sentence that includes the words *you're* and *your*.

_____

PRONOUNS

Pronouns are words that take the place of nouns (persons, places, or things). We use pronouns so that we don't have to repeat the same word over and over again.

. . . .

Section A: Pronoun Types and Reference

There are many types of pronouns. We will focus here on **personal, indefinite, reflexive,** and **intensive pronouns.**

PERSONAL PRONOUNS

Personal pronouns can play various roles in a sentence. They can be subjects, objects, or possessives.

PERSONAL PRONOUNS			
	Subject	**Object**	**Possessive**
Singular	I	me	my, mine
	you	you	your, yours
	he, she, it	him, her, it	his, her, hers, its
Plural	we	us	our, ours
	you	you	your, yours
	they	them	their, theirs

We use the subject pronouns as subjects in a sentence. They often do the action.

> *They* walked along the beach.
>
> Yesterday, *I* drove to Cincinnati.

- The pronoun *I* is always capitalized.

We use the object pronouns as objects of verbs and prepositions. They often receive the action.

> Sally appreciates *us*.   Kenneth smiled at *me*.
>
> Alan respects *her*.   We threw a party for *them*.

We use the possessive pronouns to show ownership.

> Community residents voiced *their* concerns at the meeting.
>
> We have three tickets. One is *his*. One is *hers*. One is *mine*.

- Notice that *his* and *hers* end in *-s*. *Mine* does not.

INDEFINITE PRONOUNS

Pronouns ending in *-one*, *-body*, and *-thing* are called *indefinite pronouns*.

COMMON INDEFINITE PRONOUNS			
(-one)	(-body)	(-thing)	Other
no one	nobody	nothing	any
anyone	anybody	anything	each
everyone	everybody	everything	every
someone	somebody	something	

The pronouns listed above are singular. When they are used as the subject of a sentence, the present-tense verb ends in *-s*.

> No one *wants* to leave.

- Because the pronoun *no one* is singular, we use the *-s* form: *wants*.

> Everything (on the display shelves) *is* half price.

- The words after the subject (*on the display shelves*) do not change the subject.

REFLEXIVE AND INTENSIVE PRONOUNS

Pronouns ending in *-self* and *-selves* are called reflexive and intensive pronouns.

REFLEXIVE AND INTENSIVE PRONOUNS

Singular	Plural
myself	ourselves
yourself	yourselves
himself	themselves
herself	
itself	

These pronouns show that the subject does something to or for itself:

> **The directors gave** *themselves* **a raise.**
> **I taught** *myself* **how to type.**

They also show emphasis:

> **She decided to paint the room** *herself.*
> **I** *myself* **want no part of that decision.**

If you are not emphasizing yourself or doing something to yourself, use *I* or *me*—not *myself:*

> **Keith and** *I* **took Latoya out for dinner.**
> **Peggy gave** *me* **the mail.**

Make sure you spell these words correctly:

> **They congratulated** *themselves* **when they completed the project.**

● Write *themselves*, not "theirselves" or "their selfs."

> **While lifting the lumber out of the truck, Milton hurt** *himself.*

● Write *himself*, not "hisself."

PRONOUN REFERENCE

The words or word that a pronoun refers to is called the **antecedent**.

> **Wilson keeps an extra set of keys at *his* office.**

- *His* refers to *Wilson*.
- *Wilson* is the antecedent of *his*.

Avoiding Vague Reference

When you use pronouns in your writing, make sure the pronoun's antecedent is clear. You know what word the pronoun refers to, but your reader may not.

Example 1

Vague: When Deborah told Judy what had happened, she was furious.

- Who is *she*? Was Deborah furious, or was Judy furious?

Clear: When Deborah told Judy what had happened, Judy was furious.

Example 2

Vague: When I asked about summer classes, they told me registration begins next week.

- Who is *they*? We don't know whether the writer means students in the hall, someone in the registration office, or friends in the parking lot.

Clear: When I asked about summer classes, the registrar told me registration begins next week.

Example 3

Vague: Jordan's dad often told him that he was a good driver.

- Who is the good driver: Jordan's dad or Jordan?
- Sometimes the best way to make the meaning clear is to rewrite the sentence.

Clear: Jordan's dad often told him, "Jordan, you are a good driver."

Avoiding a Shift

When we talk, we often use *you* to refer to people in general. In more formal writing, replace the general *you* with whomever you specifically mean. Use the word *you* only when you are speaking directly to the reader.

Also watch for unexpected pronoun shifts. For example, if you are writing about people, use *they*. If you are writing about yourself, use *I*. If you are writing about yourself and others, use *we*. Do not switch to the pronoun *you*.

When people work hard, ~~you~~ *they* feel a sense of accomplishment.

I buy clothes in stores rather than on the Internet because ~~you~~ *I* can see the merchandise.

• •

Exercises: Section A

⬤ **Self Test A:** Find and correct the pronoun problems in the following sentences. If a sentence is correct as is, mark it with a *C*.

1. Nicole gave a shirt to Jerry and a jacket to myself.

2. Everybody in the class agrees that the test should be postponed.

3. I assembled the gas grill by my self.

4. When I dropped the coffee cup on the glass table, it shattered into pieces.

5. Bonnie likes to visit her cousins in Atlanta because they always make you feel at home.

⬤ **Exercise 1a:** The sentences that follow are confusing because we are not sure what word the pronoun refers to. Rewrite the sentences so that the meaning is clear. Sometimes you will have to add your own words, as shown in the example.

Example

The city
~~They~~ should fix the potholes on Main Street.

1. Jeff helped Andy repave the driveway, but he did most of the work.

2. Dentists tell their patients to floss daily, but they don't do it.

3. In the halls, it says that the campus parking lot will be closed on Monday.

4. When Brenda was telling Marlene the joke, she burst out laughing.

5. Allison's sister and brother are both teachers, but it doesn't interest her.

● **Exercise 2a:** In the following sentences, replace *you* with the specific pronoun the writer needs.

Example

we

When we toured the art gallery, ~~you~~ were impressed by the power of painting.

1. I am trying to fill out the application form, but you don't understand half the questions.

2. When we looked at Jerome, you could tell he had not slept all night.

3. I want Sheila to help me with algebra because she explains things so that you can understand them.

4. When students register late, you often find that classes are filled.

5. Tony types his papers in the computer lab because you can ask the computer technician for help.

● **Exercise 3a:** In the following paragraph, correct the pronoun problems. Once you have made your corrections, you may also need to change the verb so that the new subject and verb agree.

Getting to school on time is not easy for Nikki because she lives fifty miles from campus. She always has to leave early because you can't predict how heavy the traffic will be. The traffic is even worse in summer because they do road construction and a lane is always shut down. In winter, you often can't get to the expressway because snowdrifts block the side streets. Sometimes Nikki thinks about moving closer to campus, but then you would have to face the hassle of moving.

Student writer

• •

Section B: Pronoun Agreement and Placement

Pronouns must agree with (match) their antecedents. Use singular pronouns to refer to singular nouns; use plural pronouns to refer to plural nouns.

AGREEMENT WITH SINGULAR AND PLURAL

If the noun is singular, the pronoun that refers to it must be singular.

> **Karen will type *her* paper sometime tonight.**
>
> • Because *Karen* is singular, the pronoun is singular.

If the noun is plural, the pronoun that refers to it must be plural.

> **My cousins are determined to pay *their* bills on time.**
>
> • Because the word *cousins* is plural, the pronoun is plural.

A Common Problem

Be careful not to use a plural pronoun to refer to a singular noun.

> **Incorrect:** If a *student* wants a parking permit, *they* need to register on Monday.
>
> • *Student* is singular; *they* is plural. The noun and pronoun do not match.

Solution 1

Change the pronoun.

> **Correct:** If a *student* wants a parking permit, *he or she* needs to register on Monday.
>
> • Because *student* is singular, we need a singular pronoun. If we write *he*, we could offend women. If we write *she*, we could offend men. We need to cover both genders by including both pronouns.

Solution 2

Change the noun.

> **Correct:** If *students* want a parking permit, *they* need to register on Monday.

- Changing the noun to plural is the easiest solution. If we write *students*, we don't need to choose between masculine and feminine. The pronoun *they* refers to both genders.

RECOGNIZING SUBJECT AND OBJECT

If the pronoun is doing the action, choose a subject pronoun: *I, you, he, she, it, we, they*.

> *He* walked five miles yesterday.

If the pronoun is receiving the action, choose an object pronoun: *me, you, him, her, us, them*.

> **Chelsea hugged *him*.**

A Common Problem

If another noun (person, place, or thing) is added, the pronoun remains the same. Make sure you use the correct pronoun.

> **Correct:** The manager gave *me* a raise.

> **Correct:** The manager gave *Daniel* and *me* a raise.

- Adding *Daniel* does not change the correct pronoun.

> **Incorrect:** The manager gave Daniel and I a raise.

Solution

If English is your native language, you can find the correct pronoun by temporarily removing the person's name from the sentence. Once that name is removed, you will be able to see what pronoun to use. Then return the person's name to the sentence.

Example 1

Incorrect: The mail was addressed to ~~Fred and~~ she.

- Temporarily remove *Fred*. The sentence now reads *The mail was addressed to she*. We wouldn't say *she*; we would say *her*. Now that we know the correct pronoun, we can return *Fred* to the sentence.

Correct: The mail was addressed to Fred and her.

Example 2

Incorrect: ~~My friends and~~ me went shopping.

- Temporarily remove *my friends*. The sentence now reads *Me went shopping*. We wouldn't say *me*; we would say *I*. We can now return *my friends* to the sentence.

Correct: My friends and I went shopping.

Example 3

Incorrect: There is a big difference between ~~my brother and~~ I.

- Temporarily remove *my brother*. Even though the preposition *between* needs two objects, you can hear the problem with *between I. Between me* sounds better.

Correct: There is a big difference between my brother and me.

PRONOUN PLACEMENT

When you are using the pronoun *I* along with the name of someone else, it is considered polite to name the other person first.

Incorrect: Me and Monica are planning a party.

- There are two problems here. First, the wrong pronoun is used: We need *I*, not *me*. Second, we need to put the noun (*Monica*) first.

Correct: Monica and I are planning a party.

Exercises: Section B

● **Self Test B:** Read each sentence and decide whether the pronoun is used correctly. If the pronoun is correct, mark the sentence with a *C*. If the pronoun is incorrect, mark the sentence with a checkmark (✓) and correct it.

1. My neighbor and him did not get along.

2. A taxpayer must pay their taxes no later than April 15.

3. My sister and 1 called Mom to wish her a happy birthday.

4. Many car thefts occur because the driver leaves their keys in the ignition.

5. I am happy that me and Crystal will be in the same class.

6. Just between you and I, this English class is easy.

7. A writer can improve their vocabulary by reading.

8. Me and Josh will set up the picnic tables.

9. At the end of August, Brent and her will take a two-week vacation.

10. The instructor asked Rick and me to lead the discussion.

● **Exercise 1b:** Some of the following sentences use pronouns incorrectly. Find and correct the errors. If the sentence is correct, mark it with a *C*.

Example

Me and Janet went to the concert.
Janet and I went to the concert.

1. Stanley is willing to help Helen and me paint the living room.

2. Dennis met Alicia and her in the bookstore.

3. Roy and her walked five miles yesterday.

4. We want Brandon and he to go with us.

5. Family members always turn to my husband and I for advice.

6. Me and my brother will go shopping this weekend.

7. Sally and him are good friends.

8. Chris and her gave a surprise party for Justin and I.

9. The job will give Paula and I financial security.

10. The doctor talked to my mother and me about the test results.

● **Exercise 2b:** In the following sentences, the noun and the pronoun do not match. Correct the problem by changing the singular noun to a plural noun. In most cases, you will also have to change the verb so that the new subject and verb agree.

Example

A loyal friend is there when we need them.
Loyal friends are there when we need them.

1. A renter needs to pay for one month's rent before they move in.

2. A person can compare prices of products on the Internet before they decide what they want to buy.

3. A student will receive their grades in the mail.

4. In many companies, an employee can have their paychecks deposited directly into their checking accounts.

5. If a resident wants to learn CPR (cardiopulmonary resuscitation), they can take a free course at the local hospital.

⬤ **Exercise 3b:** Find and correct the pronoun errors in the following paragraph.

For the past three months, me and Jerry have been looking for an apartment. We now have the process down to a science. My sister Betty reads the Sunday newspaper and circles apartments that look promising. Because she knows what we want, she saves Jerry and I valuable time. During the week, Jerry and her then drive by the apartments to check out the neighborhoods. If a neighborhood is attractive, me and Jerry make an appointment with the landlord. After we see the apartment, we take one more step. We always try to talk with tenants, who so far have given us important information. For example, last week me and Jerry found a place we thought was perfect. But by talking to the tenants we met in the parking lot, we learned that the landlord takes months to repair broken appliances. This three-step process has taught Jerry and me that finding a place to call home will take time.

Student writer

PART 3

FINE-TUNING SENTENCES

CLARITY

. . . .

Section A: Choosing Words Carefully

Talking takes place on the spot, giving us little time to revise and edit. We say words as they come to us, fill in the silent spaces with words to keep the conversation going, and often ramble. Writing is different. We have time to correct our errors, choose our words carefully, and replace empty words that carry little meaning with specific words. We have time to make every word count. This chapter will show you how to fine-tune your words to make your writing more effective.

AVOIDING A SHIFT IN TENSE

Yesterday, we were nervous. Today, we are more relaxed. Tomorrow, we will be confident. The verbs in these sentences change tense from past (*were*) to present (*are*) to future (*will be*) to show the difference between yesterday, today, and tomorrow. These changes in tense are necessary. Often, however, writers make the mistake of changing verb tense when there is no change in time.

When you are writing about events that happened in the past, do not switch from past tense to present tense in the middle of the story. We often do this when talking, but when writing, you should change the tense of your verbs only when you want to show a specific change in time.

Incorrect

> I *was standing* outside my apartment when my neighbor *approached*
> me. She *seemed* uneasy as she *said* hello. Slowly, she *took* a deep
> breath and *says* that she *wants* to talk to me. I *replied,* "Sure," and
> *walked* with her toward her apartment. As we *approached* her door, she
> *has* this strange look on her face. Obviously, she *is* afraid of something
> or someone. Her hands *begin* to shake as she *searches* for her keys.

- The passage begins with the past tense (*was standing, approached, seemed, said, took*) and switches to present tense (*says, wants*). It then returns to past tense (*replied, walked, approached*) and flips again to present tense (*has, is, begin, searches*).

The events all occurred in the past, so the verbs should all be past tense. When you write, keep the tense consistent unless you are indicating a time change in the events you are describing. Choose either past or present and stay with it. The following paragraph is written correctly.

Correct

> I *was standing* outside my apartment when my neighbor *approached*
> me. She *seemed* uneasy as she *said* hello. Slowly, she *took* a deep
> breath and *said* that she *wanted* to talk to me. I *replied,* "Sure," and
> *walked* with her toward her apartment. As we *approached* her door, she
> *had* this strange look on her face. Obviously, she *was* afraid of
> something or someone. Her hands *began* to shake as she *searched* for
> her keys.

OMITTING DOUBLE NEGATIVES

In standard English, do not use more than one negative term in a negative statement. Negative terms are words like *not, n't* (contraction), *hardly, barely, scarcely,* and *nothing.*

> **Incorrect:** *Nobody* did *nothing.*
> **Correct:** *Nobody* did *anything.*

> **Incorrect:** Edwin *couldn't scarcely* breathe.
> **Correct:** Edwin *could scarcely* breathe.
> **Correct:** Edwin *couldn't* breathe.

> **Incorrect:** Pat *can't hardly* walk straight.
> **Correct:** Pat *can hardly* walk straight.
> **Correct:** Pat *can't* walk straight.

> **Incorrect:** My choir teacher *didn't* take *no* excuses.
> **Correct:** My choir teacher *didn't* take *any* excuses.
> **Correct:** My choir teacher *took no* excuses.

OMITTING UNNECESSARY WORDS

When you edit your papers, make sure you avoid repeating the subject, delete empty words, get straight to the point, replace wordy phrases, and combine and condense your sentences.

Avoid Repeating the Subject

When we talk, we often announce the subject and immediately repeat it by using the pronouns *he, she, it, that,* or *they.* For example, we might say, "My sister she has a dentist appointment tomorrow." We announce that the subject is *sister,* and then we immediately repeat that subject with *she.* When we write, we need to avoid the repetition and write one clear subject.

> My sister ~~she~~ has a dentist appointment tomorrow.
> The fans who arrived early ~~they~~ got the best seats.

Delete Empty Words

The following words and phrases are "empty" because they give no information. As you edit your writing, delete them.

The thing is . . . you know . . . well . . . like I mean . . . kind of . . . anyway . . .
(We often use these "fillers" when talking. Omit them from your writing.)

I am going to write about . . . Let me give you an example . . .
(Don't say what you are going to do. Just do it.)

As you can see from what I've written . . . I guess you can tell that . . . Like I said . . .
(Omit. Readers will understand your point if you give them enough specific information.)

I could go on and on about this.
(Omit. These words actually lead readers to believe you have run out of ideas.)

Get Straight to the Point

Do not pad your writing with empty words that exhaust readers. Effective writing gets straight to the point. If you want or need to make your paper longer, add specific examples or details that prove your point.

Empty Words: In the modern-day world of this day and age, I would venture to say that we people in these United States, each and every one of us, in my opinion, drive in our automobiles along the roads and highways of our land too fast.

- *In the modern-day world of this day and age* means today. If we use a present-tense verb, we don't need this string of words. *I would venture to say that* tells us nothing, so we can delete it. *We people in these United States* means Americans, so let's use *Americans. Each and every one of us* is unnecessary. *In my opinion* is unnecessary because readers already know that this statement is the writer's opinion. The words *in our automobiles along the roads and highways of our land* include only one word of substance: *automobiles.* And we don't need *automobiles* because the preceding sentence uses *drive.*

Direct Words: Americans drive too fast.

- Once we delete the padding, we have a clear, direct statement.

Replace Wordy Phrases

Wordy phrases are groups of words that can be replaced by more concise words.

Wordy	Concise
in spite of the fact that	although
the question as to whether	whether
he is a man who	he
until such a time as	until
at this point in time	now
for the purpose of	for
because of the fact	because
due to the fact that	because
the reason why is that	because
the reason being	because
in the event that	if
owing to the fact that	since
last but not least	finally

Combine and Condense Sentences

Look for sentences that would be more effective if they were combined and unnecessary words deleted.

Example 1

Choppy: The hurricane had a lot of effects. There were mudslides. In addition to mudslides, there were floods.

Concise: The hurricane produced mudslides and floods.

- By omitting unnecessary words, we have combined three sentences into one sentence.

Example 2

Choppy: A fence surrounded the garden of roses and wildflowers. The fence wasn't painted.

Concise: An unpainted fence surrounded the garden of roses and wildflowers.

- Sometimes a more exact word can replace two or more words. Notice that *unpainted* gives the same information as *wasn't painted* but with fewer words.

• •

Exercises: Section A

◯ **Self Test A:** Rewrite each item so that it is a correct and direct sentence. When there are two sentences, condense them into one sentence. You will need to delete words, correct words, and use concise replacements.

Example

~~The reason why~~ I have chosen nursing as a career ~~is~~ because I want to help people.

I have chosen nursing as a career because I want to help people.

Example

~~This paper is going to be about how I feel about recycling. I guess you could say that it is important because~~ recycling ~~a lot of things like~~ paper and aluminum cans helps protect ~~the quality of~~ our environment ~~in this world that we live in today~~.

Recycling paper and aluminum cans helps protect our environment.

1. I am going to write about our financial problems. They were a nightmare.

_____

2. In my opinion, if people want to succeed, I mean really want to succeed, they need to know their priorities.

_____

3. In spite of the fact that Mr. Henrickson is strict, the thing is that he is someone who is fair.

_____

4. I want to give you an example of what I believe. I believe that children are affected by the violence that is portrayed in movies in this day and age that we live in.

_____

5. My goal is to become independent. I could go on and on about this because being independent is the goal I have set for my future, and I want to achieve this goal of independence in three years.

_____

● **Exercise 1a:** In each of the following sentences, find and omit the repeated subjects.

Last summer's work schedule ~~it~~ gave me time to relax.

1. Too many drivers they run red lights.

2. My Tuesday evening class it is my favorite class.

3. Taking care of my family and going to school they are both important to me.

4. Mark's graduation that was a day we will always remember.

5. Getting an *A* on that paper it made my day.

● **Exercise 2a:** The following paragraph describes an event that happened in the past. Therefore, all the verbs should be in past tense. In a few places, the writer incorrectly switches to present tense. Find those verbs and change them to past tense.

As the bus began to pick up speed, a green light flashed a warning sign. The marine driver shouts, "The brakes failed!" He tried to keep control of the bus and maneuvered past the van in front of us, but the straight road soon changed into a series of curves as it twisted down the mountain. The bus is out of control. We made a left turn, flipped on the right side, and skidded seventy feet down the road's shallow slope. I jump out of my seat to grab the overhead hand rail, but I was slammed into the ceiling of the bus. Finally, we come to a stop. Everything moves in slow motion. It was an eerie feeling.

Student writer

● **Exercise 3a:** Combine each set of sentences into one sentence by omitting unnecessary words.

Our community firemen and paramedics are volunteers. They are dedicated.

Our community firemen and paramedics are dedicated volunteers.

1. I went to a movie last night. Vicki went with me. That movie was frightening.

   _____

2. Each graduate walked across the stage. Every single one of them walked slowly and proudly.

   _____

3. We enjoyed the scenery of the mountains. We also liked the silence there.

   _____

4. Information about federal agencies is available. It is on the Internet. You can also get information about state agencies on the Internet.

   _____

5. The ambassador said that global warming is a problem with consequences. The problem is long-term. The consequences are political and economic.

   _____

• •

Section B: Using Specific Words

Specific words create vivid pictures in readers' minds. To help readers see, hear, smell, and feel what you are describing, replace general words with specific ones.

Replace general nouns with more specific nouns.

General	Specific
flowers	daisies, daffodils, roses, tulips, marigolds
breakfast	pancakes with maple syrup, orange juice, scrambled eggs
road	State Street, expressway, dirt path, side street

Rather than use *very* to intensify the meaning of another word, such as *scary*, find a word that means *very scary*.

General	Specific
very scary movie	terrifying, horrifying, hair-raising, frightening, bone-chilling
very nice person	cheerful, generous, caring, gentle, supportive
I was *very happy*	delighted, excited, thrilled, elated, ecstatic

Replace general verbs with more specific verbs.

General	Specific
said	whispered, explained, warned, advised, asked
made a noise	blared, crackled, gurgled, rattled, screeched
looked	stared, gazed, glanced, watched, peeked

Compare something you are writing about to something else. You can use *like* or *as* to make the comparison (simile) or omit these words (metaphor).

Example 1

Marianne is as gentle as a summer breeze.

- The words *summer breeze* help us imagine Marianne as a soft, smooth, and refreshing person.
- If you compare two things by using the words *like* or *as*, you are using a simile.

Example 2

Marianne is a gentle summer breeze.

- We know that Marianne is not really a summer breeze; the words help us visualize her.
- If you omit the words *like* or *as*, you are using a metaphor.

Try using everyday words in new ways. Use words that usually describe one thing to describe something else.

The instructor put my paper on an autopsy table.

● ●

Exercises: Section B

⬤ **Self Test B:** Read the following excerpts from Gary Soto's *Jesse* and underline the words and parts of sentences that help you see, hear, or feel the scene.

Example

> My only company was a kitchen sink with a <u>drippy faucet</u> and a <u>bluish fly beating the windowsill</u> where the <u>sunlight crouched in a yellowish blaze</u>. The house <u>creaked</u>, especially the living room, and the air was <u>heavy with the moisture of a new day</u> (38).

1. That night Glenda came over with her baby and a bag of doughnuts, which all four of us ate on the small patch of itchy lawn. We looked at the stars, our hands cupped around our eyes like blinders (33).

2. The day moved slowly; the crucifixlike shadow of the telephone pole crawled across the road (49).

3. "Where is everyone?" I asked. My words were picked up by the April wind and rushed away, maybe dropped in the yellow weeds where snakes and gophers struggled over a meager living (71).

4. The tires whined on the road. Wind whistled through the wing window and diesel trucks whizzed by, rocking our car. I was saved from boredom by the landscape, which I recognized from days chopping cotton and picking grapes. It kicked in a dusty memory of the time I worked on my knees nine hours— one hundred seventy-eight trays of grapes—so I could buy my mom an umbrella, one I had spotted hanging from the limp arm of a mannequin in a window (100).

5. When we pulled over to the side of the road, gravel crunching beneath the tires, I was amazed because it was the spot where Abel and I had gotten stuck hitchhiking to Pismo Beach. . . . I walked over to where Abel and I had slept. The grass was growing back, covering up the evidence that we had camped our loneliness there. I raked back the grass and discovered two apple cores,

whittled down to brown rot by ants. I remembered when Abel and I had eaten those apples. It had been dark, and neither of us could see the other's jaws going up and down on the sweetness of apple. We shivered that night and tried to convince each other that it was a learning experience to sleep in a field within earshot of a highway. We told stories, too, but mostly we just sat, cross-legged under the weight of stars and the push of time (100–01).

● **Exercise 1b:** Read each sentence and then answer the question that follows.

Example

> **Insects click in the field. —Richard Rodriguez, "To the Border"**
> **What unusual word describes insects?** *click*

1. Moonbeams splash and spill wildly in the rain. —Virginia Woolf, "A Haunted House"

 What unusual words describe moonbeams?

 _____

2. The smile faded slowly from his face. —Conrad Aiken, "Silent Snow, Secret Snow"

 What unusual word describes the smile?

 _____

3. He walks through streets that seem like hallways. —Carmen Naranjo, "Walls"

 The image of hallways tells us that the streets are _____

4. Hold fast to dreams, for if dreams die, life is a broken-winged bird that cannot fly. —Langston Hughes

 Without dreams, life _____

5. Her smile was a two-line checkerboard of white and gold. —Maya Angelou, *Gather Together in My Name*

 Imagine a checkerboard. Now imagine just two lines of it, and the colors in this checkerboard are white and gold. What is Maya Angelou describing here?

 _____

● **Exercise 2b:** The following excerpt is taken from Rick Bragg's *All Over but the Shoutin'*. In this book, Rick Bragg tells the story of his life. Underline the words he has used that help you picture the scene.

I was sitting in a cramped living room in a crumbling housing project, listening to a hollow-eyed and pitiful young woman tell how her little boy had been killed one morning by a stray bullet as he stood in the doorway, his book satchel in his hand, like a little man going to work. She told me how the Dr. Seuss and Winnie the Pooh just fell out on the stoop, how the boy looked up at her after the bullet hit, wide-eyed, wondering. And as she talked, her two surviving children rode tight circles around the couch on their bicycles, because she was afraid to let them play outside in the killing ground of the project courtyard. As I left, shaking her limp hand, she thanked me. I usually just nod my head politely and move on, struck anew every time by the graciousness of people in such a soul-killing time. But this time, I had to ask why. Why thank me for scribbling down her hopeless story for the benefit of people who live so far and safely away from this place where the gunfire twinkles like lightning bugs after dark? She answered by pulling out a scrapbook of her baby's death, cut from the local newspaper. "Peoples remembers it," she said. "People forgets if it ain't wrote down (xiii–xiv)."

CHAPTER 13

PARALLEL STRUCTURES

Sentences with **parallel structures** flow smoothly. They have balance and a pleasing rhythm.

> Pat has been *taking* notes, *completing* assignments, and *studying* hard.

- The items flow smoothly because they all begin with *-ing* verb forms.

> We pay far more attention to *what people do* than *what people say*.

- The items flow smoothly because they have the same *what people . . .* structure.

Words and phrases are parallel when they have similar forms and when they all fit the basic setup. Let's look at what this means.

● ●

Similar Forms

The items in a pair (two things) or in a series (more than two things) must match each other. Therefore, put the items in similar form—all nouns, all adjectives, all present-tense verbs, and so on.

Before the professor *begins* to talk, he *blinks* his eyes, *adjusts* his glasses, and *nods* his head.

- Each item is a present-tense verb.

The elderly couple walked *down the path*, *over the bridge*, and *into the park*.

- Each item is a prepositional phrase.

Sometimes, you may need to change the wording:

fax machines.

We live in a fast-paced world of computers, cell phones, and ~~machines that fax documents.~~

understanding.

Nick is strong, intelligent, and ~~has the ability to understand other people.~~

• •

Basic Setup

Make sure each item fits the setup. To do this, look for the basic setup of the sentence. Then read the setup with each item separately to see whether each one makes sense.

Example 1

Correct: Juan's friends are responsible, kind, and loyal.

The setup is *Juan's friends are*.

- Juan's friends are   responsible
                                     kind
                                     loyal

The setup fits each item.

- Juan's friends are responsible.
- Juan's friends are kind.
- Juan's friends are loyal.

Example 2

Incorrect: We need to fill the gas tank, check the tires, and the oil must be changed.

The setup is *We need to.*

- We need to
  - fill the gas tank
  - check the tires
  - the oil must be changed.

The last item does not make sense in this setup. We must change the wording.

- We need to fill the gas tank, check the tires, and change the oil.

Paired Words

Either . . . or, neither . . . nor, and *not only . . . but also* work together. They set up words that need to be in similar form.

EITHER ... OR

When you use the *either . . . or* pattern, the words following *either* and *or* must match.

Angela will *either* **take a walk** *or* **listen to music.**
We *either* **heard it on the news** *or* **saw it in the newspaper.**

NEITHER ... NOR

The *neither . . . nor* pattern is similar to the *either . . . or* pattern. The only difference is the addition of *-n,* which gives the sentence a negative meaning.

Angela will *neither* **take a walk** *nor* **listen to music.** (She will not take a walk, and she will not listen to music.)
We *neither* **heard it on the news** *nor* **saw it in the newspaper.** (We did not hear it on the news, and we did not see it in the newspaper.)

NOT ONLY ... BUT ALSO

When you use the *not only . . . but also* pattern, make sure the items match.

I gained *not only* **confidence,** *but also* **experience.**

• •

Exercises

⬤ **Self Test:** Each sentence is written in parallel form. Underline the groups of words that are parallel.

Example

They ordered pizza with <u>pepperoni</u>, <u>green peppers</u>, and <u>mushrooms</u>.

Example

Andy's grandmother likes to <u>crochet afghans for her children</u> and <u>knit sweaters for her grandchildren</u>.

1. The Italian restaurant is famous for its antipasto salad, tomato-cheese bread, pasta, and dessert.

2. Before buying a car, talk to your friends, do research on the Internet, and visit a number of dealers.

3. In one afternoon, we were able to paint the walls and install the kitchen counter.

4. I have searched the car, the closet, the garage, and the driveway, and I still cannot find my keys.

5. Scholarship applicants will be judged by academic achievement, financial need, and community involvement.

⬤ **Exercise 1:** Each group has one item that is not parallel to the other items because it does not have the same form. Find that item and change it so that it matches the others.

Example

cool evenings.

sunny days, warm breezes, ~~evenings that are cool~~

1. manager, supervisor, plumbing, teacher

2. listens to the music, skips across the room, dancing in the hall

3. reasonable prices, good service, the food is delicious

4. swollen feet, aching back, muscles that are sore

5. washing the car, mowing the lawn, preparation of the meals, paying the bills

● **Exercise 2:** Each sentence has one item that is not parallel to the other items because it does not have the same form. Find that item and change it so that it matches the others.

Example

mail
We can send the information by fax, e-mail, or ~~by mailing it~~.

1. The cousins were loyal, confident, and being happy.

2. Francisco has a positive attitude and who has many friends.

3. In last winter's storm, the bridge trembles, swayed, and buckled.

4. The lab technician told me to turn on the machine, review the manual, and followed the directions.

5. At the end of the day, the nine-year-old's pockets were stuffed with dead bugs, crumbled flowers, brown leaves, and grass that was dried.

● **Exercise 3:** Complete each of the following sentences by filling in the blanks with parallel words.

1. People must learn to _____ and _____ each other.

2. In five years, I will _____, _____, and _____.

3. Successful students not only _____ but also _____.

4. _____ and _____ will get you nowhere.

5. I am a _____, not a _____.

● **Exercise 4:** Below each quoted sentence is a similar sentence with blanks. Replace the highlighted words in the models with your own words. Be creative; the words you choose can entirely change the meaning of the sentence.

Example

I watch *tiny bat wings flutter across the moon,* listen to *the tinkling bell buoy a mile offshore,* and smell *the incoming sea as it laps thickly across the rocks.* —Elizabeth Lemke, "An Open Window on My Private World"

I watch <u>my mother stir the ingredients,</u> listen to <u>the clattering pots and</u> <u>pans,</u> and smell <u>the warmth of chocolate as the brownies cook in the oven.</u>

1. He crept *to the door* and squinted *through the fogged plate glass.*
    —Richard Wright, "The Man Who Lived Underground"

    He crept _____ and squinted _____.

2. Neither *intelligence* nor *integrity* can be imposed by law. —Carl Becker

    Neither _____ nor _____ can be imposed by law.

3. After nine claustrophobic days in our tents, we were tired of *gin rummy,* disgusted with *paperback novels,* and intolerant of *even the best cowboy stories.*
    —Todd Skinner, "Storming the Tower"

    After nine claustrophobic days in our tents, we were tired of _____,

    disgusted with _____, and intolerant of _____.

4. I sat in my bright kitchen *wondering what to do, knowing I would never sleep.*
    —Alice Munro, "How I Met My Husband"

    I sat in my bright kitchen _____, _____.

5. I want a *wife* who *will plan the menus, do the necessary grocery shopping, prepare the meals, serve them pleasantly,* and then *do the cleaning up* while *I do my studying.* —Judy Brady, "I Want a Wife"

    I want a _____ who will_____, _____,

    _____, _____, and then _____ while I

    _____.

SENTENCE VARIETY

Most writing consists of basic sentences because they are straight to the point. Yet a whole paper of basic sentences can be monotonous. If all of our sentences are the same length and have the same pattern, readers may become bored. We need to create sentence variety by occasionally changing the pattern. One of the best ways to do this is by using additions. As explained in previous chapters, we can place additions (baskets) on the front, in the middle, or on the back of a sentence (bike).

Section A: Additions on the Front

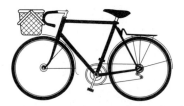

Additions on the front of the bike are not new to us. We have already written sentences beginning with dependent clauses:

> *If Nathan gets off work in time*, he will be at the party.
> *When I arrived home*, I realized that I had left my notebook at school.
> *As the world's demand for seafood grows*, the supply cannot keep pace.
> *Wherever Sarah goes*, she keeps in touch with family.

We will now look at other additions we can place at the beginning of a sentence: prepositional phrases, **infinitive phrases,** and *-ing* additions.*

PREPOSITIONAL PHRASES

One way to achieve sentence variety is to begin a sentence with a prepositional phrase. (See page 17 to review prepositional phrases.)

> *With a quick but penetrating glance,* **the coach revealed his approval.**
>
> *On many campuses,* **students can register and pay for classes over the Internet.**
>
> *In addition to strengthening bones,* **lifting weights can lower cholesterol levels.**
>
> *For three straight nights last November,* **fans lined up to see the concert.**

Often you can use a prepositional phrase in a sentence you have already written. If you need sentence variety, read each sentence and look for a prepositional phrase that would make sense at the beginning of that sentence. If you find one, move it to the beginning of the sentence and mark it with a comma so that readers know where it ends and the basic sentence begins.

Example 1

Before: The bookstore opens at 7:30 a.m. on Tuesdays and Thursdays.

- Take the prepositional phrase *on Tuesdays and Thursdays* and move it to the beginning of the sentence.

After: *On Tuesdays and Thursdays,* the bookstore opens at 7:30 a.m.

Example 2

Before: We decided to quit smoking on a rainy night last April.

- Move the prepositional phrase *on a rainy night last April* to the beginning of the sentence.

After: On a rainy night last April, *we decided to quit smoking.*

---

*Another term for *-ing* additions is **present participial phrases.**

INFINITIVE PHRASES

An infinitive phrase begins with an infinitive (a two-word verb, such as *to walk*, *to run*, *to see*). When you begin a sentence with an infinitive phrase, place a comma at the end of it so that readers can see where it ends and the basic sentence begins.

> *To get there early,* we need to leave before rush hour.
>
> *To stimulate economic activity,* the Federal Reserve reduced borrowing costs.
>
> *To understand the chapter,* you need to read it at least three times.
>
> *To relax after work,* my uncle puts on his headphones and walks around the block.

If your sentences are short and choppy, look for two sentences that could be combined into one by beginning with an infinitive phrase.

Example 1

> **Choppy:** We count our blessings daily. ~~We do this~~ to keep problems in perspective.

- The second sentence includes an infinitive phrase: *to keep problems in perspective.* Take this phrase out of the second sentence and use it to start the first sentence.

> **Concise:** *To keep problems in perspective,* we count our blessings daily.

Example 2

> **Choppy:** Trisha needs to take summer classes. ~~She wants~~ to graduate in two years.

- The second sentence includes an infinitive phrase: *to graduate in two years.* Move this phrase to the beginning of the first sentence.

> **Concise:** *To graduate in two years,* Trisha needs to take summer classes.

-*ING* ADDITIONS

We can also begin a sentence with an -*ing* addition. First, let's review some information about verbs. Every verb has an -*ing* form, such as *running, thinking, singing*. We usually use these -*ing* forms as part of the main verb in a sentence: *I am running, he was thinking, they are singing*. We can also use the -*ing* form as an addition.

> *Rocking in her chair,* **Grandma whistled her favorite tunes.**
>
> *Drinking coffee and munching on doughnuts,* **we read the newspaper.**
>
> *Hearing his name called,* **Chris walked proudly across the stage to receive his diploma.**
>
> *Speaking calmly and patiently,* **the instructor taught the jittery driver how to parallel park.**

An -*ing* addition is an excellent way to create sentence variety. Look for two sentences that could be combined by changing one of them to an -*ing* addition.

Example 1

Choppy: The child quietly opens a box of cookies. ~~She is~~ hoping no one hears her.

- Change the second sentence to an -*ing* addition: *hoping no one hears her.* Then place the addition at the front of the first sentence. Mark it with a comma so that readers can see where it ends and the basic sentence begins.

Concise: *Hoping no one hears her,* the child quietly opens a box of cookies.

Example 2

wiping

Choppy: Martin began his story. ~~He wiped~~ the perspiration from his forehead.

- Because the verb in the second sentence does not end in -*ing*, we have to change it from *wiped* to *wiping*. Now we can use this -*ing* verb as part of the addition.

Concise: *Wiping the perspiration from his forehead,* Martin began his story.

Helpful Hint: Make sure the addition describes the word that follows. If it doesn't, you will have what is called a **dangling modifier.**

> **Dangling modifier:** Driving to school today, flames poured out of the vacant building on Main Street.

- Flames don't drive to school. This sentence doesn't make sense.

> **Correct:** Driving to school this morning, I saw flames pouring out of the vacant building on Main Street.

· ·

Exercises: Section A

● **Self Test A:** Rewrite each sentence so that it begins with a prepositional phrase. The prepositional phrase or phrases you need to move are in italics. (Remember to mark the end of the phrase or phrases with a comma.)

Example

The lights went out *in the middle of the movie.*
In the middle of the movie, the lights went out.

1. The moon hid the sun for over two minutes *during the last total solar eclipse.*

_____

2. Laurence offered to help *without waiting for us to ask.*

_____

3. Traffic lights trembled *in the seventy-mile-per-hour wind.*

_____

4. Local farmers sell their vegetables *throughout the summer months* at the Farmers' Market.

_____

5. Student enrollment in elementary and high schools is expected to increase *during the next decade.*

_____

⬤ **Exercise 1a:** For each pair of sentences, change the second sentence to an infinitive phrase. Then place the phrase at the beginning of the preceding sentence and mark it with a comma. The infinitive phrase you need to move is in italics for the first three items.

Example

The airlines are raising their ticket prices. ~~The prices are being raised~~ to offset higher fuel prices.

To offset higher fuel prices, the airlines are raising their ticket prices.

1. We canceled our credit cards. We wanted *to get our finances under control.*

_____

2. People around the globe are learning to use the Internet. They want *to communicate in a technological world.*

_____

3. The museum staff is gathering sculptures and jewelry. The staff is working *to prepare for an Egyptian exhibit.*

_____

4. We had to sign a one-year contract. This was the requirement if we wanted to get a lower rate.

_____

5. The senior center is offering free cholesterol screening. The senior center wants to better serve the community.

_____

⬤ **Exercise 2a:** Change the second sentence into an *-ing* addition. Then place this basket at the beginning of the preceding sentence and mark it with a comma. To create the *-ing* addition, you will need to change the underlined verb to its *-ing* form. Hints are provided in parentheses for the first three items.

Example

taking
Tiffany began to relax. ~~She took~~ a series of deep breaths.

(Change *took* to *taking*.)

Taking a series of deep breaths, Tiffany began to relax.

1. The wind sandblasted the freshly painted car. The wind *ripped* across the open field.   (Change *ripped* to *ripping*.)

_____

2. Many states have set academic standards for student achievement. Many states *hope to improve students' test scores.*   (Change *hope* to *hoping.*)

_____

3. The ski resort has sixty miles of trails. The ski resort *rests on the western slope of Mount Washington.*   (Change *rests* to *resting.*)

_____

4. The campers saw deer in the distance. The campers *gazed* through the morning mist.

_____

5. The parents and their children named every flower they recognized. They *walked* through the forest preserve.

_____

○ **Exercise 3a:** The commas marking the end of the additions have been deleted from the following paragraph. First, read the paragraph to understand its meaning; then replace the commas.

I have finally learned how to deal with stress. When school and family responsibilities pile up I jog. When unexpected expenses eat up my paycheck I jog. When I feel depressed and am not even sure why I jog. I come home, put on my headphones, and begin running. In less than a mile I can feel the tension in my arms and legs melt away. My mind is clear. I feel like no one else is around, almost like I'm on an island with the wind blowing through my hair and the sand sifting through my toes. I am relaxed and ready to face the world again. Without jogging I don't think I would be taking this English class. I'd probably be sleeping or trying to escape by partying. Jogging has given me a way out of stress and into success.

Student writer

Section B: Additions in the Middle

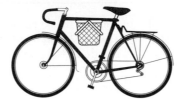

We can also place additions (baskets) in the middle of the sentence (bike). We have already written sentences with some of these additions: dependent clauses beginning with *who*, *which*, and *that*.

> **Brent and Dana, *who usually have a great sense of humor,* didn't even smile.**
>
> **The remodeling, *which started six months ago,* includes moving walls.**
>
> **The chairs *that we want to buy* are now on sale.**

We will now look at two more additions: **appositives** and *-ing* additions.

APPOSITIVES

An appositive is a "definition addition." It is a basket that defines another word in a sentence, and it goes next to the word it defines.

> **Rico, *my sister's boyfriend,* rang the doorbell.**
>
> **Judith, *a friend from grade school,* wants to be a computer engineer.**
>
> **The park, *a natural sanctuary in the heart of the city,* closes at dusk.**
>
> **Frank and Beth, *a young couple from Utah,* spoke at the conference.**

- Notice the commas on both sides of the addition. We mark both sides with commas so that readers can see where the addition begins and ends.

Look for sentences in your writing that give a definition. A sentence that defines or describes another word can often be condensed into an addition.

Example 1

Choppy: Henry understands the importance of teamwork. ~~He is~~ one of ten children.

- Change the second sentence to an addition by deleting the subject (*He*) and the *be* verb (*is*). We now have the definition: *one of ten children*.
- Place the addition after the word it describes: *Henry*.

Concise: Henry, *one of ten children*, understands the importance of teamwork.

Example 2

Choppy: Stanley's Steakhouse now has take-out service. ~~It is~~ the most popular restaurant in town.

- Change the second sentence to an addition: *the most popular restaurant in town*. Then place the addition after the words it describes: *Stanley's Steakhouse*.

Concise: Stanley's Steakhouse, *the most popular restaurant in town*, now has take-out service.

An appositive is often a shorter version of a dependent clause beginning with *who* or *which*. Both sentence patterns are effective.

Example 1

Dependent clause: Dr. Schultz, who has been our family doctor for many years, will retire in June.

Appositive: Dr. Schultz, our family doctor for many years, will retire in June.

Example 2

Dependent clause: Peanuts and almonds, which are my favorite snack food, are high in protein.

Appositive: Peanuts and almonds, my favorite snack food, are high in protein.

-*ING* ADDITIONS

Earlier in this chapter, we used *-ing* additions as baskets on the front of a bike. We can also place them in the middle of a bike after the word they describe.

> The bikers, *escaping the heat and mosquitoes,* traveled after dark.
>
> Fifty volunteers, *hoping to improve their community,* planted trees last Saturday.
>
> Tourists, *walking along the boardwalk,* watched snapping turtles and alligators.
>
> The choir director, *recognizing that we had busy schedules,* let us out early.

If your sentences sound choppy, look for two sentences that could be combined by changing one to an *-ing* addition. If the verb in the sentence does not end in *-ing,* change the verb to its *-ing* form.

Example 1

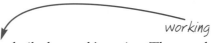

working

Choppy: Zach and Harold rebuilt the truck's engine. ~~They worked~~ late nights and many weekends.

- Change the second sentence to an *-ing* addition by changing *worked* to *working.* Then place the addition after the words it describes: *Zach and Harold.* Mark it with commas so that readers can keep track of the basic sentence.

Concise: Zach and Harold, *working late nights and many weekends,* rebuilt the truck's engine.

Example 2

forgetting

Choppy: The children tracked mud all over the living room carpet. ~~They had forgotten~~ to take off their shoes.

- Change the second sentence to an *-ing* addition by changing *had forgotten* to its *-ing* form: *forgetting.* Then add the addition after the word it describes: *children.*

Concise: The children, *forgetting to take off their shoes,* tracked mud all over the living room carpet.

Exercises: Section B

● **Self Test B:** Change the second sentence to an appositive. Then add that basket to the preceding sentence, placing it after the word it describes. The appositive is in italics for the first three items.

Vernon and Mario like chicken on their pizza. ~~They are~~ **my twin brothers.**

Vernon and Mario, my twin brothers, like chicken on their pizza.

- Notice that the addition does not include the verb *are*. Remember to delete forms of the verb *be*, such as *is*, *are*, *was*, and *were*.

1. Jerome and Conner will design homes in the new development. They are *architects with thirty years of experience.*

   _____

2. I still remember Mrs. Shank because she made me feel important. She was *my second grade teacher.*

   _____

3. The Everglades National Park is located at the southern tip of Florida. This park is *a paradise for plants and wildlife.*

   _____

4. Mr. Arlington has dedicated his life to public service. He is a respected volunteer and family man.

   _____

5. Mr. Fredrickson encouraged me to go to college. Mr. Fredrickson was my high school history teacher.

   _____

● **Exercise 1b:** Change the second sentence to an *-ing* addition and place it after the word it describes in the first sentence. The *-ing* addition is in italics for the first three items.

Example

My little cousin smiled. ~~He was~~ listening to his favorite song.

My little cousin, listening to his favorite song, smiled.

1. Katie and Daryl fell asleep. They were *listening to their relatives talk in the living room.*

   _____

2. The lost puppy made friends with everyone. The puppy was *wandering through the neighborhood.*

   _____

3. Emily waved and shouted, "Harry!" She *recognized a familiar face in the crowd.* (Change *recognized* to *recognizing*.)

   _____

4. The motivational speaker inspired all of us. He walked up and down the aisles.
   (Change *walked* to *walking*.)

   _____

5. The commuters waited for the morning train. They stood elbow to elbow with strangers.
   (Change *stood* to *standing*.)

   _____

● **Exercise 2b:** Because an addition is extra information added to a basic sentence, there must be a basic sentence outside the addition to support it. In each sentence, identify the addition and the basic sentence. Then write your answers to the questions that follow.

Example

The alarm clock, shattering the silence, shocked us awake.
What is the addition? *shattering the silence*
What is the basic sentence? *The alarm clock shocked us awake.*

1. The sleepy driver, peering through the foggy windshield, had trouble reading the signs ahead.

   What is the addition? ——————————————————————

   What is the basic sentence? ——————————————————

2. The hybrid car, the result of years of research and development, gets up to seventy miles to the gallon.

   What is the addition? ——————————————————————

   What is the basic sentence? ——————————————————

3. Juan and I, hoping to get an *A* on the exam, studied all weekend.

   What is the addition? ——————————————————————

   What is the basic sentence? ——————————————————

4. Medical Technology 101, which is offered on campus this summer, is a prerequisite for the nursing program.

   What is the addition? ——————————————————————

   What is the basic sentence? ——————————————————

5. The pilot, who saw turbulence ahead, told passengers to fasten their seat belts.

   What is the addition? ——————————————————————

   What is the basic sentence? ——————————————————

● **Exercise 3b:** Complete the additions by filling in the blanks with your own words.

1. Shoppers, wandering ————————————, searched for bargains.

2. Shoppers, tossing ————————————, searched for bargains.

3. Shoppers, who ————————————, searched for bargains.

4. Shoppers, adults and children with ——————, searched for bargains.

5. Shoppers, dragging ————————————, went home.

Section C: Additions on the Back

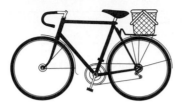

We can also place additions on the back of a bike. We have already written sentences with these additions. In Chapter 2, we attached dependent clauses beginning with words such as *when* and *because*. In Chapter 3, we attached dependent clauses beginning with *who, which,* or *that.* In Chapter 4, we corrected fragments by attaching them to the end of a preceding sentence. Here are a few examples of the kinds of sentences we wrote in those chapters:

> I make mistakes *whenever I try to do things quickly.*
>
> Natalie was late *because her car would not start.*
>
> I need to get in touch with Randy Martinez, *who is the new manager.*
>
> Johnny is majoring in geriatrics, *which involves the health needs of elderly people.*
>
> We need plants *that grow well in the shade.*
>
> The obstacle course was easy, *especially for my older brother.*
>
> My friends want to travel to someplace warm, *such as Mexico or Belize.*
>
> The campers sat by the fire, *telling stories and playing card games.*

The preceding sentences cover the main ways additions are attached at the end of a sentence. Because previous chapters cover these additions, we will now close this chapter by looking at the overall effect of using sentence variety.

Summary

Using additions helps you connect your ideas so that your sentences flow smoothly. When you are working on improving the sentences in a paper you are writing, concentrate first on particular sentences. Then read the whole paragraph out loud so that you can hear how the sentences sound together. You want your sentences to connect and flow smoothly, as in the following paragraph. Read it out loud, notice the additions highlighted in italics, and listen to the smooth sound of the sentences.

Working as a nurse's aide in a home health care program gave my life direction. One of my jobs was to visit elderly patients in their homes and assist them with daily activities, *such as bathing, dressing, and eating.* I remember particularly one patient, *a frail woman who was always propped up by pillows.* *One afternoon when I entered her room,* she was trying to hold back tears. She was staring helplessly at a tray of food in front of her, *unable to hold a fork because of her stroke.* I began to feed her slowly, and her "thank you" after each tiny spoonful went straight to my heart. Another patient, *who was in her nineties,* always greeted me at her door with freshly cut roses from her garden. Her gifts of flowers brightened my days. *The night before she passed away,* I was called to her house to bathe her. *After I bathed her,* she looked at me with tears streaming down her cheeks and said, "Thank you. *Now, when I meet God,* I will be clean." She thanked me, yet I was really the grateful one. I had discovered what I want to do with my life. I want to be a nurse.

Student writer

• •

Exercises: Section C

⬤ **Self Test C:** Read the following paragraphs for an overview of their meaning. Then focus on each sentence separately and put parentheses around any additions.

Baseball has taught me the importance of mental concentration. When I am able to block out distractions, I am a good pitcher. For example, in the Ohio Valley Regional Baseball Tournament, I was pitching against Kentucky. As soon as the game started, it began to drizzle. The ball soon became slippery, which made it harder to control. The field turned to mud, clogging up my cleats and making it harder to push off the mound. I made errors; my team made errors. Finally, I blocked out the mistakes and focused my energy on my fastball pitch. We won 7–0.

Our game against Kankakee Valley High School is another example of the power of concentration. I was facing an undefeated team. Kankakee was known for being loud and annoying, especially when it was batting. We were winning 3–2 in the seventh inning, and the whole Kankakee team was shouting. Rather than being distracted by the screaming, I used it to pump myself up for the last inning. I stepped off the mound and pointed to Kankakee Valley's dugout, waving the team on as if to say, "I'm ready. Bring it on." When Kankakee's best hitters came to bat, I was ready. Because I had learned to focus my attention, I pitched the best game of my life. Mental concentration is the key to success.

Student writer

● **Exercise 1c:** In the following sentences, the commas around the additions have been omitted. Read each sentence to find the addition, and then mark that addition with a comma or commas.

Example

> **A woman of few words Lynn pours all her extra time into drawing and painting.**
>
> *A woman of few words, Lynn pours all her extra time into drawing and painting.*

Example

> **My computer which had been making strange noises crashed.**
>
> *My computer, which had been making strange noises, crashed.*

1. Looking through the picture album the grandparents reminisced about their younger days.

2. The savings and loan which has been in the community for years offers competitive mortgage rates.

3. We drove along Rivergrove Road a cracked two-lane highway on the outskirts of town.

4. To expand their science program the university built a new research laboratory.

5. I stared at the phone for at least ten minutes trying to get the courage to call.

6. Perched on a stand near the stage the director talked with the actors.

7. Hoping to see a sign for a gas station we peered into the distance.

8. Frank Williams an elderly man on the second floor is organizing potluck dinners for residents in the apartment.

9. After taking our last final exam we decided to celebrate at Papa Joe's our favorite restaurant.

10. For people living on the island winter is a quiet and lonely time.

● **Exercise 2c:** Take the paper you are currently working on and look for sentences that could be combined by changing one into an addition.

PART 4

PUNCTUATION AND MECHANICS

CHAPTER 15

APOSTROPHES AND QUOTATION MARKS

Section A: Apostrophes

An apostrophe has two purposes: to show that letters are missing (contraction) and to show ownership (**possession**).

CONTRACTION

Some words contract, squeezing together to form one word. In the process, one or more letters pop out. Put the apostrophe where the missing letters used to be.

could not = couldn't	you will = you'll	you are = you're
should not = shouldn't	we are = we're	it is = it's (meaning *it is* or *it has*)
did not = didn't	they are = they're	let us = let's

Sometimes, in more casual writing, writers contract the subject and the verb *is*. Notice how in the following examples the apostrophe replaces the letter *-i*.

>The food is in the refrigerator. = The food's in the refrigerator.
>
>She is working weekends. = She's working weekends.

- Contractions are considered casual. For formal writing and most college writing, use both words rather than the contraction.

Helpful Hint: Remembering contractions will help you with several easily confused words.

>*You're* always means *you are*.
>
>*They're* always means *they are*.
>
>*We're* always means *we are*.
>
>*It's* always means *it is* or *it has*.
>
>*Who's* always means *who is* or *who has*.

POSSESSION

An apostrophe is also used to show ownership. When people or things "own" something mentioned right after their names, add an apostrophe and the letter *-s* to the owner. This is easy to understand if you imagine putting the owner in a box and adding an apostrophe and *-s* after the box.

The [ ]**'s** dreams came true.	[Justin]**'s** dreams came true.
One [woman]**'s** dreams came true.	[Lois]**'s** dreams came true.
Many [women]**'s** dreams came true.	[Everyone]**'s** dreams came true.
One [person]**'s** dreams came true.	Many [people]**'s** dreams came true.

Let's look at how this works:

1. Find the owner. If you are not sure you are dealing with ownership, turn the words into an *of* phrase.

>**The doctor's handwriting is hard to read.**

- Ask yourself, "Do I mean the handwriting of the doctor?" If the answer is yes, the doctor is the owner.

>**My car's bumper is dented.**

- Ask yourself, "Do I mean the bumper of my car?" If the answer is yes, the car is the owner.

2. Add an apostrophe and -*s* to the owner.

The children's crayons melted in the summer sun.

- The children own the crayons. Therefore, we add an apostrophe and -*s* after the owner (*children*): *children's.*

Karla listened carefully to her mother's advice.

- The mother owns the advice. Therefore we put an apostrophe and -*s* after *mother: mother's.*

3. Make sure the owners "own" the word or words that come after them.

Marlon's new camera was expensive.

- Marlon owns the words that come after his name: *new camera.* Therefore, we add an apostrophe and -*s* after *Marlon: Marlon's.*

Marlon likes his new camera.

- The word that comes after *Marlon* is *likes.* We do not add apostrophe and -*s* to *Marlon* because he does not own the word that follows his name. Although we know that he owns the new camera, an apostrophe and -*s* are not added because *new camera* does not follow his name.

4. If the owner is a plural noun that already ends in -*s*, just add an apostrophe. We do this because people would have difficulty saying two -*s* sounds.

All the pizzas' toppings burned.

- All the toppings of the pizzas burned. The pizzas own the toppings, so we add an apostrophe after *pizzas: pizzas'.* We don't add another -*s* because readers would stumble over the double -*s* sounds in *pizzas's.*

The musicians' performance is sold out.

- The musicians own the performance. We do not add another -*s* because readers would have difficulty saying the double -*s* sounds in *musicians's.*

5. Read the word to the left of the apostrophe to see who the owner is.

The student's grades were excellent.

- Reading the letters to the left of the apostrophe will tell us who had excellent grades: one student.

The students' grades were excellent.

- Reading the letters to the left of the apostrophe will tell us who had excellent grades: two or more students.

HOW TO USE *-S* AND AN APOSTROPHE CORRECTLY

The letter *-s* can be confusing because the same letter is used for three different things. We add *-s* to make nouns plural. We also add *-s* to present-tense verbs. Plus, we add *-s* with an apostrophe to show possession. Although we are using the same letter, these three uses have nothing to do with each other.

Here it is in a nutshell: Use just the letter *-s* for plural nouns and present-tense verbs. Use an apostrophe and the letter *-s* when you want to show possession.

Add the letter *-s* to most nouns to make them plural.

two pencils, three friends, many books

Add the letter *-s* to present-tense verbs when the subject is *he* (or any male), *she* (or any female), and *it* (or anything that is an *it*).

she listens, the student understands, the drum beats

Do not add an apostrophe and *-s* unless you are dealing with possession. When people or things own the word that comes after them, add an apostrophe and *-s* to the owner.

the truck's tire, Frank's goals, the choir's schedule

Helpful hint: There are three places where we do not use apostrophes: verbs, plural nouns, and possessive pronouns.

1. Do not use an apostrophe in verbs. Present-tense verbs end in the letter *-s* (*talks*, *walks*, *sleeps*, *laughs*), but not an apostrophe and *-s*.

   Incorrect: Nancy ~~live's~~ next door.

   Correct: Nancy lives next door.

2. Do not use an apostrophe to make nouns plural. We add the letter *-s* to make many nouns plural: *cars*, *books*, *flowers*, *shirts*. We add the *-s*, but we don't add an apostrophe.

   Incorrect: We are saving ~~coupon's~~ from the Sunday paper.

   Correct: We are saving coupons from the Sunday paper.

3. Do not add an apostrophe to possessive pronouns (*its*, *his*, *her*, *hers*, *my*, *mine*, *ours*, *yours*, *their*, and *theirs*). The most common error is made with *its*.

   Incorrect: The dogs licked it's paws.

   • *It's* means either *it is* or *it has*. This sentence does not mean "The dog licked it is paws."

   Correct: The dog licked its paws.

   • Use *its* to show ownership.

• •

Exercises: Section A

◉ **Self Test A:** Correct the apostrophe errors in the following sentences. If a sentence is correct as is, mark it with a *C*.

1. Phil run's two mile's every day.

2. The weeks before graduation were filled with activities.

3. Everyone loves my mother apple pie's.

4. The wolf can survive harsh winters because of it's thick fur.

5. The childrens' party will begin at noon.

◉ **Exercise 1a:** Read each sentence and answer the question that follows. A helpful hint: Reading the letters to the left of the apostrophe will tell you who the "owner" is.

Example

> The organization's goals are to preserve national forests and combat global warming.
>
> How many organizations have the goal? *One*

1. The store's sales begin today.

   How many stores are having a sale? _____

2. The stores' sales begin today.

   How many stores are having a sale? _____

3. The manager announced the employee's raise.

   How many employees received a raise? _____

4. The manager announced the employees' raise.

   How many employees received a raise? _____

5. The fans loved the player's positive attitude and spirit.

How many players have a positive attitude and spirit? _____

● **Exercise 2a:** Correct the apostrophe errors in the following sentences. The errors involve omitting an apostrophe, omitting an apostrophe and the letter -*s*, or placing an apostrophe where it does not belong. If a sentence has no errors, mark it with a *C*.

1. We are trying to protect the earth environment.

2. The first mistake was Richard's fault. The second mistake was my fault.

3. The policeman clocked my cars speed at eighty miles an hour.

4. We saw videos of Denise vacation.

5. Parents' should know who their children friends are.

● **Exercise 3a:** Rewrite each pair of sentences as one sentence by adding an apostrophe and -*s* to the owner.

Example

Ashley has a new computer. It is faster than mine.
Ashley's new computer is faster than mine.

Example

Martin left his jacket on the porch. The porch belongs to his neighbor.
Martin left his jacket on his neighbor's porch.

1. Jake has a garage. It is stuffed with unopened boxes and motorcycle engines.

_____

2. The attorney had evidence. The evidence proved that his client was not guilty.

_____

3. Katrina has an apartment. It is small but inexpensive.

_____

4. The teacher patiently answered the questions. They were the questions of the children.

_____

5. The jury asked for a copy of the instructions. The instructions were given by the judge.

_____

⊙ **Exercise 4a:** Read the following paragraph for an overview of its meaning. Then find the two words that need an apostrophe to show possession.

Many students decide to go to college to become successful or independent, but I decided to attend college for a different reason. I want to teach children who are deaf or hearing impaired to learn to communicate. When I was in sixth grade, my dads girlfriend inspired me. She was a sign language teacher, and she took me to meet her students. Within two hours, I was in love with those kids. They had so much passion to learn, and they all wanted to talk to me. I knew nothing about communicating with them, but they taught me a few of their hand signs. I was captivated by all the different signs, and I went home and practiced the few they had taught me. That was long ago, but I knew then I wanted to teach disabled children and make a difference in someones life. Going to college to become a sign language teacher is the best decision I have ever made.

Student writer

Exercise 5a: Find and correct the errors made with apostrophes.

My brothers addiction to drug's has affected both him and me. His desire for drug's has changed from a thirsty want to a dying need. Although he work's five days a week, he throws his paycheck away on drugs. He would rather get high than buy decent clothes or a pair of shoes. Whenever he is at home, he always wear's the same dirty clothes' that reek of cigarettes. His skin color has darkened, and his eyes' are yellow.

His addiction has also affected me. Throughout my childhood, my oldest brother was like a father to me. He talked to me, listened to me, gave me advice, and took me places. I respected him and could always trust him. That world has now crumbled. My brother, my counselor, and my friend is a drug addict and see's nothing wrong with it. I love him for being there for me in the past, but I cant count on him to be there for me in the future. Drug's destroy.

Student writer

- -

Section B: Quotation Marks

Quotation marks are used to indicate short works of art and direct quotations.

SHORT WORKS OF ART

Put quotation marks around the titles of short works of art.

> Article in a newspaper or magazine: "Our Rediscovered Universe"
> Poem: "Journey of the Magi"
> Short story: "The Rocking-Horse Winner"
> Song: "Paradise Is Here"
> Chapter of a book: "How Language Works"

Longer works of art are treated differently. If you are typing, place them in italics; if you are writing longhand, underline them.

> Book: *Beloved*   Play: *King Lear*
> Newspaper: *New York Times*   Film: *Casablanca*
> Magazine: *Newsweek*   Television program: *60 Minutes*

DIRECT QUOTATIONS

When writing about what someone said, you have two choices: You can state exactly what that person said, word for word (**direct quotation**). Or you can give a summary of what that person said (**indirect quotation**).

Example 1

> **Exact words:** Connie said, "I found my wallet."
> **Summary:** Connie said that she found her wallet.

- Notice the quotation marks in the first sentence. Quotation marks are signs that these are the person's exact words. If we had a tape recorder running, these would be the words on the tape.

- In the second sentence, notice the word *that*. The word *that* often introduces a summary of what someone said, not the exact words. We also know these are not the exact words because Connie would not refer to herself as *she* and *her*.

Example 2

Exact words: Nick explained, "My neighbor wants to drive me to the airport."

Summary: Nick explained that his neighbor wants to drive him to the airport.

- The quotation marks in the first sentence tell us that this is exactly what Nick said, word for word.

- In the second sentence, the word *that* gives us our first clue that this is a summary, not the exact words. Plus, we know these couldn't be Nick's exact words because he would not refer to himself as *his* and *him*.

Follow these guidelines if you are quoting a person's exact words.

1. Enclose the person's exact words in quotation marks. Put the first quotation mark before the first word spoken. Place the last quotation mark after the last word spoken. If the person says more than one sentence, do not mark each separate sentence. Mark the beginning and the end of what was said.

> Antonio said, "I tried calling home, but no one answered. If I have a minute between classes, I'll try calling again."

2. Separate the person talking from that person's words with a comma.

> The child whispered, "Let's go home now."

3. Capitalize the first word of a quoted sentence.

> The flight attendant announced, "Buckle your seat belts."

4. When you have finished the quotation, place the period or comma inside quotation marks.

> Marilyn walked into class and stated, "I am early."
>
> "Congratulations," one classmate responded.

5. If the person's exact words are a question, let readers know by placing a question mark inside the quotation marks.

> The bank teller asked, "Do you have a deposit slip?"

6. You can place the speaker before, after, or in the middle of the quoted words.

> **Before:** Gerald reminded me, "It's never too late to start over."
>
> **After:** "It's never too late to start over," Gerald reminded me.
>
> **Middle:** "It's never too late," Gerald reminded me, "to start over."

• •

Exercises: Section B

● **Self Test B:** Each sentence contains a summary of what the person said. Imagine what the exact words might have been and rewrite the sentence using a direct quotation.

> **Example**

Mary Jo told us we could borrow her car if we got it back to her by noon.

Mary Jo said, "You can borrow my car if you get it back to me by noon."

1. Michael said that he agrees with me.

   _____

2. Kimberly said that she would call me later.

   _____

3. The doctor's secretary announced that they no longer submit insurance forms.

   _____

4. Ryan asked whether we wanted to meet him for lunch on Wednesday.

   _____

5. Deborah mumbled that she needed a cup of coffee.

   _____

● **Exercise 1b:** As in the preceding exercise, imagine what the person might have said and rewrite the sentence using a direct quotation.

1. My sister told me to slow down and watch where I'm going.

   _____

2. Gordon asked me whether I needed a ride to class.

_____

3. The car mechanic said that I could pick up my car on Thursday.

_____

4. The instructor said that our research project is due at the end of October.

_____

5. Carmen asked us whether we are voting tomorrow.

_____

⬤ **Exercise 2b:** Read the following paragraph and add quotation marks around the direct quotations.

Yolanda's encouraging words changed my life. When I faced going back to school to get my high school diploma, I was filled with doubt. As soon as I muttered my fears, Yolanda jumped all over me, saying, I am tired of you always putting yourself down. I believe in you. You can do it. Because of her encouraging words, I went back to school, took the test, and passed. Her life-changing words returned when I thought about attending college. Again, I was filled with self-doubt. I felt I wasn't smart enough. I didn't have the courage to try and then fail. My mind paced back and forth until the day Yolanda pulled into my driveway. Although I tried to hide my anger and frustration, she saw through it and said, You did it once. You can do it again. You can do it, Dorothy. Yolanda has made a big difference in my life. Because of her life-changing words, I have my high school diploma, I am in college, and I have confidence.

Student writer

CHAPTER 16

CAPITALIZATION AND MORE PUNCTUATION

Capital Letters

PROPER AND COMMON NOUNS

The name of a specific person, place, or thing is capitalized. These specific names are called **proper nouns** and include words such as *Charlie*, *Boston*, and *Ford*. The general name is not capitalized. These general names are called **common nouns** and include words such as *man*, *city*, and *car*.

Proper nouns (Specific)	Common nouns (General)
People	
Jennifer	sister
Walter	brother
Mother, Father	my mother, her father
Aunt Margaret	aunt
Uncle George	uncle
Dr. Jameson	doctor

Professor Adams	professor
Pastor Smith	pastor
President Roosevelt	president
Senator Douglas	senator
Democrat, Republican	political party member

Places

Chicago, Miami	city
Montana, Florida	state
Switzerland, Germany	country
Atlantic Ocean	ocean
Halsted Street, Elm Avenue	street, avenue
North, South, East, West, Midwest	areas of the country
Columbia College, Harvard University	college, university
Lawrence High School	high school
Bennie's Grill	restaurant
Carlton Hardware	store
Everglades National Park	park

Things

Psychology 101	psychology course
Reston Insurance Company	insurance company
Museum of Science and Industry	museum
Raisin Bran	cereal
General Motors	company
Frontline	television program
Grapes of Wrath	book
Time, Sports Illustrated	magazine
Thanksgiving, Independence Day	holiday
Wednesday, Saturday	day
July, August	summer
October, November	fall
January, February	winter
April, May	spring
Middle Ages	historical time
English, French, Spanish	language
Judaism, Buddhism, Christianity	religion
God, Allah, Vishnu, Yahweh	deity

Compass Directions

Capitalize *north*, *south*, *east*, and *west* only when they refer to a geographical region.

Example

They drove south on Main Street and forgot to turn on Landon Avenue.

- Because *south* does not refer to an area of the United States in this sentence, it is not capitalized.

They drove to the South for the winter.

- In this sentence, *South* refers to an area of the United States. Therefore, it is capitalized.

Buildings

Capitalize the name of a building when it is the building's specific name, the name that would be written on a sign in front of the building.

Example

After graduating from Thornton High School, we went to Oakland College.

- The signs outside these buildings are "Thornton High School" and "Oakland College." Because these are the specific names of the schools, they are capitalized.

After graduating from high school, we went to college.

- The signs outside these buildings do not read "High School" and "College." These words refer to a general category of schools, not the specific name of the school. Therefore, they are not capitalized.

Titles

Capitalize titles, such as *doctor* and *professor*, only when they are part of a person's specific name.

Example 1

Ramon has an appointment with Dr. Hendrix tomorrow.

- Imagine a sign is outside the doctor's office. The sign would read, "Dr. Hendrix." That is the doctor's specific name. Because the title *Dr.* is part of the person's name, it is capitalized.

Ramon has an appointment with the doctor tomorrow.

- Because *doctor* is not part of a specific name, it is not capitalized.

Example 2

Ramon has an appointment with Professor Matthews tomorrow.

- The title *professor* is part of the person's specific name. Therefore, it is capitalized.

Ramon has an appointment with his professor tomorrow.

- Because the title *professor* is not part of a specific name, it is not capitalized.

Family Relationships

Do not capitalize a family name when there is a pronoun in front of it. For example, write *my father, his mother, our sister, her brother, their uncle,* and *your aunt.*

Example

If she has time, my mom will meet us for lunch.

- The word *mom* is not capitalized because the pronoun *my* is in front of it.

Capitalize a family name only when you are using it instead of the person's specific name, such as Brenda or George.

If she has time, Mom will meet us for lunch.

- *Mom* is capitalized because it is used as a specific name, such as *Brenda*.

- When we replace *Mom* with *Brenda*, the sentence makes sense: *If she has time, Brenda will meet us for lunch.* Therefore, we know we should capitalize *Mom*.

CAPITALIZING ADDITIONAL NOUNS

A few other words are capitalized.

Abbreviations for People and Organizations

Mr. Ms. Jr. Dr. Rev.

USA or U.S.A. FBI NATO UN NFL UPS

- Abbreviations for organizations are capitalized. They usually do not include periods.

Abbreviations for Time

Abbreviations for morning and afternoon include periods. They can be written in capital or lowercase letters.

a.m. (A.M. or AM)   p.m. (P.M. or PM)

Words in Titles

Capitalize the first, last, and all major words in titles of works of art.

Charles Dickens wrote *A Tale of Two Cities*. (Books are italicized or underlined.)

Gabriel García Márquez wrote "Eyes of a Blue Dog." (Short stories are placed in quotation marks.)

The crowd sang "America the Beautiful." (Songs are placed in quotation marks.)

• •

More Punctuation Marks

COMMAS—ADDITIONAL USES

Commas help readers navigate our sentences. Chapter 15 explains how to use commas to mark direct quotations. Chapter 6 focuses on the comma's main uses: to separate items in a series, to connect two sentences with a coordinating conjunction, and to mark additions. In this chapter, we see how commas separate two adjectives, open and close a letter, set off parts of a date, set off parts of an address, and set off numbers.

Separating Two Adjectives

Use a comma to separate two adjectives if the word *and* would make sense between them.

> **I need new blue jeans.**

- We wouldn't say "new and blue jeans." Therefore, do not put a comma between *new* and *blue*.

> **We are looking for a large, inexpensive house.**

- We would say "large and inexpensive house." Therefore, put a comma between *large* and *inexpensive*.

Opening and Closing a Letter

> Dear Mr. Lightheart,
> Sincerely yours,

Setting Off Parts of a Date

> They celebrated their fiftieth anniversary on June 1, 2004, with a trip to Hawaii.

- Notice the comma after 2004. When the date is in the middle of a sentence, place a comma after the year.

Setting Off Parts of an Address

We will move to 267 Bellevue Avenue, Monclair, New Jersey, in a few weeks.

We will move to 267 Bellevue Avenue, Monclair, New Jersey 07043, in a few weeks.

- Use a comma after each part of an address, including the state if no zip code is given.

Setting Off Numbers

The town's population rose from 22,000 to 47,500 in ten years.

COLONS

The colon (:) is like an announcement that says important information is coming. Use it to introduce a list or an explanation. There is just one requirement: The colon must follow a complete sentence.

Lists

You can use a colon to introduce a list, but there must be a complete sentence before the list.

The advertised apartment has what we want: two bedrooms, two bathrooms, and new appliances.

- A colon is used because it follows a sentence: *The advertised apartment has what we want.*

The advertised apartment has two bedrooms, two bathrooms, and new appliances.

- A colon is not used because there is not a sentence before the list. *The advertised apartment has* is not a sentence.

Explanations

You can use a colon to announce an explanation or a definition if the colon follows a complete sentence.

> I have two goals: to graduate from college and to take care of my family.

- We can use a colon because it follows a sentence: *I have two goals.*

> My two goals are to graduate from college and to take care of my family.

- We cannot use a colon because there is not a sentence in front of it. *My two goals are* is not a sentence.

DASHES

Dashes (— or two hyphens together) can be used to emphasize a dramatic pause or to set off an appositive that contains commas.

> After finishing the final exam, we walked out—smiling.
>
> Everything in our freezer—the meat, casseroles, ice cream, and éclairs—was ruined when the electricity went out.

Do not overuse dashes, or they will lose their effect.

EXCLAMATION POINTS

Use an exclamation point (!) to express a strong emotion.

> We won the game!

PARENTHESES

Use parentheses ( ) to insert incidental information that some of your readers might want to know.

> The section on home financing in our textbook (pages 55–64) explains what to look for when shopping for a mortgage.

Be careful not to use parentheses too often.

QUESTION MARKS

Use a question mark (?) at the end of a direct question.

> **Did you hear that strange noise?**
> **Should everyone take vitamins?**

Do not use a question mark at the end of an indirect question. An indirect question makes a statement about a question.

> **Friends asked me whether I heard that strange noise.**
> **Sometimes I wonder whether everyone should take vitamins.**

• •

Exercises

Self Test: Find and correct the errors in capitalization and punctuation in the following sentences. If a sentence has no errors, mark it with a *C*.

1. The doctors in the new Medical building will begin office hours in January.

2. My Father's brother, who grew up in brazil, can speak spanish, english, and portuguese.

3. Our grandparents were married April 18 1965 in Jamaica.

4. We have everything we need for winter driving: jumper cables, a shovel, a bag of sand, and a flashlight.

5. Spring and Winter are my Grandfather's favorite Seasons.

6. After Miguel graduates from college, he wants to work for an insurance agency or an advertising firm.

7. I wonder why Nancy has not called?

8. Jack London, an American novelist and short-story writer, is best known for his book *The Call of the Wild*.

9. Some good sources of protein are: beans, cheese, fish, meats, and nuts.

10. Please send the package to George Doughtery at 900 Spindell Road Tarrington New York.

◯ **Exercise 1:** Find and correct the errors in capitalization and punctuation in the following sentences. If a sentence has no errors, mark it with a *C*.

1. The lab opens at 6:30 am and closes at 8:30 pm.

2. Before she graduates, Gloria wants to take a psychology course.

3. The tutor asked me whether I needed help.

4. The home that they bought on July 28 1998 is now for sale.

5. My niece was born in the midwest and has never seen the pacific ocean.

6. The best Teacher I had in High School was Mr. Fuentes.

7. We avoided the construction by driving North on Ridge road and then West on Greenview street.

8. Anthony has three favorite sports basketball, football, and soccer.

9. Anthony's favorite sports are basketball, football, and soccer.

10. Next summer, uncle stephen and aunt alice want to visit yellowstone national park.

◯ **Exercise 2:** In the following paragraph, correct the errors made with capital letters.

Attending Parkview College has benefited both my Mother and me. My Mother dropped out of High School when she was a teenager, and she has always regretted that. My decision to go to college inspired my Mom to complete her Education. Last Summer, she returned to School and received her High School Diploma. This past Fall, she enrolled in College, beginning with a Math Course and a Reading Course. Both of us are now taking a full load of classes and spend our weekends studying. Instead of watching television, we have our eyes glued to Textbooks. The rewards are worth it. Our Professors have given us good grades, but our self-satisfaction beats any passing grade.

Student writer

● **Exercise 3:** The left column lists common nouns. Fill in the blanks in the right column by writing a corresponding proper noun. The first one is done for you.

Common noun (general)   **Proper noun (specific)**

1. aunt................................. *Aunt Madeline*

2. doctor .... _____

3. senator .... _____

4. city .... _____

5. state............................... _____

6. college............................ _____

7. high school .... _____

8. restaurant....................... _____

9. store .... _____

10. college class .... _____

11. television program .... _____

12. book.............................. _____

13. magazine........................ _____

14. language......................... _____

15. religion .... _____

PART 5

. . . .

WRITING PARAGRAPHS
AND ESSAYS

THE WRITING PROCESS

Paragraphs in books and magazines look perfect, as if the authors simply sat down and let their ideas flow easily, almost magically, onto paper. But that is not how it happened. All writers struggle to find words for their ideas. We just don't see their frustration. We only see the final product—not the process they used to get there. In this chapter, we look at the process experienced writers use so that you, too, will know how to write a polished paper. Then, in Chapter 18, we look at the qualities of a good paper so that you will have a clear idea of what to aim for. Chapter 19, which builds on these two chapters, covers essays.

Whether you are writing a one-paragraph paper or an essay, it's important to understand the writing process. This process involves discovering, organizing, drafting, revising, and editing. These are not do-it-once-and-it's-over steps. They are more like loops. Writing is a back-and-forth process that takes time. Be patient with the process, and keep in mind the rewards. Yes, getting a good grade on a paper is important. Yet equally important is the satisfaction of finding words for your ideas—and the pride of knowing that your words have the power to change what people think, how they feel, and what they do.

. . . .

Discovering Ideas

Discovering ideas is like shopping for food. Imagine trying to make dinner when nothing is in the cabinets, refrigerator, or freezer. You need to have ingredients to cook a meal, just as you do to write a paper. You need to go grocery shopping, roaming up and down the aisles, filling your cart with food.

As you prepare to shop for ideas for your paper, think about your topic and answer the question, *Who wants to know?* For example, let's say you have been assigned to write about your best or worst job. Are you writing for your instructor and classmates to explain what you think and why? Are you writing for the manager so that he or she can improve the working conditions? Or are you writing for prospective employees to tell them what to expect? Deciding who will read your paper (audience) and why you are writing (purpose) will help you decide what to put in your cart as you shop.

Writing begins by getting something—anything—on paper. Write down whatever ideas come to you. If your ideas come in isolated words, jot down those words. If your ideas flow in sentences, write down those sentences. Do not worry about spelling or grammar—don't worry about anything. Just write as if you were talking. Let the thoughts and feelings that fill your mind flow without judging them, and keep writing until you have nothing more to say. Remember that writers write to discover what they think—they don't know when they start out.

Organizing Ideas

Let's return to the food-shopping analogy. After filling your cart with food, you return home, unpack the bags on the kitchen table, and take a look at what you bought. So, look at your discovery writing and circle the words and sentences that might fit in the paper you are currently writing. Look for words and sentences where your response is, "Yeah, that's good" or "That might work." Take the ideas you have circled and list them on a clean sheet of paper.

Here are the ideas a student writer gathered about the topic "your best or worst job":

Example

Current job—Bellagina's

being a waiter—bad
Raymond in the kitchen—fun—good sense of humor
but hours bad—too long
do nothing but work
no time for what I want to do
no partying—I'm working
don't see friends—don't know what's going on
cleaning up—filthy customers
food all over—bread crumbs
spaghetti sauce—napkins on floor

they don't care—isn't their home

other waiters disgusted

screaming babies

once in a while a good tip—not enough

behind in schoolwork—too tired

girlfriend just broke up with me

nothing to do

feel like I'm going nowhere

not making much money

can't quit

FINDING A MAIN IDEA AND SUPPORT

The next step is to find a main idea and support for that idea. Begin by looking at the items on your list and putting similar details together in groups. This is like putting grocery items in groups—cereal boxes in one group, milk and eggs in another, frozen foods in another, and so on. When you are finished, look at your groups and ask yourself, *What is the main idea here? What am I trying to say?* Finding a main idea and support for that idea usually happens simultaneously. It is a back-and-forth process, a trial-and-error process, of seeing how ideas fit together. You probably won't use everything on your list; if you come across a good idea that you can't use in your current paper, save it for a future one. You may also find that you don't have everything you need. In that case, you may have to do more discovery writing, just as you would return to the grocery store to pick up additional items.

Once you have a sense of your main idea, write it in a sentence. Keep working on it until you have two parts: the topic (*who or what*) and your point about that topic (*what about it*). Under your main idea, list the proof you will use to make your idea real for readers. You will then be ready to sketch an outline.

Example

When the student writer discussed earlier looked at his list and asked, *What am I trying to say?*, he knew his main idea: Bellagina's is his worst job. He then began putting details into groups. He did not include all the details, and he may have added a few later, but he had a clear sense of how to prove his main idea:

Working as a waiter at Bellagina's is the worst job I have ever had.

1. **Work schedule is exhausting.**
2. **Customers are messy.**

You can see the sketch outline of this paper on page 212.

SKETCHING AN OUTLINE

An outline is similar to a map. Before taking a trip, we need to know where we are going and how to get there. A sketch outline shows where you are going (the main idea) and how you will get there (the evidence). Making an outline takes time, but it is time well spent. If you start your draft without an outline, you may wander off the road, go in circles, and get lost.

Sometimes writers write their draft first and then outline after they are done by looking at the draft. That process is fine. You just need to make sure you are organized, that you don't take side trips, and that you don't repeat ideas. The only way to know this for sure is to outline—either before or after you draft. A sample outline for a one- to two-paragraph paper follows. If you are writing an essay, please see the sample essay outline on page 248.

HOW TO OUTLINE A PARAGRAPH

Write your main idea in a sentence.

List the evidence that proves that idea.

Put your ideas in order so each one leads logically to the next.

Main idea: *Working as a waiter at Bellagina's is the worst job I have ever had.*

1. Work schedule is exhausting.
   - long hours: 3:30 to midnight
   - home: collapse until alarm wakes me up
   - no time for partying, studying, relaxing

2. Customers are messy.
   - careless
   - napkins on floor, breadcrumbs on chairs, spaghetti on tables

   • The map is flexible. You may have more or less evidence than what is listed here.

You can see this paragraph on page 236.

Drafting

Drafting is writing your ideas in paragraphs. A paragraph is a group of sentences that work together to make a point. Paragraphs let readers see ideas in packages so that they know what belongs together. Without paragraphs, readers would be overwhelmed by nonstop sentences.

Using your outline as a guide, write your ideas in sentences. When you begin a new point, begin a new paragraph. A first draft is a trial run, so relax. The first draft is supposed to be messy. You don't need to worry about how it looks. If you come to a dead end and don't know what to write next, read the helpful hints in *How to Bypass Roadblocks*.

HOW TO BYPASS ROADBLOCKS

1. If you are having trouble getting started, write as if you were talking to a friend. Write whatever you are thinking; begin wherever the energy is. You do not need to start at the beginning. In fact, the beginning is often the last part writers write.

2. If you are having difficulty writing one part of your paper, leave that section and work on another part that is easier. Then, later on, return to that difficult section. Often, after working on something different, ideas that were once jammed flow more easily.

3. If you find yourself going in circles, if you are confused and don't know where you are going, or if you don't even know what you are thinking, choose one or more of these options:

   - Walk away from your paper and, if possible, go to another room. Pick up a clean piece of paper and ask yourself, *What am I trying to say?* Imagine that you are talking to a fourth grader so you keep it simple. Then, list in short, simple sentences what you are trying to say.

   - Reread what you have written and leave. Take a break: Go for a walk or do something that doesn't involve thinking. In fact, don't even think about your paper. Let your unconscious do the work. If you give yourself time, usually ideas fall into place and insights pop up unexpectedly. Therefore, keep a pencil and scrap of paper handy so when an insight comes, you can jot it down.

   - Talk about your ideas with a friend or talk to yourself. Often just saying our words out loud helps us keep track of what we are thinking.

4. If your mind is blank, use these methods to discover ideas:

- Start over by rereading what you have already written. Often this process of going back will put you on track, and new ideas will emerge.

- Ask the reporter's questions: *Who? What? Where? When? Why? How?* Not every question will apply to the paper you are writing, but at least one will lead you to valuable details.

5. If you are struggling for the right words, read something similar to the paper you want to write. For example, if you are trying to describe something, read a short story or novel that uses vivid words. If you are writing about a current event, read a newspaper article. If you are writing a paper for another course, such as psychology, read your textbook or an assigned article. Whatever you have chosen to read, pay attention to the words the writers use and jot down words you would like to use in your paper.

The goal here is to become familiar with vocabulary words that will help you put your ideas into words—not to copy the specific phrases and sentences another writer has used, which is plagiarism. Plagiarism has serious consequences, so if you want to use another writer's exact phrases or sentences, you need to give full credit to your sources.

Revising

After you have finished your first draft, print it out and let it sit overnight. You need to give yourself a break so you can read it with a clear mind. Then, pick up your draft and imagine you are a stranger reading it for the first time. Ask yourself the questions listed in *How to Revise*. These questions will help you see what you need to work on in your next draft. Keep drafting, following the same process of writing, printing the draft out, and letting it sit for a while.

Ernest Hemingway, a famous American author, rewrote the ending of *A Farewell to Arms* forty-four times. Experienced authors rewrite and continue to rewrite.

HOW TO REVISE

Read your paper, asking and answering the following questions.

The main idea

- Underline the main idea. Does it include both a *who or what* and a *what about it*?

The evidence

- Does all evidence support the main idea? If not, should you delete any of it or connect it more clearly?
- Have you included enough support to convince readers of your point?
- Are your details specific?
- Have you arranged your ideas in logical order?
- Will readers be able to follow your thoughts? Do you need transition words to connect any ideas?

The conclusion

- Does your conclusion give readers something to think about? Does it tie the ideas in the paper together?

Editing

After you have written a number of drafts and are satisfied that your ideas will be clear to readers, it is time to edit. Editing is looking at the smaller details, such as spelling, punctuation, and word choice. Use the *How to Edit* chart as a guide.

HOW TO EDIT

1. Go over past papers to see what kinds of errors you made. Look for those errors in your current paper.

2. Read your paper out loud, slowly, saying every word exactly as you have written it.
   - Listen for where your voice goes down in pitch and stops: This usually means the end of a sentence.
   - Watch for any words you may have left out.

3. Check for words that begin dependent clauses, such as *because, when, if,* and *which*. Remember that those clauses need to be attached to a basic sentence.

4. See if all your sentences are in the same pattern. If so, look for sentences that would flow more smoothly if one of them were changed to an addition and placed at the beginning, middle, or end of another sentence.

5. Look for general words that could be replaced with more specific words (e.g., *roses* for *flowers*).

6. Check the verbs, specifically looking for the following:
   - *-s* and *-ed* endings
   - subject-verb agreement
   - irregular verb forms
   - unnecessary switching of tenses

7. See if you have used the correct words, specifically looking for the following:
   - easily confused words
   - contractions and possessives
   - correct pronoun choice

8. Check your spelling by using a dictionary or the spell-check program on your computer. Be aware that the spell-checker will not catch correctly spelled words used incorrectly, such as using *their* when you should have written *there*.

Using Standard Format

If your instructor has not asked you to submit your paper in a specific style, use this standard college essay format:

- Use double-spaced, twelve-point Times New Roman or a similar font. Make sure no extra line spaces appear between paragraphs.

- In the upper left-hand corner of your paper, type the following information on separate lines: your name, your instructor's name, the course name and number, and the date.

- Center the title of your paper. Capitalize the first word, the last word, and all other important words. Do not underline your title or put it in quotation marks or italics.

- Indent the first sentence of each paragraph by using the tab key or five spaces.

- Use one-inch margins on all sides.

- Unless your instructor requires a folder, just staple the pages of your paper together.

Before turning in your paper, give it one final reading, which is called proofreading. Read out loud every word you have written, slowly and carefully, checking for errors. Keep in mind that although printed papers look perfect, they often contain errors.

CHAPTER 18

CHECKPOINTS FOR PAPERS

We write all the time. We make lists of what we need to do or buy. We write letters or e-mail. We write personal messages at the bottom of greeting cards. There are many kinds of writing. In this class, we focus on one kind: the writing used in college and the working world.

College papers, like business letters and memos, have three parts: a beginning, a middle, and an end. If your paper is short, those parts will be in one paragraph. If your paper is more developed, those parts will be in many paragraphs. Regardless of the length of your paper, readers will be looking for a beginning where you state the main idea, a middle where you support that idea, and an end where you conclude that idea. More specifically, readers will be looking for the following:

- ✓ The main idea
- ✓ Convincing support
- ✓ Organized support
- ✓ Connected support
- ✓ The conclusion

• •

The Main Idea

The main idea is your way of looking at things. Main ideas aren't anything new—we use them all the time. Anytime you say, "I've had a good day" or "I've had a bad day," you are giving a main idea. Take last Saturday as an example. Imagine that you made a list of everything you did that day, from the moment you woke up to the time you went to sleep. With that list of details, you would need to stand back and decide what you want to say about the day, how you want to sum it up. You could write about Saturday being a good (or bad) day or, looking at the list from other perspectives, you could write about any of the following:

> expected or unexpected events
>
> what you accomplished
>
> decisions you made
>
> your positive attitude and how it helped you get through the day
>
> responsibilities you have—as a family member, friend, student, or employee
>
> what you learned about yourself, others, or life

Main ideas are important in a paper because they answer a question every reader has: *What's this paper about?* Readers need to know the topic (*who or what*) and your point about that topic (*what about it*). Therefore, keep working on your main idea until you have both parts in one sentence.

Who or what	What about it
Randy	is a loyal friend.
Automatic teller machines	have advantages and disadvantages.
Going to college	has taught me to organize my time.
Used cars	are better bargains than new cars.

As you work on writing your main idea, avoid the following weak formats.

Weak: I am going to write about my friend's car accident.

- This sentence has only one bit of information: *car accident*. The words *I am going to write about* are unnecessary. Do not tell readers what you are going to write about—just do it.

Weak: The effects of my friend's accident.

- Readers know that the paper will be about the effects of the accident, but they will wonder, What about the effects? Are they good or bad, and who is affected—the writer, the writer's friend, family?

Weak: How I was affected by my friend's accident.

● Avoid using the word *how* in a main idea. The word usually indicates a title, not a main idea. Readers still wonder how the writer was affected.

Strong: My friend's car accident has taught me to value life.

● Readers now have a clear idea of *who or what* (*my friend's car accident*) and *what about it* (*has taught me to value life*). The word *affected* has been replaced with *has taught me to value life*, which names a more specific effect.

Convincing Support

A main idea is a general statement. You then need to make that idea real by giving readers specific evidence, such as details, examples, reasons, and facts. An excellent way to find that evidence is to answer the reporter's questions: *Who? What? Where? When? Why? How?* Another way is to imagine that a film director is making a movie of what you write. Someone has a video camera and will film only what you write down on paper. You need to create the scene.

Remember that readers do not know what you know; they cannot read your mind. You need to include enough proof to explain your idea and to convince readers that you know what you are talking about.

Example 1

Whenever I take a test, I panic. I freeze because I am so scared. I sit there and can't remember anything. I hate tests. I get nervous just thinking about them.

Student writer

Example 2

Whenever I take a test, I panic. I sit in the back of the room, feeling disconnected from the real world. My heart starts pounding. Yet in spite of my speeding pulse rate, I feel frozen, as if I am going in slow motion. I try breathing slowly and deeply, but the minute the tests are passed down the row, panic takes over. As the exam approaches the end of the row, my palms become sweaty, my nerves jumpy, and I am short of breath. Finally, when the test sheet is on my desk, I stare at it with disbelieving eyes. I know that I studied all night for this test, yet I look at it as if it is in another language. My mind goes blank. I can't remember anything. Last week, I saw a notice in the hall for a one-hour workshop on taking exams. I have overcome all kinds of obstacles in my life. I am ready to take that workshop and overcome my terror of tests.

Student writer

- The first example lacks specific details. A person with a video camera would have nothing to film. In the second example, the writer gives us enough specific details to make the panic real.

Organized Support

We need to arrange our ideas in logical order so that readers can follow our thinking. Two of the most common ways of ordering ideas are by time and by importance.

USING TIME ORDER

When arranging ideas according to time, begin with the events that occurred first. If you were writing about a game, you could choose before the game, during the game, and after the game. If you were writing about your life, you could choose childhood, adolescence, and adulthood—or elementary school, middle school, and high school. In the following example, the writer uses time order to explain why his current job is his best job.

My best job is the one I currently have. I am an orderly in an operating room at a Chicago hospital. My main responsibility is transporting patients to and from surgery. I take pride in this job because bringing a smile to the sick comes easily to me, as naturally as slipping my feet into an old pair of comfortable shoes. Each day, I know that I will be saying, "Good morning," to patients who are scared. Their anxiety is apparent, sometimes in rigid frowns, sometimes in droplets of sweat running down their foreheads. As I position the stretcher next to their beds, their eyes are wide and glassy, and their body movements are slow, reminding me of fighters not yet ready to answer the bell. When I secure the patients, our eyes meet and they seem to cry out, "Help me." I smile, rub their shoulders, and try to assure them that everything will be all right. I tell little jokes, and for a minute, they forget their fear and chuckle. As I roll the stretcher down the cold halls with lights overhead whizzing by, I sometimes hold their hands, as a father might hold his child's hand before crossing the street. When we reach the destination, their anxiety resurfaces. I smile, hold their eyes gently in mine, and again reassure them everything will be all right. Their eyes respond with thanks and gratitude. It warms my heart, and I go home proud that I have helped someone, that in some small way I matter to other people. I love what I do. It's not a job; it's a career. It's my calling.

Student writer

USING ORDER OF IMPORTANCE

You can also order your ideas by importance, usually saving the best for last. If you were writing about why you believe or deserve something, you could begin with the least important reason and move toward the most important one. Saving the best for last is a good way to end with power. In the following example, the writer makes three points to support her main idea that her grandfather was very giving: Her family depended on him; he spoiled her brother and her; and most importantly, he would take them out to lunch.

My grandfather was the most giving person I have ever known. My whole family depended on him. Whenever anyone of us was sick, he helped out. If we had a cold, he brought us chicken soup. If we needed a ride to the doctor, he drove us. He also spoiled my brother and me by giving us things we wanted but didn't need. For example, when he realized that we wanted roller blades, he tucked money in our pockets, saying, "Now, just go ahead and buy them." He told us to consider this an early birthday gift, but when our birthdays rolled around three months later, he still gave each of us a wonderful present. The best gift he gave us, even more than the birthday presents, was taking us out to lunch. He used to surprise us by showing up spontaneously, knocking on the door, and announcing that we were going out for pizza, just the three of us. It was never near anyone's birthday or holiday. He just wanted to be with us. My grandfather wasn't good to us because he wanted to impress anyone. He did it, he said, because it brought him joy.

Student writer

STICKING TO THE POINT

Readers must be able to follow your train of thought, so make sure you don't take any side trips. Let's take the main idea *The car mechanic finally diagnosed my car's problem*. It may be true that the car mechanic plays basketball on weekends, but the writer cannot use this fact to prove that the mechanic correctly diagnosed his or her car's problem. A main idea is similar to a promise to take a friend on a journey. If you say you are going to the beach, don't take a side trip and go to the movies.

Example 1

My parents always told me that during life you only get one chance, that you can never go back. My response to that was, "Yeah, whatever," but now I wish I could go back and redo high school. I never studied or tried hard in my classes. I always did just enough to get by. My response to assignments and tests was, "School is not going to take me where I want to go. Baseball will." I was wrong. During my senior year, I realized that college coaches were looking for grades, and mine weren't there. ~~My worst grades were in English because I never turned in my papers.~~ Every college coach ignored me because I had only half of the perfect package. My parents were right.

Student writer

- The crossed-out sentence may be true, but it wanders from the writer's main idea.

Make sure you do what you say you are going to do. If you say you are going to class, then to work, and then to Maria's house, do all three and in that order. In other words, if your main idea states you are going to write about A, B, and C, make sure you cover those three points and in that order, writing about A, then B, and then C—not B, C, and A.

Example 2

Main idea: Shopping for clothes is physically, mentally, and financially exhausting.

    Point 1: Shopping for clothes exhausts me physically.

    Point 2: I am also worn out mentally.

    Point 3: The physical and the mental exhaustion pass, but the financial drain remains.

- The main idea says that the writer will write about physical exhaustion first, mental exhaustion second, and financial exhaustion last.

The writer's points follow that order. The first point tells us this section will be about the physical exhaustion. The second point tells us this section will explain the mental exhaustion. The third point tells us this section will be about the financial drain. The main idea and the points match.

Connected Support

Readers need to see how your ideas connect. Here are three ways to provide that connection:

1. Use transition words, such as *also*, *in addition*, and *finally*.

2. Weave the main idea through the paper by repeating key (significant) words from the main idea.

3. Write a transition sentence that refers to the preceding idea.

TRANSITION WORDS

You can use transition words, such as those listed in the following chart, to help readers see the relationship between your ideas.

TRANSITION WORDS

To introduce ideas

also	besides	first	in addition	next	similarly
as well as	finally	furthermore	last	second	

To introduce an example

for example	for instance	specifically

To introduce a result or a cause

accordingly	because	since	then	thus
as a result	consequently	so	therefore	

To show time

after	during	first	meanwhile	then
as	eventually	gradually	next	when
before	finally	later	soon	while

To show a change in direction

although	however	nevertheless	yet
but	in contrast	on the contrary	
conversely	instead	on the other hand	

To indicate importance

above all	equally important	more important
best	especially	most significant

In the example that follows, the transition words are in bold.

A few years ago, our financial problems were a nightmare. Our debts began the day we married. The bills from the rehearsal dinner, wedding, and honeymoon were paid by charging them. We **also** charged our furniture and appliances. **After** equipping our apartment, we charged vacations and entertainment. **Then, when** we needed a new car, we financed our car loan through a finance company. Slowly, we were digging ourselves into debt. **As** the high interest rates and late fees of credit card companies continued to grow, we borrowed from one credit card to pay the others. **When** that no longer covered us, we got cash advances from one charge card to carry us from one payday to the next. **Eventually,** we were exhausted by the telephone calls and letters from collection agencies. We were **finally** forced to face the truth. The nightmare was not a passing dream. The nightmare was a reality that we were creating.

Student writer

KEY WORDS OR IDEAS

You can weave the main idea through your paper by repeating key words. In the following sketch outline, the main idea includes the word *taught*. The writer repeats that key idea in the first and second points with the word *learned* and in the third point with the word *taught*.

Main idea: My friend's car accident **taught** me to value life.

    Point 1: I **learned** how valuable friends are.

    Point 2: In addition, I **learned** how much my family means to me.

    Point 3: Most importantly, my friend's accident **taught** me to take my life seriously.

TRANSITION SENTENCES

You can also use transition sentences to refer back to the preceding idea and forward to the next. The sketch outline that follows is identical to the preceding one, except for the third point, which is now a transition sentence. The words *not only friends and family* refer to the first and second points. The words *but also my own life* tell us what the third point is.

Main idea: My friend's car accident taught me to value life.

    Point 1: I learned how valuable friends are.

    Point 2: In addition, I learned how much my family means to me.

    Point 3: I learned to value **not only friends and family but also my own life**.

The Conclusion

A conclusion wraps up the ideas presented. It ties your paper together by returning to the main idea, bringing your paper full circle. The following guidelines will help you write an effective conclusion.

HOW TO WRITE A CONCLUSION

What to do

1. Read what you have written and see what idea emerges. Write down whatever comes to mind without worrying about how good it is. Once you have something on paper, you can go back and work with it.

2. Read your paper and ask yourself, *So what? Why is this important?* Answering these questions will help you discover an insight.

3. Repeat or refer to key (significant) words from your main idea.

4. Restate the main idea in different words and from a slightly different angle.

What not to do

1. Do not repeat the main idea word for word. This tells readers you can't think of anything else to write.

2. Do not simply tell readers what they just read. For example, do not write, "From what I have written, you can see that . . ." or "Now you can tell that . . ." This tells readers you have run out of ideas.

3. Do not conclude with an idea that you did not previously mention. An entirely new idea will confuse readers.

4. Do not give readers the moral of the story. Let's compare this to a movie. At the end of a movie, the director does not appear on screen to give us advice or tell what we should have learned. Instead, the director makes the story so real that we experience what the characters experience. It's the same with writing. Work on making your main idea real. If you have given readers specific evidence, they will understand your point. Then at the end, state the facts or the truth as you see it—from your point of view.

• •

Exercises

⬤ **Self Test:** As you read each of the following main ideas, identify the *who or what* (the topic) and the *what about it* (the point about the topic).

Example

My brother is my hero.

Who or what: *My brother*
What about it: *is my hero*

1. Money can't buy happiness.
   Who or what: _____
   What about it: _____

2. My high school coach gave me confidence.
   Who or what: _____
   What about it: _____

3. Working while going to college is difficult.
   Who or what: _____
   What about it: _____

4. Sunday is the best day of the week.
   Who or what: _____
   What about it: _____

5. Top Notch is the best restaurant in town.
   Who or what: _____
   What about it: _____

6. I need a vacation.
   Who or what: _____
   What about it: _____

7. Living in a large city has advantages.
   Who or what: _____
   What about it: _____

8. Little things irritate me.

Who or what: _____

What about it: _____

9. Lauren is a loyal friend.

Who or what: _____

What about it: _____

10. College is not what I had expected.

Who or what: _____

What about it: _____

○ **Exercise 1:** An effective paper has three parts: a beginning that states the main idea, a middle that supports that main idea, and an ending that wraps up the paper. The following paragraphs are good examples of this three-part structure. Read each one and answer the questions that follow.

Paragraph A

My children, Nicolas and Melissa, have made me feel that I am a good mother. They love to see me volunteer at their grade school. Both of them are proud that their mom helps out in the library, bakes for parties, attends field trips, works the book fair, and most of all decorates the bulletin boards for each season. I can hear them whisper to their friends, "That's my mom." When we are at home and I am cooking or folding laundry, they often walk through the kitchen, casually commenting, "Love you, Mom." I am amazed that, although they are just third and fourth graders, they manage to speak the words of encouragement that every adult wants to hear. I know that my journey of motherhood is far from over, but I also know that they have given me a priceless gift. They have taught me that, so far, I have done something well: I am a good mother.

Student writer

1. Underline the sentence that states the main idea.
2. What specific details does the writer include to prove the main idea?

_____

3. What key words in the conclusion refer back to the main idea, giving you a sense of completion?

_____

Paragraph B

I have made many mistakes, but because I am determined, I have not stayed stuck. When I graduated from high school, I went to college out of state, and I blew it. I was young, away from home for the first time, and free to party all night and sleep all day. I lacked the focus to study, and I soon flunked out. For the next ten years, I jumped from job to job, and from state to state, often commuting three to four hours a day. Deep down inside was a slow burn. I knew I had the ability to do something more with my life, but because I worked full time and had to pay my bills, I did not have the time or the money to go to college. The slow burn soon spread and began to destroy me. I became less productive at work, and I knew I would soon be fired. So I swallowed my pride, called my mother, and asked if I could come home to reach a goal. When she said yes, I put all my belongings in storage, moved back home, and registered at a local community college. I am now a first-semester student, determined to do it right this time.

Student writer

1. Underline the main idea.
2. What kind of order did the writer use to organize his details: time order or order of importance?

Paragraph C

The winter vacation I spent with my grandfather when I was six years old is still vivid in my mind. Most of our time was spent working in the garage, Grandpa's favorite pastime. I spent countless hours sitting on a bench watching him rebuild engines with the mastery of a surgeon. Whether he was replacing spark plugs or rebuilding pistons, I sat there fascinated. At the end of every afternoon, he would say to me, "We both made this go again, Kurt."

On snowy days, we journeyed to the snow hill. Smoking his cigar, Grandpa huffed and puffed his way to the top of the hill, towing me behind him. Then we rested at the top and watched the other kids slide their way to the bottom. When my turn came closer, as I sat on the round saucer, I felt a strong force pushing behind me, rocking me closer to the edge. Just as the saucer tipped over the side of the hill, that strong force jumped onto the saucer behind me. Grandpa would scream and laugh with intense joy all the way to the bottom of the hill. We always ended up rolling around in the snow, making snow angels and laughing. I can hear him today, laughing. The memory of my grandfather stays with me, constantly reminding me what a wonderful man he was. Memories last a lifetime.

Student writer

1. Underline the main idea.

2. What specific details help you see and hear what the writer remembers?

Paragraph D

Working as a waiter at Bellagina's is the worst job I have ever had. First, the work schedule is exhausting. Every day except Sunday, I work from 3:30 p.m. until midnight. When I get home at 1:15 a.m., I collapse into bed until the alarm clock blasts me awake at 7:00 a.m. for my morning classes. I have no time to party, little time to study, and no time to relax. Second, the customers are messy. I think that when people go out to eat, they are extra sloppy because they know someone else has to clean up. Filthy paper napkins are thrown on the floor; bread and food crumbs are stuck to the chairs; spaghetti sauce is slopped all over the tables. I have often thought of quitting, but the long hours and messy customers have taught me an important lesson: I don't want to be a waiter for the rest of my life. I'm sticking with this job so I can pay for tuition and get my college degree, which is my ticket to better opportunities.

Student writer

1. Underline the main idea.
2. The writer makes two points. Underline the two sentences that give those points.
3. Read the paragraph again and decide where you think the conclusion begins.

_____

Paragraph E

Four years ago, I was misjudged and mislabeled. I worked in the shipping and receiving department of a warehouse. There were twenty male employees and one female. I was the female. Because I was female, the supervisor labeled me incompetent. Actually, he made a bet with some of the other supervisors that I would not be able to handle the pressure and harassment from the male workers and truck drivers. He predicted that I would not last three months in the department. But I knew I was competent; I was determined not only to survive but to succeed.

Before the year was over, I had motivated the male workers and drivers with my skills, patience, intelligence, and sense of humor. The men respected and supported me, and we all worked hard. We had a healthy and supportive team spirit. Because of my work performance, relationships with coworkers, and overall commitment to the job, I received a promotion and a raise. Realizing he had misjudged me, the male supervisor finally apologized, saying, "I was wrong, but I just didn't think a woman could do it." His apology made me feel good, but what made me feel even better was that I knew I could do anything I put my mind to—even in a man's world. I have a new label now: female, determined, and successful.

Student writer

1. The writer uses time order to tell her story. Read the first sentence of each paragraph and underline the words that give us the time frame.

2. In the main idea, the writer states that she was misjudged and mislabeled. What label was she given?

_____

3. In the conclusion, she states that because of her job performance, the label had changed. What new label was she given?

_____

Writing Prompts for One- to Two-Paragraph Papers

Ideas to spark your thinking are listed on the following pages. Whatever topic you choose, remember to use the writing process. Readers do not know what you know—you have to convince them.

GROUP 1

1. The best (strangest, most unusual) gift I have ever received is . . .

2. My favorite city (vacation spot, car, sport, possession) is . . .

3. The happiest time in my childhood was when . . . (or) My best year in elementary school (high school) was . . .

4. The person I admired (feared) most when I was younger was . . .

5. Describe yourself from your best friend's point of view, an enemy's point of view, your employer's point of view, your favorite (least favorite) relative's point of view, your pet's point of view, or your favorite (least favorite) teacher's point of view.

6. Imagine you are a newspaper reporter. Describe your neighborhood or college.

7. My favorite family tradition (holiday celebration) is . . .

8. The best (worst) job I ever had was . . .

9. The best (worst) class I ever had was . . .

10. Write about an object that will give the reader insight into who you are. Think of objects in your home (room, car, pockets). Describe that object and explain how it reveals something about your character.

GROUP 2

1. The first time I drove a car (got a ticket, got caught in a lie, performed on stage, played in a tournament), I . . .

2. I learned a valuable lesson about life when . . .

3. My proudest achievement is . . .

4. I felt like an outsider when . . .

5. A friend (coach, teacher, relative) who has inspired me is . . .

6. _____ has made a difference in my life.

7. The easiest (most difficult) decision I ever made was . . .

8. My most embarrassing (exciting, rewarding, memorable) experience was . . .

9. My life changed when I . . .

10. I have learned that . . .

GROUP 3

1. Like most people, little things irritate me.

2. Being a mother (father, sister, brother, only child) can be frustrating (rewarding).

3. Write about someone who is honest (faithful, determined, willing to listen, forgiving, kind, sensitive, courageous, trustworthy, dependable, creative, energetic, loyal, optimistic, patient). You can choose someone you know well or yourself. In your main idea, name the person and the quality. Support your main idea with one or more examples.

4. People have become increasingly rude.

5. Living in a small town (city, big city) has advantages (disadvantages). (or) Leaving home and renting an apartment has advantages (disadvantages).

6. _____ respects (does not respect) _____.

7. Returning to college as an older adult (Attending college immediately after high school) has advantages (disadvantages).

8. Many teenagers are role models for younger children.

9. The qualities of a good parent (college student, friend) are . . .

10. I am investing (wasting) my time by . . .

GROUP 4

1. I believe that . . .

2. If I could change one thing about my life, I would . . .

3. _____ needs to be changed.

4. The best (worst) decision I ever made was to . . .

5. I deserve a raise (a promotion at my job, an *A* in a course).

6. I need a vacation.

7. I want a college degree for two (three) reasons.

8. Teenagers drop out of high school for two (three) reasons.

9. College is (is not) what I had expected.

10. What is your most prized possession? Explain why.

GROUP 5

In your main idea, state the topic and name its effect. For example, for item 1, your main idea could be *My religious faith has given me confidence.*

1. The effects of a religious faith

2. The effects of accomplishing a goal (receiving an award)

3. The effects of a positive mental attitude

4. The effects of getting (losing) a job

5. The effects of drug abuse

6. The effects of going to college (dropping out of school)

7. The effects of marriage (divorce, becoming a parent)

8. The effects of a change in law (school policy, company policy)

9. The effects of residents becoming involved in their community

10. The effects of gaining (losing) small businesses in a community

GROUP 6

In your main idea, state both the topic and the point you want to make about that topic. For example, your main idea for item 1 could be *Students can succeed in college when they put their education first.*

1. How to succeed in college (get an *A* in a particular course)

2. How to mend a broken relationship

3. How to break a bad habit

4. How your college can improve students' college experience

5. How your workplace can improve customer service (employee morale)

6. How to respond to an angry person

7. How to buy a car (television, cell phone)

8. How to present yourself positively in an interview

9. How you accomplished something you are proud of

10. How to live nonviolently in a violent society

CHAPTER 19

ESSAYS

Writing an essay is similar to writing a one- or two-paragraph paper. The difference is that you have more ideas to work with. This chapter builds on what you learned in Chapters 17 and 18 and shows you how ideas are organized in an essay.

An essay is a paper of several paragraphs that explain a main idea. As discussed earlier, papers have three parts: a beginning where you state the main idea, a middle where you support that idea, and an end where you conclude that idea. In an essay, the introductory paragraph contains the main idea; the supporting paragraphs, the evidence; and the final paragraph, the conclusion. You can see how these parts connect in the Essay Diagram that follows.

• •

Essay Diagram

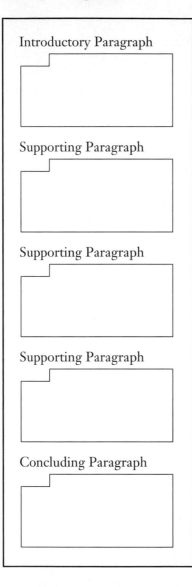

Introductory Paragraph

Include your main idea (thesis statement).

Supporting Paragraph

Explain your first point (topic sentence).

Supporting Paragraph

Explain your next point (topic sentence).

Supporting Paragraph

Explain your last point (topic sentence).

Concluding Paragraph

Return to the main idea in the introductory paragraph, bringing your paper full circle.

- Essays can have fewer than or more than three supporting paragraphs. Paragraphs let readers see ideas in sections so that they know what ideas belong together. Therefore, begin a new paragraph when you are moving to a new point.

Introductory Paragraph

The introductory paragraph has two purposes: to give the main idea and to spark the readers' interest. The main idea of an essay is called a *thesis statement*. You can place the thesis statement at the beginning or end of the paragraph.

A thesis statement has two parts: the topic (*who or what*) and your point about that topic (*what about it*). Make sure you have two parts; a topic alone will not do.

Topic	Point about that topic
Television programs	do not give a realistic picture of life in America.
My mother's common sense	has helped me survive.
Honesty and loyalty	are essential to a healthy relationship.
Self-discipline	is the most important ingredient for success.

You can attract readers' attention in a number of ways:

- Begin with a broad statement about your main idea, and then move toward your specific thesis statement.

- Give background information that readers need in order to understand your topic.

- Describe the situation, scene, or person.

- Begin with something you and readers have in common.

- Make a comparison to something familiar to readers.

- Ask a thought-provoking question, which the paper then answers.

Helpful hint: Although the introductory paragraph is the first part to be read, it is often the last part to be written. Do not worry about writing the introduction until you have written the first draft. Once you see how your supporting paragraphs work together, you will have a better idea of how to interest readers in your essay. In fact, often a short section later in a draft can be moved and used in the introduction.

• •

Supporting Paragraphs

The supporting paragraphs explain, or support, the main idea. Each one begins with a sentence that tells readers what that paragraph will be about. This sentence, the main idea of a paragraph, is called a *topic sentence*.

To find your topic sentences, use the writing process described in Chapter 17. As part of this process, ask yourself, *How would I explain my main idea to someone who does not know what I know?* Jot down your immediate answers, and work with them until you have figured out your main points. Write each point in a separate sentence. These points are your topic sentences.

ORDERING IDEAS

Put these points in order so that readers can follow your thinking. You can order your ideas according to time, importance, or category.

Time Order

To order your ideas according to time, begin with the events that occurred first and move toward the events that occurred last.

Thesis statement: Gaining confidence is similar to climbing a ladder. It's a step-by-step process that takes time.

> Point 1: When I was in grade school, the ladder was easy to climb.
>
> Point 2: When I entered middle school, the climb became more difficult. For each two steps forward, I took one step back.
>
> Point 3: In high school, I realized that I was gaining ground. I was moving up the ladder.
>
> Point 4: Now that I am older, I can look back and see how far I have come.

Order of Importance

Ordering your ideas by importance usually means saving the best point for last.

Thesis statement: My supervisor, Mr. Collins, respects his employees.

Point 1: Mr. Collins is always available to listen to our concerns.

Point 2: He also values our suggestions.

Point 3: Above all, Mr. Collins allows us flexible hours as long as we get the job completed on time.

Categories

You can also organize your ideas in categories. For example, if you were thinking about the effects of something, you could write about *who* is affected: *yourself, family, friends,* and/or *community.* If you were thinking about *how* people are affected, you could write about the *physical, financial, emotional,* and/or *spiritual* effects.

Thesis statement: My volunteer work has benefited the community, my family, and me.

Point 1: I help my community take care of people in need.

Point 2: My family members also benefit because they realize the value of serving others.

Point 3: I too benefit because I am improving my job opportunities.

- Notice that the thesis statement and points match. As explained in Chapter 18, if your main idea states that you are going to write about A, B, and C, make sure you cover those three points and in that order.

Helpful hint: The thesis statement and topic sentences are the backbone of an essay. If a total stranger reads just your thesis statement and the first sentence of each supporting paragraph, that person should have a clear summary of your paper.

OUTLINING IDEAS

Once you have your main points, sketch those ideas in an outline so you can make sure your ideas are organized logically.

HOW TO OUTLINE AN ESSAY

Write the main idea in one or two sentences: the thesis statement.

Write the supporting points: the topic sentences.

Under each topic sentence, list the details you will include in that paragraph.

Main idea of the paper (thesis statement):
I want to be more organized, stop procrastinating, and have a positive attitude.

Point 1 (topic sentence): *I want to be more organized.*

detail: *Always late. Scattered.*
detail: *Need to work ahead. Before bed: lunch, keys, set alarm.*
detail: *Then no last minute stuff, slamming doors.*

Point 2 (topic sentence): *I want to face responsibilities on time.*

detail: *Stop procrastinating. Do homework, fill gas tank, pay bills.*
detail: *Putting things off makes life worse, solves nothing.*

Point 3 (topic sentence): *I want to have a positive attitude.*

detail: *Start out on good note, on time.*
detail: *Want to concentrate in school, be calm on job.*
detail: *Have perspective on what happens, be positive.*

- The map is flexible. You can have fewer than or more than three points and accompanying details.

This essay appears on page 252.

Concluding Paragraph

A concluding paragraph wraps up your essay, bringing it full circle. When readers read your conclusion, they should sense that all the ideas in the essay are now tied together. A good conclusion flows out of what you have already written, giving readers something to think about. The suggestions in the *How to Write a Conclusion* chart on page 231 will help you end your essay effectively.

Exercises

● **Self Test:** Read the following student essay and answer the questions that follow.

(1)   Walk through any bookstore or glance at the magazine racks in any supermarket, and you will see countless promises for success: Three steps to strong biceps. Five steps to a healthy heart. Ten steps to succeeding in business. For years, I glanced at those follow-the-steps titles and thought, "Who cares? Who needs a bunch of steps?" Surprisingly, I did. I owe my life to a twelve-step program.

(2)   I was once helpless and hopeless. For too many years, I was trapped by drugs. My daily routine was chasing drugs, day after day, just to keep from feeling or facing the wreckage of my life. I lost cars, my home, my job, my friends, and my family. Locked in the prison of addiction, I finally hit bottom.

(3)   I was ready to give up, but I gave life one more chance and sought help. On a dreary Tuesday afternoon, thumbing through the yellow pages, I found Narcotics Anonymous and called them. That night, someone picked me up and drove me to my first meeting. At first, I was scared and insecure, wobbling in my fear of facing people and facing myself. But at that meeting, people told their stories, and I realized I was not alone. There were many suggestions on how to stay drug free. The ones that have helped me the most are in a twelve-step book.

(4)   The twelve-step book has been my door to freedom. The book begins by explaining the who, what, and why of the addict. Reading it, I saw my life as if for the first time. And as I continued reading, I discovered the steps and how to implement them for recovery. So far, I have completed three of them, and these three steps have given me my life. Step one is recognizing that I am powerless over drugs and that my life had become unmanageable. The second step is coming to believe that a power greater than mine can restore me to sanity. The third step is making a decision to turn my will and my life over to God, as I understand God. These steps and attending the meetings have changed my life.

(5)   Today I have turned my will and life over to God. My obsession to use drugs has changed into an obsession to live as a productive member of society. My compulsion now is to chase after my dream of becoming an X-ray technician and to live my life one day at a time. I have been drug free for two years now, and I have been restored to enough sanity to know there is hope.

(6)   My old lifestyle is gone. I am close to my family once again. My children's fear that I will fall back into drugs is slowly being replaced with trust. I attend college full time and am working hard to get *A*'s—not an easy task for someone who has been out of school for fifteen years. I am an active member of church and live my sobriety by giving to others. I even have a car, a luxury I lost years ago, along with my license. But most importantly, I know who I am, and I have the twelve steps to thank for that.

Student writer

1. In the introductory paragraph, how does the writer attract our attention?

   _____

2. Underline the thesis statement.

3. List the four topic sentences.

   a. _____

   b. _____

   c. _____

   d. _____

4. The student's concluding paragraph describes the benefits of the writer's drug-free life. What sentence explains the greatest benefit, and what words in that sentence refer back to the thesis statement?

   _____

⬤ **Exercise 1:** Read the following student essays and answer the questions that follow.

Essay A

(1)   The obstacles I face are surmountable. They are not huge problems beyond my control but little problems I know I can overcome. I want to be more organized, stop procrastinating, and have a positive attitude.

(2)   I need to be more organized. Right now, I am constantly playing catch-up, always running late and always scattered. I would be more organized if I worked ahead of time. Before I go to bed, I

could make my sandwich for the next day's lunch so I don't stain my work clothes with mustard or mayonnaise. I could also set out clothes for the next day, put the car keys on my bureau, and make sure the alarm clock is turned on. These small steps will help me avoid my current morning routine of running in circles, changing clothes at the last minute, losing keys, slamming doors, and forgetting things.

(3)   I not only need to work ahead of time, I also need to face responsibilities on time. I must stop procrastinating. Instead of waiting until the night before class, I should work on assignments throughout the week and the weekend. I am doing poorly in school because I don't get my homework done, I turn in disorganized papers, and I blank out on exams. School is not the only problem. I should fill up the gas tank when it approaches empty, not when it hits empty, and pay my bills on time to avoid penalty payments on utilities and interest charges on my credit card. When responsibilities pile up, life gets messy. Procrastinating has not solved my problems. In fact, it has magnified and, in many cases, created them.

(4)   If I am more organized and stop procrastinating, I will be able to achieve my third goal: a positive attitude. Waking up when the

alarm rings will give me time to put my day into perspective. I can begin the day by saying to myself, "This will be a good day. I can concentrate in class and succeed. I can be calm on the job and not overreact." Plus, I will have another benefit: I will know that I have done my part in preparing and being responsible. Having this confidence will free me up to know what is my fault and what is not, to recognize what I have control over and what I have no control over. Then when I face crazy situations, rather than giving up and feeling defeated, I will be able to say to myself, "O.K., this is crazy, but take a deep breath and continue on."

(5)   Living a good life, I am finally beginning to realize, is not solving the big problems but tackling the little ones. There is much in life I cannot control. But if I can become more organized, stop procrastinating, and have a positive attitude, I will be better able to handle all of life.

Student writer

1. Read the introductory paragraph. What three points does the writer promise to cover in this essay?

_____

2. Read the point of the third paragraph. What words in this sentence refer to the point made in the preceding paragraph?

_____

3. Read the point of the fourth paragraph. What words in this sentence refer to the points made in preceding paragraphs?

_____

4. The supporting paragraphs describe the changes the writer wants to make. In the conclusion, we are told what difference these changes will make in the writer's life. What will the writer gain?

_____

Essay B

We have focused so far on essays that begin with the main idea because this is the structure used most in college papers. Sometimes you may want to state the main idea at the end of the essay, rather than at the beginning.

(1)   My childhood, like everyone's childhood, was filled with valuable lessons. Share your toys, tell the truth, be kind, be careful—these are but a few of them. By the time I became an adolescent, I felt I knew everything that was worth knowing. I was wrong.

(2)   When I was fifteen, I decided to drop out of school because life was too frustrating and difficult. I went to my father, an easygoing man with sparkling eyes who refused to let anything get him down. My father did not have an easy life. The hard calluses on his blue-collar hands and the weathered wrinkles on his face told his tale. But no matter how busy or tired this hardworking man was, he always had time for me, or as he affectionately called me, "his kid." So I went to him, explained my frustrations, and presented my case for dropping out of school. I told him I was smart enough, and I had

learned enough in school to sustain me in life. I could get a job without any problem. My final reason was that he would not have to work so hard to provide for me because I would be helping out too. This was my last-ditch effort to convince my father, my judge and my jury.

(3)   His loving eyes suddenly became cold, and the laugh lines on his face formed a frown. His reply was a straightforward answer and not at all what I had expected, "Then don't go back." Chills rippled down my spine. I had made him angry, I knew. Although he had agreed with my decision, I now realized that this is not what I had expected. Parents are supposed to argue with their kids. Somehow I found the courage to ask why he was letting me quit. With a raspy, deep-throated voice, he gave me two reasons. "If you are so smart, then you are wasting your teachers' time. There are other kids in your school who are willing to work hard. You are obviously a quitter. The others, not you, deserve the teachers' time." He continued, "And you are wasting my time. I have been working hard to give you this opportunity, and you have become a fool."

(4)   Furious, I stormed out of the room. How dare he say I was a quitter and a fool. There was no way I was going to let anyone call me a quitter. My anger fumed into a new decision. I was going to do

everything in my power to prove him wrong. I refused to quit school. I buckled down in my classes. I worked with the teachers to gain extra credit. I studied harder and even took notes, something I had always thought a waste of time. With all of the hard work, I surprised even myself. I earned a place on the honor roll. Imagine, someone who months earlier was willing to throw it all away was now an honor student. I now realize the profound wisdom in my father's words and actions. He forced me to take responsibility for my life. He taught me to grow up.

Student writer

1. When an essay tells a story, the specific thesis statement is sometimes saved until the end. Writers use the introductory paragraph to interest readers in the story by giving them a clue about the essay's main idea. What two sentences in the introductory paragraph provide this clue?

_____

_____

2. In the supporting paragraphs, the writer tells a story. What is the story about?

_____

_____

3. Read the last paragraph where the writer concludes the story. What did the father's words and actions teach the writer?

_____

_____

• •

Writing Prompts for Essays

Most of the prompts listed at the end of Chapter 18 can be developed into effective essays. Additional ideas to spark your thinking are listed on the following pages.

When looking for a topic, choose one that you can prove with specific evidence. You can explain your reasons, give examples, tell a story, or use any other method that logically explains your thinking. Whatever method you choose, make sure you use the writing process described in Chapter 17.

GROUP 1

1. I am glad that . . .

2. Write about a belief (opinion) you hold that others do not hold.

3. Write about an obstacle you once faced and how you overcame it. (or) Write about an obstacle that you currently face and what you need to overcome it.

4. I think my family should change the way it . . .

5. I used to believe that _____, but I have changed my mind.

6. The biggest challenge my community faces is . . .

7. The best advice I was ever given was . . .

8. People in my community deserve an award for . . .

9. The qualities of a healthy relationship are . . .

10. Every story has two sides.

GROUP 2

1. Honesty is (is not) always the best policy.

2. Write about a recent news story that caught your attention.

3. What do you do to cope with stress?

4. What advice would you give to a student just beginning high school (college)?

5. Working (taking care of a family) and going to school at the same time is difficult.

6. Choose a character (situation) in a movie or television program. Explain how that character (situation) is realistic (unrealistic).

7. Television teaches children that . . . Complete this sentence by naming the values (lessons about life) you think television teaches children. Prove your point by describing specific television programs or advertisements.

8. Explain why teenagers rebel (why college is difficult, why someone is jealous, why someone is angry, why there is road rage).

9. What can be done to prevent violence in public schools?

10. Write about a "before" and "after." Think about an event or an experience that changed how you think, act, or feel. Describe the "before," the experience, and the "after."

GROUP 3

1. How has your attitude toward your community (high school friends, family) changed since you have entered college?

2. If you could reclaim an item (attitude, belief) from your childhood, what would it be? Describe it and explain why.

3. Interview someone who is one or two generations older than you and ask that person what life was like when he or she was young. Ask about such things as work, transportation, education, communication, music, entertainment, and fashion. Find a word that summarizes this lifestyle, such as *easy*, *difficult*, *simple*, or *stressful*. Your main idea could be "When _____ was young, life was _____." Then prove the truth of that statement by giving specific examples or reasons.

4. Choose a type of music you know fairly well and examine it as if it were a window into our culture. What do you see? What does the music say about our concerns (values, fears)?

5. Think of a time when what you did or said did not reflect what you believed. Perhaps you did something you knew was wrong, kept silent when you should have spoken, or followed a group instead of your conscience. Describe the situation. Explain what this experience taught you.

6. Write about two or more roles you play, such as student, family member, employee, friend, neighbor, or member of an organization.

7. How does your public image differ from your private self? (or) How does the public image of someone you know differ from that person's private self?

8. Choose a problem in your college, your neighborhood, your workplace, or an organization or program you are part of. Or consider a broader societal problem, such as domestic violence or environmental pollution—or a personal problem. Name the problem, describe it so readers recognize it as a problem, and explore one or more solutions. As you brainstorm, consider the cause of the problem, the history of the problem, and who is affected by the problem.

9. What is the most important value you learned from your family? How did you learn it? What difference has that value made in your life?

10. Explain why a movie (actor, athlete, politician, instructor, religious leader, community leader, book, television program, type of music) is popular. As you brainstorm, consider who is attracted, what they seek, and what they find. Make sure you describe your topic in detail so that readers who are not familiar with your topic understand your thinking.

GROUP 4

Use one of the following sayings as your main idea and prove its truth by giving examples or telling a story. Remember to include specific details so that readers can visualize your evidence.

Whenever you include a quotation from another source, you need a sentence to transition from the quotation to your experience. For example, if you were to choose the fourth topic as your main idea, you might begin with that sentence and then include a transition sentence, such as "Lao Tzu's words of wisdom apply to my life." If the author is not given, use a transition sentence, such as "These words of wisdom apply to my life."

1. What goes around comes around.

2. Money can't buy happiness.

3. With age comes wisdom.

4. A journey of a thousand miles must begin with a single step. —Lao Tzu

5. Don't find fault. Find a remedy. —Henry Ford

6. Hold fast to dreams, for if dreams die, life is a broken-winged bird that cannot fly. —Langston Hughes

7. Any fact facing us is not as important as our attitude toward it, for that determines our success or failure. —Norman Vincent Peale

8. It is never too late to be who you might have been. —George Eliot

9. The weak can never forgive. Forgiveness is the attribute of the strong. —Mahatma Gandhi

10. Prosperity is a great teacher; adversity a greater. —William Hazlitt

GROUP 5

Choose a current controversial issue, such as one in the list that follows. Do research, either by reading or talking to others, so that you are aware of the varying positions on the issue. In your thesis, state the issue and your position on the issue.

1. Should cell phones be banned from public places, like restaurants or trains?

2. Should parents supervise what their children watch on television?

3. Should parents be held legally and financially responsible for their children's actions?

4. Should high schools put less emphasis on athletics?

5. Should the government run any gambling operations, such as riverboat casinos or lotteries?

6. Who should be responsible for teaching morals and values: families, schools, religious institutions, communities?

7. Should the main purpose of jail time be punishment for the crime?

8. Should teens accused of serious crimes be tried as adults?

9. Should an employer be allowed to read the e-mail of employees or track their activity on the Internet?

10. Are elementary and high schools adequately meeting the needs of their students?

PART 6

BASICS FOR NONNATIVE SPEAKERS

CHAPTER 20

NONNATIVE SPEAKER INFORMATION

If you are a nonnative speaker, some of the ways words are used in English may be unfamiliar and confusing. This chapter summarizes a number of those patterns.

. . . .

Nouns

English has two kinds of nouns: those that can be counted and those that cannot be counted.

COUNT NOUNS

A **count noun** can be counted, as in *one pen, two pens, three pens, four pens.* Count nouns have both singular and plural forms.

Singular	Plural
one *banana*	three *bananas*
one *dollar*	many *dollars*

NONCOUNT NOUNS

A **noncount noun** cannot be counted. It has only a singular form. Noncount nouns refer to a general category of items, such as a mass, or to abstract qualities.

Nouns that refer to a mass:

advice	fruit	grass	luggage	milk	traffic
blood	furniture	information	machinery	money	transportation
equipment	garbage	jewelry	mail	scenery	water

All the *fruit* is on sale.

The *grass* is green.

Nouns that refer to abstract qualities:

beauty	faith	health	intelligence	poverty	time
confidence	fun	honesty	knowledge	satisfaction	truth
courage	happiness	hope	love	success	wealth

***Beauty* is skin deep.**

Our *health* is important to us.

Do not use *a* or *an* with noncount nouns. Use these nouns alone, with the word *the*, with pronouns, or with quantity words, such as *much, a lot of, a great deal of, a little, some, any, less,* and *no.*

Alone	**With a quantity word**
We need *information.*	We need *a great deal of information.*
Jewelry is expensive.	*Some jewelry* is expensive.

You can use noncount nouns in a countable sense by adding words that show quantity.

I appreciate his *words of advice.*

We bought *three pieces of luggage.*

• •

Determiners

Determiners are words that identify or quantify a noun. A singular count noun must begin with a determiner.

COMMON DETERMINERS

Articles: *a/an, the*

Demonstrative pronouns: *this, that, these, those*

Possessive pronouns: *my, our, your, his, her, its, their, whose*

Indefinite pronouns: *some, any, both, each, all, every, many, much, several, enough*

Possessive nouns: *Anna's, the student's, a dog's,* etc.

Numbers: *one, two, three,* etc.

A, AN, AND *THE*

A, an, and *the* are determiners called **articles.** Use *a* before a noun that begins with a consonant sound. Use *an* before a noun that begins with a vowel sound. Deciding whether to use *a* (*an*) or *the* depends on what your readers or listeners know.

Use *a* (*an*) with a singular count noun when people cannot identify the noun, usually because you are mentioning it for the first time.

We went to *a movie* last night.

- This is the first time you mention it.

Use *the* if people know the identity or you are about to tell them. *The* is used for all known nouns, whether they are count, noncount, singular, or plural.

The movie was four hours long.

- People know what movie you mean. You have previously mentioned this movie in your paper or conversation.

We want to see *the movie* that won the Oscar award.

- People know what movie you mean because the sentence identifies the specific movie.

THIS, THAT, THESE, AND *THOSE*

This, that, these, and *those* are determiners called **demonstrative pronouns.** Use *this* or *that* with singular count or noncount nouns: *this house, that milk.* Use *these* or *those* with plural count nouns: *these friends, those cars.*

In addition to singular and plural (number), these pronouns also indicate whether something is near or far from the speaker (proximity).

Proximity	Number	
	Singular	**Plural**
Near	this	these
Distant	that	those

This and *these* refer to items close to the speaker.

- *This* pen in my pocket and *these* pens on my desk work well.

That and *those* refer to items that are a distance from the speaker.

- *That* pen on the floor and *those* pens in the wastebasket don't work.

SOME AND *ANY*

Use *some* in positive statements; use *any* in negative statements.

I'll have *some* pasta. I don't want *any* pasta.

This rule also applies to the use of *something, someone, anything,* and *anyone.*

I have *something* to do today. I don't have *anything* to do today.
I know *someone* in my math class. I don't know *anyone* in my math class.

Verbs

Verbs are often followed by infinitives (*to* plus the base form) or the *-ing* verb form. Some verbs can be followed only by the infinitive, some verbs only by the *-ing* form, and others by either one. Verbs can also be used as adjectives.

VERBS FOLLOWED BY AN INFINITIVE

agree	claim	have	offer	refuse
ask	decide	hope	plan	want
beg	expect	manage	pretend	wish
choose	fail	need	promise	

She *expects to finish* her work early.

I *need to buy* a new jacket.

We *promised to help* our neighbors paint their garage.

VERBS FOLLOWED BY AN *-ING* VERB FORM

admit	consider	dislike	keep	recall	tolerate
appreciate	delay	enjoy	miss	resist	quit
avoid	deny	finish	postpone	risk	
can't help	discuss	imagine	practice	suggest	

He *suggests leaving* early in the morning.

I *finished typing* my paper and then went to bed.

We *keep thinking* about you.

VERBS FOLLOWED BY EITHER AN INFINITIVE OR AN *-ING* VERB FORM

Some verbs can be followed by either the infinitive or the *-ing* form with little or no change in meaning.

begin	continue	hate	like	love	start

We *began to study* at noon.

We *began studying* at noon.

- Both sentences have the same meaning.

With a few verbs, the meaning changes:

forget	remember	stop	try

We *stopped to eat* lunch.

- This sentence means we ate lunch.

We *stopped eating* lunch.

- This sentence means we no longer eat lunch.

VERB FORMS USED AS ADJECTIVES

Both *-ing* verb forms (present participle) and *-ed* forms (past participles) may be used as adjectives. These two forms give different information about the nouns they describe. The *-ing* adjective tells us that the noun produces the effect on others. The *-ed* adjective tells us that the noun itself feels the effect.

The *confusing* tour director

- The tour director produces confusion in others. The people listening to the tour director are the ones who are confused.

The *confused* tour director

- The tour director is the one who is confused.

Here are some common *-ing* and *-ed* verb forms:

Noun produces the effect on others	Noun already has the effect
amazing	amazed
amusing	amused
annoying	annoyed
boring	bored
convincing	convinced
depressing	depressed
disappointing	disappointed
embarrassing	embarrassed
exciting	excited
exhausting	exhausted
satisfying	satisfied
surprising	surprised

• •

Prepositions

Specific prepositions are often used with verbs and adjectives.

PREPOSITIONS WITH VERBS

Some verbs are followed by specific prepositions. Here are some of the common ones:

apologize *to* someone *for* something

apply *for* (a position)

arrive *at* (a building or an event)

arrive *in* (a country or city)

blame someone *for* something

call *off* a scheduled appointment

call *on* someone for a visit

complain *about*

concentrate *on*

congratulate someone *on* something

consist *of*

deal *with*

depend *on*

explain something *to* someone

fill *in* individual blanks on a form

fill *out* the entire form

fill *up* a gas tank

insist *on*

interfere *with*

object *to*

reason *with*

rely *on*

reply *to*

smile *at*

specialize *in*

take advantage *of*

take care *of*

thank someone *for* something

throw something *at* someone
   (who is not expecting it)

throw something *to* someone
   (who is waiting to catch it)

worry *about*

PREPOSITIONS WITH ADJECTIVES

Adjectives are often followed by specific prepositions. Here are some common ones:

addicted *to*

afraid *of*

anxious *about*

ashamed *of*

aware *of*

confused *by*

content *with*

convenient *for*

excited *about*

fond *of*

full *of*

grateful *for* (something)

grateful *to* (someone)

happy *about*

interested *in*

jealous *of*

proud *of*

responsible *for* something

responsible *to* someone

satisfied *with*

shocked *at*

similar *to*

sorry *for*

suspicious *of*

tired *of*

• •

Order of Adjectives

When you have more than one adjective before a noun, use this numbered order:

1. judgment or opinion: *awful, beautiful, intelligent, lovely, wonderful*
2. size: *big, huge, large, short, small, tall, tiny*
3. shape: *circular, flat, round, square, thin*
4. age: *ancient, middle-aged, new, old, young, youthful*
5. color: *blue, green, orange, red, yellow*
6. nationality/location: *Italian, French, northern, southern*
7. material: *glass, iron, paper, plastic, steel, wooden*

Here are a few examples of these adjectives at work:

> A *small, round glass* table would look good in the living room.
> Demetrius wants to buy the *large old Italian* house on the river.

• •

Sentence Structure

In written English, every sentence needs a subject and a verb, even when the meaning might be clear without them. Other common sentence patterns include questions, negative statements, and sentences that use *although* or *because*.

QUESTIONS

You can turn a statement into a question by placing the helping verb before the subject.

> They *are* planning to take a vacation in August.
> *Are* they planning to take a vacation in August?

If there is no helping verb, add a form of *do* and place it before the subject.

> They watched the game.

- Notice that *watched* indicates the past tense.

Did they watch the game?

- Notice that *did* indicates the past tense.

NEGATIVES

You can form a negative statement by using one of these words:

never	nobody	no one	nowhere
no	none	not	

If you use the word *not*, place it after the first helping verb in a sentence.

The child has been running a fever.
The child has *not* been running a fever.

If there is no helping verb, add a form of *do*.

We relax on Saturdays.
We *do not* relax on Saturdays.

USING *ALTHOUGH* AND *BECAUSE*

Do not combine the subordinating conjunctions *although* and *because* with coordinating conjunctions (*but, so*) or transition words (*however, therefore*).

Incorrect: Although the rain has stopped, ~~but~~ the streets are still wet.
Correct: Although the rain has stopped, the streets are still wet.

Incorrect: Because we studied, ~~therefore~~ we knew the answers.
Correct: Because we studied, we knew the answers.

APPENDIX: ANSWERS TO SELF TESTS

Chapter 1: The Basic Sentence

● **Self Test A:** To find the subject and predicate of a sentence, read the sentence out loud and ask, *Who or what?* and *What about it?* To give you a sense of how this works, the answers to these questions are given for the first five items.

1. Tulips and daffodils / are spring flowers.

   Who or what: Tulips and daffodils

   What about it: are spring flowers

2. The National Weather Service / predicts above-normal temperatures over the Great Lakes.

   Who or what: The National Weather Service

   What about it: predicts above-normal temperatures over the Great Lakes

3. Rescue workers / carry global-positioning systems and radio equipment.

   Who or what: Rescue workers

   What about it: carry global-positioning systems and radio equipment

4. The team / stopped for pizza after practice.

   Who or what: The team

   What about it: stopped for pizza after practice

5. City planners / encouraged development of apartments and condominiums near the train station.

   Who or what: City planners

   What about it: encouraged development of apartments and condominiums near the train station

6. Friends and family members / packed the auditorium bleachers.

7. The youth organization / emphasizes character building and community service.

8. Nearly sixty percent of the best-selling prescription drugs in America's pharmacies / are based on compounds taken from nature.

9. The San Francisco French Bread Company / produces approximately two million loaves of bread each week.

10. The local hospital / is sponsoring a class to introduce young people to medical and hospital-related careers.

● Self Test B

1. The second test was ~~more~~ **easier** than the first, but the last test was the ~~most~~ **easiest.**

   The writer begins by comparing two tests: the second and the first. We use *easier* to compare two things. The writer then compares the last test to all the tests. We use *easiest* when comparing three or more things.

2. The children listened ~~careful~~ **carefully** to the instructions.

   Careful is used to describe things (nouns): *a careful person, a careful driver.* The word *carefully* is used to describe actions (verbs): *drive carefully, move carefully.* In this sentence, the word describes *listened,* so we need *carefully.*

3. The ~~confuse~~ **confused** and ~~frighten~~ **frightened** tourist stopped at the gas station and asked for directions.

   Confused and *frightened* are -*ed* adjectives that describe *tourist.*

4. **C**

5. The weather was ~~worst~~ **worse** on Friday than it was on Saturday.

   Two things are being compared here, so we need *worse.* One way to remember these words is to remember that *worse* means "badder," and *worst* means the "baddest."

Chapter 2: Dependent Clauses

● **Self Test A:** Whenever you begin a sentence with a word such as *because, if,* or *when,* readers will be looking for a comma. They need to know when the "*because* idea" is over and the basic sentence begins. If you read the sentence out loud, you will hear where the clause ends and the basic sentence begins.

1. Since the beginning of the year, life has gone smoothly for us.

2. Because I forgot to set my alarm, I was late for class.

3. Even though the price of gas has increased, commuters continue to crowd the expressways.

4. Unless we hear from you, we will meet for dinner at seven.

5. Although the electricity went out for only a split second, everything we had not saved on the computer was lost.

● Self Test B

1. a. Whenever I try to do things quickly, I make mistakes.

   b. I make mistakes whenever I try to do things quickly.

2. a. Because we could not see the stage clearly, we moved to the middle of the auditorium.

   b. We moved to the middle of the auditorium because we could not see the stage clearly.

3. a. If we want to be on time, we should leave now.

   b. We should leave now if we want to be on time.

4. a. Since I started my new job, I have had little time for shopping and no time for partying.

   b. I have had little time for shopping and no time for partying since I started my new job.

5. a. As soon as we heard that the airlines were raising their prices, we made our plane reservations.

   b. We made our plane reservations as soon as we heard that the airlines were raising their prices.

Chapter 3: More Dependent Clauses

● Self Test A

1. The <u>kids</u> *who were snapping their gum* distracted us during the movie.

2. The college is remodeling the computer <u>lab</u>, *which will open in January*.

3. <u>Participants</u> *who arrive early* will receive free lunch tickets.

4. The <u>companies</u> *that upgraded their technology* increased their sales.

5. The <u>U.S. Supreme Court</u>, *which consists of nine men and women*, debates valuable issues and interprets the law.

Self Test B

1. The two disks **that I bought yesterday** need to be formatted.

2. The clothes **that are stuffed in the suitcase** need to be washed and ironed.

3. All of the books **that Frederick bought** were on sale.

4. The workshop **that explains the new Medicare rules** is free to the public.

5. I can't read the notes **that I wrote in class yesterday**.

Chapter 4: Sentence Fragments

Self Test

1. If the weather changes.

   ✓ The word *if* makes this a fragment. *The weather changes* is a sentence, but the minute *if* is added, we set up a questionable situation. Readers wonder what will happen if the weather changes. We need to add a basic sentence: *If the weather changes, we will go ahead with the picnic.*

2. Students studying in the cafeteria.

   ✓ This is a fragment because a verb ending in *-ing* is not a complete verb. It needs a helping verb. If we add *are*, we will have a sentence: *Students are studying in the cafeteria.*

3. People who love to fish.

   ✓ The word *who* makes this a fragment. If we take out *who*, we have a sentence: *People love to fish.* Keeping the word *who* lets us write a sentence with more information. We can change this fragment to a sentence by finishing the thought: *People who love to fish enjoy being outside.*

4. I understand.

C This is a sentence. We have a *who or what* (*I*) and a *what about it* (*understand*).

5. To find out which phone companies were offering the best promotions.

✓ Ideas that begin with *to* need a basic sentence to complete the thought. Here are two options: (1) *I searched the Internet to find out which phone companies were offering the best promotions.* (2) *To find out which phone companies were offering the best promotions, I searched the Internet.*

6. Because we didn't watch the news.

✓ The word *because* sets up a questionable situation; readers wonder what happened. We need to attach this "*because* idea" to a basic sentence. Here is one example: *Because we didn't watch the news, we don't know the results of the election.*

7. Looking beyond the present moment.

✓ We know the sentence is about *looking beyond the present moment*, but what about it? We could finish the thought by adding a predicate: *Looking beyond the present moment is important.* Or we could add a subject and a helping verb: *We are looking beyond the present moment.*

8. Choosing a career is often difficult.

C We have a *who or what* (*Choosing a career*) and a *what about it* (*is often difficult*).

9. Which is the best decision we could have made.

✓ This is a fragment because the word *which* needs to refer to something already mentioned in the sentence. We have a basket, but we need a sentence to carry it: *We decided to leave on Saturday morning, which is the best decision we could have made.*

10. The hubcap that fell off my car.

✓ If we omit the word *that*, we have a sentence: *The hubcap fell off my car.* Keeping the word *that* lets us write a more mature sentence. We just need to complete the thought: *The hubcap that fell off my car was expensive.*

Chapter 5: Punctuating Sentences

⬤ Self Test

1. Ann's boss is supportive he gave her a day off.

   ✓ There are two sentences here. The first is *Ann's boss is supportive.* The second is *He gave her a day off.*

2. Our neighbors just moved from Texas, they seem friendly.

   ✓ There are two sentences here. The first is *Our neighbors just moved from Texas.* The second is *They seem friendly.*

3. When we made plans for the weekend, we did not know that Marcus would have to work.

   C This sentence is correct. It begins with a dependent clause, which is correctly marked with a comma.

4. My grandmother didn't let disappointment bother her she just kept living day by day.

   ✓ There are two sentences here. The first is *My grandmother didn't let disappointment bother her.* The second sentence is *She just kept living day by day.*

5. I can trust Serena and Valerie they don't gossip about others.

   ✓ There are two sentences here. The first is *I can trust Serena and Valerie.* The second is *They don't gossip about others.*

Chapter 6: Using Commas

⬤ Self Test A: Using the pencil test will let you know if there are two sentences.

1. The dog grabbed the ham bone and dashed out the back door.

   Who or what: the dog   *What about it:* grabbed the ham bone
   Who or what: ?   *What about it:* dashed out the door

   There is no subject for the second "sentence"—the *dog* is in the first sentence. Because we are missing a subject, we don't have two sentences. No comma.

2. The mechanic changed the oil and rotated the tires on my car.

Who or what: the mechanic   *What about it:* changed the oil

Who or what: ?   *What about it:* rotated the tires on my car

We don't have a subject for the second "sentence"—the *mechanic* is in the first sentence. We are missing a subject, so we do not have two sentences. No comma.

3. The stores will be closed on Friday and Saturday for inventory.

Who or what: the stores   *What about it:* will be closed on Friday

Who or what: Saturday for inventory   *What about it:* ?

We do not have two sentences. The *and* doesn't connect two sentences; it connects *Friday* and *Saturday*. Therefore, we do not add a comma.

4. Terry works in the garden on Saturdays, and his children help him.

Who or what: Terry   *What about it:* works in the garden on Saturdays

Who or what: his children   *What about it:* help him

We have two sentences here. Therefore, we add a comma.

5. We bought a couch last week and will pick it up next week.

Who or what: We   *What about it:* bought a couch last week

Who or what: ?   *What about it:* will pick it up next week.

The *and* does not connect two sentences. It connects two predicates: *bought a couch last week* and *will pick it up next week.* Therefore, we don't add a comma.

● **Self Test B:** An addition must be supported by a basic sentence, which has two parts: a *who or what* and a *what about it.* In the answers below, the *who or what* is *Debra.* The *what about it* is *enrolled her children in the after-school program.*

1. <u>Debra enrolled her children in the after-school program</u>, which runs throughout the year.

2. <u>Debra</u>, my neighbor across the street, <u>enrolled her children in the after-school program.</u>

3. <u>Debra enrolled her children in the after-school program</u>, a series of enrichment opportunities that include art and drama.

4. <u>Debra</u>, wanting to give her children a safe and nurturing environment, <u>enrolled her children in the after-school program</u>.

5. At the beginning of the year, <u>Debra enrolled her children in the after-school program</u>.

Chapter 7: Verbs

● Self Test

1. The game was ~~postpone~~ **postponed** because of weather.

2. I should have ~~stay~~ **stayed** in high school and ~~graduate~~ **graduated** with my class.

3. Their work schedule has been ~~shorten~~ **shortened** to four days a week.

4. For the past two months, we have ~~walk~~ **walked** three miles every day.

5. Pat was ~~hire~~ **hired** in April as an orderly in the operating room.

6. Everyone in the class has ~~practice~~ **practiced** these verb forms.

7. Technology has ~~change~~ **changed** how we live.

8. Our friends have ~~encourage~~ **encouraged** and ~~help~~ **helped** us in the past.

9. We ~~learn~~ **learned** yesterday that our medical benefits will be ~~increase~~ **increased**.

10. The soldiers have ~~serve~~ **served** their country well.

Chapter 8: Subject-Verb Agreement

● **Self Test:** The forms of *be*, *do*, and *have* can be confusing. If the subject is *he*, *she*, or *it* (or anything that is a *he*, *she*, or *it*), the present-tense verb ends in *-s*. Some students remember it this way:

One thing *is*.	A bunch of things *are*.
One thing *does*.	A bunch of things *do*.
One thing *has*.	A bunch of things *have*.

1. Both socks **have** holes in them.

2. The lawnmower **doesn't** work well because the blades need sharpening.

3. The mechanic **has** replaced the brake drums.

4. He **was** leaving when I arrived.

5. If Carla **has** the answer, she will tell us.

6. He **does** whatever he can to help our neighbors.

7. The people **were** friendly and helpful.

8. My uncle, who **has** been married for ten years, is planning an anniversary party.

9. My friends **don't** want to leave for vacation until Saturday.

10. We heard the news while we **were** walking home.

Chapter 9: Irregular Verbs

⬤ Self Test

1. Last week, we ~~buyed~~ **bought** all our school supplies because they were on sale.

2. My phone has ~~rang~~ **rung** all morning.

3. After Henry had ~~drove~~ **driven** for three hours, he asked me to take over.

4. **C**

5. We have ~~came~~ **come** too far to turn back now.

6. I have a sore throat. I think I ~~catched~~ **caught** a cold from someone.

7. Our neighbors can't babysit because they have ~~went~~ **gone** shopping.

8. **C**

9. Joanna has ~~brung~~ **brought** the food for the picnic.

10. **C**

Chapter 10: Easily Confused Words

⬤ Self Test

1. ~~Its~~ **It's** not ~~to~~ **too** late to change your ~~mine~~ **mind.**

2. I ~~no~~ **know** now that we should ~~of~~ **have** paid ~~are~~ **our** bills on time.

3. Some people get angry when ~~your~~ **you're** (or **you are**) right and ~~there~~ **they're** (or **they are**) wrong.

4. John ~~past~~ **passed** the ball to Mark who was ~~suppose~~ **supposed** to grab it.

5. I can talk faster ~~then~~ **than** I can ~~right~~ **write.**

6. **C**

7. The angry customers announced that they would take ~~there~~ **their** business elsewhere.

8. Kristin ~~an~~ **and** Kelley were ~~to~~ **too** surprised to say anything to ~~they're~~ **their** boss.

9. Because I ~~excepted~~ **accepted** responsibility ~~an~~ **and** didn't ~~quiet~~ **quit,** I succeeded.

10. After the fire, we could not ~~breath~~ **breathe** because the ~~hole~~ **whole** room was filled with smoke.

Chapter 11: Pronouns

⬤ Self Test A

1. Nicole gave a shirt to Jerry and a jacket to ~~myself~~ **me.**

   If you are not emphasizing yourself or doing something to yourself, use *I* or *me*—not *myself*.

2. Everybody in the class agrees that the test should be postponed.

   C The subject is *everybody*, which is singular. We therefore need the *-s* form: *agrees*.

3. I assembled the gas grill by ~~my self~~ **myself.**

   Myself is one word, not two.

4. When I dropped my coffee cup on the glass table, ~~it~~ **the table** shattered into pieces.

   We don't know what *it* refers to. What shattered: the coffee cup or the table?

5. Bonnie likes to visit her cousins in Atlanta because they always make ~~you~~ **her** feel at home.

   Bonnie is the person who feels at home. The sentence begins with *Bonnie* and *her*, but then incorrectly switches to *you*.

● Self Test B

1. My neighbor and ~~him~~ **he** did not get along.

✓ Here is how we know that the correct pronoun is *he*. We temporarily remove *my neighbor*, and we get *Him did not get along*. We wouldn't say *him*. We would say *he*. Now that we know to use the subject pronoun, we put *my neighbor* back in the sentence.

2. ~~A taxpayer~~ **Taxpayers** must pay their taxes no later than April 15.

✓ The noun (*taxpayer*) is singular, but the pronoun (*their*) is plural. They do not match. Changing *taxpayer* to *taxpayers* corrects the problem.

3. My sister and I called Mom to wish her a happy birthday.

C We know this sentence is correct because when we temporarily remove *my sister*, we get *I called Mom to wish her a happy birthday*. If English is your native language, this sounds right. We are using a subject pronoun.

4. Many car thefts occur because the ~~driver leaves~~ **drivers leave** their keys in the ignition.

✓ The noun (*driver*) and pronoun (*their*) do not match: One is singular and the other is plural. Changing *driver* to *drivers* corrects the problem. Notice that the verb then also changes.

5. I am happy that ~~me and Crystal~~ **Crystal and I** will be in the same class.

✓ This sentence uses the wrong pronoun in the wrong place. Temporarily removing *Crystal* gives us *I am happy that me will be in the same class*. That doesn't sound right. We need the subject pronoun *I*. We then need to put that pronoun after the name, not before it.

6. Just between you and ~~I~~ **me,** this English class is easy.

✓ *Between me* sounds better than *between I*. The correct pronoun is *me* because *between* is a preposition, and with prepositions we need an object pronoun. The phrase *you and me* is the object of the preposition.

7. ~~A writer~~ **Writers** can improve their vocabulary by reading.

✓ *A writer* refers to one, but *their* refers to more than one. We can solve the problem by using a plural noun: *writers*.

8. ~~Me and Josh~~ **Josh and I** will set up the picnic tables.

✓ There are two problems here. First, the pronoun is wrong. If we remove *Josh*, the sentence reads *Me will set up the picnic tables.* We can now see that the correct pronoun is *I.* The second problem is placement. The pronoun *I* should follow the noun *Josh*.

9. At the end of August, Brent and ~~her~~ **she** will take a two-week vacation.

✓ Temporarily removing *Brent* shows what is left: *At the end of August, her will take a two-week vacation.* We would not say *Her would take a vacation.* We need a subject pronoun here: *she.*

10. The instructor asked Rick and me to lead the discussion.

C When we temporarily remove *Rick*, we have *The instructor asked me to lead the discussion.* That sounds right. We need an object pronoun.

Chapter 12: Clarity

⬤ Self Test A

Answers will vary. Here are some possibilities:

1. Our financial problems were a nightmare.

2. If people want to succeed, they need to know their priorities.

3. Although Mr. Henrickson is strict, he is fair.

4. Children are affected by the violence in today's movies.

5. My goal is to become independent in three years.

⬤ Self Test B

Answers will vary. Trust your judgment and select words that you like.

Chapter 13: Parallel Structures

⬤ Self Test

1. The Italian restaurant is famous for its <u>antipasto salad</u>, <u>tomato-cheese bread</u>, <u>pasta</u>, and <u>dessert</u>.

2. Before buying a car, <u>talk to your friends</u>, <u>do research on the Internet</u>, and <u>visit a number of dealers</u>.

3. In one afternoon, we were able to <u>paint the walls</u> and <u>install the kitchen counter</u>.

4. I have searched <u>the car</u>, <u>the closet</u>, <u>the garage</u>, and <u>the driveway</u>, and I still cannot find my keys.

5. Scholarship applicants will be judged by <u>academic achievement</u>, <u>financial need</u>, and <u>community involvement</u>.

Chapter 14: Sentence Variety

● Self Test A

1. During the last total solar eclipse, the moon hid the sun for over two minutes.

2. Without waiting for us to ask, Laurence offered to help.

3. In the seventy-mile-per-hour wind, traffic lights trembled.

4. Throughout the summer months, local farmers sell their vegetables at the Farmers' Market.

5. During the next decade, student enrollment in elementary and high schools is expected to increase.

● Self Test B

1. Jerome and Conner, architects with thirty years of experience, will design homes in the new development.

2. I still remember Mrs. Shank, my second grade teacher, because she made me feel important.

3. The Everglades National Park, a paradise for plants and wildlife, is located at the southern tip of Florida.

4. Mr. Arlington, a respected volunteer and family man, has dedicated his life to public service.

5. Mr. Fredrickson, my high school history teacher, encouraged me to go to college.

◉ Self Test C

Baseball has taught me the importance of mental concentration. (When I am able to block out distractions), I am a good pitcher. (For example), (in the Ohio Valley Regional Baseball Tournament), I was pitching against Kentucky. (As soon as the game started), it began to drizzle. The ball soon became slippery, (which made it harder to control). The field turned to mud, (clogging up my cleats and making it harder to push off the mound). I made errors; my team made errors. (Finally), I blocked out the mistakes and focused my energy on my fastball pitch. We won 7–0.

Our game against Kankakee Valley High School is another example of the power of concentration. I was facing an undefeated team. Kankakee was known for being loud and annoying, (especially when it was batting). We were winning 3–2 in the seventh inning, and the whole Kankakee team was shouting. (Rather than being distracted by the screaming), I used it to pump myself up for the last inning. I stepped off the mound and pointed to Kankakee Valley's dugout, (waving the team on as if to say, "I'm ready. Bring it on.") (When Kankakee's best hitters came to bat), I was ready. (Because I had learned to focus my attention), I pitched the best game of my life. Mental concentration is the key to success.

Chapter 15: Apostrophes and Quotation Marks

◉ Self Test A

1. Phil **runs** two **miles** every day.

   Runs is a verb, and we don't add apostrophes to verbs. *Miles* is a plural noun, meaning more than one. We don't add an apostrophe to make nouns plural.

2. **C**

3. Everyone loves my **mother's** apple **pies.**

   The mother owns the apple pies, so we add an apostrophe and *-s* to mother: *mother's*. The pies don't own anything. The writer is talking about more than one pie: *pies.*

4. The wolf can survive harsh winters because of **its** thick fur.

   This sentence does not mean "The wolf can survive harsh winters because of it is thick fur." *It's* means either *it is* or *it has*. If we want to show ownership, we use *its*. (The pronoun *its* does not take an apostrophe: The dog wagged *its* tail; the car lost *its* muffler. See Chapter 10 for a review of *its* and *it's*.)

5. The **children's** party will begin at noon.

   Do we mean the party of the children? Yes. Therefore, we add an apostrophe and *-s* after *children: children's*. Remember to *read the word to the left of the apostrophe to see who the owner is.*

⬤ Self Test B

Answers will vary. Here are some possibilities:

1. Michael said, "I agree with you."

2. Kimberly said, "I'll call you later."

3. The doctor's secretary announced, "We no longer submit insurance forms."

4. Ryan asked, "Do you guys want to meet for lunch on Wednesday?"

5. Deborah mumbled, "I need a cup of coffee."

Chapter 16: Capitalization and More Punctuation

⬤ Self Test

1. The doctors in the new **medical** building will begin office hours in January.

2. My **father's** brother, who grew up in **Brazil,** can speak **Spanish, English,** and **Portuguese.**

3. Our grandparents were married April **18, 1965,** in Jamaica.

4. **C**

5. Spring and **winter** are my **grandfather's** favorite **seasons.**

6. **C**

7. I wonder why Nancy has not called**.** (period, not question mark)

8. **C**

9. Some good sources of protein **are beans**, cheese, fish, meats, and nuts. (no colon)

10. Please send the package to George Doughtery at 900 Spindell **Road, Tarrington,** New York.

Chapter 18: Checkpoints for Papers

⬤ Self Test

1. *Who or what:* Money *What about it:* can't buy happiness

2. *Who or what:* My high school coach *What about it:* gave me confidence

3. *Who or what:* Working while going to college *What about it:* is difficult

4. *Who or what:* Sunday *What about it:* is the best day of the week

5. *Who or what:* Top Notch   *What about it:* is the best restaurant in town

6. *Who or what:* I   *What about it:* need a vacation

7. *Who or what:* Living in a large city   *What about it:* has advantages

8. *Who or what:* Little things   *What about it:* irritate me

9. *Who or what:* Lauren   *What about it:* is a loyal friend

10. *Who or what:* College   *What about it:* is not what I had expected

Chapter 19: Essays

Self Test

1. The writer gives examples of something familiar to us: magazine and book titles that promise success.

2. I owe my life to a twelve-step program.

3. a. I was once helpless and hopeless.

   b. I was ready to give up, but I gave life one more chance and sought help.

   c. The twelve-step book has been my door to freedom.

   d. Today I have turned my will and life over to God.

4. But most importantly, I know who I am, and I have the **twelve steps** to thank for that.

GLOSSARY OF GRAMMATICAL TERMS

For a more thorough explanation of the terms listed here, check the index for page references.

active voice A relationship between the subject and verb in which the subject performs the action. Jackson *replaced* the blinking fluorescent lights in the cafeteria. See also *passive voice*.

adjective A word that describes a noun: *quiet* night, *happy* child, *easy* test. Most adjectives have comparative and superlative forms: *quieter/quietest, happier/happiest, easier/easiest*.

adverb A word that describes a verb. Most adverbs end in *-ly: slowly, quickly, carefully*. These adverbs tell *how* about the verb. Other adverbs add information about time (*soon, now, then, tomorrow, today, yesterday*), place (*here, there, somewhere*), or frequency (*often, sometimes, rarely, never, always*).

antecedent The word(s) that a pronoun refers to. *Tanya* talked to *her* friends.

appositive A "definition addition" that renames or identifies another noun. Mrs. Santori, *a teaching assistant*, helps individual students after school.

article The determiners *a, an,* and *the*. *The* sun is shining.

base form The form of the verb listed in dictionaries. In all verbs except *be*, the base form is the present tense: *see, listen, walk*.

basic sentence A subject and predicate that can stand alone as a sentence; an independent clause.

clause A group of words containing a subject and a predicate. See also *dependent clause; independent clause*.

comma splice See *run-on sentence*.

common noun See *noun*.

comparative The form of an adjective that compares two things: *stronger, softer*.

complex sentence A sentence that includes at least one dependent clause. *When I finish this paper, I will breathe a sigh of relief.*

compound predicate A predicate that includes more than one verb. We *talked about our childhood* and *laughed at ourselves.*

compound sentence Two sentences connected by a coordinating conjunction (*and, but, or, nor, for, yet*) or a semicolon. *I wanted to go home, but Billie didn't. I wanted to go home; Billie didn't.*

compound subject Two or more subjects connected by a coordinating conjunction. *Gary* and *Dawn* will meet us at noon. Both *the pumpkin pie* and *the chocolate cake* look good.

contraction Two words that have been squeezed together (contracted) to form one word. In the process, one or more letters have been omitted. An apostrophe marks where the letters have been omitted: *doesn't, they're, I'm*.

coordinating conjunction A word that connects two sentences or structures within a sentence as equals: *and, but, or, nor, for, yet*.

count noun A noun that can be counted: one *car*, five *books*, seven *miles*. See also *noncount noun*.

dangling modifier Words that do not logically modify the word they are meant to describe. *At the age of ten*, my family moved to Arizona. (The family was not ten when they moved.) *Crossing the street this morning*, a car almost hit me. (The car was not crossing the street.) Corrections: When I was ten, my family moved to Arizona. Crossing the street this morning, I was almost hit by a car.

demonstrative pronoun The pronouns *this* (plural *these*) and *that* (plural *those*). *This* and *these* refer to items near the speaker. *That* and *those* refer to items at a distance. *This* car is a better buy than *that* one over there.

dependent clause A clause that plays a part in another sentence; it begins with a subordinating conjunction or a relative pronoun. I missed class today *because I was sick*. The woman *who lives next door* sometimes bakes cookies for me. See also *independent clause*.

determiner Words that signal a noun: *a* class, *the* computer, *many* friends, *some* homework.

direct quotation A quotation that states exactly what a person said, word for word, set off by quotation marks. *Bobby asked, "Do you want to go to a Sox game on Wednesday?"* See also *indirect quotation*.

fragment A part of a sentence that is punctuated as if it were a complete sentence. It may lack a subject (*Always tries to understand my point of view*) or a predicate (*Students who study*), or it may be a dependent clause (*Whenever I hear that song*).

fused sentence See *run-on sentence*.

gerund An *-ing* verb functioning as a noun. *Swimming* is good exercise.

helping verb A verb that combines with the base form, the past participle, or the present participle. Helping verbs include the various forms of *be*, *do*, and *have*, and the words *may*, *might*, *must*, *can*, *could*, *will*, *would*, *shall*, *should*, and *ought to*. Also called an auxiliary verb.

indefinite pronoun A pronoun that does not refer to a specific person or thing: *some*, *several*, *many*, *all*, *everyone*, *everything*, *someone*, *anyone*, *nothing*.

independent clause A clause that can stand alone as a sentence; a basic sentence. See also *dependent clause*.

indirect quotation A summary of what a person said, rather than the exact words. It does not take quotation marks. *Bobby asked whether I wanted to go to a Sox game on Wednesday*. See also *direct quotation*.

infinitive The base form of the verb preceded by *to*: *to sing*, *to dance*, *to study*.

infinitive phrase A group of words consisting of an infinitive and related words. *To get to my house*, take the first right on Main Street.

intensive pronoun A pronoun ending in *-self* or *-selves* that shows emphasis. I painted that room *myself*.

irregular verb A verb that does not form its past tense or past participle by adding *-d* or *-ed* to the base form. We *went* to Daniel's house last night. We have *gone* there often. See also *past participle*.

main verb The verb that carries the central meaning in the predicate. Joe has *worked* all morning. The students have been *doing* their homework. We *were* too tired to go bowling. I *have* one goal for this week. See also *helping verb*.

noncount noun A noun that cannot be counted. It has only a singular form. The *equipment* is new. The *water* is pure. See also *count noun*.

noun A word that names people, places, and things. Nouns can be common (*girl*, *city*) or proper (*Jennie*, *Chicago*). Most nouns have a plural form (*girls*, *cities*).

object of a preposition The word or phrase that follows a preposition to form a prepositional phrase. I slept (for *eight hours*). The roads are filled (with *weekend tourists*). He gave it (to *me*).

parallel structure A compound structure in which the parts have the same grammatical form—all nouns, all adjectives, all present-tense verb forms, and so on. I enjoy *swimming* and *hiking*.

passive voice A relationship between the subject and verb in which the subject receives the action. The blinking fluorescent lights in the cafeteria *were replaced*. See also *active voice*.

past participle The form of verbs used with the helping verb *have*. In regular verbs, such as *finish*, the past participle has the same form (*-ed*) as the past tense: I have *finished* my homework. Irregular verbs have a variety of irregular forms, including *-en* (*driven, seen, taken, written*): I have *written* three papers this week.

past tense The *-ed* form of regular verbs. Irregular verbs have irregular forms (*saw, ran, went*). Past-tense verbs refer to past actions. Yesterday we *walked* to the art fair and *bought* a painting.

personal pronoun A pronoun that refers to a specific person or thing. Personal pronouns can be subjects, objects, or possessives. *They* drove home. Jake respects *her*. Christy listened to *our* advice.

phrase A group of words that functions as a single unit in a sentence. See also *prepositional phrase*.

plural The form of a noun or pronoun that refers to more than one person or thing: *apples, movies, these, they*.

possession A feature of nouns and pronouns, indicating ownership: *Nellie's* motorcycle, the *child's* dreams, the *students'* attitudes, *my* friend.

predicate The verb part of a sentence that makes a comment about the subject, telling *what about it*. The children in the doctor's office *played with the toys*.

prepositional phrase A group of words that consists of a preposition (a word such as *in, on,* or *with*) and its object, usually a noun or pronoun: *in the middle, with ketchup and mustard, on us*.

present participial phrase A group of words that begins with an *-ing* verb form. When the phrase gives extra information about a noun, it is marked with commas: Sergio, *trying to get my attention*, whistled and waved his arms. When the phrase identifies the noun, the commas are omitted: The child *standing on the corner* looks confused.

present participle The *-ing* form of a verb: *seeing, living, talking*.

present tense The base form and the *-s* form of the verb: *laugh, laughs*. Present-tense verbs refer to events that occur in the present (*I understand your point*) or on a regular basis (*I work out at the gym*), or explain general truths (*Vegetables are good for us*).

pronoun A word used in place of a noun: *he, her, their, someone, it, that*.

proper noun See *noun*.

reflexive pronoun A pronoun ending in *-self* or *-selves* that indicates the subject does something to or for itself. We are taking good care of *ourselves*.

regular verb A verb that forms its past tense and past participle by adding *-d* or *-ed* to the base form. In regular verbs, these two forms are always identical. I *talked* to Cheryl. I have *talked* to Cheryl every day this week.

relative pronoun The pronouns *who, whose, whom, which,* and *that* when they introduce dependent clauses that describe nouns. The man *whose car I borrowed* lives next door. The graduation ceremony, *which I want to attend*, begins at noon.

run-on sentence An error resulting from two sentences that run into each other because of incorrect punctuation. If there is no punctuation, the run-on is called a *fused sentence*. If the two sentences are separated by a comma, the run-on is called a *comma splice*.

-s form The present-tense verb form that is used when the subject is *he, she,* or *it*, or anything that can be substituted by *he, she,* or *it*. Andrew *smiles;* the child *giggles;* the sun *shines*.

sentence A complete statement containing a subject and a predicate. The written sentence begins with a capital letter and ends with a period, question mark, or exclamation point.

simple subject See *subject*.

singular The form of a noun or pronoun that refers to one person or thing: *apple, movie, this, it*.

subject The noun or pronoun and related words that tell *who or what* the sentence is about. (*The children in the doctor's office played with the toys.*) The *simple subject* is the noun or pronoun. (The *children* in the doctor's office played with the toys.)

subject-verb agreement A condition wherein subjects and verbs match in form. When the subject is *he*, *she*, or *it*, or anything that is a *he*, *she*, or *it*, the present-tense verb ends in -*s*. (The computer *works*.) When the subject is plural, the verb does not end in -*s*. (The computers *work*.)

subordinating conjunction A word that introduces a dependent clause. *Because* it was raining, the game was cancelled. Let's go to the mall *if* we get out of class early.

superlative The form of an adjective that compares three or more things: *strongest, easiest.*

tense A feature of verbs relating to time. They *listened* carefully (past tense). We *will go* soon (future tense).

verb A word indicating action, feeling, or being. Any word that makes sense following the statement "I like to . . ." is a verb. All verbs have an -*s* and an -*ing* ending. See also *regular verb, irregular verb.*

WORKS CITED

Bragg, Rick. *All Over but the Shoutin'*. New York: Vintage Books, A division of Random House, Inc., 1997.

Buscaglia, Leo. *Personhood: The Art of Being Fully Human*. New York: Fawcett Columbine, 1978.

"Chicago Marathon Weather." *Chicago Tribune*. 13 Oct. 2002: 12.

Conover, Ted. "Peru's Long Haul." *National Geographic*. June 2003.

Iyer, Pico. "In Praise of the Humble Comma." *Time*. 13 June 1988.

Soto, Gary. *Jesse*. San Diego: Harcourt Brace & Company, 1994.

Staples, Brent. "The Runaway Son." from *Family: American Writers Remember Their Own*. Eds. Sharon Sloan Figger and Steve Fiffer. New York: Pantheon Books, 1996.

"Weather Report." *New York Times*. 12 Feb. 2004: C22.

INDEX